CardioPulmonary Exercise Testing

Physiologic Principles and Clinical Applications

KARL T. WEBER, M.D.

Harold H. Hines, Jr.
Professor of Medicine
Director
Cardiovascular Institute
   and Division of Cardiology

JOSEPH S. JANICKI, Ph.D.

Professor of Medicine
Associate Director
Cardiovascular Institute
Division of Cardiology

Michael Reese Hospital and Medical Center
Pritzker School of Medicine
University of Chicago
Chicago, Illinois

1986 W.B. SAUNDERS COMPANY

Philadelphia ☐ London ☐ Toronto ☐ Mexico City
Rio de Janeiro ☐ Sydney ☐ Tokyo ☐ Hong Kong

W. B. Saunders Company: West Washington Square
Philadelphia, PA 19105

Library of Congress Cataloging-in-Publication Data

Weber, Karl T., Janicki, Joseph S.

Cardiopulmonary exercise testing.

1. Exercise tests.   2. Heart function tests.
   3. Pulmonary function tests.   4. Heart—Diseases—
   Diagnosis.   5. Lungs—Diseases—Diagnosis.
   I. Title. [DNLM: 1. Cardiovascular Diseases—diagno-
   sis.   2. Cardiovascular Diseases—rehabilitation.
   WG 141.5.F9 W374c]

RC683.5.E94W43 1986   616.1'07'5   85–25019

ISBN 0–7216–1300–4

Editor: Dana Dreibelbis
Designer: Terri Siegel
Production Manager: Bob Butler
Manuscript Editor: Wynette Kommer
Illustration Coordinator: Walt Verbitski
Indexer: Dennis Dolan

Cardiopulmonary Exercise Testing: Physiologic Principles and Clinical Applications   ISBN   0–7216–1300–4

Last digit is the print number: 9   8   7   6   5   4   3   2   1

We dedicate this book to our parents:

Karl T. and Hedwig R. Weber
and the late
Bernard M. and Stella A. Janicki

Contributors

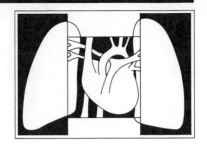

LARRY C. CASEY, M.D.
Assistant Professor of Medicine
Division of Pulmonary Medicine

ANDREW C. EISENHAUER, M.D.
Assistant Professor of Medicine
Director, Cardiac Catheterization Laboratory
Division of Cardiology

JOSEPH S. JANICKI, Ph.D.
Professor of Medicine
Associate Director, Cardiovascular Institute
Division of Cardiology

CAROL S. MASKIN, M.D.
Assistant Professor of Medicine
Director, Cardiac Rehabilitation
Division of Cardiology

PATRICIA A. McELROY, M.D.
Instructor in Medicine
Division of Cardiology

DAVID A. MEYERSON, M.D.
Assistant Professor of Medicine
Director, Cardiac Surveillance Center
Division of Cardiology

SANJEEV G. SHROFF, Ph.D.
Assistant Professor of Medicine
Director, Cardiac Mechanics Laboratory
Division of Cardiology

J. PETER SZIDON, M.D.
Professor of Medicine
Director, Pulmonary Medicine
Division of Medicine

KARL. T. WEBER, M.D.
Harold H. Hines, Jr., Professor of Medicine
Director, Cardiovascular Institute and Division
   of Cardiology

Michael Reese Hospital and Medical Center
Pritzker School of Medicine
University of Chicago, Chicago, Illinois

Foreword

Every high school student of Elementary Mammalian Biology knows that the cardiovascular and pulmonary systems function as a unit to take up oxygen from the atmosphere and deliver it to the metabolizing cells, while transporting carbon dioxide produced by these cells to the lungs and discharging it to the atmosphere. An enormous array of human diseases interferes with this exchange of gases in one way or another. These disorders are as diverse as bronchial asthma, interstitial lung disease, primary pulmonary hypertension, numerous disorders of cardiac structure and function, as well as disturbed regulation of systemic vascular resistance, i.e., essential hypertension.

Despite the logic inherent in considering the cardiovascular and pulmonary systems as a unit, why is this so rarely done? Largely, I believe, because the subspecialties of internal medicine have become too focused on the details of their organ systems, sometimes to the exclusion of the larger picture.

Cardiology and Pulmonology, in particular, have been too far apart for too long. These two subspecialties of Internal Medicine developed early during this century, Cardiology largely as a consequence of the development of the electrocardiograph, and Pulmonology as an outgrowth of the specialized care of the patient with pulmonary tuberculosis. These two important specialties intersected in a major way in the laboratory of André Cournand and Dickinson Richards at Bellevue Hospital, where I was privileged to receive a portion of my training. These two Nobel laureates established a *Cardiopulmonary* Laboratory, which considered the heart and lungs as a single integrated system and in which disorders affecting gas exchange and transport were studied, without concern about the traditional boundaries between Cardiology and Pulmonology. Alfred P. Fishman was a major investigator in the Bellevue Laboratory and one of the few clinical investigators in America to carry the "cardiopulmonary" torch. After an extensive and productive association with Fishman, Karl Weber has continued to champion the concept of considering the cardiovascular and pulmonary systems as a unit designed for gas exchange and transport. Dr. Weber and his colleagues have carried out investigation of great clinical significance during the past decade. In particular, they have used exercise to study disorders of the system as a whole and of its components. Along the way they have developed and standardized techniques that have become powerful tools in clinical investigation.

Now Weber and his associates have put their concepts together into this truly important book. First, they present the anatomic and physiologic principles of the cardiopulmonary system in a clear, logical, and straightforward manner, emphasizing the integration among the airways, lungs, pulmonary circulation, heart, and peripheral vascular bed throughout. What is unique about this effort is the broad perspective it offers, one that is not found among the best cardiac *or* pulmonary pathophysiologists who focus attention on one *or* the other system. The section on cardiopulmonary exercise testing not only provides a theoretic construct for using this physiologic stress to study the cardiopulmonary system but it also offers sufficient technical detail and even description of equipment to allow the reader to establish a similar laboratory and carry out similar studies. Then, Weber describes carefully and clearly the results of challenging the cardiopulmonary system with a systematically applied exercise stress in the major classes of diseases involving the heart and lungs. He provides a series of case reports that illuminate how cardiopulmonary exercise testing may be of inestimable value in identifying the nature of the disorder, determining its physiologic consequences and severity, developing a therapeutic strategy, and assessing the efficacy of therapy.

This is an exceptionally well written book. Just as its underlying theme is the integration of the cardiopulmonary system, so is this book well integrated internally. Dr. Weber and his colleagues have rendered a major service by presenting their thoughts and experiences on many important issues in Cardiopulmonary Pathophysiology in a lucid manner, describing their own extensive experience and presenting it in the context of the work of other investigators. This book should be of enormous interest to clinicians, investigators, and trainees in Cardiology and Pulmonology and should aid in lowering what has become, I believe, an inappropriate barrier between these two important subspecialties.

EUGENE BRAUNWALD, M.D.
Harvard Medical School
Brigham and Women's Hospital
Beth Israel Hospital
Boston, Massachusetts

Foreword

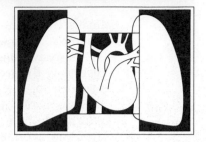

Muscular exercise is such a regular feature of daily life that no one pays much heed to it until discomfort sets in. In essence, the body acts like a well-oiled machine until it is pushed to its limit. The limit may be reached quickly, as by sprinting, or gradually, as by steady state exercise. In sprinting for short distances, such as a 100-yard dash, it is muscular performance that counts since the breath can be held throughout the dash and all metabolic debts repaid during recovery. In contrast, running the mile requires close integration of the respiration, circulation, and oxygen delivery to muscles to complete the distance.

After World War I, Morgan and Murray pictured in a four-quadrant diagram the interplay that was involved in accomplishing the smooth transfer of oxygen into the bloodstream, its uptake by the blood in the lungs, and its delivery to the exercising muscles. This picture of integrated performance— which could be drawn for gas exchange in the tissues as well as in the lungs— implied that failure on the part of any component of the cardiorespiratory system might throw a monkey wrench into the coordinated performance of the system as a whole. Since then, others have explored how individual disturbances of the circulatory and respiratory systems would affect the interplay. As a result, much has been learned about the nature of the integrating mechanisms, the respective roles played by each component part, compensating mechanisms, and the limits of performance. Another dimension to the picture of integrated performance operating within physiologic boundaries was added by Bannister when he set the world record for the mile run. He pointed out that limits of performance could be stretched by the urge to win—i.e., by psychologic behavior.

Not until after World War II, with the advent and standardization of cardiac catheterization for hemodynamic measurements during rest and exercise, could the parameters involved in the Morgan-Murray type of diagram be determined. It was then that cardiopulmonary physiology and medicine became distinct entities, operating within their own conceptual and practical frameworks. However, in the 1950s and 1960s, under the stimulus of discoveries relating predominantly to cardiology on the one hand and pulmonary disease on the other, "cardiopulmonary" began to lose its identity, its two components barely held together by the threads of pulmonary hypertension, pulmonary edema, adult respiratory distress syndrome, and cardiothoracic surgery. In this volume, Weber and Janicki forge another link by depicting an approach to exercise testing that is anchored in the coordinated interplay among respiration, circulation, and metabolism. The book begins with a consideration of the physiologic principles underlying the integrated performance of the respiratory and circulatory systems. The next section applies the physiologic principles to practical clinical assessment. The final section caps the volume by looking ahead to the potential uses of exercise in diagnosis, treatment, and rehabilitation.

A prevailing undercurrent to the Morgan-Murray approach to exercise testing is the fact that the human organism is a complex hierarchic system, made up of a wide array of parts, ranging from cells to organs, that execute their functions in a predetermined way. This flexible system, which operates effortlessly in normal individuals at rest, during sleep, and during exercise, could not work without remarkable mechanisms for the transfer of information from one part to another. The information system operates at different levels: at one extreme is the visible network of nerves supplemented by humoral substances in the blood—that is, the neurohumoral system; at the other extreme are molecular mechanisms tht convey their messages at a cellular or molecular level. This integrated system of communication is responsible for the coordinated responses of the living organism for a lifetime spent at different levels of activity. It is not difficult to imagine disease as a failure of integration or as an overresponse of one part of the system. Clearly, damage to a vital component, such as the heart, will interfere with the integrated behavior of the entire system and lower the limit of exercise performance.

Bainbridge began his classic volume on muscular exercise more than a half-century ago with the following perspective:

A man, who is performing hard physical work, may use 8 or 10 times as much oxygen as during rest, and the burden of meeting this demand for oxygen falls upon the respiratory and circulatory systems, which, for this purpose, are indissolubly linked together. Every increase in the requirements in the body for oxygen is accompanied by adaptive changes in the circulation and the respiration, which enable oxygen to be transferred more rapidly from the lungs to the tissues; and the rapid, deep breathing, the powerfully beating heart, the high blood-pressure, and the frequent pulse, present in the man who is engaged in violent exercise, are just as much a part of the exercise, and just as vital to its effective performance, as the movements of the muscles themselves. Violent exercise taxes the resources of the circulatory and respiratory systems equally with those of the muscles; and, partly because it is called upon to maintain an adequate supply of oxygen to the brain as well as to the muscles, partly, perhaps, owing to the larger number and greater complexity of the adjustments required for this purpose, the heart, as a rule, reaches the limit of its powers earlier than the skeletal muscles, and its functional capacity determines a man's capability for exertion. It is clear, then, that, apart from the changes taking place in the muscles themselves, the activities of the rest of the body are largely directed during exercise to the provision of an adequate supply of oxygen for the muscles, the heart, and the brain; hence any picture of muscular exercise must include the full range of these activities.*

With this statement, Bainbridge underscored enduring challenge to those who aspire to understand the coordinated performance of complex, hierarchic living systems that engage in different levels of activity for a lifetime. The present volume depicts how far physiologists, bioengineers, and physicians have come in unraveling the responses and adaptations to muscular exercise and how the accrued knowledge can be turned to practical advantage in testing physical capabilities.

ALFRED P. FISHMAN, M.D.

*William Maul Measey Professor of Medicine
Director, Cardiovascular-Pulmonary Division
Department of Medicine
University of Pennsylvania
Philadelphia, Pennsylvania*

---

*Bainbridge FA. The Physiology of Muscular Exercise. 3rd edition, rewritten by Boch AV, Dill DB. London, Longmans, Green & Company, 1931, p 2.

Preface

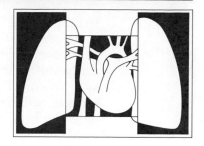

The rapid explosion of technology and scientific information in the sub-specialties of cardiovascular and pulmonary medicine has accelerated the growth of each of these disciplines. At the same time, however, it has had a negative impact on our intellectual growth and development by polarizing the two fields. The prevalence of coronary artery disease and systemic hypertension and their predominant involvement of the left heart has served to narrow the cardiologist's focus to the left ventricle. Similarly, the incidence of chronic bronchitis and emphysema has restricted the pulmonologist to the airways. Lost to this process of specialization is the fact that the heart and lungs work together to form a highly integrated cardiopulmonary unit, subservient to the body's need for oxygen.

Physical activity increases the oxygen utilized and the carbon dioxide produced by the working muscles. As a result, the cardiopulmonary unit is placed under a physiologic stress. Overt and even subclinical defects within the unit will become evident during exercise in a manner that is inversely proportional to the severity of the underlying disorder: the greater the defects, the lighter the work load required to elicit the abnormality. Hence, exercise testing is a physiologic stress that can be used to evaluate the integrity of the diseased cardiopulmonary unit and at the same time objectively establish the functional capacity of the patient.

The measurement of expired oxygen and carbon dioxide, together with air flow, during an exercise test provides a noninvasive evaluation of both the cardiocirculatory and respiratory systems. We have therefore viewed this approach as representing a *cardiopulmonary exercise (CPX) test.*

Until recently, however, exercise testing in most clinical laboratories has been narrowly focused. The traditionally trained cardiologist uses an exercise test for the sole purpose of evaluating myocardial perfusion in patients with coronary artery disease. Here the assessment of exercise is focused solely on the response in heart rate, arterial pressure, and the electrocardiogram. Accordingly, CPX represents a new concept and a new technique to physicians for which they have received little training. Concepts of respiratory gas exchange, albeit fundamental to the Fick cardiac output determination, may have been forgotten, inasmuch as a greater reliance is placed on dye dilution and thermodilution methods. Consequently, the measurement of respiratory gases is perceived by the cardiologist to fall under the purview of the pulmonary specialist. The pulmonologist, on the other hand, relies on the exercise test primarily to detect gas transfer abnormalities in the patient with chronic lung disease. In addition, the cumbersome techniques associated with the collection of expired air and the tedium inherent in measuring its oxygen and carbon dioxide content have throttled the level of enthusiasm among both subspecialists. However, as emphasized in the text, current instrumentation alleviates these concerns. Presently, oxygen uptake, carbon dioxide production, minute ventilation, tidal volume, and respiratory rate during exercise can be determined easily on an intermittent or breath-by-breath basis. Commercially available systems are "user friendly," and results can be obtained in digital and graphic formats both during the CPX test and immediately afterward. The electrocardiogram, heart rate, and blood pressure also can be monitored, thus providing a comprehensive evaluation of the exercise response.

This comprehensive evaluation should appeal to the cardiologist or the pulmonologist who seeks to evaluate various disorders of the cardiopulmonary unit. In addition, physicians in occupational or industrial medicine who are faced with issues relevant to the determination of work capacity or disability will find CPX a useful and objective guide. The same is true for writing an individualized exercise prescription for patients or normal individuals interested in a program of rehabilitation. CPX also provides the physician in sports medicine with objective information central to monitoring the progress of an exercise training or rehabilitation program.

Finally, many in cardiology, pulmonology, sports medicine, or occupational and industrial medicine may wonder whether CPX testing is justified when cost containment is mandated on all fronts of today's health care system. Would not current, more familiar, tests provide equivalent information? In the pages that follow, this issue is addressed in a practical, understandable manner, and it becomes evident quickly that the answer is no! The tremendous potential of CPX in the evaluation and management of patients with various disorders of the cardiopulmonary unit, including chronic heart failure (Chapter 11), valvular heart disease (Chapter 12), pulmonary (Chapter 13) and systemic hypertension (Chapter 14), chronotropic dysfunction of the heart (Chapter 15), lung disease and chest wall deformity (Chapter 16), and the patient with exertional dyspnea who may have coexistent heart and lung disease (Chapter 17) is stressed throughout. CPX is cost effective because it is objective and more directly targeted to the issues than are most conventional tests. The costlier radionuclide ejection fraction determination, for example, does not predict the functional or aerobic capacity, the cardiac reserve, or the severity of disease.

This text has been written entirely by faculty members in cardiology and pulmonary medicine at Michael Reese Hospital and Medical Center, University of Chicago. It has been structured to provide practical insights into cardiopulmonary physiology (Chapters 1 through 6), setting up a cardiopulmonary exercise laboratory (Chapters 7, 8, and 9), and the application of CPX testing to clinical practice (Chapters 10 through 21). We have drawn heavily on our own experience with CPX over the past decade to support our viewpoint and recommendations. We have deliberately avoided long bibliographies and have cited reviews and monographs wherever possible. Moreover, we have not been shy to tackle issues that are admittedly in question and to make projections, even though the clinical experience with CPX in the evaluation of various disorders is still very much in evolution. Notwithstanding our boldness, we have attempted to present the issues in a style that is not overly dogmatic. We fully expect that as our understanding of CPX continues to grow, some of our viewpoints will require revision, correction, or even dismissal.

Credit must be given to our talented colleagues who joined us in preparing this text. We are indebted to their commitment to scholarship, their patience, and their loyalty. Finally, the preparation of this book would not have been possible without the dedicated assistance of several very special individuals: Lester Shelton, Thomas Nusbickel and James Morgan, who were responsible for the day-to-day operation of the Cardiopulmonary Evaluation Laboratory; David Ward, who provided valued editorial assistance and the overall organization of each chapter; the nursing staff of our Clinical Pharmacology Unit: Carolyn Blakely, Cynthia Class, Jean DeBoo, Jean Hughes, and Elizabeth Manglal-lan; Thelma Joyce Johnson, who prepared the illustrative material; and Joyce Chisom, Connie Duplessis, and Marceine Lamb, whose dedicated secretarial assistance in preparing draft after draft was clearly the glue that held this effort together. We are extremely grateful to these individuals. The skillful assistance of our friends at W. B. Saunders is also deeply appreciated.

KARL T. WEBER
JOSEPH S. JANICKI

Contents

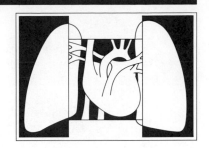

SECTION I

PHYSIOLOGIC PRINCIPLES

KARL T. WEBER

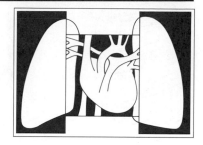

Anatomic Characteristics of the Cardiopulmonary Unit

The cardiopulmonary unit is contained within the thorax. This chapter is devoted to describing the anatomic characteristics of the thorax, the heart, and the ventilatory system, and to introducing the manner in which these features contribute to the dynamic behavior of the cardiopulmonary unit at rest and during exercise.

THE THORAX, OR RESPIRATORY PUMP

The thorax is formed by the 12 thoracic vertebrae with their cushion-like intervertebral discs and the 12 ribs, which have pliable cartilaginous attachments to the sternum and seventh rib. Its inner membranous lining, the parietal pleura, and the intercostal muscles aid in sealing and protecting the contents of the thorax from the atmosphere. Aside from protecting the heart and lungs, the bony thorax serves several other important functions, each of which is relevant to gas transport. Various muscle groups, including those of the neck, upper limb, chest wall, back, and abdomen, and the diaphragm are attached to it. The contraction of these muscle groups, together with the elasticity of the bony thorax, creates a bellows-like chamber of variable volume, which has been termed the respiratory pump. An increase in intrathoracic volume, for example, enhances the movement of air into the lungs and blood into the right heart. In addition, the marrow of the ribs and sternum is a principal site of red blood cell production and thereby the body's hemoglobin pool.

The Configuration of the Respiratory Pump

The thoracic cage of the adult has a conical shape, being narrower at the thoracic inlet and larger at the thoracic outlet (Fig. 1–1). The infant's thorax, on the other hand, is more barrel-shaped. In the adult the transverse diameter of the thorax is approximately 25 per cent greater than its anteroposterior dimension while the curvature of the thoracic spine indents the cavity posteriorly. The configuration of the thorax is altered in three dimensions with *inspiration*; these include the anteroposterior, transverse, and longitudinal directions (Fig. 1–2). The contractions of various muscle groups, such as the intercostals, the scalene group (anterior, middle, and posterior scalenes), the diaphragm, and the posterior superior serratus, increase the internal

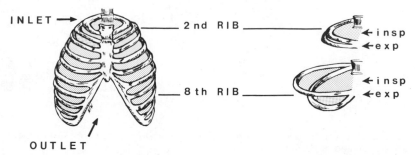

FIGURE 1–1. The configuration of the adult thorax and its motion during the respiratory cycle.

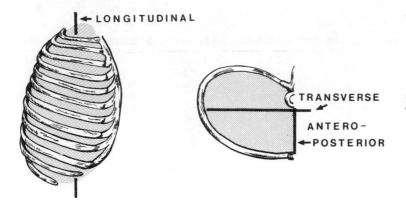

←LONGITUDINAL

TRANSVERSE

ANTERO-
←POSTERIOR

FIGURE 1–2. The dimensions of the adult thorax.

dimensions of the thoracic cage. The direction of motion of the ribs during the contraction of any of these muscle groups depends on their curvature; their anatomic attachments to the thoracic vertebrae, the sternum, and the other ribs (Fig. 1–3); and the direction of muscle contraction. Most ribs, for example, move upward and outward during inspiration.

The scalene muscles arise from the cervical vertebrae and insert on the anterior end of the first and second ribs. Their action is to raise these ribs upward and outward as well as to stabilize the upper portion of the rib cage. This facilitates the contraction of the intercostal muscles, which are attached to the first through sixth ribs. An upward and forward movement of the first to sixth ribs occurs as the intercostal muscles contract to

increase the anteroposterior dimension of the upper thorax. The outward movement of the first four ribs, however, is minimal because they have a small radius of curvature. The fifth and sixth ribs, on the other hand, which have larger radii of curvature, are lifted upward and outward to a much greater extent by the intercostal muscles. The transverse dimension of the thorax is increased at the level of the seventh to tenth ribs by the contraction of their intercostal muscles. The intercostals also serve to maintain the space between ribs by exerting an upward pull on each rib while providing a resistance to inward displacement or outward expansion of the thoracic contents. A further increase in the transverse diameter of the lower third of the thorax, as well as its longitudinal dimension, occurs with diaphragmatic contraction.

INSPIRATORY   EXPIRATORY

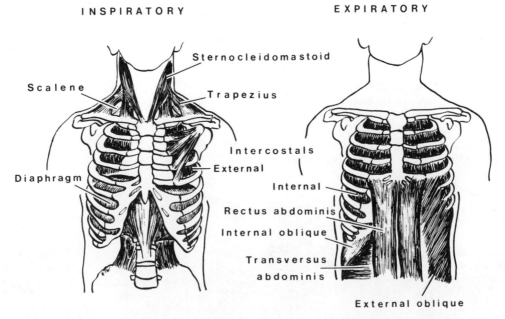

Sternocleidomastoid

Scalene

Trapezius

Intercostals

External

Diaphragm

Internal

Rectus abdominis

Internal oblique

Transversus
abdominis

External oblique

FIGURE 1–3. The muscles of the neck, chest, and abdomen that are used to alter the dimensions of the thorax during inspiration and expiration.

Expiration occurs with the relaxation of the various muscle groups of the thorax—the diaphragm in particular—and with the elastic recoil of the lungs. The thorax assumes a smaller configuration, and its volume is reduced with expiration. A forced expiration elicits the contraction of the abdominal muscles and resultant depression of the lower ribs. The contraction of these abdominal muscles, which normally do not participate in the respiratory movement of the thorax, also raises intrathoracic pressure by restraining the outward motion of the abdominal wall, making it more rigid and thereby retarding the dissipation of intrathoracic pressure into the abdominal cavity.

The Innervation and Blood Supply of the Respiratory Pump

The thoracic intercostal nerves arise from the first six thoracic spinal nerves to supply the external and internal intercostal muscles, the posterior superior serratus, and the subcostal and transverse thoracic muscles. The thoracoabdominal intercostal nerves of the seventh to eleventh thoracic spinal nerves supply the abdominal muscles that are used in forced expiration. The scalene group of muscles, which raises the first and second ribs, is innervated by the cervical plexus, which is composed of cervical nerves 1 to 4. The phrenic nerve is responsible for the innervation of the diaphragm. It too is derived from the cervical plexus, predominantly cervical nerve four, with variable contributions from cervical nerves 3 and 5.

The intercostal arteries of the thoracic aorta supply most of the intercostal muscles. The first two intercostal muscles derive their vascular supply from the costocervical trunk of the subclavian artery while the internal mammary artery, which also arises from the subclavian artery, provides the musculophrenic and pericardiacophrenic arteries supplying the superior surface of the diaphragm. Anterior intercostal arteries of the internal mammary artery supply the first six intercostal muscles and similar branches from the musculophrenic artery vascularize the anterior segments of the seventh to eleventh intercostal muscles. The inferior surface of the diaphragm derives its blood supply from the phrenic artery of the abdominal aorta.

THE HEART

The heart is located in the thorax, where it is coupled to the arterial, venous, and pulmonic circulations. Its contraction provides the propulsive force that sustains the circulation of blood through each vascular segment of the body and lungs and thereby guarantees gas transport to and from the metabolizing tissues. The heart normally pumps 4 to 6 liters of arterial blood to the tissues each minute while the body is at rest, consuming an average quantity of 200 to 250 ml/min of oxygen. The heart receives 4 to 6 liters of venous blood for delivery to the lungs in the resting state, where carbon dioxide production ranges from 140 to 180 ml/min. Cardiac output, venous return, and pulmonary blood flow are each increased proportionally during exercise to a level that is commensurate with the oxidative metabolism of working muscle. During vigorous physical activity, for example, each may rise to 20 liters/min or more.

The Pericardium and Chambers of the Heart

Not unlike the pleura, which is invaginated by the lungs, the pericardium is a serous sac that encloses the heart and the roots of the venae cavae, pulmonary artery, and ascending aorta. The external fibrous layer of the pericardium fuses with the central tendon of the diaphragm inferiorly and the adventitia of the great vessels superiorly. During inspiration the descent of the diaphragm creates a downward radial traction on the pericardium, reducing its distensibility and perhaps retarding the ability of the ventricles to be filled.

Situated in the middle mediastinum, which has also been termed the cardiac fossa,[1] the pericardium is in contact with and has several attachments to various components of the thorax. It is attached to the sternum by ligaments that traverse the anterior mediastinum. On its lateral surfaces, which are in contact with the mediastinal pleura and the lungs, course the phrenic nerves. The posterior surface of the pericardium forms the anterior boundary of the posterior mediastinum, which contains the esophagus and thoracic aorta.

The human heart is composed of four chambers, including two atria and two ventricles. Each chamber is separated from the other despite their close approximation. The atria receive blood that they subsequently transfer to the ventricles. The ventricles, in turn, propel blood into the pulmonic and systemic circulations. A coordinated sequence of alternating contraction and relaxation between the atria and ventricles—termed systole and diastole, respectively—and the presence of one-way valves within the heart ensure that blood flow is unidirectional, proceeding through the right heart, the pulmonary circulation, and then the left heart and aorta. As the musculature of the atria and the myocardium surrounding each ventricle are electrically depolarized, they contract, ejecting the blood contained within their respective chambers. During the electromechanical systole of the ventricles, the right and left atria are in a relaxed state and are being passively filled from the venae cavae and pulmonary venous circulation, respectively. As the ventricles relax, their pressure falls below that in the atria, thus permitting the blood they contain to passively enter the ventricles. This is the diastolic phase of the cardiac cycle for both the atria and ventricles. Atrial depolarization and subsequent contraction precedes ventricular depolarization by approximately 120 to 180 milliseconds; this provides an additional volume of blood to each relaxed ventricle prior to contraction.

Systemic venous return from the inferior and superior venae cavae enters the right atrium. The right atrium also receives the heart's venous drainage via the coronary sinus and anterior cardiac veins. The contents of the right atrium traverse the tricuspid valve to fill the right ventricle. The subsequent contraction of the myocardium raises the pressure within the right ventricular chamber, thereby closing the tricuspid valve and preventing the regurgitation of blood into the right atrium. When right ventricular pressure exceeds that in the pulmonary artery, venous blood is propelled from the ventricle across the pulmonic valve into this vessel. Right ventricular pressure falls with myocardial relaxation; the pulmonic valve closes and its chamber is once again filled from the right atrium when ventricular pressure is less than that in the atrium. Closure of the pulmonic valve sustains the pressure within the pulmonary artery. This diastolic pulmonary artery pressure continues to drive blood forward into the capillaries surrounding the gas exchange surface of the alveoli. Together, the right atrium and right ventricle represent the venous blood pump, which is responsible for receiving and propelling venous blood into the pulmonary circulation for the exchange of oxygen and carbon dioxide.

After oxygenation, arterial blood leaves the lungs by traversing the four pulmonary veins to enter the left atrium. From the left atrial reservoir, arterial blood enters the relaxed left ventricle via the mitral valve. The contraction of the myocardium raises left ventricular chamber pressure, thereby closing the mitral valve and preventing the regurgitation of blood into the left atrium. As left ventricular pressure rises to exceed aortic pressure, blood is propelled across the aortic valve into the ascending aorta. Left ventricular ejection ceases with myocardial relaxation. The subsequent decline in left ventricular pressure permits closure of the aortic valve and a diastolic pressure to be sustained within the aorta, ensuring the continued forward direction of blood flow into the peripheral arterial circulation throughout the cardiac cycle. The left atrium and ventricle represent the arterial blood pump, which is responsible for the transport of oxygen and other nutrients and substrates to the metabolizing tissues.

The Valves of the Heart

Blood flow through the heart and circulatory system is unidirectional because of the differences in driving pressure, described in more detail in Chapter 2. It is sustained by the alternating sequence of atrial and ventricular contraction and the presence of one-way valves within the heart. The tricuspid and mitral valves separate the right atrium and right ventricle and the left atrium and left ventricle, respectively, and are termed atrioventricular valves. Each atrioventricular valve has a parachute-like configuration. Their pliable leaflets—three in the case of the tricuspid valve and two for the mitral valve—are attached to the heart's fibrous skeleton at the atrioventricular groove. On the other end of the leaflets are stringlike chordae tendineae, which insert into the head of the papillary muscles; the other end of these muscles is derived from the endomyocardium (Fig. 1–4). The contraction of the papillary muscles ensures the closure of the mitral and tricuspid valves. The proper mechanical function of the atrioventricular valves is based not only on these leaflets but also on the anatomic integrity of the chordae and their attachment to the papillary muscles and the muscles' insertion into the underlying endomyocardium.

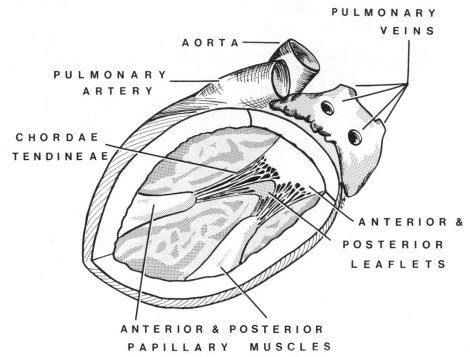

FIGURE 1–4. The mitral valve apparatus, including its leaflets, chordae tendineae, and anterior and posterior papillary muscles.

The semilunar pulmonic and aortic valves are quite similar to one another and consist of three leaflets formed from the heart's fibrous skeleton at the roots of the pulmonary artery and aorta, respectively. They have no chordal attachments. Their superior surface is convex toward the lumen of the respective vessels, which assures their opening into the vessel and the forward direction of blood flow. Their closure seals each vessel from its respective ventricle. The orifice, or cross-sectional area, of these valves is 2 to 4 cm² and roughly one half that of the atrioventricular valves (Fig. 1–5). The larger valve area of the atrioventricular valves permits blood to enter the ventricles from the relatively small gradient in driving pressure that exists between the atrium and ventricle they separate. The contraction of the myocardium creates a large driving pressure to sustain blood flow across the smaller orifice of the aortic and pulmonic valves.

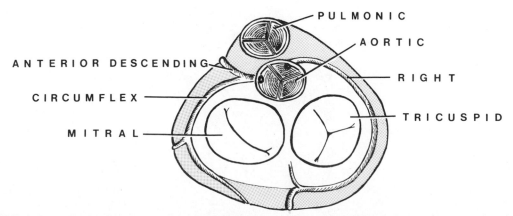

FIGURE 1–5. A superior view of the base of the heart depicting the four valves (tricuspid, pulmonic, mitral, and aortic) and the major segments of the coronary circulation, including the right, left main anterior descending, and circumflex coronary arteries.

The Heart's Muscular Wall: The Myocardium

The ventricular chambers are formed by the myocardium, which is attached to the fibrous skeleton of the heart. Each chamber has a free wall of myocardium and a common wall formed by the interventricular septum. Like the free walls, the septum is also muscular throughout its length except near its upper and posterior portions, where it is a thin, fibrous membrane. The membranous septum separates the left ventricle from the lower part of the right atrium and the upper portion of the right ventricle near the septal leaflet of the tricuspid valve.

The myocardium is composed of cardiac muscle, connective tissue, and the coronary circulation. Each muscle fiber consists of numerous myofibrils and their constituent subunits, termed myocytes. It is the contraction of these myocytes and the tension they generate within the myofibrils and muscle fibers that leads to the development of pressure within each ventricular chamber. The myocytes are depolarized in a sequential order; they do not contract simultaneously. Wiggers described the sequence of muscle fiber contraction as a series of rapidly summated fractionate contractions.[2] Electrical depolarization, for example, begins high in the interventricular septum and extends downward through the septum toward the apex of the left ventricle. Thereafter, the remainder of the left and right ventricular free walls is depolarized in a sequence that proceeds from the apex to the base of the heart. Thus, after the septum has been activated, ventricular contraction proceeds from the apex toward the base, resembling a peristaltic pump. An ordered sequence of contraction aids in ventricular emptying.

The mass of myocardium surrounding each ventricle is proportional to the amount of pressure work each chamber is required to generate. In the adult human heart, left ventricular muscle mass is three to four times that of the right ventricle because of the differences in pressure work that the ventricles must perform (see Chapter 2). Myocardial mass will increase if the resistance opposing the ejection of blood from either ventricle is increased and the pressure it must generate is enhanced.

In the past, it was thought that the muscle fibers of the myocardium were arranged in discrete bundles and separated from one another by distinct planes of cleavage. These conclusions were drawn from a technique based on the teasing or tearing apart of the postmortem myocardium. This approach, however, created artificial distinctions in fiber orientation and hence the notion that they were arranged as discrete bundles. More recently, Streeter and colleagues have used a light microscopic assessment to indicate that muscle fibers are actually arranged as a continuum, which can be described with respect to the angle they describe in the circumferential direction.[3] Figure 1–6 depicts the fiber alignment of the canine heart from its epicardium to endocardium. These observa-

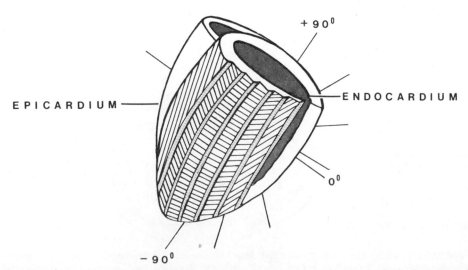

FIGURE 1–6. The alignment of heart muscle fibers within the myocardium of the left ventricle. The majority of fibers, occupying the midwall, are aligned in the circumferential direction whereas those fibers near the epicardium and endocardium have a nearly vertical alignment.

WEAVE and TENDONS

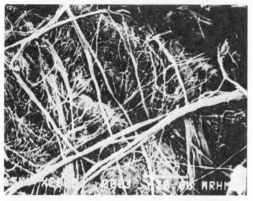

STRUTS

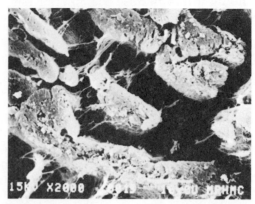

FIGURE 1–7. The ultrastructure of the primate heart depicted by the scanning electron microscope. Individual myocytes are grouped together by a weave of collagen having tendinous insertions while a fine reticular network of collagen joins individual myocytes together and to their capillaries (not shown).

tions have recently been confirmed in our laboratory by Pearlman et al for the normal human myocardium.[4]

It is also important to recognize that the myocardium is not simply muscle. Myocytes are tethered within and supported by a connective tissue network composed largely of collagen (Fig. 1–7). Using the scanning electron microscope, Borg and Caulfield have described the morphologic characteristics of this network.[5] There are several components of the heart's collagen matrix: (a) a complex weave of collagen bundles that surrounds myocytes, sequestering them into groups, which includes long, tendon-like strands of collagen that insert into the weave; and (b) a finer network of collagen that joins individual myocytes together and to their capillaries. The collagenous weave and intermyocyte connections maintain the alignment of myocytes throughout the cardiac cycle, permitting reversible interdigitation, on the one hand, and limiting the degree of slippage between myocytes on the other. Moreover, as a composite material composed of muscle and collagen, the viscoelasticity of the myocardium will be a function of the viscoelasticity of muscle and collagen and their relative proportions (see Chapter 4).

The Heart's Blood Supply

Two coronary arteries arise from the sinuses of the ascending aorta to supply arterial blood to the atria and myocardium. The right coronary artery arises from the right aortic sinus (see Fig. 1–5) where one of its earliest branches, in approximately 55 per cent of the human population, is the sinus node artery. The right coronary artery courses along the atrioventricular groove to the posterior surface of the heart, giving off branches to the right atrium and right ventricular myocardium along the way. At the confluence of the atrioventricular groove and posterior interventricular sulcus, termed the crux of the heart, the atrioventricular nodal artery arises from the right coronary artery. This occurs in 90 per cent or more of human hearts and determines whether or not the right coronary artery is considered "dominant." The continuation of the right coronary artery in the interventricular groove beyond the crux supplies the inferior and posterior surfaces of the left ventricle and its posterior papillary muscle. The right coronary artery also gives rise to a posterior descending artery, which courses within the posterior interventricular sulcus to the posterior half of the interventricular septum and the apex of the heart. Anastomoses between the posterior and anterior descending coronary arteries are present at the apex.

The left main coronary artery arises from the left aortic sinus. After a short distance it bifurcates into the left anterior descending and left circumflex coronary arteries (see Fig. 1–5), which course down the anterior interventricular sulcus and atrioventricular groove, respectively. The left circumflex coronary artery may anastomose with the right coronary artery on the posterior surface of the left ventricle. The anterior descending and circumflex coronary arteries, and their diagonal and marginal arteries, supply the majority of the left ventricular myocardium, left atrium, and anterior papillary muscle, while septal branches of the anterior descending artery perfuse the anterior half of the interventricular septum.

The veins draining the heart course parallel to the coronary arteries. They, however, bear different names than the arteries. The major terminus for the veins is the coronary sinus. It is situated at the posterior portion of the atrioventricular groove, and its ostia drains into the right atrium near its junction with the inferior vena cava. The veins that empty into the coronary sinus include the great and middle cardiac veins, which traverse the anterior and posterior interventricular sulci, respectively, and the lesser veins from the left ventricle. Several anterior cardiac veins arise from the anterior surface of the right ventricle to empty directly into the right atrium. Thus, the venous blood of the coronary sinus is primarily, but not exclusively, representative of the drainage of the left ventricular myocardium. This fact, together with the accessibility of the coronary sinus ostia to catheterization, has made the coronary sinus a prime site for monitoring the energy requirements and metabolic activity of the left ventricular myocardium.

The Heart's Conduction System and Innervation

The heart beats automatically because of its specialized pacemaker tissue and conduction system, which initiate and transmit electrical impulses that depolarize the myocardium. Aside from its inherent rhythmicity, the heart is also under the influence of nerves and ganglia that can alter the frequency of its contraction.

As previously noted, the myocardium is depolarized in an orderly fashion: the atria followed by the ventricles. The sinoatrial (SA) node, located at the junction of the superior vena cava and right atrium, has the greatest intrinsic automaticity and therefore initiates the heart's contraction. This occurs approximately 70 times per minute in the resting state. The impulse of the sinoatrial node is propagated within the atria and to the atrioventricular (AV) node. The AV node is situated in the septal wall of the right atrium above the opening of the coronary sinus. Once stimulated, the AV node transmits the impulse to the specialized conduction tissue of the myocardium. This tissue includes the bundle of His and its two major ramifications, the right and left bundles, which

course down the interventricular septum to terminate in the Purkinje fibers that are responsible for myocardial depolarization.

The higher intrinsic automaticity of the SA node dictates that it is the dominant pacemaker of the heart and responsible for the heart's contraction frequency. Loss of normal SA node automaticity or an inability of its impulse to escape the node requires that the AV node or the remaining conduction system assume the role of dominant pacemaker and initiate the impulses that will depolarize the myocardium. The AV node, having a slower inherent automaticity than the SA node, will assume rhythmic control under these circumstances. However, the heart is now stimulated at a reduced rate of approximately 40 times per minute. The impulses from the AV node disrupt the ordered sequence of contraction between atria and ventricles. As a result, the contribution of right and left atrial contraction to right and left ventricular filling is lost. This may account for a reduction in ventricular filling volume of up to 20 per cent.

The heart's conduction system is innervated by sympathetic and parasympathetic nerves that modulate the intrinsic rhythmicity of the heart. The right vagus, representing the parasympathetic system, and right sympathetic branches of the cardiac plexus innervate the SA node whereas the AV node is chiefly innervated by their counterparts on the left. Stimulation of the sympathetic nerves increases heart rate, the rate of impulse conduction, and the force of myocardial contraction. Parasympathetic stimulation, on the other hand, slows the heart rate and the conduction rate. Uncertainty exists as to whether or not vagal stimulation will influence the force of ventricular contraction.

The innervation of the coronary arteries is less clear. The low density of alpha receptors on the coronary arteries appears to prevent their constriction during the heightened adrenergic stimulation that accompanies hemorrhagic shock or heart failure. However, direct stimulation of sympathetic ganglia or the intravenous infusion of ergonovine may elicit coronary artery constriction. Visceral efferent fibers of the vagus and sympathetic nerves, which emanate from the heart and coronary arteries, end in the first four cervical segments of the spinal cord. The modulation of this reflex arc is thought to accelerate or decelerate heart rate and contractile force, as well as to elicit the sensation of angina pectoris during myocardial ischemia. An indirect activation of the cervical plexus may occur during myocardial ischemia to account for the sensation of the neck, jaw, or left arm pain.

THE VENTILATORY SYSTEM

The oxygen requirements of single cellular organisms are met by the simple diffusion of atmospheric air across their cell membrane. In humans, however, the metabolizing cells are located at some distance from the atmosphere. Simple diffusion across the skin, for example, becomes an entirely inadequate source of oxygen. As a result, other processes must be available to ensure the transfer of oxygen from the atmosphere to the metabolizing cells. At the same time, nearly equal quantities of carbon dioxide must be eliminated into the atmosphere. Two forms of respiration are present; each still relies on gas diffusion to satisfy oxygen and carbon dioxide transfer. The interchange of these respiratory gases between the air brought into the lungs and its alveoli with the blood in the alveolar capillaries has been termed external respiration. Internal respiration, on the other hand, is the interchange or diffusion of these gases between the systemic capillaries and the metabolizing cells; here the cell's membrane serves as the gas exchange surface.

The movement of air into and out of the alveoli is accomplished by the muscular contraction of the respiratory pump. Air is brought into and out of the lungs as a result of intrathoracic pressure being cyclically lowered with respect to atmospheric pressure. A specialized conductance network facilitates the flow of air to and from the alveoli, as well as warming, humidifying, and cleansing the air brought to the alveoli.

The Conductance Network

The nasal and oral cavities, pharynx, larynx, trachea, and bronchi represent a highly vascularized, semirigid conduit that permits the alveolus to gain access to the atmosphere. This conductance network, however, does not participate in the gas exchange process. Hence, the movement of air into and out of the conduit has been considered as "wasted" or dead space ventilation. Nevertheless, this dead space ventilation serves several important functions, each of which facilitate gas exchange. These include (a) transforming atmospheric air, at its ambient temperature, to body temperature; (b) humidifying the inspired air; and (c) filtering and entrapping particulate matter contained within atmospheric air.

The primary conduits that bring air to the lungs are the trachea and bronchi (Fig. 1–8). Bronchioles and alveolar ducts are further subdivisions of the bronchi that permit the admixture of inspired and alveolar air. The rigidity of the trachea and bronchi, provided by semicircular rings of cartilage, facilitates airflow to and from the alveoli. The blood supply of the trachea, bronchi, and respiratory bronchioles is provided by the bronchial arteries, which arise from the thoracic aorta and upper intercostal arteries. Bronchial veins drain these regions and empty into the azygos vein and the hemiazygos or superior intercostal vein. Bronchial venous drainage from the terminal portions of the bronchial tree is returned to the left atrium via the pulmonary veins. This small volume of venous drainage represents a physiologic ve-

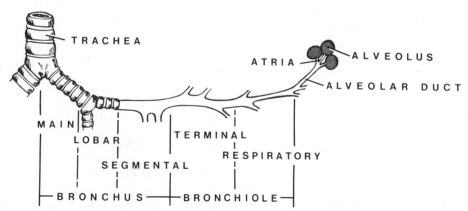

FIGURE 1–8. The components of the bronchial tree, including the various subdivisions of the bronchus and bronchiole.

nous admixture with the oxygenated blood of the pulmonary veins. Another physiologic source of venous admixture occurs within the left ventricle where a small volume of venous drainage of the coronary circulation empties directly into its chamber through the thebesian veins. The venous admixture from the bronchial and thebesian veins does not significantly alter the oxygen content of arterial blood perfusing the systemic circulation. The perfusion of poorly ventilated segments of the lung represents a major source of venous admixture, which can become clinically significant as will be discussed in Chapter 16.

The innervation of the tracheobronchial tree includes parasympathetic and sympathetic components. Vagal innervation provides constrictor fibers to the bronchial musculature and secretory fibers to its mucous glands. Bronchodilatation and reduced glandular secretion occur with sympathetic stimulation.

The Lungs

The atmosphere is brought into contact with capillary blood within the lungs and their alveoli. The lungs are light in weight, easily compressible, and highly elastic. Their external surface is smooth as a result of covering by the visceral pleura. This permits the lungs to glide effortlessly along the bony thorax during inflation and deflation. Because of their compressibility, the shape of the lungs is determined by contiguous neighboring structures. The configuration of the thorax and its own elasticity dictates the lateral limit to lung expansion, and the position of the diaphragm determines the inferior boundary for lung expansion. Medially, the heart creates an impression on each lung, which is larger and deeper on the left because of the heart's position within the left hemithorax. Although this discussion has emphasized the lung's compressibility, the lung too contributes to the configuration of contiguous structures. For example, the cardiac fossa is formed by the lungs. During inflation, the lungs may determine the limits of cardiac expansion.[1] In patients with advanced airway disease the hyperinflated lungs flatten the curvature of the diaphragm.

Several fissures divide the lungs into lobes. The oblique fissure of each lung creates a superior and inferior lobe; the horizontal fissure of the right lung produces a third lobe called the middle lobe. Each lobe has discrete segments supplied by branches of the secondary lobar bronchi. These smaller subdivisions are called the bronchopulmonary segments. Secondary bronchi are located within the substance of the lung; their subdivisions are called bronchioles (see Fig. 1–8). Their terminal subdivisions, or lobular bronchioles, resemble the major and minor bronchi. They function as conduits for air and do not participate in gas exchange. The terminal bronchioles give rise to yet further subdivisions, called the respiratory bronchioles. The alveolar ducts arise from the respiratory bronchioles. Single alveoli arise from respiratory bronchioles whereas numerous alveolar sacs originate from alveolar ducts. Alveolar ducts and respiratory bronchioles differ in that the ducts are completely alveolarized and ciliated epithelium is absent. Small communications or pores, called atria, exist between alveolar ducts and the alveoli to foster the further interchange of respiratory gases between adjacent alveoli.

The Alveoli

The alveoli are thin, membranous sacs, 250 μm in diameter, which are highly vascularized by the capillaries of the pulmonary circulation that surround each alveolus (Fig. 1–9). Thus, a rich vascular network exists for the diffusion of oxygen into the capillaries and for the transfer of the highly diffusible carbon dioxide from the capillaries into the alveoli. It is estimated that in the adult lung there are several hundred million alveoli comprising a surface area of 80 square meters, of which 90 per cent is covered by capillaries. The highly elastic nature of the alveoli and the expansive capability of the lung itself, enhanced by its numerous infoldings, aid in creating the enormous surface area. The alveolar-capillary membrane is the site of respiratory gas exchange. The alveolar-capillary membrane is composed of the alveolar epithelium and the capillary endothelium and is separated by an interstitial space composed of basement membrane and connective tissue. The interstitium facing the alveolus is stretched out and thinned by capillaries which course from one alveolus to another. Gas exchange occurs across the thinner segment of the interstial space while liquid and solute exchange take place across its thicker segment.

At rest, the movement of 6 liters of air each minute is adequate to maintain the oxygenation of blood and eucapnia. During vigorous exercise, minute ventilation may

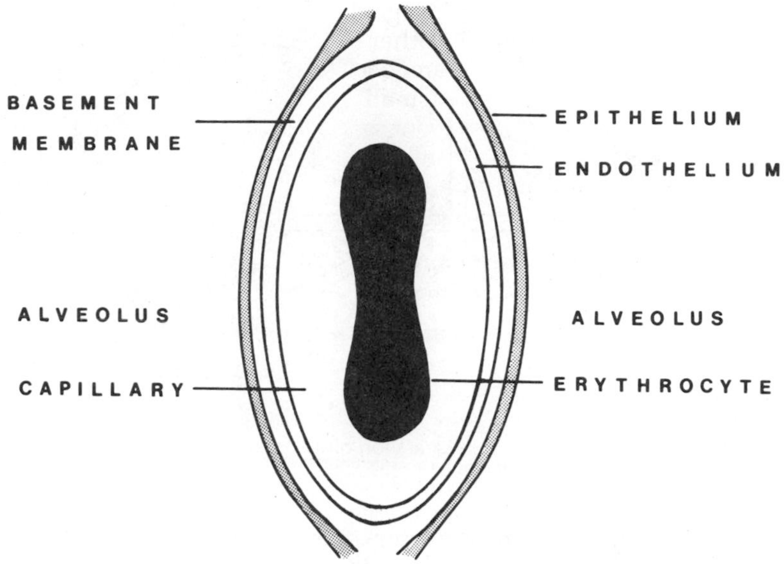

FIGURE 1–9. A schematic representation of the alveolus and a capillary of the pulmonary circulation. The interalveolar septum is lined on each side by epithelium and the capillary containing the erythrocyte by endothelium. Each epithelial layer rests on basement membranes that are separated by an interstitial space.

BASEMENT
MEMBRANE

EPITHELIUM

ENDOTHELIUM

ALVEOLUS

ALVEOLUS

CAPILLARY

ERYTHROCYTE

rise to 100 liters/min in order to sustain appropriate gas exchange. In the absence of lung disease, ventilation itself poses no limit to the individual's capacity for exercise, even at strenuous or maximal levels of physical activity. This is not the case for the heart, which has a finite limit to its ability to circulate blood (i.e., the cardiac reserve).

The Pulmonary Circulation

The pulmonary artery, which arises from the right ventricle, receives all the systemic venous blood from the body's various circulatory beds. It is therefore described as containing truly "mixed" venous blood. The main pulmonary artery divides into a right and left pulmonary artery, with the right being larger and longer. Each further divides to supply the lobes of the right and left lung, respectively. Additional branching of each pulmonary artery takes place in accordance with these subdivisions to accompany respiratory bronchioles, alveolar ducts, and alveoli. The capillaries of the pulmonary circulation traverse each alveolus. In the adult, the pulmonary arteries that accompany terminal and respiratory bronchioles have a muscular media; at birth, however, only a small portion of these vessels possesses any smooth muscle. In general, three different types of pulmonary arteries can be identified in the adult. Each of these vessels bears a relationship to the branching pattern of the airways. Elastic pulmonary arteries, which have an elastic fiber bounding smooth muscle, are more than 1000 μm in external di-

ameter and are part of the proximal portion of the pulmonary circulation (that is, the main artery, its branches, and all extralobular arteries). The muscular pulmonary arteries are smaller in diameter (100 to 1000 μm); each of these vessels has an elastic lamina that surrounds both sides of smooth muscle (i.e., internal and external elastic laminae). Muscular arteries accompany bronchioles within each lobule. Finally, pulmonary arterioles are the terminal branches of the pulmonary arterial circulation. They are less than 100 μm in diameter and supply alveolar ducts and alveoli. A muscular wall can be found in the arterioles that originates from muscular arteries, whereas terminally these vessels contain only endothelium and an elastic lamina.

Other branches of the pulmonary artery, called supernumerary arteries, do not follow the airways. These vessels can be found at the hilum and as far distally as the end of the respiratory bronchioles.[6] Near the hilum they comprise 25 per cent of the total cross-sectional area of the pulmonary circulation, whereas at the periphery they account for 40 per cent of the vasculature. These supernumerary vessels provide a rich collateral network and additional source of blood to the gas exchange surface while fostering the low impedance profile of the pulmonary circulation.

The pulmonary veins are formed by the confluence of the venules, which unite to form larger venous channels draining the various bronchopulmonary segments. There are more of these smaller veins than arteries,

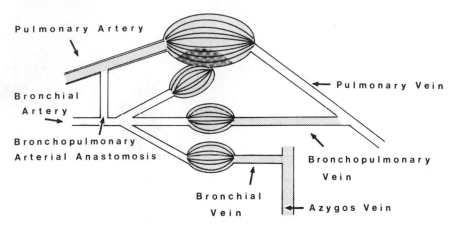

FIGURE 1–10. A schematic representation of the interrelationship between the pulmonary and bronchial circulations.

which is related to the greater number of supernumerary veins; these veins do not have a muscular coat and therefore their impediment to pulmonary blood flow is less than that of the arterial circulation. From these veins a single pulmonary vein is formed that drains each lobe. The pulmonary vein draining the right middle lobe joins that of the right inferior lobe; therefore, in humans there are four pulmonary veins that empty into the left atrium.

The veins and arteries of the pulmonary circulation have parasympathetic and sympathetic innervation. Vagal innervation is vasodilatory, whereas sympathetic innervation is vasoconstrictor in nature.

The Bronchial Circulation

The arterial blood supply to the lung itself, its nerves, ganglia, arteries and veins, lymph nodes, and visceral pleura, is provided by the bronchial circulation. The bronchial circulation receives 1 to 2 per cent of the cardiac output. The interrelationship between the bronchial and pulmonary circulations is depicted in Figure 1–10. In humans, a single bronchial artery to the right lung arises from the upper right intercostal artery, the right subclavian artery, or the internal mammary artery. In the left lung, two bronchial arteries are present, which arise directly from the upper portion of the thoracic aorta. Within the parenchyma of the lung, the bronchial arteries course along the bronchi where they branch into several arteries that anastomose with one another to form a peribronchial plexus. This plexus accompanies each subdivision of the conducting airways. At the terminal bronchioles the bronchial arterioles form a network of capillaries that anastomose with the capillary network of the alveoli.

The return of bronchial venous blood to the heart occurs through bronchial veins that are formed from the plexus vessels originating around lobar and segmental bronchi and the visceral pleura. These bronchial veins drain into the azygos, hemiazygos or intercostal veins, from which the venous blood return eventually reaches the right atrium. Bronchial veins that originate from bronchial capillaries, on the other hand, join the pulmonary veins and are called bronchopulmonary veins. Their venous blood reaches the left atrium and represents a venous admixture of arterial blood. The relative proportions of bronchial venous blood that reaches the right and left atrium are 30 and 70 per cent, respectively.

REFERENCES

1. Butler J. The heart is in good hands. Circulation 67:1163–1168, 1983.
2. Wiggers CJ. The interpretation of the intraventricular pressure curve on the basis of rapidly summated fractionate contractions. Am J Physiol 80:1–11, 1927.
3. Streeter DD, Spotnitz HM, Patel DJ, Ross J, Sonnenblick EH. Fiber orientation in the canine left ventricle during diastole and systole. Circ Res 24:339–347, 1969.
4. Pearlman ES, Weber KT, Janicki JS, Pietra G, Fishman AP. Muscle fiber orientation and collagen content in the hypertrophied human heart. Lab Invest 46:158–164, 1982.
5. Borg TK, Caulfield JB: The collagen matrix of the heart, in Weber KT, Hawthorne EW (eds): Symposium on Cardiac Shape and Structure. Fed Proc 40:2037–2041, 1981.
6. Murray JF: The Normal Lung; The Basis for Diagnosis and Treatment of Pulmonary Disease. WB Saunders, Philadelphia, 1976.

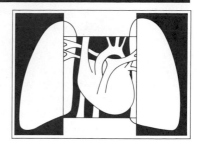

Gas Transport and the Cardiopulmonary Unit

The functional integration of the heart and lungs into a metabolic gas transport unit is accomplished through their anatomic arrangement, as we have just reviewed in Chapter 1, through their mechanical interplay, and by a complex neurohumoral control system. The integration of the gas transport system is particularly evident during physiologic or pathophysiologic forms of stress, (e.g., exercise, fever, hyperthyroidism, anemia, and elevations in ambient temperature), in which the oxygen consumed and the carbon dioxide produced by the body are increased, and thereby the demands for gas transport are increased.

Isotonic exercise, for example, is a physiologic stress that is an integral part of daily living. With exercise, the integrated function of the cardiopulmonary unit must be precise and the functional integrity of each of its components intact if the oxygen and carbon dioxide transport requirements are to be satisfied in a manner that is commensurate with prevailing metabolic activity of the tissues. During strenuous levels of muscular work, for example, oxygen utilization may rise tenfold to 2500 ml/min. Accompanying this increase in $\dot{V}O_2$ there is a proportional increase in carbon dioxide production to 1800 ml/min. This CO_2 must be eliminated into the atmosphere if a person is to remain eucapnic. Cardiovascular or pulmonary disease may disrupt the functional integrity of the unit and thereby compromise its performance. With severe expressions of cardiopulmonary disease, the abnormality in gas transport may be apparent even when a person is at rest and the body's oxygen requirements are modest. With less severe expressions of disease, cardiopulmonary function at rest may be normal or only minimally impaired. However, when the unit is stressed by an elevation in oxygen uptake, such as that evoked with muscular work, the abnormality in gas transport becomes apparent. To understand how cardiopulmonary disease will alter the gas transport function of the unit, it is first necessary to have a working knowledge of its normal behavior.

This chapter is devoted to describing the gas transport function of the normal cardiopulmonary unit and how it serves the body's oxygen requirements, both at rest and during isotonic and isometric exercise. The chapter begins by first examining the oxygen utilization of the body and its various organs. Next, the oxygen transport function of the unit is reviewed in relation to oxygen uptake, followed by a consideration of carbon dioxide production and transport. Finally, the hemodynamic characteristics of the unit relative to oxygen and carbon dioxide are reviewed at rest and during exercise.

OXYGEN UTILIZATION AND TRANSPORT

The oxidation of carbohydrates, fats, and proteins is the principal source of energy for cells to maintain their various biologic functions, including life itself. Human beings, for all intents and purposes, are obligate aerobic organisms. It is therefore essential that the oxygen available to the tissues is matched with their oxygen demand. Anaerobic sources of energy are inadequate and inefficient. Thus, the cells must be linked to the atmosphere and its supply of oxygen.

The Evolution of Mammalian Oxygen Requirements

The needs for oxygen were altered as animal life evolved from water to a terrestrial existence.[1] This evolutionary process not only altered the source of oxygen from water to air but also changed the pattern of ventilation. On land, oxygen was less likely to be available through processes of diffusion or convection. In addition, and quite importantly, the overall need for oxygen was increased as land-living animals became warm-blooded. The oxygen uptake ($\dot{V}O_2$) of resting warm-blooded mammals (3.5 to 8.0 ml/min/kg), for example, is eight to ten times that of fish (0.5 to 1.0 ml/min/kg). The mobility and survival of these land-living mammals depended on their capacity to perform muscular work and to use oxidative metabolism as an energy source. A system of oxygen transport was therefore needed to accommodate the terrestrial existence and to meet the enhanced aerobic requirements of the tissues, as well as to do so on a moment-to-moment basis according to prevailing need. The heart and lungs, together with hemoglobin, have evolved to serve as the body's oxygen transport system.

The oxygen transport requirements of the mammalian cardiopulmonary unit are considerable. Given that the resting $\dot{V}O_2$ of humans is roughly eight to ten times that of fish, humans had to have a greater cardiac output (70 to 150 versus 10 to 40 ml/min/kg). Similarly, minute ventilation had to be greater. The performance of the heart and the lungs is controlled by the metabolizing tissues and their need for oxygen. The controls are quite precise in ensuring oxygen availability. The control logic of the oxygen transport system, however, is not well understood. Input signals to the cardiopulmonary unit, and its individual components, appear to originate from a whole host of sources, including working skeletal muscle, the sympathetic nervous system, and the cardiovascular, respiratory, and central nervous systems.[2-5]

Oxidative Metabolism

The chemical energy from which cells and tissues derive their ability to conduct their many functions is obtained from the oxidation of carbohydrates, fats, and proteins. The energy in these basic components of food becomes available to the cell through a series of complex, enzymatically-controlled biochemical reactions, which occur within each cell and involve the generation of adenosine triphosphate (ATP). ATP is a storage site of potential energy and is often referred to as a high-energy phosphate. The chemical energy required to perform biologic work is derived from the hydrolysis of ATP. Only a small quantity of ATP, however, is stored within the cell, a circumstance which requires its continuous replenishment. Maximum exercise that depends on the intracellular stores of ATP can be performed only for several seconds. The hydrolysis of ATP and the formation of adenosine diphosphate (ADP) as a result, however, serves as a stimulus to the breakdown of stored nutrients within the cell and thereby the provision of additional energy for ATP resynthesis. Creatine phosphate (CP), another intracellular high-energy phosphate compound, provides a rapid supply of phosphate for ATP resynthesis, even in the absence of oxygen. The intracellular concentration of the CP reservoir is three to five times that of ATP.

Cellular oxidation is the chemical process in which electrons are transferred from hydrogen to oxygen via catalytic enzymes termed dehydrogenases and carrier proteins called cytochromes. The mitochondria are the primary site of cellular oxidation. Oxidative phosphorylation refers to the ATP that is formed during the transfer of electrons from one dehydrogenase to another. Over 90 per cent of the cell's ATP source is derived by these oxidative reactions. Hence, the resynthesis of ATP requires that donor electrons be available from the dehydrogenases, that oxygen be available as the hydrogen acceptor, and that the appropriate enzymes are present to sustain each chemical reaction. Oxygen therefore plays a central role in energy metabolism by serving as the final hydrogen acceptor. To sustain mitochondrial aerobic metabolism, oxygen must be available to accept hydrogen electrons and thereby form water. Water is one of the end-products of aerobic metabolism.

Muscular work places a large demand on the body's energy stores. The intensity and duration of exercise determine the energy that has to be transferred from potential stores and whether or not aerobic metabolism can sustain the necessary energy requirements.

Resting Oxygen Utilization

The concepts relevant to the discussion of oxygen utilization, as well as those of the

Table 2–1. Concepts and Calculations Pertaining to Oxygen Utilization, Content, Transport, and Extraction

$$\frac{\text{O}_2 \text{ utilization}}{250 \text{ ml/min}} \quad \begin{cases} = \text{Cardiac output} \cdot (\text{arterial O}_2 \text{ content} - \text{venous O}_2 \text{ content}) \\ = 5000 \text{ ml/min} \quad \cdot (19 \text{ ml/dl} - 14 \text{ ml/dl}) \end{cases}$$

$$\frac{\text{Arterial O}_2 \text{ content}}{19 \text{ ml/dl}} \quad \begin{cases} = \text{Hemoglobin} \quad \cdot \% \text{ saturation} \cdot \text{O}_2 \text{ combining capacity} \\ = 14 \text{ gm/dl} \quad \cdot 0.96 \quad \cdot 1.34 \text{ ml/gm} \end{cases}$$

$$\frac{\text{Venous O}_2 \text{ content}}{14 \text{ ml/dl}} \quad = 14 \text{ gm/dl} \quad \cdot 0.75 \quad \cdot 1.34 \text{ ml/gm}$$

$$\frac{\text{Arteriovenous O}_2 \text{ difference}}{5 \text{ ml/dl}} \quad \begin{cases} = \text{Arterial O}_2 \text{ content} - \text{venous O}_2 \text{ content} \\ = 19 \text{ ml/dl} - 14 \text{ ml/dl} \end{cases}$$

$$\frac{\text{O}_2 \text{ transport}}{950 \text{ ml/min}} \quad \begin{cases} = \text{Cardiac output} \cdot \text{arterial O}_2 \text{ content} \\ = 5000 \text{ ml/min} \quad \cdot 19 \text{ ml/dl} \end{cases}$$

$$\frac{\text{O}_2 \text{ extraction}}{25\%} \quad \begin{cases} = \dfrac{\text{Arteriovenous O}_2 \text{ difference}}{\text{Arterial O}_2 \text{ content}} \cdot 100\% \\ \\ = \dfrac{19 - 14}{19} \cdot 100\% \end{cases}$$

oxygen content of blood, oxygen transport to the tissues, and oxygen extraction by the tissues, are reviewed in Table 2–1. The resting $\dot{V}O_2$ and O_2 extraction by the body's various organs are summarized in Table 2–2 according to their apportionment of systemic blood flow. These data have been adapted from the classic work of Wade and Bishop.[6] Collectively, the abdominal viscera, skeletal muscle, and kidneys receive 65 per cent of the cardiac output. From Table 2–2, it should be apparent, however, that blood flow distribution bears little relation to oxygen utilization. Wide variations in $\dot{V}O_2$ exist among the body's organs; these variations are disparate from the percentage of systemic blood flow they receive. For example, in filtering blood, exchanging salts and water, and excreting urea, the kidneys do not utilize as much oxygen as does the heart. To perform their biologic task, however, the kidneys

must receive 20 per cent of the cardiac output. Thus the necessity of maintaining the osmotic pressure of the extracellular space demanded a high glomerular filtration rate; correspondingly, a high renal blood flow became the top priority of the kidney over that of its $\dot{V}O_2$. On the other hand, skeletal muscle occupies a large portion of the total body weight and is critical to the mobility—and thereby the survival—of mammals. During physical activity, the $\dot{V}O_2$ of muscles can be enormous, and hence they need to receive a large percentage of the cardiac output. The differences in $\dot{V}O_2$ among the tissues, however, becomes more disparate throughout the day as the body's needs for various functions are altered (e.g., digestion, sweating, or walking).

Each tissue meets its need for oxygen by extracting a certain amount of oxygen from the arterial blood it receives (Table 2–2).

Table 2–2. Oxygen Utilization, Transport, and Extraction in Normal Human Subjects at Rest

	Blood Flow (l/min)	Blood Flow (% Total)	Arteriovenous O₂ Difference (ml/dl)	O₂ Extraction* (%)	O₂ Uptake (ml/min)	O₂ Uptake (ml/min/100 gm)	O₂ Uptake (% Total)
Viscera	1.40	24	4.1	21	58	2.3	25
Skeletal Muscle	1.20	21	8.0	41	70	0.2	30
Kidneys	1.10	19	1.3	7	16	5.3	7
Brain	0.75	13	6.3	31	46	3.1	20
Skin	0.50	8	1.0	5	5	0.2	2
Other Organs	0.60	10	3.0	15	12		5
Heart	0.25	3	11.4	59	27	9.0	11
OVERALL	5.80	—	4.0	25	234	3.5	—

*Using assumed arterial O_2 content of 19.4 vols % and body surface area of 1.75 m²
(Adapted from Wade OL, Bishop JM. Cardiac Output and Regional Blood Flow. FA Davis, Philadelphia, 1962.)

Collectively, the tissues extract 25 per cent of the arterial oxygen content (18 to 20 vols %); therefore, the difference in oxygen content between arterial blood and the mixed venous blood of the pulmonary artery, termed the systemic arteriovenous O_2 difference, is 4 to 5 ml/dl. The level of oxygen extraction among the tissues, however, is quite variable and is based on their apportionment of the cardiac output and their given level of $\dot{V}O_2$. Because the kidneys consume a small quantity of oxygen relative to their receiving 19 per cent of systemic blood flow, their extraction of oxygen is quite small at 7 per cent. The heart, on the other hand, which works continuously but receives only 3 per cent of the cardiac output, must extract more than 50 per cent of its oxygen supply to meet its prevailing oxygen requirements. If necessary, each tissue is capable of extracting 80 to 90 per cent of its arterial oxygen content. Once the extraction of oxygen by an organ has reached its physiologic limit, however, any further need for oxygen must be met solely by enhanced blood flow. Such an increment in oxygen delivery is accomplished by the vasodilation of the organ's arterial circulation, thereby capturing a greater apportionment of the systemic blood flow. This metabolically based augmentation in flow is termed *autoregulation*. In most organs, both oxygen extraction and autoregulation occur simultaneously to satisfy oxygen requirements.[7–10]

Resting Oxygen Transport

The heart and lungs must satisfy the metabolic requirements of each tissue. They must do so as the needs of each tissue are altered on a moment-to-moment basis throughout the day and according to physiologic priorities. It is the tissues which dictate that the lungs ventilate a certain volume of air and that the heart circulate a given volume of oxygenated blood per unit of time. In an average-sized, resting individual, $\dot{V}O_2$ averages 250 ml/min or 3.5 ml/min/kg of body weight. To sustain resting metabolism, 8 to 10 liters/min of air must be brought to the alveoli while 4 to 6 liters/min of blood must be circulated through the lungs and delivered to the tissues.

The quantity of oxygen which is bound to hemoglobin at the gas exchange surface of the alveoli determines the per cent saturation of hemoglobin and thereby the oxygen content (see Table 2–1). Oxygen is delivered to

the tissues by the heart's contraction and propulsion of blood into the arterial circulation. Oxygen transport, also termed oxygen delivery, is therefore the product of the arterial oxygen content and the cardiac output (see Table 2–1). In our calculation of arterial oxygen content given in Table 2–1, we have purposely excluded the small quantity of oxygen that is dissolved in blood. The amount of dissolved oxygen, for example, when arterial oxygen tension is 100 mm Hg, is 0.31 ml/dl. The importance of arterial oxygen tension is based on the fact that it determines the degree of hemoglobin oxygen saturation. In accordance with the oxyhemoglobin dissociation curve given in Figure 2–1 and the normal range of arterial oxygen tension (70 to 100 mm Hg) seen in the adult population ranging in age from 20 to 80 years, the per cent saturation of hemoglobin ranges from 92 to 97. When arterial oxygen tension falls below 60 mm Hg, there is a marked decline in hemoglobin oxygen saturation. Thus, the metabolizing tissues are protected from major changes in arterial oxygen content over the normal range of arterial oxygen tensions of 70 to 95 mm Hg. Tissue oxygen delivery is therefore generally 730 to 1040 ml/min for a cardiac output of 4 to 6 liters/min and arterial O_2 content of 19 ml/dl.

In the venous circulation, the oxygen con-

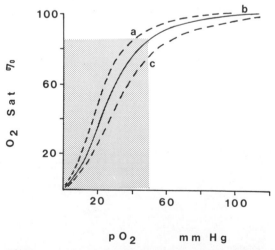

FIGURE 2–1. The O_2 dissociation curve of human hemoglobin at various values of pH and arterial CO_2 tension. Line *b* is the curve for normal pH (7.40) and pCO_2 (40 mm Hg). Lines *a* and *c* are for more alkaline (pH 7.60; pCO_2 20 mm Hg) or acidic (pH 7.20; pCO_2 60 mm Hg) conditions, respectively. The shaded area indicates the portion of the normal curve where a slight reduction in O_2 tension is associated with a marked fall in O_2 saturation.

Table 2–3. Oxygen Content, Saturation, and Tension in Various Segments of the Human Circulation at Rest

	Brachial Artery	Pulmonary Artery	Coronary Sinus	Renal Vein	Hepatic Vein
O_2 content (ml/dl)	19	15	6	15	13
	(18–22)	(12–16)	(4–7)	(14–17)	(7–17)
O_2 saturation (%)	96	77	34	77	73
	(90–98)	(69–82)	(29–38)		(56–83)
O_2 tension (mm Hg)	96	39	20	39	38
	(86–107)	(34–49)	(18–22)		(28–47)

(Adapted from Altman PL, Dittmer DS (eds). Respiration and Circulation. FASEB, Bethesda, MD, 1971.)

tent is much lower since the tissues have extracted a portion of the oxygen from the arterial blood (Table 2–3). The average mixed venous oxygen tension is 40 mm Hg, which falls on the steep portion of the oxyhemoglobin dissociation curve. From Figure 2–1 it appears that this would mean that the per cent saturation of oxygen in venous blood is less than 80 per cent; in the pulmonary artery, oxygen saturation averages 77 per cent. Variations in tissue oxygen extraction and blood flow will significantly alter the venous oxygen content and thereby the arteriovenous oxygen difference of each organ or segment of the circulation (Table 2–4). Because venous blood leaving the capillaries falls on the steep portion of the oxyhemoglobin dissociation curve, the monitoring of mixed venous (i.e., pulmonary artery) oxygen saturation serves as as useful measure of oxygen extraction and cardiac output. This

Table 2–4. Arteriovenous Oxygen Difference and Oxygen Extraction of Various Segments of the Human Circulation at Rest

	Arteriovenous O_2 Difference (ml/dl)	O_2 Extraction (%)
Brachial artery— pulmonary artery	4.5 ± 0.8	23
Brachial artery— antecubital vein	4.2 ± 0.9	22
Brachial artery— femoral vein	9.8 ± 1.4	51
Femoral artery— internal jugular vein	7.0 ± 0.3	36
Brachial artery— coronary sinus	11.4 ± 0.5	59
Femoral artery— renal vein	1.4 ± 0.4	7

(Adapted from Altman PL, Dittmer DS (eds). Respiration and Circulation. FASEB, Bethesda, MD, 1971.)

subject is considered more fully in subsequent chapters.

Given that the overall $\dot{V}O_2$ of the body at rest is 3.5 ml/min/kg, or 250 ml/min in a 70 kg individual, the oxygen delivered (950 ml/min) is more than adequate to meet the prevailing need. An excess of 700 ml of oxygen is delivered each minute. Consequently, oxygen extraction averages 25 per cent. During physiologic (e.g., exercise) or pathophysiologic (e.g., fever or hyperthyroidism) increments in $\dot{V}O_2$, oxygen delivery must increase to a degree that is proportional to the nature and severity of the elevation in $\dot{V}O_2$. On the other hand, whenever oxygen delivery is severely reduced so that it fails to match $\dot{V}O_2$, oxygen extraction must increase if anaerobic metabolism with lactate production is to be avoided. Therefore, the factors that normally determine oxygen availability are the cardiac output, the hemoglobin concentration, the per cent saturation of hemoglobin, oxygen extraction, and autoregulation.

A detailed discussion of oxygen transport and the regional responses that are evoked to protect cellular oxygen availability will be considered in more detail in subsequent chapters. A brief discussion, however, may be useful. The ratio of $\dot{V}O_2$ to oxygen delivery represents a demand-to-supply ratio. As shown in Table 2–5, this relation can be further separated into its individual components. By factoring out cardiac output, these terms reduce to the arteriovenous oxygen difference divided by the arterial oxygen content or oxygen extraction. Reserves in cardiac output and oxygen extraction ensure oxygen availability under a variety of circumstances. If the cardiac output were to remain constant at 5 liters/min during increments in $\dot{V}O_2$, tissue oxygen extraction alone would have to account for oxygen availability. A threefold increase in oxygen extraction raises the arte-

Table 2–5. Oxygen Transport, Utilization, and Demand to Supply Ratio

$$O_2 \text{ transport} = \underset{(CO)}{\text{Cardiac output}} \cdot \underset{(Art\ O_2)}{\text{Arterial } O_2 \text{ content}}$$

$$\underset{(\dot{V}O_2)}{O_2 \text{ utilization}} = \underset{(CO)}{\text{Cardiac output}} \cdot \underset{(AVO_2)}{\text{(Arteriovenous } O_2 \text{ difference)}}$$

$$\frac{O_2 \text{ demand}}{O_2 \text{ supply}} = \frac{O_2 \text{ utilization}}{O_2 \text{ transport}}$$

$$= \frac{CO \cdot AVO_2}{CO \cdot Art\ O_2}$$

$$= \frac{AVO_2}{Art\ O_2}$$

$$= O_2 \text{ extraction}$$

$$= 25\%$$

riovenous oxygen difference to 15 ml/dl, and thereby oxygen uptake can be sustained up to 750 ml/min, or 5 liter/min • 15 ml/dl. An elevation in $\dot{V}O_2$ beyond 750 ml/min, however, must be accompanied by an increase in cardiac output if oxidative metabolism is to remain the dominant source of energy. Contrariwise, if resting cardiac output falls from its normal resting value of 5 to 2 liters/min, while resting $\dot{V}O_2$ is constant, oxygen delivery is still adequate to sustain aerobic metabolism. With a cardiac output below 1.5 liters/min, however, lactate production occurs, which leads to a metabolic acidosis incompatible with life if sustained. Thus, reserves in oxygen transport and oxygen extraction guarantee a ninefold margin in resting oxygen availability to prevent lactic acidosis. These concepts of oxygen delivery, however, do not consider the other important consequences of a reduced cardiac output, such as the inability of the kidney to sustain its normal excretion of urea.

Oxygen Uptake and Transport During Exercise

Muscular work raises the $\dot{V}O_2$ of the body, and in particular the $\dot{V}O_2$ of skeletal muscle. Minute ventilation and oxygen delivery must each rise proportionately at a rate commensurate with the level of $\dot{V}O_2$ to sustain aerobic skeletal muscle metabolism. With strenuous work, minute ventilation will rise to eight times its resting level (Fig. 2–2). Rarely does ventilation pose any limitation to the ability to carry out all levels of aerobic work.[11]

Compared with minute ventilation, the rate and extent to which the cardiac output rises during progressive work is much less dramatic (Fig. 2–2). For every 100 ml/min

increment in $\dot{V}O_2$ above its resting value, cardiac output will rise 600 ml/min. This is the normal "gain" setting of the cardiac output control system. In untrained individuals, cardiac output increases only four- or fivefold above its resting value. Thus, unlike the lungs, the heart poses a limitation to the ability to perform aerobic work. Fortunately, additional mechanisms are present to ensure oxygen availability to working muscle. Enhanced oxygen extraction and circulatory autoregulation play a very important role in

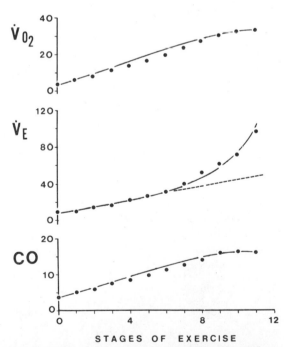

FIGURE 2–2. The response in cardiac output (CO; liters/min) and minute ventilation ($\dot{V}_E$; liters/min) to incremental isotonic exercise and increasing O_2 uptake ($\dot{V}O_2$; ml/min/kg) performed on the treadmill by a normal subject.

ensuring oxygen availability during physical activity. Reflexive and humoral influences, which produce a vasoconstriction in less metabolically active tissues (e.g. kidney and splanchnic circulations), permit a greater apportionment of the blood flow to be delivered to exercising muscle. The metabolically mediated vasodilation present in the circulation of working muscle overrides any competing vasoconstrictive neurohumoral stimulus (e.g., plasma norepinephrine) and thus ensures its oxygen availability.

Physiologic limits to the elevation above resting cardiac output (i.e., a cardiac reserve of approximately 20 to 25 liters/min) and oxygen extraction (approximately 75 to 80 per cent) dictate the aerobic capacity of untrained subjects. Beyond these physiologic limits, any additional increment in work will not be accompanied by an elevation in oxygen utilization. Accordingly, a plateau in oxygen uptake is attained during vigorous incremental exercise, which has been termed the *maximal oxygen uptake*; it is abbreviated $\dot{V}O_2$ *max*. The $\dot{V}O_2$ max attained by an individual during a progressive exercise test, therefore, not only reflects aerobic capacity but also the physiologic capacity of the cardiovascular system to deliver oxygen.[12] In the average-sized untrained individual whose maximum cardiac output is 20 liters/min and whose maximum level of oxygen extraction is 75 per cent (i.e., an arteriovenous oxygen difference of 14 ml/dl), a $\dot{V}O_2$ max of 2800 ml/min would be expected. In athletes, a greater cardiac reserve and an enhanced capacity for oxidative metabolism by trained muscle are available.[13] As a result, greater levels of $\dot{V}O_2$ max can be achieved. In contrast, as we will discuss in later chapters, patients with heart disease will have a reduction in aerobic capacity according to their heart's inability to raise cardiac output sufficiently during exercise.

CARBON DIOXIDE PRODUCTION AND TRANSPORT

Carbon dioxide production ($\dot{V}CO_2$) is an end-result of oxidative metabolism. The cardiopulmonary unit, via its right heart and gas exchange surface of the alveoli, accepts this metabolic end-product and eliminates it into the atmosphere. An abnormal elevation in carbon dioxide creates a respiratory acidosis that has dire consequences on the body and its cellular viability. Fortunately, carbon

dioxide is a major respiratory stimulant, and any accumulation quickly evokes a heightened level of ventilation to maintain the eucapnic state.

Oxidative Metabolism

During oxidative metabolism, oxygen is consumed while carbon dioxide is produced. In normal individuals consuming an average diet of carbohydrates and fats, 75 to 80 per cent of the oxygen consumed (250 ml/min) is converted to carbon dioxide. Accordingly, 190 ml of carbon dioxide are returned to the right heart each minute by the venous blood. The right ventricle delivers this carbon dioxide to the lungs for elimination into the atmosphere. The carbon dioxide produced by oxidative metabolism of the tissues is considered to represent the *metabolic* source of carbon dioxide. The ratio of $\dot{V}CO_2$ to $\dot{V}O_2$, $\dot{V}CO_2/\dot{V}O_2$, is termed the respiratory gas exchange ratio, or R. R, therefore, normally equals 0.75 to 0.85. The absolute value of R depends on the proportion of carbohydrates and fats available from the diet to be utilized in supporting ATP stores and caloric production (Table 2–6). For example, in a fasting individual using only body fat for energy, R = 0.70. The R value measured at rest is preserved during physical activity as long as the tissues are performing aerobic work and an adequate amount of oxygen is available to sustain oxidative metabolism. Anaerobic metabolism and the buffering of lactate increase $\dot{V}CO_2$, as we will discuss subsequently. Minute ventilation ($\dot{V}_E$) may increase to 80 liters/min or more during strenuous aerobic exercise (see Figure 2–2). A corresponding increment in alveolar ventilation

Table 2–6. Respiratory Gas Exchange Ratio (R) and Its Relationship to Food Fuels and Total Caloric Output

R	% O_2 Uptake		% Total Caloric Production	
	CHO	*Fats*	*CHO*	*Fats*
0.70	0	100	0	100
0.75	14.7	85.3	14.6	84.4
0.80	31.7	68.3	33.4	66.6
0.85	48.8	51.2	50.7	49.3
0.90	65.9	34.1	67.5	32.5
1.00	100	0	100	0

CHO, carbohydrates.
(Adapted from Harris T, Benedict J. A biometric study of basal metabolism in man. Publication 279 of the Carnegie Institute, Washington, DC, 1919.)

and carbon dioxide elimination must therefore also occur to maintain eucapnia.

From Table 2–6 it is apparent that the amount of carbon dioxide produced relative to the oxygen consumed is a function of the amount of carbohydrate (CHO) and fat that is utilized in providing the total caloric production. Even though the breakdown of CHO and fat is designed to generate ATP, the biochemical processes involved in each degradation are different, the needs for oxygen are different, and the amount of energy produced is quite different.

Glucose is derived from CHO. The degradation of glucose within the cell yields carbon dioxide and water and a maximum of 686 kcal of chemical energy. In skeletal muscle only 260 kcal or 38 per cent of the available energy is transferred into 36 moles of ATP; the remaining 62 per cent is lost as heat. Glucose degradation yields two molecules of pyruvic acid by anaerobic reactions termed glycolysis. Glycolytic reactions occur intracellularly, but outside the mitochondria. The aerobic breakdown of pyruvic acid to carbon dioxide and water, which involves electron transport and oxidative phosphorylation, takes place within mitochondria. Only 5 per cent of the total ATP formed by the cell occurs during glycolysis. However, the rate of the glycolytic reactions is such that they provide a rapid source of energy, and the reactions can occur in the absence of oxygen. Under such anaerobic circumstances, the electrons released during glycolysis can be taken up by pyruvate to form lactic acid. The rapid diffusion of lactate from the cell to the intravascular space prevents any negative feedback on further glycolytic reactions and thereby a continuous, albeit modest, source of energy by ATP resynthesis is provided. Lactic acid, however, may lead to a reduction in the muscles' ability to sustain work because it inactivates other enzymes and thereby leads to the sensation of fatigue.

The remaining 95 per cent of the ATP derived from CHO occurs when pyruvic acid is converted to acetyl-CoA by the Krebs or citric acid cycle; these biochemical events occur within mitochondria. Once again, carbon dioxide and hydrogen are the end-products of this series of reactions. Two carbon dioxide molecules and four pairs of hydrogen atoms are formed from pyruvic acid, whereas four carbon dioxide molecules result from acetyl-CoA. The electron transport and oxidative phosphorylation reactions proceed under aerobic conditions to yield 32 moles of ATP.

Unlike carbohydrate, stored fat in adipose tissue of the body represents an enormous source of energy, yielding roughly 100,000 kcal. Free fatty acids and glycerol are cleaved from triglycerides of adipose tissue. Glycerol can proceed through anaerobic reactions of glycolysis to yield pyruvic acid and subsequent oxidation within the Krebs cycle. Twenty-two molecules of ATP are synthesized in this manner. Free fatty acids, on the other hand, undergo oxidative transformation to acetyl-CoA within the mitochondria, where it then enters the Krebs cycle and oxidative phosphorylation. Aerobic conditions must again prevail for these reactions to proceed. A total of 463 molecules of ATP are formed from the breakdown of glycerol (22 molecules) and free fatty acids (441 molecules), nearly 13 times the ATP derived from CHO. The utilization of fats by muscle, however, proceeds with approximately the same efficiency (i.e., 40 per cent) as that seen for CHO.

Anaerobic Metabolism

Muscular work and the consumption of oxygen may rise more quickly or to an extent whereby the cardiovascular system is not able to provide oxygen at a commensurate rate. Consequently, oxygen availability to the tissues is inadequate. Skeletal muscle must therefore utilize less efficient anaerobic metabolism to derive its energy. Anaerobic muscle produces lactate. Because of its low dissociation constant, intracellular lactate is rapidly buffered by bicarbonate, which leads to the production of carbonic acid and eventually carbon dioxide and water. This *nonmetabolic* source of carbon dioxide represents an additional source of $\dot{V}CO_2$, which raises the respiratory gas exchange ratio in excess of that associated with aerobic metabolism. The onset of anaerobic metabolism during a progressive exercise test, therefore, can be detected by the disproportionate rise in R (Fig. 2–3). This topic will be discussed in greater detail in Chapter 10. Because this extra carbon dioxide must also be eliminated into the atmosphere, alveolar ventilation must increase in order to maintain eucapnia. This is easily accomplished by the heightened chemical drive (via carbon dioxide) to respiration mediated by the carotid bodies. The corresponding level of work or $\dot{V}O_2$, at which time anaerobic metabolism occurs, has been termed the *anaerobic threshold*.[14] Anaerobiosis normally occurs when 60 per cent or more of the subject's aerobic capacity has been attained.

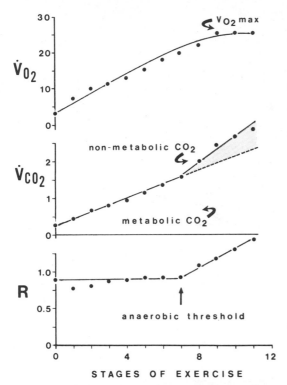

FIGURE 2–3. The response in CO_2 production ($\dot{V}CO_2$; liters/min), O_2 uptake ($\dot{V}O_2$; ml/min/kg). The respiratory gas exchange ratio (R) to progressive isotonic treadmill exercise and increasing O_2 uptake ($\dot{V}O_2$; ml/min/kg) for a normal subject. The metabolic and nonmetabolic (stippled area) components of the $\dot{V}CO_2$ response are indicated, and the onset of anaerobic metabolism is identified by the response in R (arrow) as the anaerobic threshold.

HEMODYNAMIC BEHAVIOR OF THE UNIT AT REST

To gain a perspective of the hemodynamic behavior of the cardiopulmonary unit relative to its gas transport function, we will begin by tracing the flow of venous blood from the tissues to the lung. After its oxygen content has been restored and part of its carbon dioxide content eliminated in the lung, we will then follow the course of blood back to the tissues. We will begin by examining the hemodynamic behavior of the unit when the body is at rest.

The Return of Venous Blood to the Lung

Venous blood, from both the lower and upper extremities, the abdomen, and the head, flows toward the thorax. Hence the thorax more or less divides the body into two, though not equivalent, metabolic segments. Venous flow toward the thorax is promoted by the gradient in venous pressure that exists between the periphery and each vena cava. In addition to this gradient in venous pressure, the contraction of skeletal muscle displacing blood from its veins, the presence of one-way valves in the veins, and the negative pressure within the thorax all serve to promote blood flow toward the thorax.

The various attachments between the venous circulation and the right heart, the right heart and pulmonary circulation, pulmonary circulation and the left heart, and the left heart and arterial circulation are each contained within the confines of the thorax, as shown in Figure 2–4. Consequently, the pressure within the thorax, termed *intrathoracic or pleural pressure,* surrounds the cardiopulmonary unit and each of these circulatory attachments. Pleural pressure averages -3 cm H_2O at end-expiration and -6 cm H_2O during inspiration. Because the various segments of the heart and circulation are surrounded by this negative pressure, their hemodynamic behavior is influenced by pleural pressure.[15] For example, the pressure with which these vessels and chambers of the heart are distended is related to the difference in intravascular and intrathoracic pressures, or the difference in pressure between the interior and exterior of the vessel or chamber, which is termed the *transmural pressure.* The transmural pressure is the true distending pressure of the intrathoracic vessels and cardiac chambers. The physiologic importance of transmural pressure can be demonstrated by considering its influence on inferior vena cava distention and filling. The normal intravascular pressure in this vessel is 5 mm Hg (Table 2–7). However, the transmural pressure on the vena cava at end-inspiration is 9 mm Hg, or $5-(-4)$ mm Hg. Thus the cava is filled by a distending pressure greater than 5 mm Hg and therefore pleural pressure aids in promoting venous return into the thorax.

An additional role of pleural pressure on the flow of venous blood to the thorax can be demonstrated by considering its influence on the large capacitance venous circulation. The major part of the venous circulation is located entirely outside the thorax. As depicted in Figure 2–5, it serves as the filling reservoir of the right heart.[16] The normal intravascular filling pressure gradient for the return of venous blood to the right atrium is 5 mm Hg, or the difference in pressure between the extrathoracic veins (10 mm Hg) and the intrathoracic veins and right atrium

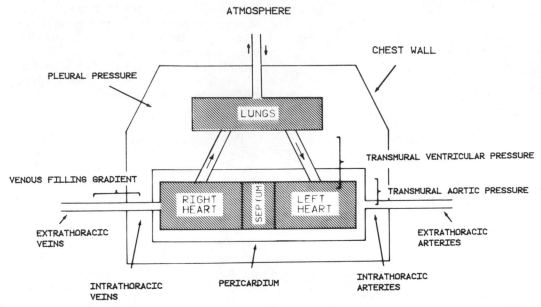

FIGURE 2–4. The cardiopulmonary unit with its intra- and extrathoracic attachments to the venous and arterial circulations. (From Weber KT, Janicki JS, Shroff SG, Fishman AP. Contractile mechanics and interaction of the right and left ventricles. Am J Cardiol 47:686–695, 1981.)

(5 mm Hg). The reduction in intrathoracic pressure accentuates this transthoracic pressure gradient. Thus, the respiratory motion of the thorax and the accompanying fluctuation in intrathoracic pressure not only aid the flow of air into and out of the lungs, but they also assist in the return of 5 liters of venous blood to the right heart each minute.

To this point, we have traced the flow of venous blood to the right atrium. Commenc-ing with myocardial relaxation, right ventricular pressure falls. When pressure falls below 5 mm Hg, the tricuspid valve opens, permitting venous blood to rapidly fill the right ventricular chamber. A period of slower filling, called diastasis, follows. The final event in ventricular filling is atrial contraction, which adds an additional, albeit small, volume of blood to the right ventricle. Myocardial depolarization normally follows atrial

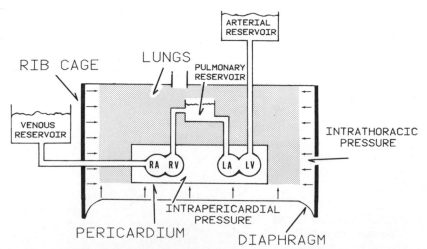

FIGURE 2–5. The functional coupling that exists between the heart and circulation. Shown are the relationships between the venous circulation (or reservoir) and the right heart; the pulmonary circulation, with its blood volume, to the left heart; and the arterial reservoir, which is filled by the left heart. The connection between the arterial and venous reservoirs is not shown. Intrapleural pressure surrounds the entire heart-lung unit while intrapericardial pressure acts only on the heart. (From Weber KT, Janicki JS, Shroff SG, Likoff MJ, St John Sutton MG. The right ventricle: physiologic and pathophysiologic considerations. Crit Care Med 11:323–328, 1983.)

Table 2–7. Normal Hemodynamic Values for the Human Cardiopulmonary Unit at Rest

	mm Hg
Venae cavae	10
Right atrium (RAP)	5
Right ventricle	30/5
Pulmonary artery (PAP)	30/12 (mean 18)
Left atrium	12
Left ventricle	120/12
Aorta (AP)	120/70 (mean 80)
Arteries	80
Arterioles	60
Capillaries	40
Veins	10
Cardiac output (CO)	5 liters/min

$$\text{Pulmonary vascular resistance (PVR; dynes} \cdot \text{sec} \cdot \text{cm}^{-5}) = \frac{PA - PCW}{CO} \cdot 80$$

$$96 = \frac{18 - 12}{5} \cdot 80$$

$$\text{Systemic vascular resistance (SVR; dynes} \cdot \text{sec} \cdot \text{cm}^{-5}) = \frac{AP - RAP}{CO} \cdot 80$$

$$1200 = \frac{80 - 5}{5} \cdot 80$$

depolarization within 120 to 180 msec. The depolarized myocardium begins to generate tension within its muscle fibers. As a result, the right ventricular chamber and its blood are compressed; right ventricular pressure rises. To eject venous blood into the pulmonary circulation, the right ventricle has to generate at least 12 mm Hg of pressure to open the pulmonic valve. Once this occurs, blood flows into the pulmonary artery. To eject blood into the pulmonary circulation, right ventricular systolic pressure rises on the average to a peak of 30 mm Hg while the mean pressure throughout ejection averages 20 mm Hg. These modest levels of systolic pressure are all that are required to sustain a pulmonary blood flow of 5 liters/min. This is in sharp contrast to the left ventricle, which has to generate a systolic pressure four times as high to sustain a cardiac output of 5 liters per minute into the arterial circulation. The impedance characteristics of the pulmonary circulation are therefore quite modest. This is true because it is possible to recruit previously collapsed vessels and to further distend already patent vessels within the air-filled lungs. Even if venous return were to increase three- to four-fold, as seen during vigorous physical activity, the right ventricle never has to develop more than 40 to 50 mm Hg of systolic pressure. The right ventricle, therefore, may be viewed as a volume displacement pump. Accordingly, the mass of right ventricular myocardium never achieves the proportions found for the left ventricle; its mass (60 gm) and wall thickness are one third that of the left ventricle.

Because the pressure-generating requirements of the right ventricle are modest, its functional significance in sustaining the circulation has been questioned. Experimental studies in which a massive destruction of the right ventricular free wall was created, without an adverse effect on cardiac output or central venous pressure,[17] are often cited in support of this argument. However, when the gradient in right heart filling is reduced or pulmonary vascular resistance is elevated, the presence of a pulsatile right ventricle is critical to sustaining pulmonary blood flow. When the elevation in vascular resistance is prolonged, the right ventricular myocardium will hypertrophy so that it too is capable of behaving as a pressure-generating pump. The hypertrophied right ventricular myocardium will have the mass and thickness of the left ventricle, and it is capable of generating systemic or even suprasystemic levels of systolic pressure, as we shall discuss in Chapter 13.

Pulmonary Blood Flow

Blood flow through any segment of the lung is the result of the difference in pressure between the pulmonary artery and the downstream smaller pulmonary vessels. Mean pulmonary artery pressure averages 18 mm Hg. Because the vasculature is contained within the lung parenchyma, its vessels are subjected to external forces that compress, tether, and dilate their lumina (Fig. 2–6). For example, when lung volume is low, the radial traction on extra-alveolar vessels falls and they collapse; alveolar vessels, however, are pulled open by the elastic recoil of small alveoli. At larger lung volumes, the alveolar vessels are compressed whereas the lumina of the extra-alveolar vessels are tethered open. Blood flow will depend, therefore, on these pressures and the relative differences in pressure between the arterial, alveolar, and venous portions of the pulmonary circulation.

In segments of the lung where alveolar pressure exceeds venous pressure, termed Zone II, blood flow resembles a vascular waterfall in that it is independent of the downstream venous pressure (Fig. 2–7). In the more dependent portions of the lungs,

EXTRA-ALVEOLAR VESSELS

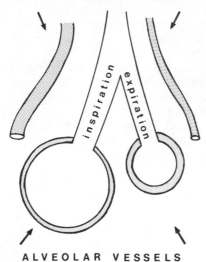

ALVEOLAR VESSELS

FIGURE 2–6. Within the lung the pulmonary circulation can be described as representing alveolar and extra-alveolar vessels. The external forces applied to each of these vessels will be a function of the respiratory cycle. See text for discussion.

or Zone III, where venous pressure exceeds alveolar pressure, blood flow is related to the difference in each of these intravascular pressures. Hence, in Zone III blood flow is related to the difference in pulmonary artery and venous pressures. In segments where alveolar pressure actually exceeds pulmonary arterial pressure, there is no blood flow. This is termed Zone I, and it is rare in normal human lungs. Zone I segments, however, may accompany the oligemic, hyperinflated lungs seen in obstructive airway disease.

In evaluating the pressure-flow relation of the normal human pulmonary circulation during upright exercise, we have found the downstream pressure to be adequately represented by the occlusive wedge pressure[18] (see Chapter 13). Hence, pulmonary vascular resistance may be simply represented by calculating the gradient in pressure between the pulmonary artery (mean pressure, 18 mm Hg) and the venous bed or left atrium (12 mm Hg) and dividing it by pulmonary blood flow (5 liters/min); this value is then converted to standard units of vascular resistance (dynes · sec · cm^{-5}) by multiplying by 80, where 1 mm Hg/liter/min = 80 dynes · sec · cm^{-5} (see Table 2–7). The average normal range of vascular resistance of the pulmonary circulation is 140 ± 60 dynes · sec · cm^{-5}. Pulmonary vascular resistance is further discussed in Chapter 13.

The Flow of Oxygenated Blood to the Tissues

Venous blood is oxygenated in the lung. The pulmonary blood volume, which is the filling reservoir for the left atrium, is located entirely within the thorax (see Fig. 2–5). Therefore, and quite unlike the filling reservoir for the right heart, variations in pleural pressure simultaneously influence the left atrium and its filling reservoir. Consequently, fluctuations in pleural pressure have lesser influence on determining left heart filling and the filling pressure gradient between this reservoir and the left atrium. Left atrial pressure averages 5 to 12 mm Hg. This pressure drives oxygenated blood into the relaxed left ventricle in diastole. Once again, a period of rapid left ventricular filling is followed by diastasis and finally left atrial contraction. Atrial contraction provides an additional 10 to 20 per cent to the filling volume of the left ventricle.

The ejection of oxygenated blood from the depolarized left ventricle into the ascending aorta and arterial circulation requires that at least 70 mm Hg be generated to open the aortic valve. Peak systolic and mean ejection pressures of 120 and 90 mm Hg, respectively, are required to propel blood to the tissues through the high impedance arterial circulation (Fig. 2–8). Thus, the left ventricle must

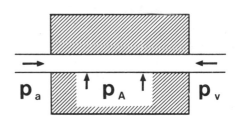

ZONE 1 : $P_A > P_a > P_v$

ZONE 2 : $P_a > P_A > P_v$

ZONE 3 : $P_a > P_v > P_A$

FIGURE 2–7. The pulmonary circulation traverses the lung (shaded area) where it is subjected to external forces as reflected by alveolar pressure (P_A). The gradient in pressure between the pulmonary artery (P_a) and a downstream site, such as the alveolus or venous circulation (P_v), will determine pulmonary blood flow. The lung has been designated as having three zones, depending on the relationship between these three pressures, P_a, P_A and P_v. See text for details.

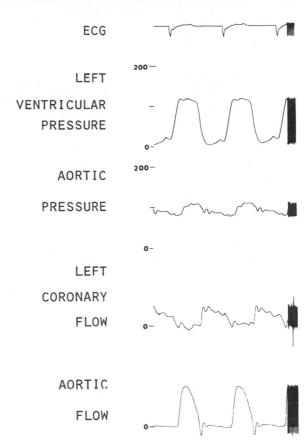

FIGURE 2–8. Measurements of left ventricular and aortic pressures, together with left main and ascending aorta blood flow and the electrocardiogram, are shown for a conscious instrumented calf. The ejection of blood from the left ventricle into the aorta occurs when ventricular pressure exceeds aortic pressure. Blood flow through the left coronary circulation is essentially confined in diastole because of the throttling of coronary flow by the rise in left ventricular systolic pressure.

generate four times the pressure of the right ventricle in sustaining the cardiac output. As a result, the mass of left ventricular myocardium is three times (180 gm) that of the right ventricle (Fig. 2–9). These differences in myocardial mass between ventricles impart a substantial difference in the compliance of their respective chambers. The right ventricle is normally twice as distensible as the left ventricle.

The human left ventricular chamber normally contains 100 to 150 ml of blood at end-diastole; 60 to 90 ml of this diastolic volume are ejected. The ratio of the volume ejected, or *stroke volume*, to the ventricle's diastolic filling volume is termed the *ejection fraction*. For the normal left ventricle, the ejection fraction averages 60 ± 5 per cent. A residual or end-systolic volume of 40 to 60 ml, therefore, remains in the left ventricle at end-ejection. In untrained normal individuals, heart rate averages 70 beats/minute, which produces an average cardiac output (i.e., stroke volume · heart rate) of 4 to 6 liters/min. For a steady state balance of blood flow between the lungs and the tissues, pulmonary blood flow and right ventricular output

must match left ventricular output. Because of differences in shape of the right ventricle relative to the truncated ellipsoid configuration of the left ventricle, its ejection fraction is between 52 and 57 per cent.

A mean aortic pressure of 80 mm Hg drives arterial blood into the systemic circulation throughout the cardiac cycle. Much of this pressure is dissipated in the perfusion of the distal arterial circulation where its muscular arterioles offer a significant resistance to blood flow (Fig. 2–10). Fifty millimeters of mercury pressure are lost as blood flow traverses these resistance vessels. The vascular resistance of the systemic circulation may be approximated by calculating the difference between mean aortic pressure (80 mm Hg) and right atrial pressure (5 mm Hg) and dividing this gradient by the cardiac output (5 liters/min). After the appropriate conversion, systemic vascular resistance is found to average 1200 ± 200 dynes · sec · cm^{-5}. Thus, systemic vascular resistance is roughly ten times that of the pulmonary circulation.

The capillaries of the body's various organs are perfused with a pressure of 40 mm Hg. A further drop in circulatory pressure occurs

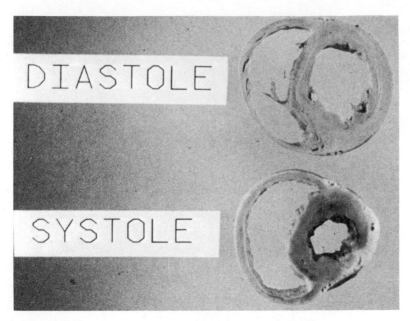

FIGURE 2–9. The left ventricle is a pressure pump; the right ventricle is a volume pump. The differences in systolic pressure that each ventricle must generate account for the differences in their muscle mass and wall thickness. The left ventricle has three to four times the mass of the right ventricle. See text. (Adapted from Weber KT, Janicki JS, Shroff SG, Likoff MJ, St John Sutton MG. The right ventricle: physiologic and pathophysiologic considerations. Crit Care Med *11*:323–328, 1983.)

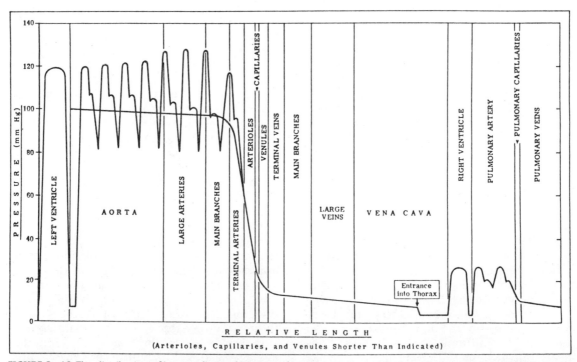

FIGURE 2–10. The distribution of intracardiac and intravascular pressures across the heart and circulation. The differences in pressure, which are responsible for sustaining systemic blood flow and venous return, are described in the text. (From Selkurt EE. Physiology. Little, Brown and Co, Boston, 1962.)

as blood crosses the capillaries, leaving 5 to 10 mm Hg as the range of pressure within the venous circulation. This venous pressure becomes the driving pressure for the return of venous blood to the thorax. This circulatory pressure has been found to average 7 mm Hg and is determined by the elasticity of the circulation and the volume of blood it contains.[19]

HEMODYNAMIC BEHAVIOR OF THE UNIT DURING EXERCISE

Muscular work may be isotonic or isometric. *Isotonic* exercise is defined as muscular work in which muscle groups are able to alter their length during contraction while the force they exert is constant. *Isometric* exercise occurs when muscle groups contract from a constant muscle length while the force of their contraction may be maximal or less than maximum for the muscle length. A *maximum voluntary contraction* refers to the maximal tension that a muscle or group of muscles can attain during an isometric contraction at constant muscle length. Most isometric contractions are at some fraction (e.g., 20, 40, or 60 per cent) of this maximum contraction. Light isometric exercise is at 10 to 25 per cent of maximum, whereas more than 25 per cent of maximum is considered to be heavy exercise. The cardiovascular or hemodynamic responses to isotonic and isometric work are quite different. We will begin by reviewing the impact of isotonic and isometric exercise on the cardiovascular system.

Isotonic Exercise

During isotonic muscular work, the $\dot{V}O_2$ of the exercising muscles is increased but the $\dot{V}O_2$ of nonworking muscle is not significantly altered. The isotonic contraction of muscle(s) elicits a host of responses that ultimately lead to an increase in cardiac output. Many of these responses remain poorly understood, but in all likelihood they include reflexes elicited from within the contracting muscles as well as the central and peripheral nervous systems. The release of vasoactive and neuroendocrine substances, such as norepinephrine and epinephrine, may also be a factor. Kotchen et al have examined the response of the adrenergic nervous system during progressive isotonic exercise in military recruits.[18] They observed that plasma

norepinephrine rose during exercise, but only at higher levels of work corresponding to 75 per cent or more of the subject's aerobic capacity. Plasma epinephrine also rose, but only at $\dot{V}O_2$ max. Thus, circulating catecholamines do not appear to play a major role in mediating the cardiac output response during submaximal aerobic levels of work. Similar observations were also reported for the renin-angiotensin-aldosterone system.[20]

A number of mechanical events influence the hemodynamic behavior of the cardiopulmonary unit during isotonic exercise. Muscular contraction compresses the venous circulation, thereby raising venous return. In addition, the fall in intrathoracic pressure that accompanies the increase in minute ventilation augments venous return. The resultant increment in ventricular filling will distend the myocardium and through its Frank-Starling mechanism raise the cardiac output. A one- to twofold increase in stroke volume accompanies the rise in cardiac output seen during low levels of upright work. This is not the case for supine work, where the legs are raised and intrathoracic blood volume is increased at rest. As a result, stroke volume does not rise above its resting level in the supine position. As higher work loads (more than 50 per cent $\dot{V}O_2$ max) are achieved in the upright posture, the increment in stroke volume is modest. The explanation for this relative plateau in the stroke volume response at higher loads is considered in more detail later, but we feel it may be related to the pericardium and its restraint on ventricular filling. Therefore, stroke volume plays a lesser role in augmenting cardiac output than does heart rate, which rises throughout progressive isotonic exercise (Fig. 2–11).

The response in heart rate is mediated by a variety of mechanisms that appear to depend on the level of muscular work. Certainly, an increment in venous return is known to elicit an increase in heart rate through an activation of the Bainbridge reflex, which originates from stretch or neuronally activated receptors located in the central venous circulation. At low levels of work there is withdrawal of the parasympathetic nervous system, whereas at higher work loads there is an activation of the sympathetic nervous system. Together, these responses create the milieu for a progressive elevation in heart rate during incremental exercise. Hence, heart rate will rise to a level that is appropriate for the work load and is a function of age. It may reach values of 170

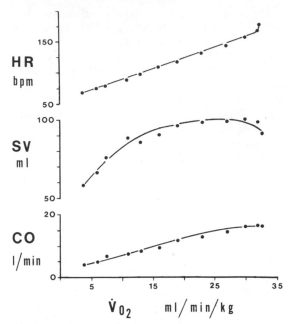

FIGURE 2–11. The normal response in heart rate, stroke volume, and cardiac output to upright incremental treadmill exercise. Heart rate rises throughout exercise whereas stroke volume is increased primarily during the transition from rest to moderate levels of muscular work. Thereafter, the rise in stroke volume is modest. Eventually, cardiac output fails to rise further despite continued incremental work.

to five fold without requiring an equivalent rise in right ventricular systolic pressure. Pulmonary vascular resistance, which averages 96 dynes · sec · cm^{-5} at rest, falls to 60 dynes · sec · cm^{-5} with exercise. This reduction in pulmonary vascular resistance occurs because of the great distensibility of the pulmonary circulation and the recruitment of previously collapsed vessels.

The rise in left ventricular systolic pressure during exercise is more apparent than that seen in the right ventricle because the vascular impedance of the systemic circulation is significantly greater than that of the pulmonary circulation. Left ventricular systolic pressure may rise to 170 mm Hg with maximal exercise. In the aorta, systolic pressure mirrors that of the left ventricle. During diastole, an enhanced run-off into the dilated circulation of working skeletal muscle permits aortic diastolic pressure to remain within several millimeters of mercury of its resting value (70 mm Hg). Hence, a widened pulse pressure is characteristic of the response in aortic pressure during isotonic exercise.

As noted, the response in systemic vascular resistance is determined by the vasodilation of working skeletal muscle; this occurs

beats/min or more, representing a two- or threefold increase above that present at rest. As a result, for most forms of work the major determinant of the increase in exercise cardiac output is mediated by an elevation in heart rate. Maximum heart rate can be predicted from the formula: 220 − age in years.

Throughout incremental isotonic exercise, right atrial pressure rises modestly from its resting value of 5 mm Hg. This imperceptible rise in atrial pressure early in exercise is the result of the large distensibility of the central venous system and the fact that it is subjected to negative levels of intrathoracic pressure. In similar fashion, right ventricular diastolic pressure does not rise until higher levels of exercise are attained (Fig. 2–12).

Right ventricular systolic pressure rises gradually and modestly during progressive isotonic exercise. The same is true for the systolic pressure in the pulmonary artery. Pulmonary artery diastolic pressure also rises to a limited extent (approximately 10 mm Hg or less), which is most apparent at higher work loads when pulmonary blood flow has quadrupled its resting value (Fig. 2–13). The low impedance of the pulmonary circulation permits pulmonary blood flow to rise four-

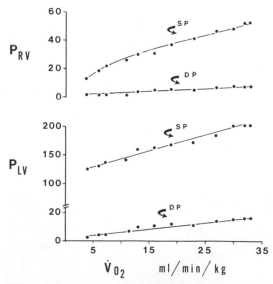

FIGURE 2–12. The normal response in systolic (SP) and diastolic (DP) pressures of the right and left ventricles to upright incremental treadmill exercise. For the right ventricle, systolic pressure rarely exceeds 50 mm Hg even during vigorous work when cardiac output exceeds 20 liters/min. Left ventricular systolic pressure, on the other hand, may rise 50 per cent, to 180 mm Hg or more. These differences in systolic pressure are accounted for by the differences between the impedance of the systemic and pulmonary circulations. Nevertheless, for either ventricle, isotonic exercise is primarily a volume load.

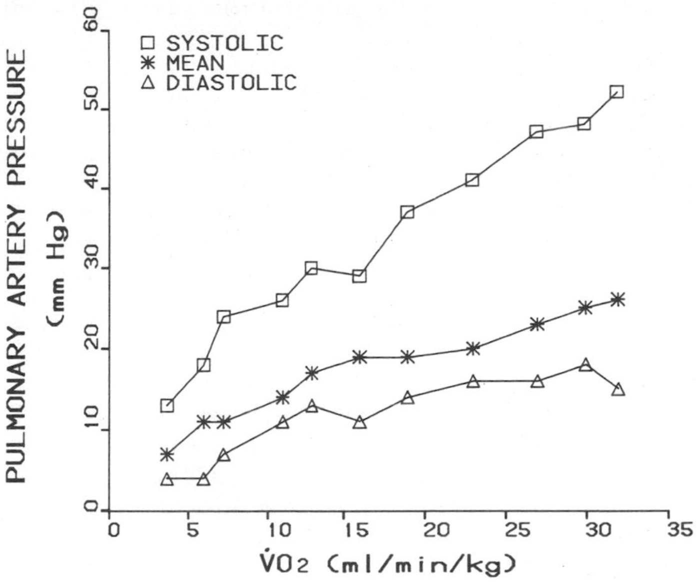

FIGURE 2–13. The normal response in pulmonary artery pressure to upright incremental treadmill exercise.

as metabolic end-products, such as adenosine, accumulate around blood vessels. As a result, blood flow and oxygen are redistributed to these muscles and away from less metabolically active muscles and other tissues. This redistribution of blood toward working muscle is accomplished by the vasodilation of working muscle and a vasoconstriction of less metabolically active circulations, such as that of the intestines and kidneys. Blood flow to the lower limbs may rise from 600 ml/min at rest to over 6000 ml/min with running: a tenfold increase in blood flow, which represents 25 per cent of the cardiac output. As a result of this vasodilation in muscle, systemic vascular resistance falls progressively during incremental exercise, reaching values as low as 600 dynes · sec · cm^{-5}. Even so, the dilated vascular resistance of the systemic circulation is still ten times that of the pulmonary circulation. The redistribution of blood flow within the systemic circulation that occurs during exercise is given in Table 2–8.

Isometric Exercise

In addition to isotonic forms of exercise, in which muscle length changes during the course of physical activity and the tension exerted by muscle is more or less constant (for example, walking, running, and swimming), isometric exercise occupies a certain portion of daily living. With isometric exercise, muscle length does not change, but the tension developed by muscle is increased to accommodate the load (for example, lifting or carrying or moving heavy objects). This form of exercise is often termed *static* work. The response of the cardiopulmonary unit to

Table 2–8. Oxygen Transport in Normal Human Subjects at Rest and During Light, Moderate, and Maximum Exercise

	Blood Flow (Liters/min/% Total)			
	Resting	*Light*	*Moderate*	*Maximum*
Viscera	1.4/24	1.1/11	0.60/3	0.30/1
Skeletal muscle	1.2/21	4.50/47	12.50/71	22.00/88
Kidneys	1.1/19	0.90/10	0.60/3	0.25/1
Brain	0.7/13	0.75/8	0.75/4	0.75/3
Skin	0.5/8	1.50/15	1.90/12	0.60/2
Other organs	0.6/10	0.40/4	0.40/3	0.10/1
Heart	0.3/3	0.35/4	0.75/4	1.00/4
Overall	5.8	9.50	17.50	25.00

(Adapted from Wade OL, Bishop JM. Cardiac Output and Regional Blood Flow. FA Davis, Philadelphia, 1962; and Falls HB (ed). Exercise Physiology. Academic Press, New York, 1968.)

isometric exercise is quite different from that seen with isotonic exercise.[21]

Isotonic exercise represents a volume challenge to the heart, in which its pumping function must increase in a manner commensurate with both the heightened venous return and peripheral demands for oxygen delivery. Isometric exercise, on the other hand, represents a pressure challenge to the left ventricle (Fig. 2–14). Because blood flow to isometrically contracting muscle is partially or totally throttled, depending on the proportion of a maximum isometric contraction that is evoked by static work, systemic vascular resistance does not fall from its resting value. The isometric contraction, however, squeezes veins, increasing venous return. Heart rate also increases. As a result, the increment in cardiac output seen with isometric exercise causes an elevation in both arterial systolic and diastolic pressures. The elevation in heart rate is mediated by the withdrawal of vagal tone and an enhanced response of the adrenergic nervous system as a result of reflexes elicited from mechanoreceptors in muscle or the central nervous system.

The absolute extent to which arterial pressure and heart rate rise during static exercise appears to be a function of the weight that is being lifted, or the per cent of maximal voluntary contraction that a given muscle group must exert, and the mass of muscle involved. Lind and McNicol, for example, found that in right-handed normal men the rise in mean arterial pressure and heart rate was greater when a 20 kg weight was lifted by the left arm rather than the right arm.[22]

The left arm, presumed to be weaker in these individuals, had to contract at a greater proportion of its maximal tension. In addition, the pressor response to simultaneous contractions of both arms was determined by the muscle group exerting the greatest tension. When fatiguing exercise was compared with nonfatiguing work, the blood pressure response was different. For lighter loads, a steady state rise in pressure was reached, whereas a continual rise in pressure was seen with fatiguing exercise.

Bonde-Petersen and coworkers have indicated that because muscle blood flow is throttled during an isometric contraction, the duration of static exercise will be limited by the magnitude of the contraction.[23] A maximal contraction can be performed only for a very short period of time (in seconds), whereas at 50 per cent of maximum the work can be performed for several minutes. Thus, even though cardiac output rises, the ability of the working muscles to receive oxygen is limited; therefore, less efficient anaerobic sources, such as the breakdown of stored ATP, CP, and glycogen, must be utilized for energy during isometric exercise. The result is a short-lived contraction of muscle prior to its becoming fatigued. The isometric contraction elicits cardiovascular responses that resemble those seen with ischemia. Because systemic flow is not delivered to isometrically contracting muscles, the work of the cardiopulmonary unit is wasted, and more oxygen will be delivered to less metabolically active tissues. Consequently, the arteriovenous oxygen difference remains unchanged or may even fall, depending on the degree of this "shunting." Thus, isometric exercise is a rather inefficient form of muscular work.

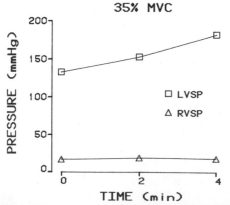

FIGURE 2–14. Isometric exercise represents a pressure load on the left ventricle. Systolic left ventricular pressure (LVSP) may normally exceed 200 mm Hg during heavy isometric work loads. The right ventricle does not have a major elevation in its systolic pressure (RVSP) with isometric exercise. MVC = maximal voluntary contraction.

REFERENCES

1. Harris P. Evolution of the cardiac patient. Cardiovasc Res 17:315–319, 373—378, 437–445, 1983.
2. Mitchell JH, Blomqvist CG, Lind AR, Saltin B, Shepherd JT. Static (isometric) exercise: Cardiovascular responses and neural control mechanisams. Circ Res 48:(Suppl I), 1981.
3. Smith EE, Guyton AC, Manning D, White RJ. Integrated mechanisms of cardiovascular response and control during exercise in the normal human. Prog Cardiovasc Dis 18:421–443, 1976.
4. Murray JF. The Normal Lung; The Basis for Diagnosis and Treatment of Pulmonary Disease. WB Saunders, Philadelphia, 1976.
5. Wasserman K. Breathing during exercise. N Engl J Med 298:785–789, 1978.
6. Wade OL, Bishop JM. Cardiac Output and Regional Blood Flow. FA Davis, Philadelphia, 1962.

7. Weber KT, Kinasewitz GT, Janicki JS, Fishman AP. Oxygen utilization and ventilation during exercise in patients with chronic cardiac failure. Circulation 65:1212–1223, 1982.

8. Wilson JR, Martin JL, Ferraro N, Weber KT. Effect of hydralazine on perfusion and metabolism in the leg during upright bicycle exercise in patients with heart failure. Circulation 68:425–432, 1983.

9. Weber KT, Janicki JS, Fishman AP. The aerobic limit of the heart perfused at constant pressure. Am J Physiol 238:118–125, 1980.

10. Feigl EO. Coronary physiology. Physiolog Rev 63:1–205, 1983.

11. Freedman S. Sustained maximum voluntary ventilation. Resp Physiol 8:230–244, 1970.

12. Mitchell JE, Sproule BJ, Chapman CG. The physiological meaning of maximal oxygen intake test. J Clin Invest 37:538–545, 1958.

13. Holloszy JO, Adaptations of muscular tissue to training. Prog Cardiovasc Dis 18:445–458, 1976.

14. Wasserman K, McIlroy MB. Detecting the threshold of anaerobic metabolism in cardiac patients during exercise. Am J Cardiol 14:844–850, 1964.

15. Weber KT, Janicki JS, Shroff SG, Fishman AP. Contractile mechanics and interaction of the right and left ventricles. Am J Cardiol 47:686–695, 1981.

16. Weber KT, Janicki JS, Shroff SG, Likoff MJ, St John Sutton MG. The right ventricle: Physiologic and pathophysiologic considerations. Crit Care Med 11:323–328, 1983.

17. Starr I, Jeffers WA, Meade RH. The absence of conspicuous increments of venous pressure after severe damage to the right ventricle of the dog. With a discussion of the relation between clinical congestive failure and heart disease. Am Heart J 3:291–302, 1943.

18. Janicki JS, Weber KT, Likoff MJ, Fishman AP. The pressure-flow response of the hypertensive pulmonary circulation. Circulation 72:1270–1278, 1985.

19. Guyton AC, Jones CE, Coleman TG. Circulatory Physiology: Cardiac Output and Its Regulation. WB Saunders, Philadelphia, 1973.

20. Kotchen TA, Hartley LH, Rice TW, Mogey EH, Jones LG, Mason JW. Renin, norepinephrine, and epinephrine responses to graded exercise. J Appl Physiol 31:178–184, 1971.

21. Asmussen E. Similarities and dissimilarities between static and dynamic exercise. Circ Res 48:(Suppl 1) I3–10, 1981.

22. Lind AR, McNicol GW. Cardiovascular responses to holding and carrying weights by hand and by shoulder harness. J Appl Physiol 15:261–267, 1968.

23. Bonde-Petersen F, Mork AL, Nielsen E. Local muscle blood flow and sustained contractions of human arm and back muscles. Eur J Appl Physiol 34:43–50, 1975.

3

KARL T. WEBER
JOSEPH S. JANICKI
SANJEEV G. SHROFF

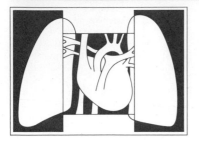

The Heart as a Mechanical Pump

In reviewing the concept of respiratory gas transport, the central role played by the heart and its pumping function in the delivery of oxygen and carbon dioxide should be apparent. The manner in which the right and left heart generate pulmonic and systemic blood flow, respectively, and the factors that influence their ability to accept and displace blood will be the focus of this chapter. We will begin by reviewing the mechanical properties of the ventricular chamber, first in diastole as the ventricle is filled and then in systole as blood is ejected. These mechanical properties play a key role in the determination of pump function. Also, we will consider several factors, both intrinsic and extrinsic to the ventricles, that influence their mechanical properties or their systolic performance or both. For example, intrinsic factors include alterations in the structural and/or biochemical composition of the myocardium, whereas extrinsic factors include the mechanical interplay and interdependence of the right and the left heart, of the heart and the lungs, and finally, of the heart and the circulation. Each of these topics has received considerable attention over the years. In this chapter, we will draw heavily on our own work to highlight various topics of interest, and we make no attempt to provide an exhaustive review of the subject. For this purpose, the interested reader is referred elsewhere.[1-4]

THE MECHANICAL PROPERTIES OF THE PUMP

The myocardium consists of a syncytium of muscle fibers and blood vessels that are tethered within a connective tissue matrix composed largely of collagen (see Chapter 1). As a composite material consisting of muscle and collagen, the mechanical properties of the myocardium will be a function of the mechanical properties of each element and the proportion of the myocardium that they represent. Consequently, whenever a stress is applied to the heart, whether during the filling of the ventricles in diastole or during the ejection of blood in systole, the myocardium is deformed in accordance with the *composite* mechanical properties of cardiac muscle and collagen. Even though collagen occupies a small fraction (2 to 3 per cent) of normal myocardium,[5] its stiffness, relative to that of muscle, dictates that the myocardium will be less compliant than if it were composed solely of muscle. Collagen, however, serves an important purpose in maintaining muscle fiber alignment throughout the cardiac cycle, thereby permitting reversible interdigitation of the fibers while preventing their slippage. The connective tissue network also maintains the overall configuration of the myocardium; without collagen, the myocardium would resemble a "floppy bag."

Stress-Strain Versus Pressure-Volume Relations

At this point, it is appropriate to distinguish the mechanical properties of the ventricular chamber from those of the myocardium. The *chamber* mechanical properties are generally computed from the pressure-volume relation of the ventricle. On the other hand, the *myocardial* properties are computed from its stress-strain relation. It should be noted that direct measurements of myocardial stress and strain in an intact heart are not possible at present; instead, they are computed indirectly from the measurements

34

of ventricular pressure, volume, and geometry. The primary goal of assessing the stress-strain relation is to obtain a measure of the intrinsic mechanical properties of the myocardium that are independent of the shape and size of the ventricle and also of the external forces (eg, pericardial pressure and intrathoracic pressure). Consequently, the evaluation of the stress-strain relation is the only meaningful way to compare hearts among patients with varying volumes, shapes, and myocardial masses. Since myocardial stress and strain are indirectly calculated from ventricular pressure and volume, it is critical that an appropriate structural and geometric model of the ventricle be used. A number of limitations are inherent in the current methodology used to compute stress and strain. These will be discussed in the subsequent section.

The pressure-volume relation of the ventricle is relatively easy to obtain. In addition, it is useful in assessing acute changes in the chamber mechanical properties of a given heart and also in quantitating the coupling of the heart to its circulation.

Elastic and Viscous Properties

A purely elastic system will deform and completely recover from its deformation independent of the rate with which the deforming stress is applied (Fig. 3–1). The *elastic* behavior of the ventricular chamber and the myocardium can be quantitated by the pressure-volume and stress-strain (or tension-length) relations, respectively. Like most biologic tissue, however, the myocardium does not demonstrate purely elastic behavior. The heart also exhibits a *viscous* property that dictates that the mechanical behavior of the heart is also dependent on flow or strain rate (Fig. 3–2). The elastic and viscous properties together determine the extent and the rate of shortening in response to a given transmural pressure or stress.[6] The viscous properties are often ignored, especially at end-diastole and end-systole, when the rate processes (flow or strain rate) are usually quite small. However, under those circumstances wherein the rate processes are significant (eg, rapid filling phase of diastole and ejection period of systole), the computations of elastic properties based solely on a purely elastic model will be in substantial error.

Concept of Stress and Strain

Myocardial *stress* is defined as force per unit area of the myocardium. A complete description of stress at a given location in the myocardium consists of specifying both its magnitude and direction. Stress is generally resolved into components that act normal (normal stress) or parallel (shearing stress) to the cross-sectional area under consideration. Owing to the three-dimensional nature of the ventricle, the most general description of

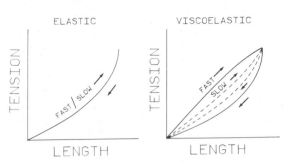

FIGURE 3–2. The mechanical properties of the myocardium include elastic and viscoelastic behavior. If the myocardium were purely elastic (left panel), its tension and length with rapid or slow stretching and shortening would be identical. However, a viscous component that resists deformation must also be taken into account. The viscous drag produces a somewhat higher tension than does a purely elastic system as the myocardium is slowly elongated (right panel; broken lines, short arrows). The same drag prevents length from decreasing as quickly as tension is falling during shortening. With faster rates of lengthening and shortening (solid lines, long arrows), the viscous, or resistive, component introduces an even greater discrepancy. (Adapted from Weber KT, Hawthorne EW. Descriptors and determinants of cardiac shape, *in* Weber KT, Hawthorne EW (eds). Symposium on Cardiac Shape and Structure. Fed Proc 40:2005–2010, 1981.)

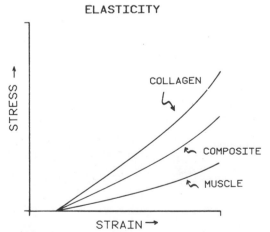

FIGURE 3–1. The myocardium is a composite material consisting of muscle and connective tissue. Its stress-strain relation will be determined by the stress-strain relation of each structural element and the proportion of the myocardium that it occupies.

stress consists of nine components: three normal stress (circumferential, longitudinal, and radial) and six shearing stress components. In most cases, owing to the symmetry of the stress-strain relation, the six shearing stresses can be reduced to three. In the computation of stress from the measurements of pressure and volume, one often assumes that the myocardium is homogeneous and isotropic. The assumption of homogeneity implies that the smallest element cut from the myocardium exhibits the same specific physical properties as the original organ, whereas the assumption of isotropy implies that the physical properties are the same in all directions. For certain locations in the myocardium (eg, midwall region in the equatorial plane), the results based on the assumptions of isotropy and homogeneity are qualitatively in agreement with those obtained by more general theories.[7] A number of equations have been developed to compute myocardial stress from pressure and volume.[3, 7] A specific example of this procedure is presented in Chapter 4. These equations differ with respect to the assumptions of geometry (eg, spheroid, prolate spheroid, ellipsoid of revolution), thin or thick wall, isotropy, homogeneity, and fiber orientation. A comprehen-

sive discussion of the usefulness and limits of these formulas can be found elsewhere.[3, 7]

Deformation can be quantified in terms of *strain*, defined either as the ratio of instantaneous length (L) or change in length (△L) with respect to "reference" length. The choice of reference length is quite arbitrary. The passive, unstressed (ie, zero transmural end-diastolic pressure) state is often chosen to represent this reference state. Similar to the stress representation, a complete description of strain consists of resolving it into nine components: three dilatational (circumferential, longitudinal, and radial) and six shearing strains. Figure 3–3 depicts the three dilatational strains with and without shearing. Once again, similar to the shearing stresses, the six shearing strains can be reduced to three. Finally, a general description of the elastic properties of the myocardium is comprised of the relation between the six stress and strain components via the respective elastic moduli. In practice, however, the midwall region of the equatorial plane is chosen for analysis, and only circumferential stress-strain relations are assessed because of the predominantly circumferential orientation of the muscle fibers in this region (see subsequent discussion).

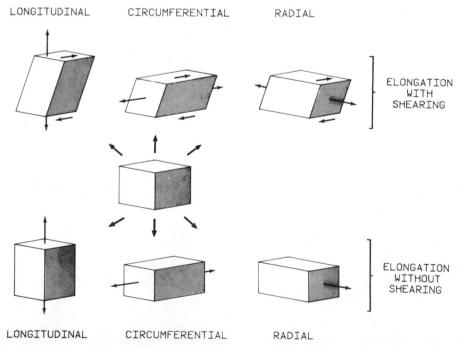

FIGURE 3–3. A schematic representation of a segment of myocardium, together with the three directions of pure dilatational (elongational) strains (longitudinal, circumferential, and radial) in the lower half of the figure. In the upper half of the figure the same strains are shown with a superimposed shearing strain. (From Weber KT, Hawthorne EW. Descriptors and determinants of cardiac shape, *in* Weber KT, Hawthorne EW (eds). Symposium on Cardiac Shape and Structure. Fed Proc *40.*2005–2010, 1981.)

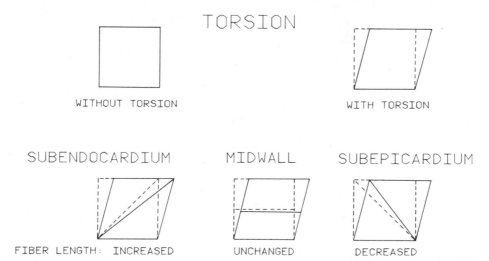

FIGURE 3–4. A rotational deformation, or torsion, imparts a shearing strain on the myocardium and its constituent muscle fibers, as shown in Figure 3–3. Torsion may also permit uniform fiber shortening by promoting different length changes across the myocardium. With torsion, for example, muscle fiber length (represented by a diagonal line in the square of myocardium) will increase in the subendocardium, whereas fiber length in the midwall remains unchanged. (From Weber KT, Hawthorne EW. Descriptors and determinants of cardiac shape, *in* Weber KT, Hawthorne EW (eds). Symposium on Cardiac Shape and Structure. Fed Proc *40*:2005–2010, 1981.)

Effect of Muscle Fiber Orientation

The wall of the myocardium is composed of muscle fibers with varying orientation across the wall,[8] which results in a significant anisotropic behavior. As indicated in Chapter 1, the subepicardial and subendocardial fibers are nearly meridional, whereas the midwall fibers are predominantly circumferential.[8, 9] Thus, it is appropriate to analyze stress and strain at a given location in the direction of the local orientation of the muscle fibers. For example, the midwall fibers in the equatorial plane will exhibit predominantly circumferential stress and strain, whereas the subendocardial and subepicardial fibers will predominantly deform in the meridional direction. However, one can simplify the analysis by assessing the stress and strain for an equivalent area of the myocardium that represents the average stress and strain across the full thickness of the wall. Such an area is found in an equatorial plane approximately halfway through the wall. Thus, one can consider this area as behaving in an isotropic manner and thereby can compute average circumferential stress and strain.

Finally, owing to the helical arrangement of fibers, a twisting deformation or *torsion* of the left ventricle has been observed during ejection.[10, 11] It has been postulated that torsion results in the equalization of fiber strain across the wall.[10, 11] In the absence of torsion, the subendocardial fibers would have to shorten considerably more during ejection than would the subepicardial fibers. As shown in Figure 3–4, torsion has different effects on fiber strain, depending on the location and orientation of the fiber within the myocardium. For example, fiber length would be decreased in the subepicardium, whereas it would be increased in the subendocardium; fiber length in the midwall would remain unchanged. This is exactly the kind of differential action needed to counterbalance the tendency for greater endocardial shortening that would otherwise (ie, without torsion) be present. The magnitude of this rotational shearing does not need to be large (eg, less than 10 degrees) to produce equalization of fiber strains across the wall.

Mechanical Properties in Diastole

The diastolic portion of the cardiac cycle begins when the ejection of blood from the ventricle has ceased, or just prior to aortic valve closure; it terminates when the myocardium is depolarized. The diastolic period is divided into five phases as shown in Figure 3–5: protodiastole, isovolumetric relaxation, rapid filling, diastasis, and atrial contraction, labeled 1 to 5 in Figure 3–5. After the contraction of the atria, there is a point when atrial and ventricular pressures are essentially equal. This connotes the hemodynamic end-point of diastole. Generally, ventricular filling at end-diastole is complete and, consequently, the viscous effects (proportional

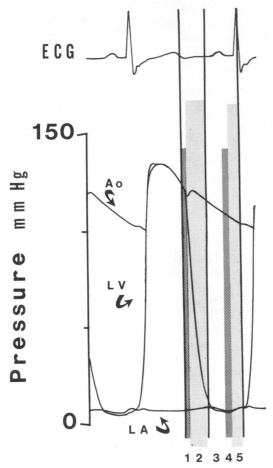

FIGURE 3–5. The five phases of diastole are depicted from the pressure tracings of the left ventricle (LV), aorta (Ao), and left atrium (LA). See text for discussion.

ing a monoexponential curve-fitting routine to analyze the end-diastolic pressure-volume data (usually for end-diastolic pressure greater than 5 mm Hg), the slope or chamber stiffness can be linearly related to the chamber pressure.[12] The slope of this linear relation is termed the *chamber stiffness constant*. An increase in the steepness of the pressure-volume relation will result in an increase in the chamber stiffness constant, although a rightward parallel shift in the pressure-volume relation will not affect the chamber stiffness constant.

As noted before, the information obtained from the pressure-volume relation alone is not useful in comparing hearts of varying size, shape, and myocardial mass.[12] Therefore, for an intact heart one computes a myocardial stress-strain relation based on a preselected structural and geometric model of the ventricle. This process results in a nonlinear and monoexponential stress-strain relation for the myocardium. *Myocardial stiffness* can then be computed as the slope of the stress-strain relation. Once again, owing to the nonlinear stress-strain relation, the slope of myocardial stiffness varies with the level of stress, and this variation can be represented as a linear function.[3, 12] The slope of this linear relation is defined as the *myocardial stiffness constant*. Unlike the chamber stiffness constant, the myocardial stiffness constant is expected to represent the intrinsic

to flow or strain rate) are minimal. Thus, at end-diastole the pressure-volume relation primarily reflects the elastic behavior of the myocardium. In contrast, the pressure-volume relation obtained throughout the filling period (ie, from the onset of rapid filling period to end-diastole) is influenced by both the elastic and viscous properties. In the following discussion, we will focus our attention only on the mechanical properties at end-diastole and not on the instantaneous pressure-volume or stress-strain relations throughout diastole.

The end-diastolic pressure-volume relation is typically nonlinear for filling pressures greater than 5 mm Hg. The slope of this relation ($\Delta P/\Delta V$) is a measure of the static *chamber stiffness* (inverse of chamber compliance or distensibility, $\Delta V/\Delta P$). Because of the nonlinear nature of the pressure-volume relation (Fig. 3–6), chamber stiffness varies with filling or end-diastolic pressure. By us-

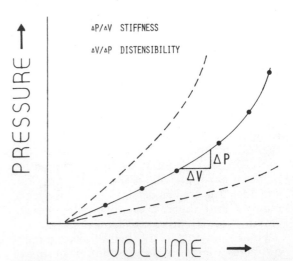

FIGURE 3–6. The end-diastolic pressure-volume (P-V) relation for the left ventricle. Chamber stiffness is quantitated by the slope ($\Delta P/\Delta V$) of this relation by using a monoexponential curve fitting routine. An increase or decrease in chamber stiffness is depicted by the relations (broken lines) shown above or below a normal curve (solid line).

material property wherein the effects of chamber geometry, muscle mass, and external (eg, pericardial and intrathoracic) forces have been appropriately taken into account.

Factors Influencing Mechanical Properties in Diastole

By definition, in order to induce changes in *myocardial mechanical properties,* the composition of the myocardium must change. Cardiac disease may induce a change in myocardial stiffness through a variety of mechanisms (eg, ischemia, increased collagen, and fibrosis). These intrinsic alterations of the myocardium must be distinguished from the extrinsic factors (eg, the pericardium or the interplay between the ventricles) that will alter only *chamber* stiffness or the pressure-volume relation or both.[13] In the latter case, the myocardium is not diseased; only the chamber stiffness is altered. Such a situation frequently presents itself for the left ventricle when the right heart is enlarged. As we will discuss more fully later in the chapter, the left ventricle as a chamber may appear stiffer under these circumstances because the position of the interventricular septum is altered, thereby altering the geometry of the left ventricle.

Finally, it should be noted that with cardiac disease there may be a change in myocardial mass and chamber size and shape, which is expected to affect chamber stiffness. Thus, assessment of the stress-strain relation is the only meaningful approach to comparing different hearts for their diastolic mechanical properties. Peterson and colleagues[14] have taken this approach in evaluating patients with left ventricular hypertrophy secondary to aortic valvular stenosis. They found that one group of patients had normal chamber and myocardial stiffness, while another group had an increased stiffness of both the chamber and the myocardium. This was true even though there was no difference between groups in muscle mass, wall thickness, or the ratio of diastolic left ventricular volume to muscle mass. An elevated left ventricular end-diastolic pressure was seen in patients either with increased muscle mass and normal myocardial stiffness or with abnormal myocardial stiffness. These differences in myocardial stiffness may be a result of discrete areas of myocardial fibrosis or diffuse increase in collagen concentration that accompany the hypertrophic process.

Hess and associates[15] have been able to demonstrate a close relationship between myocardial stiffness and the degree of fibrosis measured morphometrically. We have also found that there is an increase in collagen volume fraction in hypertrophied left ventricle owing to systemic hypertension.[9] Moreover, the appearance of clinical heart failure in hypertension was found to be accompanied by an even greater increase in myocardial collagen. At present it is not clear whether the increase in collagen is a normal component of myocardial growth, much like the remodeling of bone, or whether there is an intrinsic condition within the pressure-overloaded myocardium that favors collagen formation. Gaasch and colleagues[16] have found myocardial stiffness to be altered in patients with either aortic stenosis or aortic regurgitation. The importance of myocardial stiffness and its relationship to myocardial collagen should be examined in greater detail in the future, particularly since they may be relevant to the timing of surgical valve replacement.

We will now discuss those extramyocardial factors that primarily influence the *ventricular pressure-volume relationship* or *chamber stiffness.*[13] These include heart rate, level of left ventricular ejection pressure, coronary blood volume, and pericardium.

Increases in *heart rate* shorten diastole, and as a result, systole occupies a greater percentage of the cardiac cycle. Below 170 beats per minute, the diastolic pressure-volume relation is insensitive to this reduction in diastolic interval. Above 170 beats per minute relaxation is incomplete, which causes an elevated ventricular pressure for any given end-diastolic volume. Consequently, the end-diastolic pressure-volume relation is shifted to the left. In circumstances in which the mitral or tricuspid valve is diseased and its orifice for ventricular filling is narrowed, elevations in heart rate above 100 to 120 beats per minute may prohibit the adequate filling of the ventricle, while leading to acute atrial distension.

Studies in our laboratory[17] have indicated that the end-diastolic pressure-volume relation of the left ventricle is also altered by the level of its *ejection pressure* (Fig. 3–7). From a constant filling volume, an increase in ejection pressure results in a decline in end-diastolic pressure. The magnitude of the change in filling pressure is dependent on the absolute increment in ejection pressure and the ventricular chamber volume before

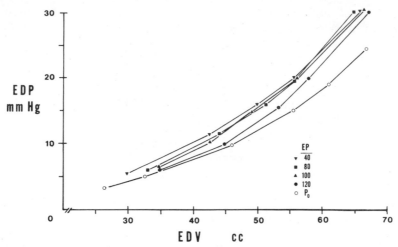

FIGURE 3–7. End-diastolic pressure (EDP) versus end-diastolic volume (EDV) relations obtained at four constant ejection pressures (EP, solid symbols) and also for the isovolumetric state (P_o, open circles). As ejection pressure is increased, the EDP-EDV relation is shifted downward or to the right, with the lowest curve corresponding to the isovolumetric state (that is, with the ventricle contracting isovolumetrically the maximum systolic pressure is attained for any given EDV). Thus, variations in arterial pressure will influence the diastolic pressure-volume relation (From Janicki JS, Weber KT. Ejection pressure and the diastolic left ventricular pressure-volume relation. Am J Physiol 232:H545–H552, 1977. Fed Proc 39:133–140, 1980.)

the perturbation in pressure. The fact that end-diastolic pressure falls following an elevation in ejection pressure indicates that the pressure-volume relation is shifted to the right. These observations leave little doubt that alterations in diastolic distensibility occur with increments in arterial pressure and serve to explain similar observations noted with interventions that are unavoidably accompanied by increments in arterial pressure (eg, catecholamines and paired pacing).

Another factor that will alter the diastolic properties of the chamber is the *coronary blood volume.* A modest increment in the end-diastolic pressure-volume relation is observed with an elevation in coronary perfusion pressure and a greater distention of the coronary circulation. This swelling of the myocardium, termed the "erectile" response, accounts for a decline in chamber distensibility.

To this point, the physiologic factors that we have reviewed have a minor effect on diastolic chamber stiffness. Other factors, such as the pericardium and the mechanical interplay between ventricles, play a more important role.[13, 18] Each of these factors is considered in more detail elsewhere in this chapter. In brief, however, the parietal *pericardium,* which forms a discrete sac surrounding the ventricles and atria, will significantly influence the pressure-volume relation of each chamber. The effect of the pericardium is demonstrated in Figure 3–8, in which the diastolic pressure-volume relation for each ventricle is presented before and after pericardiectomy. In order to minimize the effects of right and left ventricular interaction (vide infra), these data have been presented when the filling pressure in the contralateral ventricle was zero. Removal of the pericardium

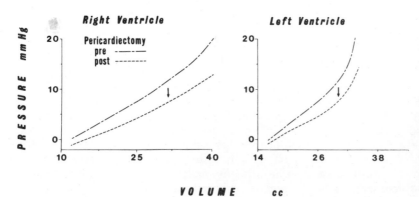

FIGURE 3–8. The parietal pericardium, which is contiguous with both ventricles, will significantly influence the diastolic pressure-volume relation of each ventricle. Removal of the pericardium results in a downward, nonparallel shift of the end-diastolic pressure-volume curves. (From Janicki JS, Weber KT. Factors influencing the diastolic pressure-volume relation of the cardiac ventricles. Fed Proc 39:133–140, 1980.)

resulted in a significant decrease in chamber stiffness. The decrease in chamber stiffness following pericardiectomy is a function of the ventricle's filling volume; the greatest reduction is noted at higher filling volumes. With the pericardium intact, each ventricular chamber appears to be stiffer. Thus, the pericardium can be viewed as restraining the acute distension of the ventricles and the atria. More gradual increments in heart size, as occur in growth from infancy to adulthood or in the failing heart, are not constrained by the pericardium; in fact, the pericardial space is increased and the pericardial pressure-volume relation shifts to the right.

Mechanical Properties in Systole

In the following discussion, we will present primarily the methods for quantitating the *chamber* mechanical properties of the ventricle during systole. Limited data are available regarding the computation of *myocardial* mechanical properties in systole from the measurements of pressure, volume, and flow. Therefore, our discussion regarding the systolic myocardial properties will be limited to identifying both current problems and directions for future research.

The instantaneous ventricular systolic pressure is primarily a function of the time during systole, chamber volume, flow, and contractile state. Chamber *elastance* (mm Hg/ml) describes the relationship between chamber pressure and volume. In a manner analogous to this relationship in an elastic bag, the higher the volume in the chamber, the greater the pressure in the chamber. However, unlike the elastance of a passive elastic bag, the chamber elastance during systole is not constant; instead, it increases with time in systole. This is evident from the observation that chamber pressure increases with time, even for a fixed chamber volume (ie, an isovolumetric contraction). Thus, ventricular pressure-volume relations during systole can be described in terms of a time-varying elastance. Chamber *resistance* (mmHg-sec/ml), on the other hand, describes the property of the chamber that is flow-dependent. Conceptually, the role of resistance can be viewed as subtracting from the pressure that would have existed for either a purely elastic system or a condition with zero flow.

In the case of an isovolumetric contraction, in which there is no ejection, ventricular pressure first increases and then declines.

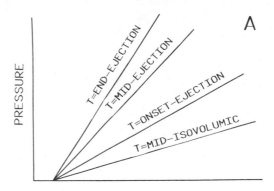

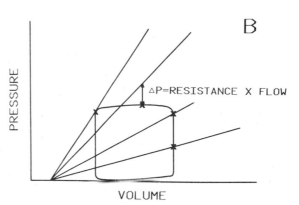

FIGURE 3–9. The systolic elastance of the pump may be described by its pressure-volume relation. *A*, If there were no flow from the ventricle, the four pressure-volume relations would pertain. *B*, During ejection, however, when flow occurs, ventricular resistance reduces the pressure (△P) that is generated, and hence the pressure-volume loop does not reach the elastic relation during this period. For the remainder of the cycle (no flow), however, the elastic behavior dominates. (From Weber KT, Janicki JS, Hunter WC, Shroff SG, Pearlman ES, Fishman AP. The contractile behavior of the heart and its functional coupling to the circulation. Prog Cardiovasc Dis *24*:375–400, 1982.)

Figure 3–9*A* illustrates pressure-volume relations for an isovolumetric contraction at various times in systole. The slope of each pressure-volume line represents ventricular elastance at a given instant in systole. An ejecting beat is superimposed on the isovolumetric pressure-volume relations and is represented by the pressure-volume loop in Figure 3–9*B*. During the isovolumic period of systole, when there is no flow, ventricular pressure is governed by the elastic behavior, and therefore, the ejecting beat pressure-volume points during this period fall on the isovolumetric pressure-volume relations. During the ejection period, however, ventricular pressure falls below that predicted by pure elastic behavior. The difference (△P) in predicted (based on pure elastic behavior) and actual pressure is due to ventricular resistive behavior. Ventricular resistance, for a given time and volume in systole, is defined as this pressure difference divided by the flow.

Experimental evidence[19–21] indicates that ventricular pressure-volume-time relations during systole can be adequately quantitated by a time-varying elastance. Furthermore, the elastance function is independent of the external loading conditions, that is, end-diastolic volume and ejection pressure. This is depicted in Figure 3–10, in which the solid curves represent ventricular elastance as a function of time for various combinations of end-diastolic volume and ejection-pressure. On the other hand, when the contractile state is raised by the catecholamine, such as dobutamine, elastance (broken curve, Fig. 3–10) is significantly altered such that it reaches a higher maximum in a shorter period of time. Ventricular elastance (especially its peak value) can be used to represent the intrinsic force generating capability of the heart, because of both its insensitivity to external loading conditions and its behaving in a predictable manner with variations in contractile state.

Similar to elastance, ventricular resistance is not constant during systole; instead, it varies throughout systole.[22, 23] However, ventricular resistance for a given combination of systolic time, volume, and contractile state is uniquely related to the corresponding isovolumetric pressure P_o (ie, for the same time, volume, and contractile state but with zero

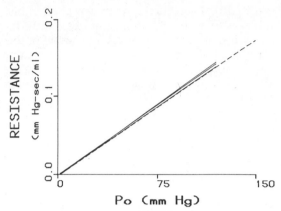

FIGURE 3–11. Left ventricular systolic resistance is a linear function of ventricular isovolumetric pressure (see text). This linear relationship is not affected by alterations in loading condition (end-diastolic volume and ejection pressure, solid lines) or contractility (broken line).

flow).[22, 23] As shown in Figure 3–11, this relationship between resistance and isovolumetric pressure is linear and independent of changes in end-diastolic volume, ejection pressure, and contractile state.[21–23]

It should be emphasized that ventricular systolic elastance and resistance are strictly phenomenologic descriptions of mechanical properties; elastance describes the volume and time dependence of pressure, whereas resistance describes the flow dependence. At present, one can only speculate as to the physical basis of these global properties. For example, elastance and resistance may be a manifestation of the force-length and force-velocity relations of the constituent muscle fibers, respectively. However, factors other than the properties of the individual muscle fibers (eg, collagen concentration, geometry, muscle mass) may also contribute to the measured values of elastance and resistance.

In a manner similar to diastolic chamber stiffness, ventricular systolic elastance and resistance represent chamber rather than myocardial properties. In order to derive the myocardial properties so as to facilitate comparisons among hearts with varying sizes and shapes, one has to appropriately normalize pressure, volume, and flow data. For this purpose, one can transform pressure, volume, and flow to stress, strain, and strain rate, respectively. However, since stress and strain have multiple components and an additional variable (strain rate) is present, this process will result in a relatively large number of relations and, therefore, may have limited practical utility. Another approach to normalization is to concentrate on specific aspects of the elastance and resistance func-

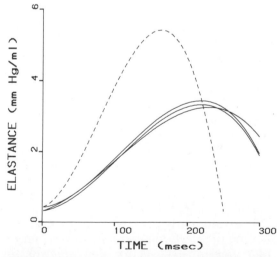

FIGURE 3–10. The time-varying systolic elastance of the left ventricle is not influenced by the variations in loading conditions (end-diastolic volume and ejection pressure, solid lines). Changes in contractility alter elastance. For example, dobutamine, a synthetic catecholamine, will raise elastance (broken curve).

tions (eg, peak elastance and the slope of resistance-pressure relationship) and derive empirical normalization factors based on simultaneous experiments performed on the intact ventricle and isolated papillary muscle from the same ventricle. These experiments have not yet been performed, and it is clear that much work needs to be done in this area.

Factors Influencing the Mechanical Properties in Systole

Since an explicit description of myocardial systolic mechanical properties is not currently available, the following discussion primarily focuses on those factors that influence the chamber mechanical properties.

The effects of various factors on ventricular elastance have generally been studied for the left ventricle in terms of two quantities that are derived from the entire elastance function: peak elastance (E_{max}) and the volume axis intercept of the peak elastance (V_d). As noted earlier, variations in arterial load or end-diastolic volume do not affect E_{max} or V_d,[21, 24] although increases in contractile state with catecholamines (eg, dobutamine) significantly increase E_{max} without altering the intercept.[19, 21] Global ischemia reduces E_{max} without altering slope,[24] whereas regional ischemia increases V_d without altering E_{max}.[24] Finally, an increase in right ventricular systolic pressure and end-diastolic volume results in a decrease in V_d without any change in E_{max}.[18] These observations suggest that an increase or decrease in E_{max} can be interpreted to represent an augmentation or a depression of contractile state, respectively. However, a change in V_d alone is difficult to interpret.

Factors influencing ventricular resistance have not been studied. However, based on our preliminary studies,[23] we believe that the rate limiting process of the contractile apparatus is one of the major determinants of the chamber ventricular resistance. In addition, it is possible that the extracellular components (eg, collagen), shearing forces between myocardial fibers, and geometric deformation during systole may contribute to chamber resistance. The relative contributions of each of these components needs further evaluation.

Factors Influencing Ventricular Systolic Performance

In the following discussion we will briefly discuss the three major factors (ejection pressure, end-diastolic volume, and contractile state) that influence ventricular performance in terms of stroke volume and stroke work. This analysis is based on the mean values of measurements, such as pressure and volume, and should be contrasted with the analysis presented in Chapter 4, in which instantaneous muscle force-length-velocity variables are used. This pressure-volume analysis will be useful in describing the coupling of the heart to the circulation, as described in the subsequent section.

The hemodynamic performance of the pump may be considered by using the mean values of ejection pressure and flow and the stroke volume. Figure 3–12 depicts the inverse relationships that exist between stroke volume and mean ejection rate with mean ejection pressure.[25] For any given end-diastolic volume, as the level of *ejection pressure* increases, the stroke volume and ejection rate fall. Eventually, ejection pressure reaches a level such that there is no ejection. This is an isovolumetric contraction, during which there is no flow or volume ejected; it is represented by the points that intersect the abscissa. The elastic properties of the pump are reflected in the slope of the relation between stroke volume and ejection pressure. As the contractile state of the pump is compromised (Fig. 3–12, right panel), systolic elastance will fall. Of equal importance is the fact that when elastance falls (eg, in the failing heart), the slope of this relation is increased so that the ventricle is influenced to a greater extent by changes in ejection pressure. Hence, the failing heart has become more sensitive to its arterial load.

For any given ejection pressure, the larger the *end-diastolic volume* the greater the stroke volume and the rate of ejection (Fig. 3–12, left panel). This volume-dependent property of the pump has been termed the Frank-Starling mechanism, after Otto Frank and Ernest Starling, who described this behavior of the ventricle at the turn of the century. If one considers the inter-relationship between ejection pressure and the volume ejected, we have a representation of systolic work, in which stroke work equals the force exerted over a unit distance. For a given diastolic volume, stroke work normally rises and falls over the physiologic range of ejection pressure. Peak work generally occurs at the expected normal range of arterial pressures (eg, 80 to 140 mm Hg). Beyond this point, stroke volume falls and work declines (Fig. 3–13). Thus, the normal ventricle operates at the peak of its work-load curve. In order for it to

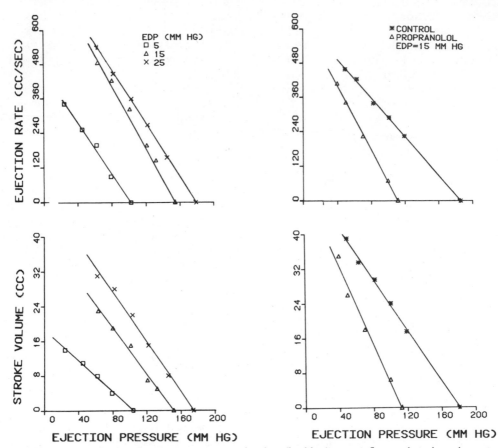

FIGURE 3–12. The behavior of the heart as a pump may be described by its mean flow and stroke volume-to-ejection pressure relations. For any given filling pressure (left panels), the greater the ejection pressure the less the stroke volume and rate of ejection. As filling pressure is raised, the flow and volume displaced from the chamber increases for any given ejection pressure. Compared with the normal heart, the failing heart (right panels; propranolol) generates less flow and displaces less volume from its chamber for any given ejection pressure. In addition, it becomes more sensitive to ejection pressure (small increments in ejection pressure will significantly reduce the stroke volume). (From Weber KT, Janicki JS, Hunter WC, Shroff SG, Pearlman ES, Fishman AP. The contractile behavior of the heart and its functional coupling to the circulation. Prog Cardiovasc Dis 24:375–400, 1982.)

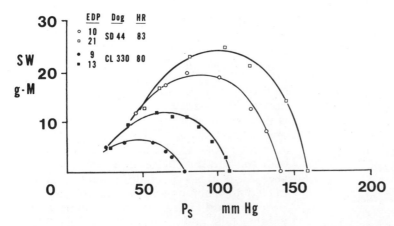

FIGURE 3–13. Influence of end-diastolic pressure (EDP) on the parabolic relation between stroke work (SW) and the ejection pressure (P_s) is shown for two different dog hearts. See text. (From Weber KT, Janicki JS, Reeves RC, Hefner LL, Reeves TJ. Determinants of stroke volume in the isolated canine heart. J Appl Physiol 37:742–747, 1974.)

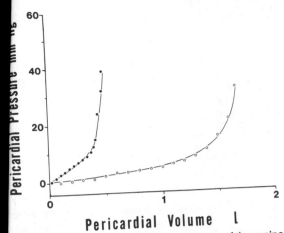

FIGURE 3–17. The pressure-volume relation of the canine pericardium. The curve on the left (solid circles) was obtained in the normal pericardium. The curve on the right (open circles) was obtained in an animal with a large and chronic pericardial effusion.

pericardium may therefore contribute to the inability of the dilated heart to raise its stroke volume during exercise. This situation only further compounds the inability of the failing heart to sustain oxygen transport during physical activity.

Pleural Pressure

Unlike intrapericardial pressure, pleural pressure surrounds both the heart and the lungs. It too contributes to the interplay of the ventricles by regulating the filling pres-

sure gradient between each ventricle and its respective filling reservoirs, the venous and pulmonary circulations (Fig. 3–18).[28-31] Pleural pressure normally ranges from −2 mmHg at end-expiration to −5 mm Hg at end-inspiration. Transmural right atrial pressure is, therefore, 5 − (−2) or 7 mm Hg at end-expiration and 5 − (− 5) or 10 mm Hg at end-inspiration. The respiratory motion of the thorax assists right heart filling by reducing intrathoracic pressure during inspiration, thereby elevating the gradient to filling between the extrathoracic and intrathoracic veins. In the case of the left ventricle, whose pulmonary blood reservoir is located within the thorax, variations in pleural pressure simultaneously affect it and its filling reservoir. During inspiration, the filling pressure gradient of the left ventricle is not increased, even though its transmural filling pressure will be. In fact, left ventricular filling may fall, because blood is pooled in the lung and right ventricle and there is an elevation in transmural aortic pressure that is felt as an increased hydrostatic load by the left ventricle. As a result of these various hemodynamic adjustments, left ventricular stroke volume falls and with it arterial systolic pressure. The effects of negative intrapleural pressure on arterial blood pressure are particularly evident during a forced inspiratory effort (Fig. 3–19), such as that associated with acute bronchospasm. In this case, the normal fall of 10 mmHg or less that occurs in arterial

perform at its peak during increments in ejection pressure, there must be a corresponding increase in diastolic volume. We will consider pump work further in Chapter 4, as we discuss the concept of mechanical efficiency, or the ratio of work performed relative to energy utilized by the myocardium.

Finally, the *contractile state* of the pump will determine the volume and rate of ejection for any given filling volume and ejection pressure (Fig. 3–12, right panel). Contractility or the contractile state is a term used to describe this property of the pump, which is independent of its filling volume and arterial load but sensitive to neurohumoral influences (such as plasma norepinephrine) and dependent on the intrinsic constituents (such as myosin isoform composition) of its myocardium. This topic will also be discussed in greater detail in Chapter 4.

THE INTERPLAY AND INTERDEPENDENCE OF THE RIGHT AND LEFT VENTRICLES

To ensure proper oxygen and carbon dioxide transport and a steady state of fluid balance and nutrient exchange across the lungs and circulation, pulmonary and systemic blood flow must be balanced relative to one another. The equilibrium that normally exists between the right and left heart is promoted by their anatomic arrangement, which, conceptually speaking, may be represented as two muscular pumps aligned in series via their mechanical coupling by the lungs (Fig. 3–14). Several anatomic and physiologic factors also provide for the interplay of the ventricles.[26] These include the muscle fibers that interconnect the ventricular free walls and interventricular septum, the mobile interventricular septum itself, the pericardium, and the intrapleural pressure. Collectively, these factors create and foster an interdependence between the ventricles.

Muscle Fibers

For many years it was thought that the myocardium was composed of discrete muscle bundles. Each ventricle was thought to have a distinct composition of several of these muscles. More recent evidence, however, indicates that these muscle bundles probably do not exist. Instead, the myocardium should be considered a continuum of

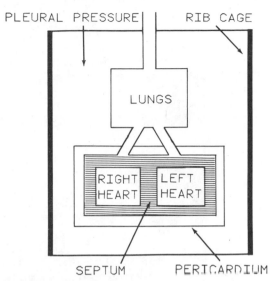

FIGURE 3–14. A schematic representation of the cardiopulmonary unit and its components. (From Weber KT, Janicki JS, Shroff SG, Likoff MJ. The cardio-pulmonary unit. The body's gas transport system. Clin Chest Med 4:101–110, 1983.)

wound muscle fibers.[8] Irrespective of one's viewpoint, the alignment of muscle fibers within the interventricular septum and ventricular free walls will determine in part the interaction of the ventricles.

In the interventricular septum muscle fiber alignment resembles that of the left ventricle, so that the left ventricular side of the septum has an orientation of fibers similar to that of the left ventricular subendocardium, whereas the right ventricular side of the septum and its fibers resemble the epicardial fibers of the left ventricular free wall.[9] Morphologically, therefore, the septum resembles the left ventricle. The concentric reduction of the left ventricular chamber during systole (Fig. 3–15) would also support the view, from a functional standpoint, that the septum and left ventricle behave as a unit. The alignment of fibers within the right ventricular free wall and its attachments to the septum and left ventricle remain undefined. Nevertheless, these attachments almost certainly would promote the interdependence of the ventricles by creating a radial force that draws the right ventricular free wall into the septum, thereby aiding in right ventricular emptying.

Interventricular Septum

The septum is a deformable structure that separates the two ventricles. Its position and curvature relative to the ventricles is deter-

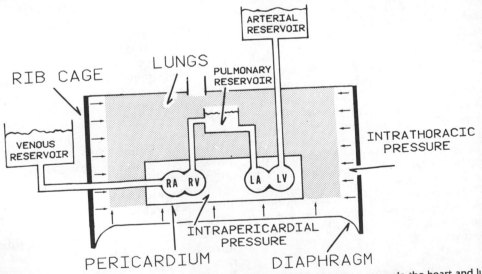

FIGURE 3–18. A diagram of the thorax and its components. Intrathoracic pressure surrounds the heart and lungs while intrapericardial pressure is applied solely to the right and left hearts. (From Weber KT, Janicki JS, Shroff SG, Likoff M St John Sutton MG. The right ventricle: physiologic and pathophysiologic considerations. Crit Care Med 11:323–328 1983.)

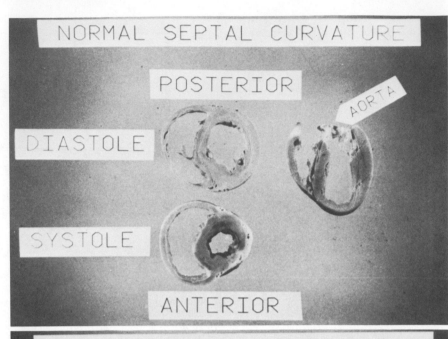

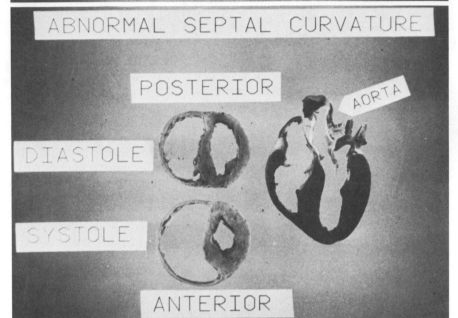

FIGURE 3–15. The normal curvature of the canine interventricular septum is shown for two canine hearts—one arrested in diastole and the other in systole. In each case, the pericardium was intact and ventricular volume fixed. The abnormal curvature of the septum that accompanies a volume overload of the right ventricle in the diastolically or systolically arrested heart is shown, as well as the change in LV geometry. (From Weber KT, Janicki, JS, Shroff SG, Likoff MJ, St John Sutton MG. The right ventricle: physiologic and pathophysiologic considerations. Crit Care Med *11*:323–328, 1983.)

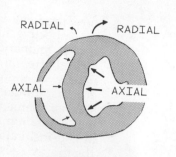

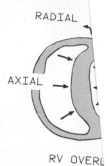

FIGURE 3–16. The relative dominance and direction of the axial and radial forces that determine the curvature of the interventricular septum are shown for a normal heart and for one in which the volume and filling pressures of the RV are increased. (From Weber KT, Janicki JS, Shroff SG, Likoff MJ, St John Sutton MG. The right ventricle: physiologic and pathophysiologic considerations. Crit Care Med *11*:323–328, 1983.)

mined by the distribution of forces across its surface (Fig. 3–16). Radial and axial forces are present on both its right and left ventricular surfaces. A radial force is created by the tethering or pulling of the muscle fibers in the septum toward the free wall of each ventricle. From the information presented earlier about the alignment of muscle fibers within the septum, this radial force will dom-

inate in the direction of the left ventricular free wall. The axial force is related to ventricular pressure and septal surface area. Normally, the difference in pressure between the ventricles creates an axial force that bows that septum toward the right ventricle.

Acute variations in right ventricular volume or pressure alter the distribution of this axial force, and thereby also alter septal po-

sition and motion (Figs. 3–15 and 3–16). For example, a forced inspiration will increase right ventricular volume transiently, moving the septum toward the left ventricle. When this occurs, the geometry of the left ventricle is distorted and the distensibility of its chamber is reduced. The left ventricle now appears to be stiffer. Left ventricular geometry and distensibility may be substantially altered in patients with right ventricular enlargement and cor pulmonale or congenital heart disease. In either setting, left ventricular filling pressure may be increased. These findings, however, should not be interpreted as indicative of left ventricular disease. Instead, it is the distensibility of the left ventricle that is reduced. This does not imply that the left ventricle cannot become involved in such patients but rather is meant to imply that an elevation in left ventricular filling pressure must be interpreted with caution in patients with right ventricular chamber enlargement. Left ventricular dysfunction can be found in patients with pulmonary hypertension secondary to chronic airway disease or pulmonary vascular disease.[27] In severe pulmonary vascular disease, the systolic pressure of the right ventricle will reach or even exceed that of the left ventricle. In such cases, the septum is hypertrophied, its motion during the cardiac cycle altered, and its diastolic position shifted leftward—particularly near its basilar portion. In this position, the septum may partially obliterate the outflow tract of the left ventricle and may therefore account for the left ventricular hypertrophy that often accompanies severe pulmonary hypertension.[28] The abnormality in septal motion seen in pulmonary hypertension may be predictive of systolic and mean pulmonary artery pressures.

Pericardium

The pericardium surrounds the heart. The viscoelastic properties of the pericardium de-

termine intrapericardial pressure given intrapericardial volume. Both and ventricles are subjected to intra dial pressure. For normal ventricu umes the pericardium imposes little physical constraint, and, therefore, pericardial and intrapleural pressur equivalent.[29] During diastole, the in between the ventricles is modestly enh by the pericardium. In systole, as c volume declines, the pericardium im no constraint on the behavior of the v cles.

During an acute increase in heart size viscoelastic limits of the pericardium brought into play. Here, intraperican pressure rises to produce a positive exter pressure on the external surfaces of b ventricles. This serves to lower the tra mural pressure of the ventricles and there to lower ventricular filling. A pericardial e fusion may also create a positive extracardia pressure. The more severe the effusion the more rapid its onset, the greater its pro pensity to compromise cardiac filling as the viscoelastic properties of the pericardium are once again introduced (Fig. 3–17). An intra pericardial pressure of 12 mmHg or more represents the point at which the pressure in each cardiac chamber will be equalized.[30] It is at this point that ventricular filling is severely compromised. As a result, cardiac output falls and systemic hypotension appears. This is the circumstance termed *cardiac tamponade*. When intrapericardial volume rises more gradually, as occurs in the period from infancy to adulthood or in the failing heart, the pericardium itself grows, and alterations in its viscoelastic properties may also occur. In these circumstances, intrapericardial and intrapleural pressures remain equal. Even here, however, an acute increase in heart size (eg, the heightened venous return of exercise in the dilated failing heart) raises pericardial pressure and restricts the further filling of the heart. The elastic limits of the perform at its peak during increments in ejection pressure, there must be a corresponding increase in diastolic volume. We will consider pump work further in Chapter 4, as we discuss the concept of mechanical efficiency, or the ratio of work performed relative to energy utilized by the myocardium.

Finally, the *contractile state* of the pump will determine the volume and rate of ejection for any given filling volume and ejection pressure (Fig. 3–12, right panel). Contractility or the contractile state is a term used to describe this property of the pump, which is independent of its filling volume and arterial load but sensitive to neurohumoral influences (such as plasma norepinephrine) and dependent on the intrinsic constituents (such as myosin isoform composition) of its myocardium. This topic will also be discussed in greater detail in Chapter 4.

THE INTERPLAY AND INTERDEPENDENCE OF THE RIGHT AND LEFT VENTRICLES

To ensure proper oxygen and carbon dioxide transport and a steady state of fluid balance and nutrient exchange across the lungs and circulation, pulmonary and systemic blood flow must be balanced relative to one another. The equilibrium that normally exists between the right and left heart is promoted by their anatomic arrangement, which, conceptually speaking, may be represented as two muscular pumps aligned in series via their mechanical coupling by the lungs (Fig. 3–14). Several anatomic and physiologic factors also provide for the interplay of the ventricles.[26] These include the muscle fibers that interconnect the ventricular free walls and interventricular septum, the mobile interventricular septum itself, the pericardium, and the intrapleural pressure. Collectively, these factors create and foster an interdependence between the ventricles.

Muscle Fibers

For many years it was thought that the myocardium was composed of discrete muscle bundles. Each ventricle was thought to have a distinct composition of several of these muscles. More recent evidence, however, indicates that these muscle bundles probably do not exist. Instead, the myocardium should be considered a continuum of

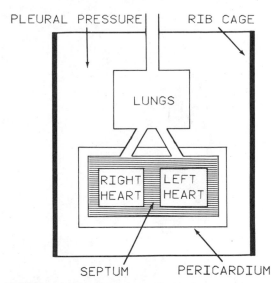

FIGURE 3–14. A schematic representation of the cardio-pulmonary unit and its components. (From Weber KT, Janicki JS, Shroff SG, Likoff MJ. The cardio-pulmonary unit. The body's gas transport system. Clin Chest Med 4:101–110, 1983.)

wound muscle fibers.[8] Irrespective of one's viewpoint, the alignment of muscle fibers within the interventricular septum and ventricular free walls will determine in part the interaction of the ventricles.

In the interventricular septum muscle fiber alignment resembles that of the left ventricle, so that the left ventricular side of the septum has an orientation of fibers similar to that of the left ventricular subendocardium, whereas the right ventricular side of the septum and its fibers resemble the epicardial fibers of the left ventricular free wall.[9] Morphologically, therefore, the septum resembles the left ventricle. The concentric reduction of the left ventricular chamber during systole (Fig. 3–15) would also support the view, from a functional standpoint, that the septum and left ventricle behave as a unit. The alignment of fibers within the right ventricular free wall and its attachments to the septum and left ventricle remain undefined. Nevertheless, these attachments almost certainly would promote the interdependence of the ventricles by creating a radial force that draws the right ventricular free wall into the septum, thereby aiding in right ventricular emptying.

Interventricular Septum

The septum is a deformable structure that separates the two ventricles. Its position and curvature relative to the ventricles is deter-

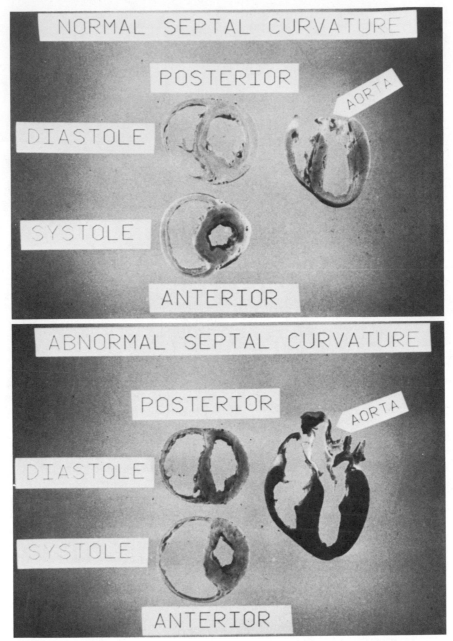

FIGURE 3–15. The normal curvature of the canine interventricular septum is shown for two canine hearts—one arrested in diastole and the other in systole. In each case, the pericardium was intact and ventricular volume fixed. The abnormal curvature of the septum that accompanies a volume overload of the right ventricle in the diastolically or systolically arrested heart is shown, as well as the change in LV geometry. (From Weber KT, Janicki, JS, Shroff SG, Likoff MJ, St John Sutton MG. The right ventricle: physiologic and pathophysiologic considerations. Crit Care Med *11*:323–328, 1983.)

mined by the distribution of forces across its surface (Fig. 3–16). Radial and axial forces are present on both its right and left ventricular surfaces. A radial force is created by the tethering or pulling of the muscle fibers in the septum toward the free wall of each ventricle. From the information presented earlier about the alignment of muscle fibers within the septum, this radial force will dom-

inate in the direction of the left ventricular free wall. The axial force is related to ventricular pressure and septal surface area. Normally, the difference in pressure between the ventricles creates an axial force that bows that septum toward the right ventricle.

Acute variations in right ventricular volume or pressure alter the distribution of this axial force, and thereby also alter septal po-

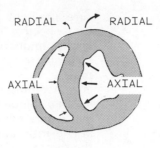

FIGURE 3–16. The relative dominance and direction of the axial and radial forces that determine the curvature of the interventricular septum are shown for a normal heart and for one in which the volume and filling pressures of the RV are increased. (From Weber KT, Janicki JS, Shroff SG, Likoff MJ, St John Sutton MG. The right ventricle: physiologic and pathophysiologic considerations. Crit Care Med 11:323–328, 1983.)

sition and motion (Figs. 3–15 and 3–16). For example, a forced inspiration will increase right ventricular volume transiently, moving the septum toward the left ventricle. When this occurs, the geometry of the left ventricle is distorted and the distensibility of its chamber is reduced. The left ventricle now appears to be stiffer. Left ventricular geometry and distensibility may be substantially altered in patients with right ventricular enlargement and cor pulmonale or congenital heart disease. In either setting, left ventricular filling pressure may be increased. These findings, however, should not be interpreted as indicative of left ventricular disease. Instead, it is the distensibility of the left ventricle that is reduced. This does not imply that the left ventricle cannot become involved in such patients but rather is meant to imply that an elevation in left ventricular filling pressure must be interpreted with caution in patients with right ventricular chamber enlargement. Left ventricular dysfunction can be found in patients with pulmonary hypertension secondary to chronic airway disease or pulmonary vascular disease.[27] In severe pulmonary vascular disease, the systolic pressure of the right ventricle will reach or even exceed that of the left ventricle. In such cases, the septum is hypertrophied, its motion during the cardiac cycle altered, and its diastolic position shifted leftward—particularly near its basilar portion. In this position, the septum may partially obliterate the outflow tract of the left ventricle and may therefore account for the left ventricular hypertrophy that often accompanies severe pulmonary hypertension.[28] The abnormality in septal motion seen in pulmonary hypertension may be predictive of systolic and mean pulmonary artery pressures.

Pericardium

The pericardium surrounds the heart. The viscoelastic properties of the pericardium de-termine intrapericardial pressure for any given intrapericardial volume. Both the atria and ventricles are subjected to intrapericardial pressure. For normal ventricular volumes the pericardium imposes little if any physical constraint, and, therefore, intrapericardial and intrapleural pressures are equivalent.[29] During diastole, the interplay between the ventricles is modestly enhanced by the pericardium. In systole, as cardiac volume declines, the pericardium imposes no constraint on the behavior of the ventricles.

During an acute increase in heart size, the viscoelastic limits of the pericardium are brought into play. Here, intrapericardial pressure rises to produce a positive external pressure on the external surfaces of both ventricles. This serves to lower the transmural pressure of the ventricles and thereby to lower ventricular filling. A pericardial effusion may also create a positive extracardiac pressure. The more severe the effusion or the more rapid its onset, the greater its propensity to compromise cardiac filling as the viscoelastic properties of the pericardium are once again introduced (Fig. 3–17). An intrapericardial pressure of 12 mmHg or more represents the point at which the pressure in each cardiac chamber will be equalized.[30] It is at this point that ventricular filling is severely compromised. As a result, cardiac output falls and systemic hypotension appears. This is the circumstance termed *cardiac tamponade.* When intrapericardial volume rises more gradually, as occurs in the period from infancy to adulthood or in the failing heart, the pericardium itself grows, and alterations in its viscoelastic properties may also occur. In these circumstances, intrapericardial and intrapleural pressures remain equal. Even here, however, an acute increase in heart size (eg, the heightened venous return of exercise in the dilated failing heart) raises pericardial pressure and restricts the further filling of the heart. The elastic limits of the

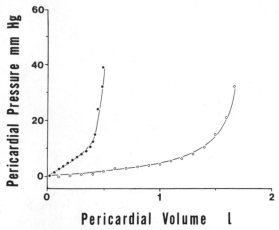

FIGURE 3–17. The pressure-volume relation of the canine pericardium. The curve on the left (solid circles) was obtained in the normal pericardium. The curve on the right (open circles) was obtained in an animal with a large and chronic pericardial effusion.

pericardium may therefore contribute to the inability of the dilated heart to raise its stroke volume during exercise. This situation only further compounds the inability of the failing heart to sustain oxygen transport during physical activity.

Pleural Pressure

Unlike intrapericardial pressure, pleural pressure surrounds both the heart and the lungs. It too contributes to the interplay of the ventricles by regulating the filling pres-

sure gradient between each ventricle and its respective filling reservoirs, the venous and pulmonary circulations (Fig. 3–18).[28–31] Pleural pressure normally ranges from −2 mmHg at end-expiration to −5 mm Hg at end-inspiration. Transmural right atrial pressure is, therefore, 5 − (−2) or 7 mm Hg at end-expiration and 5 − (− 5) or 10 mm Hg at end-inspiration. The respiratory motion of the thorax assists right heart filling by reducing intrathoracic pressure during inspiration, thereby elevating the gradient to filling between the extrathoracic and intrathoracic veins. In the case of the left ventricle, whose pulmonary blood reservoir is located within the thorax, variations in pleural pressure simultaneously affect it and its filling reservoir. During inspiration, the filling pressure gradient of the left ventricle is not increased, even though its transmural filling pressure will be. In fact, left ventricular filling may fall, because blood is pooled in the lung and right ventricle and there is an elevation in transmural aortic pressure that is felt as an increased hydrostatic load by the left ventricle. As a result of these various hemodynamic adjustments, left ventricular stroke volume falls and with it arterial systolic pressure. The effects of negative intrapleural pressure on arterial blood pressure are particularly evident during a forced inspiratory effort (Fig. 3–19), such as that associated with acute bronchospasm. In this case, the normal fall of 10 mmHg or less that occurs in arterial

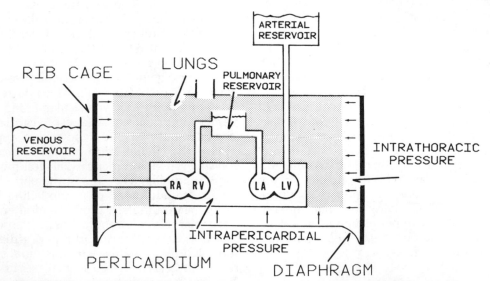

FIGURE 3–18. A diagram of the thorax and its components. Intrathoracic pressure surrounds the heart and lungs while intrapericardial pressure is applied solely to the right and left hearts. (From Weber KT, Janicki JS, Shroff SG, Likoff MJ, St John Sutton MG. The right ventricle: physiologic and pathophysiologic considerations. Crit Care Med *11*:323–328, 1983.)

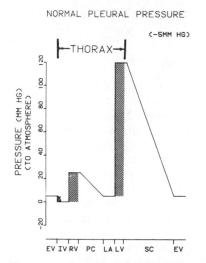
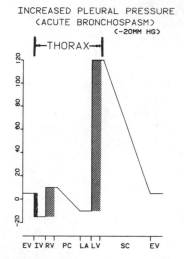
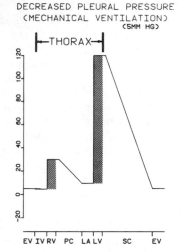

FIGURE 3–19. Variations in pleural pressure influence cardiac chamber pressures (referenced to atmosphere), their filling, and systolic behavior. *EV* and *IV*, extra- and intrathoracic veins, respectively. Included in *IV* is the right atrium; *RV*, right ventricle; *PC*, pulmonary circulation; *LA* and *LV*, left atrium and ventricle, respectively; *SC*, systemic circulation (see text). (From Weber KT, Janicki JS, Hunter WC, Shroff SG, Pearlman ES, Fishman AP. The contractile behavior of the heart and its functional coupling to the circulation. Prog Cardiovasc Dis *24*:375–400, 1982.)

systolic pressure during inspiration is accentuated, producing a "paradoxic" pulse. Thus, in patients with acute asthma, the disparate overfilling of the right ventricle, the leftward displacement of the septum, and the increase in left ventricular transmural and aortic pressure all serve to reduce left ventricular filling and emptying. This is a dramatic example of how pleural pressure affects the interplay of the ventricles.

Alternatively, an increase in pleural pressure—as occurs in the strain phase of the Valsalva maneuver, in mechanical ventilatory support, or in a pneumothorax—reduces the transmural pressure to ventricular filling (Fig. 3–19). The elevation in pleural pressure associated with mechanical ventilation may also compress the alveolar vessels, raising pulmonary vascular resistance, and thereby reducing right ventricular stroke volume and increasing right heart volume. Collectively, these effects serve to decrease left ventricular compliance.

THE INTERPLAY OF THE HEART AND LUNGS

A number of factors promote the interaction between the heart and lungs. These include airway pressure, the compliance of the thorax, lung volume, and a complex neurohumoral control system.

Airway Pressure

During inspiration, the gradient in pressure between the airways and the pleural space is termed the *transpulmonary pressure.* This pressure gradient serves to inflate the lungs. In the diseased lung, distensibility is reduced because of interstitial fibrosis or congestion. Accordingly, a greater inspiratory effort is required to lower pleural pressure and maintain transpulmonary pressure for any given tidal volume. Under these circumstances, the accessory muscles of respiration must be used to create a greater inspiratory effort. In patients with lung disease who are undergoing mechanical ventilation, the airways are pulsed with a volume of air; airway pressure rises in proportion to lung compliance. The stiffer the lungs, the greater the airway pressure for any given tidal volume delivered by the ventilator. The elevation in airway pressure compresses the pulmonary circulation and its alveolar vessels, thereby raising vascular impedance and the systolic pressure that the right ventricle must generate. A significant overloading of the right ventricle may follow, with a secondary effect on the left heart as its configuration is altered and diastolic distensibility reduced.

Changes in airway pressure during assisted ventilation will also influence the pulmonary capillary wedge pressure tracing, which is often monitored in critically ill patients. To avoid erroneous information, this intravascular pressure must be measured during the expiratory phase of assisted ventilation. During normal spontaneous respiration, pulmonary wedge pressure must be measured at end expiration, when the lung is at its functional residual capacity and pleural pressure is closest to zero, for it is at this time that pulmonary vascular resistance is minimal and pleural pressure approximates atmospheric pressure. A serious underestimation of left ventricular filling pressure can occur as a result either of measuring wedge pressure during inspiration or of electronically averaging wedge pressure throughout the respiratory cycle.

The Thorax and Its Compliance

The bellows-like action of the thorax creates variations in pleural pressure that aid lung inflation. A paralysis or weakness of the diaphragm or the respiratory muscles compromise the ability of the thoracic pump to change intrathoracic volume and pressure. A structural deformity of the chest wall, such as that seen in patients with kyphoscoliosis or pectus excavatum, will compromise thoracic compliance and, thereby, the mechanical efficiency of the lung. These abnormalities in the compliance of the thoracic pump will affect the heart by virtue of one of several mechanisms, including the following: (1) impaired ventilation with hypoxic pulmonary vasoconstriction, and attendant right-sided pressure overload; (2) a compromised capacity to lower intrathoracic pressure and thereby to assist venous return, which may be particularly evident during physical activity; and (3) an anatomic distortion of the heart and its ventricles by direct compression.

The importance of thoracic compliance in regulating intrapleural pressure has been emphasized in more recent studies of cardiopulmonary resuscitation.[32] A physical restraint of outward chest wall and abdominal motion minimizes the loss in positive pleural pressure that occurs with the compressive phase of the resuscitation effort. This approach, together with pulsed airway pressure synchronous with cardiac diastole, has been used to enhance the emptying of the intrathoracic aorta and thereby to lower the impedance to the subsequent displacement of blood from the compression of the arrested heart. These principles may also prove useful in assisting the severely failing heart to maintain systemic blood flow and oxygen delivery.

Lung Volume

The lungs are in contact with the lateral and posterior surfaces of the heart and pericardium. It has been suggested that lung inflation provides a compressive force on the myocardium.[33, 34] During positive end-expiratory pressure, for example, this compressive effect is thought to raise adversely left ventricular filling pressure. From our discussion of pericardial effusion and the 12 mm Hg of intrapericardial pressure required to reduce ventricular filling, we would surmise that the thick-walled left ventricle would be only modestly influenced by the air-filled, compressible lung. Further studies, however, are required to quantitate this effect.

THE VENTRICLES COUPLED TO THE CIRCULATION

The heart and the circulation represent two individual mechanical systems that are coupled to each other. Under the conditions of coupled equilibrium, the pressure, volume, and flow variables measured at any point in the cardiovascular system are determined by the mechanical properties of each system and their mutual interactions. In this respect, the terms *cardiac* output and *arterial* pressure, which are actually determined by the joint interaction of heart and circulation, could be misconstrued. On the surface, one might suppose that the cardiac output were determined solely by the heart and not the vasculature. Similarly, the term arterial pressure suggests that only the vasculature determines it. In reality, both these variables are determined by the mutual interaction of heart and circulation. Finally, the analysis of coupling is based on variables such as pressure, volume, and flow. Therefore, chamber mechanical properties (eg, elastance and resistance), and not the myocardial properties, are useful in such an endeavor.

Coupling to the Arterial Circulation

The following discussion is limited to the coupling of the left ventricle to the systemic arterial circulation. Conceptually, one can analyze the coupling of the right ventricle to the pulmonary arterial circulation in a similar manner.

The intrinsic chamber mechanical properties of the left ventricle are its elastance and resistance, as we have described earlier in the chapter. Similarly, the mechanical properties of the systemic arterial circulation can be represented by its input impedance spectrum, a detailed description of which can be found elsewhere.[35] In brief, the arterial circulation does not act as a pure resistance; instead, the load imposed on the left ventricle is frequency dependent. In addition, the pressure and flow events are not exactly in phase, and the phase difference is also a function of frequency. Therefore, the input impedance spectrum, which quantitates both the magnitude and phase of the load as a function of frequency, is a more complete definition of the mechanical properties of the arterial circulation.

The input impedance spectrum is often approximated by a three-element modified Windkessel[36] consisting of (1) systemic vascular resistance (Rp); (2) the collective compliance of the arterial circulation (C); and (3) characteristic impedance (Rc). Rp is primarily determined by the resistance of small vessels and arterioles, C represents the overall static compliance ($\triangle V/\triangle P$) of the arterial circulation; and Rc is primarily a property of major arteries. If one has a knowledge of ventricular elastance and resistance throughout systole and parameters Rp, C, and Rc, one can predict the entire time-course of pressure and flow that would result when these two systems are coupled. These results cannot be presented as explicit analytic equations; instead, one derives the results from numerical solution of a set of coupled differential equations. On the other hand, if one is interested only in predicting the average values of the resultant variables (eg, average arterial pressure, stroke volume, or cardiac output), and

not in the exact time-course, then one can simplify the analysis considerably. The simplified analysis results in explicit analytic expressions for pressures and flows and can also be represented graphically. One such example is discussed below.

The left ventricle and its arterial load are characterized in terms of average pressure-flow relations in Figure 3–20. For the arterial load, this relationship is represented by the line demonstrating the proportional increase in mean arterial pressure as the flow through the arteries is increased. The inverse of the slope of this relation represents systemic vascular resistance. In other words, when systemic vascular resistance is reduced, the slope becomes steeper. Similarly, the left ventricle is represented by a relationship between mean flow (ie, cardiac output) and mean ejection pressure (similar to those in Fig. 3–12) for a given end-diastolic volume and contractile state. An increase in the end-diastolic volume shifts this relationship to the right in a parallel fashion; however, an augmentation of the contractile state shifts this relationship such that the extrapolated flow axis intercept (cardiac output for zero ejection pressure) is invariant, whereas the ejection pressure axis intercept (ejection pressure for zero cardiac output) is increased. In order to couple these two relationships and establish the point of equilibrium (ie, the intersection point), one needs to have a common variable represented by the pressure axis. We have observed that there exists a linear relation between mean ejection pressure and mean arterial pressure (mean arterial pressure = K × mean ejection pressure). The proportionality coefficient (K) is dependent on the arterial load parameters Rp and C, and heart rate. However, the variation of K within the physiologic range of arterial

FIGURE 3–20. The functional coupling of the heart to the systemic arterial circulation may be represented according to the scheme that relates the flow and pressure variables of each system (left and middle panels). When coupled, cardiac output, ejection pressure, and arterial pressure are uniquely determined by the intersection of the two curves (coupled equilibrium in right panel). (From Weber KT, Janicki JS, Hunter WC, Shroff SG, Pearlman ES, Fishman AP. The contractile behavior of the heart and its functional coupling to the circulation. Prog Cardiovasc Dis 24:375–400, 1982.)

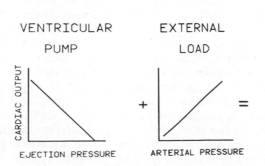

ARTERIAL COUPLING

VENTRICULAR PUMP

EXTERNAL LOAD

COUPLED EQUILIBRIUM

CARDIAC OUTPUT

EJECTION PRESSURE

ARTERIAL PRESSURE

EJECTION PRESSURE OR ARTERIAL PRESSURE

load and heart rate is small. In addition, the conceptual discussion of the coupling analysis presented here is not affected by the variations of K with arterial load.

Having converted the mean arterial pressure to mean ejection pressure, one can now calculate the equilibrium point as the intersection of the arterial and ventricular relations (Fig. 3–20). At this equilibrium point, the capability of the cardiac pump to generate pressure at a given flow balances the pressure required to force the same flow through the arterial load.

In the above example, we have purposely simplified the actual conditions and focused, in effect, on average values of pressure and flow. The pulsatile nature of cardiac contraction, however, introduces many complexities. For example, in addition to the systemic vascular resistance, arterial compliance (C) also affects cardiac output, such that cardiac output declines as C is reduced. Sunagawa and colleagues[37] have incorporated the effects of heart rate, Rp, and C in their analysis of left ventricular–arterial coupling and have derived an analytic expression for predicting the equilibrium stroke volume from the intrinsic properties of the two mechanical systems, the left ventricle and the arterial load. Finally, it should be noted that the aortic input impedance spectrum, which is a complete description of arterial load, was simplified in terms of the three elements Rp, C, and Rc. In doing so, one effectively ignores the reflected pressure and flow waves that are known to exist in the arterial system.[35] These reflections may affect cardiac output independent of the absolute magnitude of the load (ie, values of Rp, C, and Rc). The relative importance of reflected waves in determining left ventricular–arterial coupling is presently unknown.

The degree to which the left ventricle and arterial circulation interact to contribute to the generation of the equilibrium pressure and flow is determined in part by the functional state of the left ventricle itself. In other words, the amount of change in the equilibrium cardiac output for a given change in arterial load is dependent on the properties (such as the cardiac output–ejection pressure relation) of the left ventricular pump. For example, the cardiac output–ejection pressure relation for a normal ventricle is relatively more horizontal (ie, cardiac output is less sensitive to changes in ejection pressure) than that of a failing ventricle (Fig. 3–21, *left panel*). Accordingly, the interaction of the left ventricle and the arterial load is relatively modest for a normal left ventricle, whereas the failing left ventricle is quite sensitive to changes in arterial load (Fig. 3–21, *left panel*).

Coupling to the Venous Circulation

In addition to the coupling of the left ventricle and the arterial circulation, a similar coupling is present between the right ventricle and the venous circulation. The classic analysis of this venous coupling by Guyton and associates[4] follows the logic outlined earlier for the arteries. The right heart is a flow generator; the venous circulation, its filling reservoir. Each can be described by its own unique pressure-flow relation (Fig. 3–22), traditionally termed the ventricular function curve for the right ventricle and the venous return curve for the venous circulation, respectively. Cardiac output, or more specifically pulmonary blood flow, and right atrial pressure form this coupling and equilibrium point. At equilibrium, the capacity of the venous system to return flow to the right heart against a given filling pressure is balanced by the ability of the heart to generate flow when it is distended by the given filling pressure.

Sarnoff and Berglund[38] have popularized the term *ventricular function curve* to describe the relationship between the mechanical work of the ventricle and its filling volume. They have emphasized the fact that alterations in the functional state of the ventricle are best described by a "family" of such curves. In the human or the intact animal, the ventricular function curve is usually obtained during intravascular volume expansion, when arterial load will be increasing. As a result, pump output is measured under conditions of varying arterial pressure. Ideally, the ventricular function curve would be best determined for a given level of ejection pressure (see Fig. 3–21, *right panels*). The heavy, superimposed curve depicts the Frank-Starling relation and the fact that the ventricle can eject more when it is filled with a larger diastolic volume.

In addition, various other factors influence the function curve, including the diastolic properties of the chamber. For example, the more the ventricle is distended, the stiffer it becomes, and increments in filling pressure are consequently less effective in increasing diastolic volume. Increments in arterial loading diminish pump output for any given filling volume and therefore also affect the

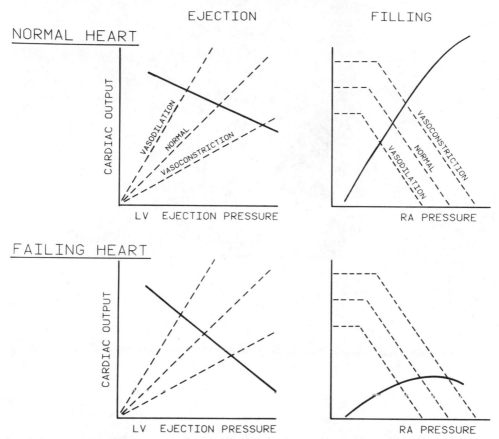

FIGURE 3–21. The coupling of the pump to the arterial (ejection) and venous (filling) circulations. The relation for the heart is represented as the heavy line, and the vasculature is the broken lines. The normal heart is primarily regulated by the venous return; arterial resistance has little effect. In the failing heart, however, arterial resistance becomes dominant (see text). (From Weber KT, Janicki JS, Hunter WC, Shroff SG, Pearlman ES, Fishman AP. The contractile behavior of the heart and its functional coupling to the circulation. Prog Cardiovasc Dis *24*:375–400, 1982.)

FIGURE 3–22. The functional coupling of the heart to the systemic venous circulation may be represented according to the scheme that relates the flow and pressure variables of each system (left and middle panels). When coupled, cardiac output, venous return, and right atrial pressure are uniquely determined by the intersection of the two curves (coupled equilibrium in right panel). (From Weber KT, Janicki JS, Hunter WC, Shroff SG, Pearlman ES, Fishman AP. The contractile behavior of the heart and its functional coupling to the circulation. Prog Cardiovasc Dis *24*:375–400, 1982.)

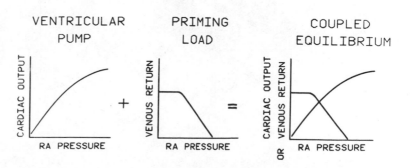

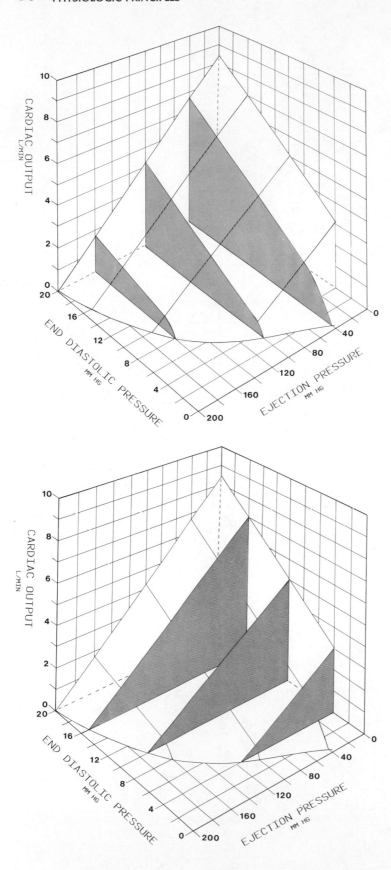

FIGURE 3–23. The three-dimensional surface depicting the interrelationship between cardiac output, left ventricular filling pressure, and ejection pressure. On the top, ventricular function curves are shown for three levels of ejection pressure (shaded areas). On the bottom, the cardiac output–ejection pressure relations are shown for three filling pressures (shaded areas). (From Weber KT, Janicki JS, Hunter WC, Shroff SG, Pearlman ES, Fishman AP. The contractile behavior of the heart and its functional coupling to the circulation. Prog Cardiovasc Dis 24:375–400, 1982.)

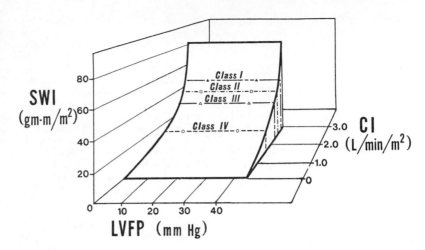

FIGURE 3–24. Hemodynamic profile of acute myocardial infarction based on stroke work index (SWI), cardiac index (CI), and left ventricular filling pressure (LVFP) presented for each clinical class. Classes I to IV connote the severity of left ventricular dysfunction that is present on clinical examination following acute myocardial infarction. Class I no failure; II, mild pulmonary congestion; III, pulmonary edema; and IV, shock. (From Weber KT, Janicki JS, Russell RO, Rackley CE. Identification of high risk subsets of acute myocardial infarction. Am J Cardiol 41:197–293, 1978.)

relation. These two factors are the primary reasons for the curvature that exists in the ventricular function curve. Additional factors that may contribute to this response include the interaction among the atria and ventricles in diastole, atrial contraction, and the pericardium.

The Heart Coupled to the Arterial and Venous Circulations

The coupling of either ventricle to its respective circulation (ie, venous and arterial) obviously occurs in similar fashion. Alterations in the coupling between either system will affect the other. To visualize this coupling, it is useful to consider the two pressure-flow relations, for a given ventricle, within a three-dimensional surface.[39] Figure 3–23 depicts left ventricular function in the plane of venous coupling (top panel) and the plane of arterial coupling (bottom panel). This three-dimensional surface reflects the fact that as a result of increases in filling pressure from 4 to 10 and to 16 mm Hg and, hence, in diastolic volume (as shown at the bottom), the curve relating ejection pressure during ejection to cardiac output is shifted upward in a parallel manner. Thus, a greater stroke volume can be generated by a more distended ventricle (ie, the Frank-Starling relation) for any systolic pressure. On the contrary, increasing systolic pressure (eg, from 40 to 100 to 160 mm Hg, as shown at the top) will depress the ventricular function curve such that at any filling pressure, cardiac output is reduced.

Thus, the three-dimensional surface integrates all of the coupling phenomena and provides a more concise summary of the pumping function of the heart. As the con-

tractile state of the pump is raised by inotropic agents or reduced by heart failure, the shape of this surface is altered. A similar approach has been taken in depicting the severity of cardiac failure following acute myocardial infarction (Fig. 3–24). In this analysis, the relationship between left ventricular stroke work and filling pressure have been examined for various degrees of left ventricular dysfunction expressed according to the level or plane of cardiac output.[40, 41] As the heart fails, its ability to generate systemic flow declines, irrespective of the level of its filling pressure. This relationship and a similar derivation for the ventricular function curve observed during upright isotonic exercise will be presented more fully in Chapter 10.

REFERENCES

1. Braunwald E, Ross J, Sonnenblick EH. Mechanisms of Contraction of the Normal and Failing Heart. Little, Brown and Co, Boston, 1976.
2. Noble MIM. The Cardiac Cycle. Blackwell Scientific Publications, Oxford, 1979.
3. Mirsky I, Ghista DN, Sandler H. Cardiac Mechanics. Physiological, Clinical and Mathematical Considerations. John Wiley and Sons, New York, 1974.
4. Guyton AC, Jones CE, Coleman TG. Circulatory Physiology: Cardiac Output and its Regulation. WB Saunders Co, Philadelphia, 1973.
5. Pearlman ES, Weber KT, Janicki JS. Quantitative histology of the hypertrophied human heart, in Weber KT, Hawthorne EW (eds). Symposium on Cardiac Shape and Structure. Fed Proc 40:2042–2047, 1981.
6. Weber KT, Hawthorne EW. Descriptors and determinants of cardiac shape, in Weber KT, Hawthorne EW (eds). Symposium on Cardiac Shape and Structure. Fed Proc 40:2005–2010, 1981.
7. Yin, FCP. Ventricular wall stress. Circ Res 49:829–842, 1981.

8. Streeter DD Jr, Sponitz HW, Patel DJ, Ross J Jr, Sonnenblick EH. Fiber orientation in canine left ventricle during diastole and systole. Circ Res 24:339–347, 1969.

9. Pearlman ES, Weber KT, Janicki JS, Pietra GG, Fishman AP. Muscle fiber orientation and connective tissue content in the hypertrophied human heart. Lab Invest 46:158–164, 1982.

10. Arts T, Reneman RS, Venstra PC. A model of the mechanics of the left ventricle. Ann Biomed Eng 7:299–318, 1979.

11. Hunter WC, Arts T, Baan J, Reneman RS. Torsion, shape and equilibrium in the left ventricular wall. Fed Proc 38:1306, 1979.

12. Gaasch WH, Bing OHL, Mirsky I. Chamber compliance and myocardial stiffness in left ventricular hypertrophy. Eur Heart J 3:139–145, 1982.

13. Janicki JS, Weber KT. Factors influencing the diastolic pressure-volume relation of the cardiac ventricles. Fed Proc 39:133–140, 1980.

14. Peterson KL, Tsuji J, Johnson A, DiDonna J, LeWinter M. Diastolic left ventricular pressure-volume and stress-strain relations in patients with valvular aortic stenosis. Circulation 58:77–89, 1978.

15. Hess OM, Schneider J, Kich R, Bambert C, Grimm J, Krayenbuehl KP. Diastolic function and myocardial structure in patients with myocardial hypertrophy: special reference to normalized viscoelastic data. Circulation 63:360–371, 1981.

16. Gaasch WH, Levine HJ, Quinones MA, Alexander JK. Left ventricular compliance: mechanisms and clinical implications. Am J Cardiol 38:645–653, 1976.

17. Janicki JS, Weber KT. Ejection pressure and the diastolic left ventricular pressure-volume relation. Am J Physiol 232:H545–H552, 1977.

18. Weber KT, Janicki JS, Shroff SG, Fishman AP. Contractile mechanics and interaction of the right and left ventricles. Am J Cardiol 47:686–695, 1981.

19. Suga H, Sagawa K, Shoukas AA. Load independence of instantaneous pressure-volume ratio of the canine left ventricle and effects of epinephrine and heart rate on the ratio. Circ Res 32:314–322, 1973.

20. Sagawa K, Suga H, Shoukas AA, Bakalar KM. End-systolic pressure/volume ratio: a new index of ventricular contractility. Am J Cardiol 40:748–753, 1977.

21. Shroff SG, Janicki JS, Weber KT. Left ventricular systolic dynamics in terms of its chamber mechanical properties. Am J Physiol 245:H110–H124, 1983.

22. Hunter WC, Janicki JS, Weber KT, Noordergraaf A. Systolic mechanical properties of the left ventricle: effects of volume and contractile state. Circ Res 52:319–327, 1983.

23. Shroff SG, Janicki JS, Weber KT. Evidence and quantitation of left ventricular systolic resistance. Am J Physiol, 249:H358–H370, 1985.

24. Maughan WL, Sunagawa K. Factors affecting the end-systolic pressure-volume relationship. Fed Proc 43:2408–2410, 1984.

25. Weber KT, Janicki JS, Reeves RC, Hefner LL. Determinants of stroke volume in isolated canine heart. J Appl Physiol 37:742–747, 1974.

26. Weber KT, Janicki JS, Shroff SG, Likoff MJ. The cardiopulmonary unit. The body's gas transport system. Clin Chest Med 4:101–110, 1983.

27. Matthay RA, Berger HJ. Noninvasive assessment of right and left ventricular function in acute and chronic respiratory failure. Crit Care Med 11:329–338, 1983.

28. Weber KT, Janicki JS, Shroff SG, Likoff MJ, St John Sutton MG. The right ventricle: physiologic and pathophysiologic considerations. Crit Care Med 11:323–328, 1983.

29. Spodick DH. Pericardial Diseases, in Brest, AN (ed). Cardiovascular Clinics, 7/3, FA Davis Co, Philadelphia, 1976.

30. Janicki JS, Shroff SG, Weber KT. Influence of extra-cardiac forces on the cardiopulmonary unit, In Yin FGP (ed). Cardiac/Vascular Coupling. Springer-Verlag, New York, in press, 1986.

31. Summer WR, Permutt S, Sagawa K. Effects of spontaneous respiration on canine left ventricular function. Circ Res 45:719–728, 1979.

32. Rudikoff MT, Maughan WL, Effron M. Mechanisms of blood flow during cardiopulmonary resuscitation. Circulation 61:345–352, 1980.

33. Cassidy SS, Eschenbacher WL, Robertson CH Jr. Cardiovascular effects of positive-pressure ventilation in normal subjects. J Appl Physiol 47:453–461, 1979.

34. Butler J. The heart is in good hands. Circulation 67:1163–1168, 1983.

35. Milnor WR. Hemodynamics. Williams and Wilkins, Baltimore, 1982.

36. Westerhof N, Elzinga G, Sipkema P. Artificial arterial system for pumping hearts. J Appl Physiol 228:776–781, 1971.

37. Sunagawa K, Sagawa K, Maughan WL. Ventricular interaction with the loading system. Ann Biomed Eng 12:163–189, 1984.

38. Sarnoff SJ, Berglund E. Ventricular function. I. Starling's law of the heart studied by means of simultaneous right and left ventricular function curves in the dog. Circulation 9:706–718, 1954.

39. Weber KT, Janicki JS, Hunter WC, Shroff SG, Pearlman ES, Fishman AP. The contractile behavior of the heart and its functional coupling to the circulation. Prog Cardiovasc Dis 24:375–400, 1982.

40. Weber KT, Ratshin RA, Janicki JS, Rackley CE, Russell RO. Left ventricular dysfunction following acute myocardial infarction: a clinicopathologic and hemodynamic profile of shock and failure. Am J Med 54:697–705, 1973.

41. Weber KT, Janicki JS, Russell RO, Rackley CE. Identification of high risk subsets of acute myocardial infarction. Am J Cardiol 41:197–293, 1978.

KARL T. WEBER
JOSEPH S. JANICKI
SANJEEV G. SHROFF

4

The Mechanics and Energetics of Ventricular Contraction

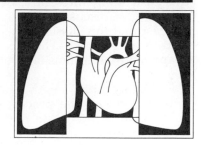

In Chapters 2 and 3, cardiac performance has been described in terms of the pumping capability of the ventricles (ie, stroke volume and stroke work). In addition, a discussion regarding the computation of chamber and myocardial mechanical properties, both in diastole and systole, has been presented in Chapter 3. In both these chapters, the ventricles were considered to be mechanical pumps, and the relevant variables in the analysis were ventricular pressure, volume, and flow. Historically, this approach emerged from the laboratories of Otto Frank and Ernest Starling at the turn of the century—a viewpoint of cardiac performance that emphasized the relationship between the diastolic volume of the ventricle and its stroke volume or stroke work.

An alternative approach to analyzing ventricular performance is based on the recognition of the fact that the ventricles are muscular pumps composed of muscle fibers, connective tissue, and blood vessels. Accordingly, the description of the performance of these muscle pumps can be made in terms of the behavior of the constituent elements. The primary motivation behind this approach was the possibility that a distinction could be made between disturbances in ventricular performance that are related to alterations in the myocardium per se (ie, its contractile state) and those that accompany abnormalities in the ventricular chamber (ie, chamber shape, size, architecture, and muscle mass). In addition, as it will become clear from the following discussion, the assessment of myocardial energetics is facilitated by this approach.

The relevant variables in this type of analysis are instantaneous muscle force (or stress), length, and velocity, with the index

of performance being the extent of fiber shortening. It should be noted that it is not possible to measure these variables directly; instead, they are computed from the measurements of ventricular pressure, volume, and flow, and of chamber geometry and muscle mass.

The main purpose of this chapter is to provide an overview of the analysis of ventricular performance, which is based on the behavior of the cardiac muscle. Specifically, the discussion focuses on the analysis of ventricular systolic performance and not on the computation of intrinsic mechanical properties (ie, myocardial stress-strain and stress-strain rate relations; see Chapter 3). In addition, a discussion of the energetics of ventricular contraction and its relationship to the mechanical behavior of the muscular pump is also presented. As in previous chapters, this review cannot be comprehensive and draws heavily on our own work. More extensive reviews can be found elsewhere.[1-3]

THE MECHANICS OF THE MUSCULAR PUMP

Because the wall that surrounds each ventricle is composed of cardiac muscle and blood vessels that are supported within a matrix of collagen, the dynamics of either ventricle may be expressed in terms of the force that the muscle fibers generate and the rate and extent of their shortening. The sequence of events that occur within the myocardium during the cardiac cycle may be described as follows. During ventricular filling, the myocardium is progressively stretched; at the end of the diastolic filling period, a force distends the muscular wall,

57

stretching its muscle fibers to a given length. In a manner analogous to isolated muscle, this distending force has been termed the *preload*. Our discussion in Chapter 3 would suggest that this diastolic wall force, or preload, is a function of chamber size, chamber shape, and the distensibility of the muscular wall.

From this initial length, muscle fibers are depolarized and the process of mechanical contraction follows. The sequence of depolarization varies topographically within the myocardium. In the case of the left ventricle, fibers within its septum and apex are depolarized first. As a result, they contract prior to those fibers situated in the free wall. Recognition of this fact led Carl Wiggers to describe the contraction process as a series of rapidly summated, fractionate contractions whose sequence was determined by the pattern of depolarization.[4] The contraction of the myocardium may therefore be likened to a peristaltic pump whose contraction proceeds sequentially in an apical to basal direction. The sequential process of depolarization also accounts for the changes in chamber configuration that occur during the isovolumic period of contraction prior to ejection. The actual pattern of regional fiber contraction, which is dependent not only on the sequence of electrical activation but also on ventricular chamber volume and fiber alignment, remains poorly understood. Nevertheless, because of these changes in chamber shape and hence in fiber length during the period between mitral valve closure and aortic valve opening, this phase of the cardiac cycle is not truly isometric (ie, a contraction from constant muscle length); therefore, it is simply considered to be the isovolumic phase of contraction.

The contraction of the excited muscle fibers generates a force within the wall, which causes the development of pressure inside the ventricular chamber. Once chamber pressure exceeds that of the aorta or pulmonary artery, ejection begins. Fiber shortening now displaces blood from the ventricle into its major blood vessel. The shortening of these muscle fibers occurs against a force, or shortening load, termed the *afterload*. As in the preload, afterload is dependent on chamber pressure, size, and shape. Because chamber configuration and pressure are changing throughout the ejection period, afterload has a time-varying value. In the normal heart, afterload peaks shortly after ejection begins and then declines throughout the remainder

of ejection. The heart is therefore able to partially unload itself. Wiggers[5] has used the term *allasotonic* to describe this contraction of variable force and to distinguish it from an isotonic contraction.

Concepts of Force, Stress, Tension, and Fiber Length for the Intact Myocardium

The direct measurements of force and length for a particular muscle fiber in the intact myocardium cannot be performed with current technology. However, a global description of muscle dynamics can be developed for the myocardium. According to this view, the total contraction of all fibers determines wall shortening and hence chamber volume displacement. For this global description, a simplified derivation of wall force and fiber length will suffice.

If we envision the ventricular chamber, containing blood under pressure, and its surrounding myocardium as being divided by an imaginary plane, as represented in Figure 4–1, then we see that a force is created on either side of the plane that tends to pull the myocardium apart. The magnitude of this force is a function of chamber pressure and the area of the chamber included in the plane. Under the condition of static equilibrium, this force must be counterbalanced by an equal and opposite force (ie, wall force) that exists within the rim of the subtended myocardium and holds the two halves of the myocardium together. It should be noted that this computed wall force is a net result of the summation of the forces generated by individual muscle fibers. Thus, even though it cannot be measured, the net wall force may be calculated as the product of chamber pressure and the cross-sectional area of the chamber included in any given plane. Hefner and colleagues[6] have validated this concept by measuring the force recorded from a strain gauge that held together two edges of a slit made in the left ventricular myocardium. They found this force to be closely related to the product of chamber area and pressure.

Each ventricle has an irregular shape. The magnitude of wall force will vary according to the cross-sectional area of the chamber subtended by any imaginary plane. For the left ventricle, which is often represented by an ellipsoid of revolution, the plane bisecting the ventricle and myocardium at the minor axis (Fig. 4–1) will have a force vector, which lies in the longitudinal direction. A plane

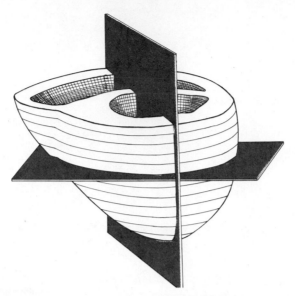

CIRCUMFERENTIAL FORCE

∝

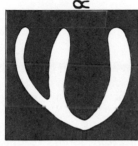

LONGITUDINAL FORCE

∝

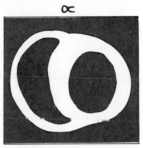

FIGURE 4–1. The ventricles and myocardium of the heart bisected by horizontal and vertical planes. For either ventricle, net wall force is a function of the pressure inside the ventricle and the cross-sectional area of its chamber included in each plane; longitudinal wall force is proportional to the chamber area subtended by the horizontal plane, whereas circumferential force is determined by the area transcribed by the vertical plane. (From Weber KT, Janicki JS, Hunter WC, Shroff SG, Pearlman ES, Fishman AP. The contractile behavior of the heart and its functional coupling to the circulation. Prog Cardiovasc Dis *24*:375–400, 1982.)

that subtends the long or major axis of the left ventricular chamber and myocardium will have a force vector in the circumferential direction. From the equation for force, the difference in magnitude between the longitudinal and circumferential forces will be related to the difference in length of the minor and major axes, respectively.

The distribution of wall force (grams) across a cross-sectional area of myocardium (cm²) represents wall *stress* (grams/cm²). In other words, wall stress is the force borne by a unit area of the myocardium. In humans, the circumferential, peak systolic wall stress averages 330 grams/cm².[7, 8] It exceeds that in the longitudinal plane (174 grams/cm²) by a factor of approximately 1.5 to 2.0, which is the ratio of the major and minor axes of the chamber. As we noted in Chapter 1, the majority of muscle fibers is located in the circumferential direction. This is fortunate,

because the larger circumferential force will be supported and normalized by the shortening and corresponding thickening of a larger number of muscle fibers, while the lesser number of oblique fibers shorten and thicken in the meridional direction against the lesser longitudinal force.

The growth of muscle is thought to be a function of muscle *tension*. Tension (grams/cm) describes the force that exists along a unit length of muscle. Because the myocardium is thick-walled, the application of the tension concept can be facilitated by considering the myocardium and its muscle fibers to be represented by a set of nested, concentric shells of finite thickness, as shown in Figure 4–2. The tension that exists at a point along the surface of any given shell can then be related to the pressure and the principal radii of curvature (R_1 and R_2) at that point.[9] Hence, for any given pressure, the

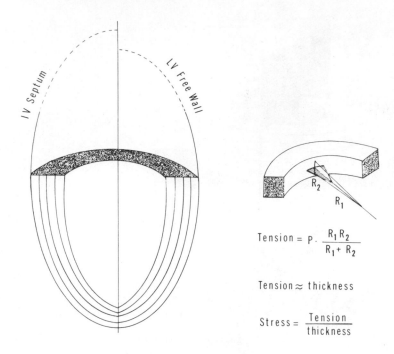

Tension $= P \cdot \dfrac{R_1 R_2}{R_1 + R_2}$

Tension $\approx$ thickness

Stress $= \dfrac{Tension}{thickness}$

FIGURE 4–2. The concept of tension is best applied to thin-walled structures. If the left ventricle is viewed as consisting of a series of nested shells of finite thickness, then the tension existing at any point along the surface of one of these shells is related to the product of chamber pressure and the two principal radii of curvature (R_1 and R_2). Because the radius of curvature is larger for the septum than for the free wall or apex of the left ventricle, septal tension and thickness must be greater than in the other regions of the ventricle. Stress expresses tension per unit wall thickness. (From Weber KT, Reichek N, Janicki JS, Shroff SG. The pressure overloaded heart: physiological and clinical correlates, *in* Strauer B (ed). The Heart in Hypertension. Springer-Verlag, Berlin, 1981.)

tension developed by a muscle fiber is a function of chamber geometry. The complex shape of the ventricle dictates that there will be differences in regional tension. For example, the tension existing along the interventricular septum, which has a large radius of curvature, would be greater than that found at the apex.

In an elegant description of this concept in 1892, Woods[10] has shown that at any point the thickness of the myocardium is proportional to tension. Given the fact that systolic loading disorders lead to ventricular hypertrophy but diastolic disorders do not, myocardial growth would appear to be most related to systolic tension. Moreover, for any systolic pressure, myocardial thickness is a function of its regional configuration. For example, the apex is thinner than the interventricular septum. The variations that exist in wall thickness of the myocardium suggest that systolic wall stress, or systolic tension per unit thickness, is uniform despite the complex shape of the ventricle. Such a homogeneous distribution of stress favors an ordered process of ventricular contraction. If stress were not uniformly distributed, the performance of the muscular pump would be compromised by a distortion in shape and wall motion at regions of higher stress. However, such a condition does exist when the myocardium is scarred secondary to myocar-

dial infarction. The result of this scarring may be an aneurysmal expansion of the wall in systole with the aneurysm bulging paradoxically away from the remainder of the wall. The effectiveness of the contraction by the viable myocardium here is compromised, as it displaces blood both into the aneurysm and out from the ventricular chamber.

It should again be emphasized that the concept of net wall force does not take into consideration either the distribution of forces among the fibers or the orientation of these fibers. The net circumferential and longitudinal wall forces are related to the respective circumferential and longitudinal muscle lengths. However, the analysis can be simplified by considering the ventricle to be a sphere; therefore, it is adequate to relate circumferential force to circumferential length only.

Finally, the midwall circumferential muscle *length* is chosen to represent the average length over the entire thickness of the myocardium. The change in circumferential length from end-diastole to end-systole is considered the *extent* to which these fibers have shortened, whereas the rate of change of length with respect to time in systole represents the *velocity* of shortening. The following discussion assumes a spheric geometry for the left ventricle, and therefore only one force-length relation is required.

The Isovolumetric Force-Length Relation

The concepts of muscle force, length, and shortening are used to describe the contractile behavior of the heart as a muscular pump.[11–15] The maximum force that the myocardium will develop for any chamber volume can be found in the isovolumetrically beating heart from which blood cannot be ejected. An isovolumetric contraction can be created in the laboratory by cross-clamping the ascending aorta or pulmonary artery, or by sewing their valve leaflets together. If the ventricle is then progressively stretched by slowly increasing its filling volume, we would find an increase in both the end-diastolic force, the preload, and the systolic force, which the ventricle will generate from its fixed volume. In Figure 4–3A, the relation between ventricular force and chamber diameter (a quantity proportional to muscle length) is depicted. This relation was derived to represent the increase in chamber volume that would occur over the physiologic range of filling pressure (ie, 1 to 25 mm Hg). Once again, force was calculated from the product of chamber pressure and the cross-sectional area of the chamber included in the plane of the measured diameter. This relation depicts a fundamental property of cardiac muscle, namely, the dependence of force on fiber length. This has also been termed the Frank-Starling relation.

Within the physiologic range of filling volumes, the peak isovolumetric force-length relation of the intact myocardium does not exhibit a maximum. This is unlike isolated cardiac muscle, in which developed isometric force peaks and then subsequently declines as muscle is progressively stretched. Pharmacologic or intrinsic alterations in the contractile state of the myocardium result in nonparallel shifts in the developed force-length relation. Positive or negative inotropic interventions, for example, raise or reduce the slope of this relation, respectively. This response is depicted in Figure 4–3B, in which dobutamine, a synthetic catecholamine, is shown to raise the force developed for any particular end-diastolic dimension. The augmentation in the maximum force-length relation is a function of the rate of the catecholamine infusion.[12] This is illustrated in Figure 4–4 by the stress-normalized length relations that are equivalent to force-length relations. Thus, this response is not an all-or-none phenomenon. A limit, however,

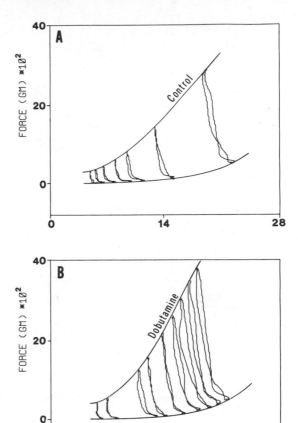

FIGURE 4–3. The maximal force-diameter relation obtained from the isovolumetrically beating left ventricle of the isolated canine heart. Chamber diameter was measured along the minor axis of the ventricle between the lateral free wall and interventricular septum, using piezoelectric crystals implanted on the endocardium and the sonomicrometry technique. A, Control data; B, following dobutamine (6 μg/min). (From Weber KT, Janicki JS. The dynamics of ventricular contraction: force, length and shortening, in Weber KT, Janicki JS (eds). Symposium on Cardiac Mechanics. Fed Proc 39:188–195, 1980.)

does exist beyond which the maximum developed force will no longer increase in response to such agents. This limit is related to myocardial oxygen availability, as we will discuss subsequently.[16]

Under physiologic conditions, the slope of the peak isovolumetric force-length relation is proportional to the contractile state of the myocardium. Parallel shifts in the force-length relation of a given ventricle, on the other hand, do not necessarily connote an alteration in myocardial contractile state. For example, a parallel upward shift is observed when the end-diastolic volume of the contralateral ventricle is raised, causing a concom-

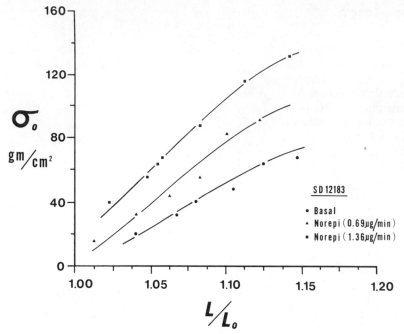

FIGURE 4–4. Manipulation of the contractile state and the maximal isovolumetric stress-length (normalized by L_o, length at zero end-diastolic pressure) relation is shown for norepinephrine. Note that the extent of this manipulation is a function of the norepinephrine infusion rate. (From Weber KT, Janicki JS, Reeves RC, Hefner LL. Factors influencing left ventricular shortenings in isolated canine heart. Am J Physiol *230*:419–426, 1976.)

itant shift in the compliance and diastolic pressure-volume relation of the ventricle under consideration.[17] In the failing heart, this relation is shifted to the right with a reduced slope, and the contractile or inotropic reserve is attenuated. Exercise represents a physiologic stress that can be used to assess the pump reserve of the heart. This approach to assessing cardiac reserve in patients with heart disease is considered further in Chapter 11.

The Limit to Fiber Shortening

The isovolumetric developed force-length relation establishes the limit to which the fibers of the ejecting ventricle will shorten and thereby be able to reduce its end-systolic volume.[13] The force that exists in the wall at end ejection is equal to the maximum developed force that end systolic length can sustain. The equivalence of the isovolumetric and end ejection force-length relations has been demonstrated in isolated cardiac muscle, the isolated heart, and the intact animal.

To illustrate this point further, several force-length loops obtained in the ejecting isolated heart are presented in Figure 4–5, along with their isovolumetric force-length relations (*dashed lines*). Force has been calculated by assuming the left ventricle to be a thick-walled sphere. In *A*, four force-length loops are given for four different afterloads. From an initial end diastolic length (point *a*)

the ventricle generates force until the onset of ejection (point *b*). Force peaks shortly after the onset of ejection and then declines during the remainder of ejection. As soon as a force is achieved that is maximum for the given systolic length, the muscle fiber no longer shortens (point *c*). The ventricle has reached its isovolumetric condition. Another contraction, which had a higher afterload, is represented by *def*. It too ceases to shorten when the maximum force-length relation is attained. In *B*, the afterload has been varied from the same onset ejection force and end-diastolic length to create three different end-systolic lengths. In each case, however, shortening ceases when the isovolumetric force-length relation is attained.

From these findings, it should be apparent that end-systolic length is independent of end-diastolic length and of the ejection force that exists at onset of ejection. These latter conditions merely serve to determine the starting points of each contraction. End-systolic length is strictly a function of end-systolic force and is insensitive to the manner in which the ventricle arrived at this end-systolic force. The equivalence of the peak isovolumetric and end-systolic force-length relations has also been verified during variations in myocardial contractile state (Fig. 4–5C). Therefore, the ejecting ventricle contracts within the confines of the diastolic and peak isovolumetric force-length relations.

The end-systolic force-length relation pro-

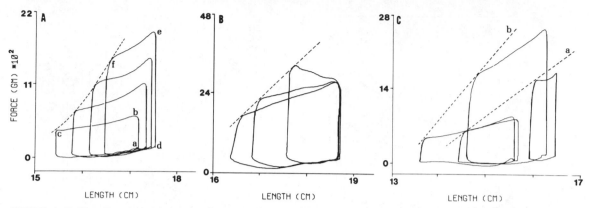

FIGURE 4–5. The close interrelationship between the isovolumetric maximal force-length relation (dotted lines) and the end-systolic force-length relation of ejecting contractions from three isolated hearts. A, Four counterclockwise force-length loops are given for an ejecting ventricle. End-diastole, onset, and end-ejection are denoted by a, b, and c and d, e, and f, respectively, in the widest and tallest loops. B, Three contractions in which end-diastole length and initial shortening load were identical. However, because the trajectory of instantaneous shortening load was varied, three different end-systolic lengths were obtained. C, The equivalence of the isovolumetric and end-ejection force-length relations is preserved following the pharmacologic depression in the contractile state (propranolol, 0.1 mg/min; line a). (From Weber KT, Janicki JS. The dynamics of ventricular contraction: force, length and shortening, in Weber KT, Janicki JS (eds): Symposium on Cardiac Mechanics. Fed Proc 39:188–195, 1980.)

vides an estimate of the peak isovolumetric force-length curve. Hence, in deriving this relation, the contractile state of the myocardium can be quantitated in the ejecting ventricle. In order to describe adequately the slope of the relation, three or more points must be obtained without altering contractile state. This may be accomplished pharmacologically with noninotropic agents such as nitroprusside, methoxamine, or phenylephrine. The changes in arterial pressure produced by these agents, however, should be modest so as not to invoke a response in arterial baroreceptor reflex and modification in contractility.

It should be noted that the data presented in the preceding discussion were obtained from the normal isolated canine heart. Therefore, we used the variables such as force and length to analyze the limit to fiber shortening and, consequently, to quantitate the acute changes in contractile state of the myocardium in terms of end-systolic force-length relation. However, it is necessary to replace force by stress (ie, force per unit area of myocardium) in the quantitation of contractile state for those conditions in which significant alterations in myocardial mass occur (eg, chronic heart disease or comparison of hearts of different individuals). Angiographic and echocardiographic techniques have been used to derive this relation in humans in order to compare differences in myocardial contractile state between patient groups.[18–20]

Determinants of Fiber Shortening

The limit to myocardial shortening has been identified as the maximal isovolumetric or end-systolic force-length relation. Moreover, shortening is independent of those conditions of length and load that exist at the onset of contraction (or end-diastole). Instead, the fibers comprising the heart's muscular wall are responsive to the shortening load that is present at each instant of ejection.[12, 14] The influence of *instantaneous shortening load* on the extent and rate of shortening has been studied extensively in both isolated cardiac muscle and the isolated heart.[12–14]

Four different afterloaded contractions are shown in Figure 4–6, along with the rate and extent of midwall circumferential fiber shortening. Each contraction begins from approximately the same preload. In A, the contractions are shown in the force-length domain together with the isovolumetric force-length relation, shown as the broken line. For each contraction, the extent of fiber shortening is determined by the instantaneous force, or afterload, opposing shortening. Shortening is greatest in beat a, having the least shortening load. The responsiveness of the velocity of shortening to instantaneous shortening load is depicted in Figure 4–6B. It can be seen that for a given muscle length, the instantaneous velocity is greatest for the contraction with smallest shortening load (ie, beat a). Consequently, the peak velocity is

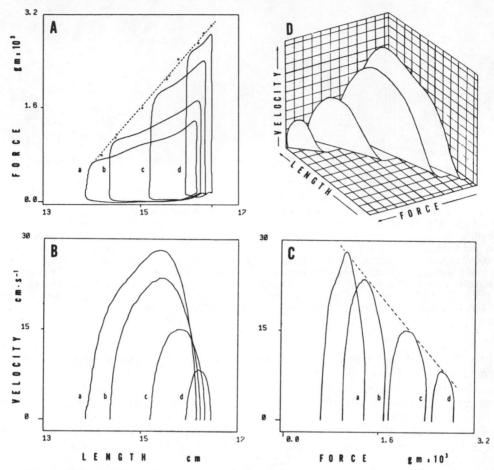

FIGURE 4–6. The importance of instantaneous shortening load for velocity and extent of shortening is demonstrated by a series of four variably afterloaded allasotonic contractions in terms of the interrelationships among force, length, and velocity of shortening. Contraction a, having the smallest instantaneous shortening load, has the greatest peak and instantaneous velocity of shortening, as well as the greatest extent (i.e., change in length) of shortening. The inverse force-velocity relation is demonstrated in panel C, using the peak velocity of shortening (see text). (From Weber KT, Janicki JS. Instantaneous force-velocity-length relations in isolated dog heart. Am J Physiol 232:H241–H249, 1977.)

inversely proportional to shortening load. This inverse force-velocity relation is depicted in C and represents a fundamental property of the muscle. Finally, D summarizes, in three dimensions, the interrelationship among shortening velocity, fiber length, and shortening load for the four contractions.

The relevance of instantaneous shortening load in regulating the performance of the muscular pump is particularly underscored in the enlarged and failing heart. As a result of a reduction in the contractile state of the failing myocardium and an increase in shortening load associated with enlarged chamber size, the extent of muscle shortening is significantly reduced. Owing to the reduced shortening, the diminution of chamber size from end-diastole to end-systole is markedly attenuated, which results in maintenance of

higher shortening load throughout the ejection period. Thus, the failing heart works at a mechanical disadvantage in that it cannot unload itself to the same extent as a normal heart.[21–22]

The myocardial hypertrophy seen with various forms of heart disease is the result of an increased systolic wall tension that accompanies a chronic elevation in ventricular chamber pressure or size or both. The hypertrophic process is compensatory and serves to distribute the greater force over a larger area of muscle. Hence, wall stress at end-diastole and the onset of ejection may be maintained within the normal range. On the other hand, the level of instantaneous systolic stress will be determined by the increment in wall thickness that occurs during ejection and the reduction in ventricular volume. One can use end-systolic stress as a useful estimate of whether or not instantaneous shortening load is normalized in the failing heart.

The second determinant of wall shortening is the *instantaneous shortening length*. In Figure 4–7, instantaneous shortening length has been raised by increasing the initial or onset contraction length, whereas instantaneous shortening load has been held constant. Consequently, each beat traverses the common trajectory within the shortening load-length domain, and thus the same end-systolic force-length point is reached (*panel A*). The rate and extend of each contraction's shortening are quite different, and a function of instantaneous shortening length. Contraction *d*, which has the greatest instantaneous shortening length, shortens with the greatest

peak and instantaneous shortening velocity (*panel B*) and to the greatest extent (*panel A*). Moreover, it is apparent that instantaneous shortening velocity is not a function of contraction duration, as each beat reaches the common velocity-length trajectory (*panel B*) at a different time during ejection. *Panel C* indicates that once the common load or force is reached, the force-velocity trajectories of all four contractions superimpose, even though the instantaneous lengths are different. Finally, in *panel D*, the inter-relationships among shortening load, length, and velocity are depicted in three dimensions.

The traditional estimate of pump function, the ventricular function curve, defined as the relation between stroke volume and the filling volume of the ventricle, may be derived from shortening load-length relationships.

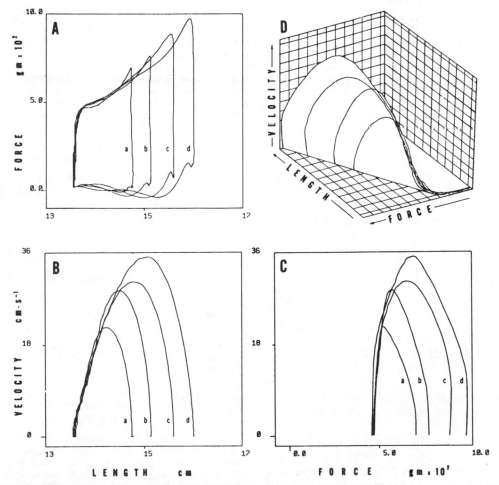

FIGURE 4–7. The importance of instantaneous shortening length for the velocity and extent of shortening is demonstrated by a series of contractions, each of which traverses an essentially identical trajectory of instantaneous shortening load. As end-diastolic fiber length is progressively raised from beats *a* to *d*, the instantaneous shortening length becomes greater. Thus, for the same shortening load, the peak and instantaneous velocity of shortening and the extent of shortening are greatest for beat *d* (see text). (From Weber KT, Janicki JS. Instantaneous force-velocity-length relations in isolated dog heart. Am J Physiol *232*:H241–H249, 1977.)

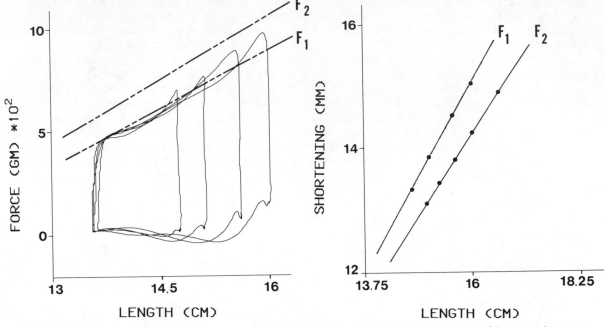

FIGURE 4–8. The ventricular function curve may be derived from the shortening-length relation of the muscular pump. In the left panel, the common instantaneous length-load trajectory has been simplified and represented by the broken line labeled F_1. Because the instantaneous shortening length has been progressively increased in these contractions that have the same shortening load, the extent of shortening will increase. This is demonstrated by the linear relation between the extent of shortening and end-diastolic length relation shown in the right panel. For a greater shortening load trajectory, F_2, the slope of the linear shortening-length relation would be reduced; hence there is less shortening for any equivalent initial length. (From Weber KT, Reichek N, Janicki JS, Shroff S. The pressure overloaded heart: physiological and clinical correlates. *In* Strauer B (ed). The Heart in Hypertension. Springer-Verlag, Berlin, 1981.)

For each constant shortening load trajectory shown in Figures 4–8 and 4–9 and labeled $F_1, F_2 \ldots F_n$, the extent of fiber shortening increases in a linear fashion as the initial (ie, end-diastolic) length is progressively raised. As the shortening load becomes greater (eg, $F_2 > F_1$), the amount of shortening is less for any equivalent length. The ventricular function curve can be derived by examining the response of stroke volume (or shortening) to increments in end-diastolic volume (or length). In an intact circulation, the shortening load progressively increases with increments in end-diastolic volume or length. Therefore, the ventricular function curve (Fig. 4–9, *broken line*) is simply the shortening-length relationship obtained at progressively increasing values of shortening load (ie, $F_1, F_2 \ldots F_n$).

For any given shortening load, a positive shift in contractile state would raise the slope of the shortening-length relation. For this augmented series of shortening-length relations, the ventricular function curve would be shifted upward or to the left. The opposite would hold true for a decline in contractility. In the failing heart, the level of shortening load may become quite elevated, and, con-

sequently, shortening actually declines as chamber size increases, leading to a "descending limb" of the function curve. Thus, the concept of a "family" of function curves,

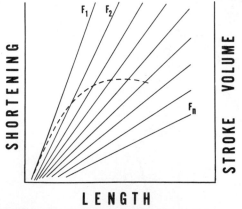

FIGURE 4–9. A series of shortening-length relations could be constructed for a range of ever-increasing shortening load trajectories, from $F_1, F_2, \ldots F_n$. In the intact animal, the derivation of the ventricular function curve during volume loading will be associated with increased intracardiac and intravascular volumes and hence for a series of increasing shortening load trajectories. (Modified from Weber KT, Reichek N, Janicki JS, Shroff S. The pressure overloaded heart: physiological and clinical correlates, *in* Strauer B (ed). The Heart in Hypertension. Springer-Verlag, Berlin, 1981.)

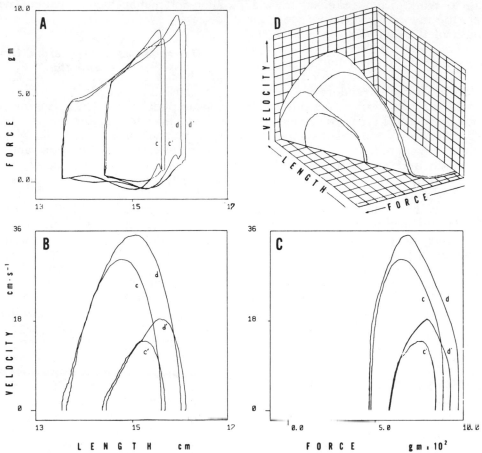

FIGURE 4–10. The interrelationship among force, length, and velocity when the contractile state of the myocardium has been pharmacologically reduced by propranolol (0.07 mg/min). Following beta blockade, the rate and extent of shortening of contractions c′ and d′ are reduced from the control beats c and d despite the similar conditions of initial length, instantaneous length, and shortening load (see text). (From Weber KT, Janicki JS. Instantaneous force-velocity-length relations in isolated dog heart. Am J Physiol 232:H241–H249, 1977.)

which has been popularized by Sarnoff and associates[23] to explain variations in ventricular performance, may in fact be derived from a series of fundamental shortening-length relationships of the muscular pump.

The third major determinant of fiber shortening is the *contractile state* of the myocardium. The decline in fiber shortening seen during a pharmacologic depression of contractile state with the beta adrenergic receptor antagonist propranolol is illustrated in Figure 4–10. The control state of contractility (beats c and d) and that following beta blockade (beats c′ and d′) are given for comparable conditions of instantaneous shortening load and length. Following propranolol, the isovolumetric force-length relation (not shown) and the end-systolic force-length relation are each shifted downward or to the right (see Fig. 4–5C). Thus, the instantaneous velocity and extent of shortening are both reduced (beats c′ and d′). On the other hand, a posi-

tive shift in contractile state (with a catecholamine, for example) would increase the rate and extent of shortening above that observed for the control state. By using the trajectories of instantaneous force, length, and shortening velocity, a three-dimensional representation of their inter-relationshp can be constructed (Fig. 4–10D). Intrinsic or pharmacologic shifts in myocardial contractile state either expand or contract this three-dimensional surface.

THE ENERGETICS OF THE MUSCULAR PUMP

The work of the heart is continuous. The myocardium is an "endurance" muscle that must generate force and shorten continuously if oxygen is to be transported and life is to be preserved. Even when the remainder of the organism is resting, the heart must continue to work. Unlike skeletal muscle, however, the myocardium cannot work for any length of time without oxygen. In the absence of oxygen, the energy production of the myocardium falters rapidly and its performance deteriorates within seconds. As a result, the heart cannot endure an oxygen debt. Thus, the heart can be considered to be an obligate aerobic organ that must continuously utilize aerobic metabolism in order to sustain its function.[24-25]

Anatomically and biochemically, the heart is well suited for continuous aerobic work. Its concentration of oxidative enzymes is the highest of any tissue in the body, and its mitochondria, which are the major sites of oxidative phosphorylation, are present in great numbers throughout the cell, composing 25 to 30 per cent of the entire cell mass. A rich vascular network provides each myocyte with a capillary, so that a large fraction of the oxygen that traverses its coronary circulation can be extracted. Unfortunately, what appears to be a comfortable reserve in oxygen availability in the normal heart may not hold true for the heart subjected to chronic elevations in work or when atherosclerotic lesions impede coronary blood flow. Sustained increments in mechanical work increase the expenditure of chemical energy by the myocardium, as well as elicit a series of responses that includes the growth of cardiac muscle, which, in turn, increase requirements for oxygen. Thus, the adjustments to chronic overloading may create a requirement for oxygen that surpasses the aerobic capacity of the heart. In this connection, the diffusion distance for oxygen from capillary to mitochondria may also be critically increased as the overall dimensions of hypertrophied myocytes are increased.

Because of its singular arterial blood supply and major efferent venous drainage site, the coronary sinus, oxygen used by the myocardium can readily be determined from a knowledge of its arteriovenous oxygen difference and coronary blood flow. This approach has been the basis of experimental and clinical studies that were designed to examine the major determinants of myocardial oxygen consumption ($M\dot{V}O_2$). Recent advances in technology, such as the coronary sinus catheter with thermistor to measure coronary sinus blood flow by thermodilution and the ability to sample coronary sinus blood, have made bedside monitoring of myocardial energetics a reality in the evaluation and management of patients with heart disease.

Determinants of Myocardial Oxygen Consumption

Because it is an obligate aerobic organ, the consumption of oxygen by the myocardium reflects its energy requirements. The oxygen used in maintaining organelle systems, the cost of electric depolarization, and the activation of the contractile process have been shown to require a modest portion of the total energy consumed by the heart. The major determinants of $M\dot{V}O_2$ include systolic wall force (as determined by both chamber pressure and volume), myocardial contractility, and heart rate. These three components of ventricular contraction represent the major determinants of myocardial $\dot{V}O_2$ or metabolic demand of the heart (Fig. 4–11).[26-27]

The relative contribution of each of these major determinants of $M\dot{V}O_2$ has been difficult to quantify. Each, however, is interrelated through their influence on systolic wall force. Thus, a uniform expression of $M\dot{V}O_2$ can be developed if the effects of a perturbation in ventricular pressure and in volume, contractile state, and heart rate are related to $M\dot{V}O_2$ through their influence on systolic wall force. Specifically, the influence of these variables include the following components of systolic wall force (Fig. 4–12): (1) the magnitude of developed force; (2) the interval during which force is developed and maintained for each contraction, or the integral of systolic force; (3) the rate of force development; and (4) the frequency with which force is developed per unit of time.[24, 26]

An increment in ventricular chamber pressure or volume will raise both the magnitude of force that the myocardium must develop and the force that it maintains during ejection, or the afterload (Table 4–1). As a result, the integral of systolic force for any given cardiac cycle is increased. Increments in filling volume and diastolic pressure raise the preload and the degree of muscle fiber stretch. As noted previously, this effect would serve to raise the rate with which force is developed prior to ejection. A reduction in diastolic chamber size, on the other hand, would serve to reduce both the integral or systolic force and the rate of force development.

Alterations in myocardial contractility exert their influence on $M\dot{V}O_2$ by changing the rate

Cellular O_2 Supply :

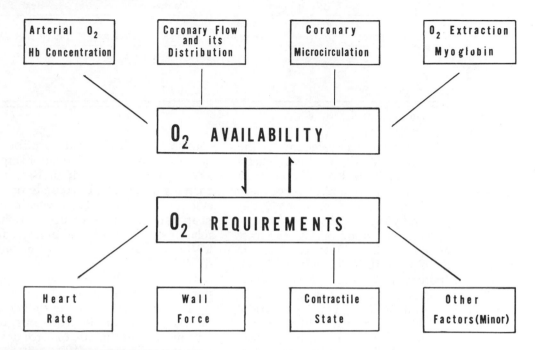

Cellular O_2 Demand :

FIGURE 4–11. The factors that regulate the demand and supply of O_2 in myocytes and thereby reflect the heart's requirements for oxygen and its availability. (From Weber KT, Janicki JS. The metabolic demand and oxygen supply of the heart: physiologic and clinical considerations. Am J Cardiol *44*:722–729, 1979.)

of force development.[27] These effects may also influence the magnitude of developed force (Table 4–1). The direction of these responses in systolic wall force are a function of whether a positive or negative shift in contractility was induced and whether this was mediated by pharmacologic agents that also had chronotropic effects or an influence on the resistance vessels of the systemic circulation. Epinephrine, for example, would raise not only the inherent rate of force development but also the frequency with which force is developed each minute (ie, heart rate). The response in the magnitude and integral of force development would also be influenced by the degree to which epinephrine induced arteriolar vasoconstriction. Hence, the overall effect of epinephrine in the normal heart would be to increase $M\dot{V}O_2$.

Increments in heart rate alone increase myocardial $\dot{V}O_2$ per *minute*.[27] An augmentation in contractile state and the rate of force development may also accompany elevations in heart rate. Under these circumstances, the integral of systolic force may actually decline,

and as a result, the oxygen used per *beat* will be determined by the magnitude of these discordant responses. If the increment in heart rate raises the rate of force development

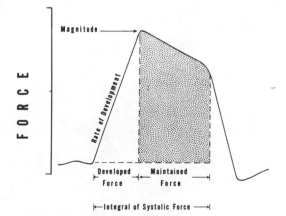

FIGURE 4–12. The major determinants of myocardial O_2 consumption expressed in relation to their influence on the components of systolic wall force. (From Weber KT, Janicki JS. The metabolic demand and oxygen supply of the heart: Physiologic and clinical considerations. Am J Cardiol *44*:722–729, 1979.)

Table 4–1. Factors Regulating the Components of Wall Force

Component of Wall Force	Chamber		Contractile State		Heart Rate	
	Pressure Increase	Volume Increase	Increase	Decrease	Increase	Decrease
Magnitude	+	+	+ or −	+	0	0
Integral	+	+	−	+	−	+
Rate of development	+	+	+	−	+	−
Frequency of development	0	0	0	0	+	−

+, increase; −, decrease; 0, no change

less than the accompanying decline in the force integral, then $\dot{M}VO_2$ per beat acually falls. Nonetheless, with tachycardia the heart must generate and sustain a given force more frequently each minute and hence $\dot{M}VO_2$ per minute is generally increased.

The interrelations among $\dot{M}VO_2$, the integral of systolic force per minute, and the rate of force development is shown in Figure 4–13. An increment in any of these components of wall force requires a nearly equivalent elevation in $\dot{M}VO_2$. Hence, we could represent $\dot{M}VO_2$ as a function of its determinants according to the following equation: $\dot{M}VO_2 = aTFI + bdF/dt + c$, where TFI is the systolic force integral per minute, dF/dt is the peak rate of force development, c represents the minor determinants of oxygen consumption, and a and b are constants. We have shown that this relationship between $\dot{M}VO_2$ and TFI and dF/dt is insensitive to changes in diastolic volume or contractile state or both.[24, 26, 27] However, increments in heart rate result in an upward shift of this relationship, so that a greater amount of $\dot{M}VO_2$ is required for any given TFI and dF/dt.[24, 26, 27]

The ultimate response in $\dot{M}VO_2$ to variations in its major determinants is dependent on the net balance of the individual contributions. For example, if the integral of force falls more than the rate of force development is increased, then $\dot{M}VO_2$ will be reduced. This is the circumstance that relates most closely to the treatment of the failing heart. Some patients with ischemic heart disease

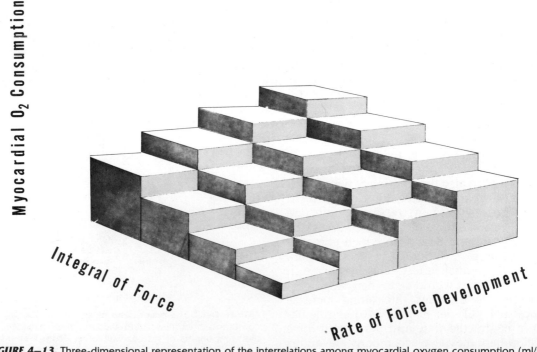

FIGURE 4–13. Three-dimensional representation of the interrelations among myocardial oxygen consumption (ml/min per 100 grams), the integral of systolic wall force per minute, and the peak rate of force development. (From Weber KT, Janicki JS. The metabolic demand and oxygen supply of the heart: Physiologic and clinical considerations. Am J Cardiol 44:722–729, 1979.)

and heart failure experience angina pectoris secondary to myocardial ischemia. The cause of the ischemia may be secondary to an augmented systolic wall stress that accompanies left ventricular dilatation and poor contractile function or subendocardial ischemia or both, because of the elevated left ventricular diastolic pressure. Irrespective of its cause, a reduction in ventricular size and filling pressure will ameliorate the angina. For this purpose, a positive inotropic agent (eg, digoxin) and a diuretic agent are used to treat the failing heart, to increase its stroke volume and reduce its filling pressure and ventricular size. The net result of such therapy is to reduce instantaneous systolic wall force and, thereby, the integral of force to a greater extent than digoxin raises the rate of force development. The net result is a reduction in $M\dot{V}O_2$ and the control of the angina.

A similar situation exists with the use of the new orally active inotropic agents in the treatment of the dilated failing heart. $M\dot{V}O_2$ has been measured in patients with heart failure, that may or may not be secondary to ischemic heart disease, using a thermistor catheter inserted into the coronary sinus to sample coronary sinus blood flow and oxygen content.[28-30] The results of these studies indicate that after the administration of the inotropic agents, $M\dot{V}O_2$ falls or remains the same (Fig. 4–14). Thus, even though contractility is increased with these drugs, their net effect on $M\dot{V}O_2$ is a favorable one because of enhanced ventricular emptying. Only dobutamine has been found to adversely raise $M\dot{V}O_2$.[31] This may be related to a wasting effect on myocardial energetics that accompanies the catecholamines, the use of excessive doses of the drug, or the fact that the left ventricle in these patients was not enlarged. The dilated ventricle and the reduction in ventricular size with positive inotropic agents are central to their reducing or sustaining $M\dot{V}O_2$.

Finally, studies of the contractile proteins of the myocardium, actin and myosin, indicate that myosin exists as different isoforms.[32] In cardiac muscle, three isomyosins have been identified: V_1, V_2, and V_3. The intrinsic velocity of fiber shortening and Ca^{++}-ATPase activity are markedly different for these isomyosins, with V_1 having the highest values for both velocity and Ca^{++}-ATPase activity and V_3 having the lowest.[33] This is analogous to the "fast-twitch" and "slow-twitch" fibers of skeletal muscle. Alpert and Mulieri[34] have indicated that the heat production per unit

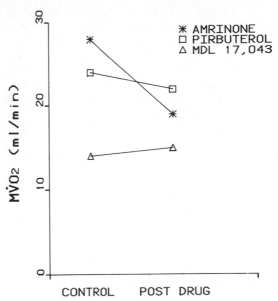

FIGURE 4–14. Clinical studies, in which myocardial O_2 consumption has been measured before and after the administration of positive inotropic agents like pirbuterol, amrinone, or MDL 17,043, do not indicate that myocardial O_2 uptake is adversely elevated with these drugs. (Adapted from Benotti JR, Grossman W, Braunwald E, Carabello BA. Effects of amrinone on myocardial energy metabolism and hemodynamics in patients with severe congestive heart failure due to coronary artery disease. Circulation 62:28–34, 1980; Rude RE, Turi Z, Brown EJ, Lorell BH, Colucci WS, Mudge GH, Taylor RC, Grossman W. Acute effects of pirbuterol on myocardial oxygen metabolism and systemic hemodynamics in chronic congestive heart failure. Circulation 64:139–145, 1981; and Martin JL, Likoff MJ, Janicki JS, Laskey WK, Hirschfeld JW, Weber KT. Myocardial energetics and clinical response to the cardiotonic agent MDL 17,043 in advanced heart failure. J Am Coll Cardiol 4:875–881, 1983.)

of tension development for V_1 isomyosin is much greater than is that of V_3 isomyosin. Accordingly, the amount of oxygen consumed per unit of tension development is much higher for V_1 isomyosin. Thus, the overall isomyosin composition (the relative amounts of V_1, V_2, and V_3) is another determinant of the myocardial oxygen consumption. At present, the relative importance of isomyosin composition in determining $M\dot{V}O_2$ of a diseased heart and its potential usefulness in choosing a therapeutic approach are unclear and need further investigation.

Metabolic Supply To The Heart

The amount of oxygen available to the myocardium and to its mitochondria in particular is determined by the following (see Fig. 4–11): (1) the oxygen delivered to the myocardium, which is a function of the arterial oxygen saturation, hemoglobin concentration, and coronary blood flow; (2) the anatomic characteristics of the coronary macro- and microcirculation, and in particular the relation of the capillaries to myocytes, which determines the diffusion distance for oxygen; and (3) the portion of the delivered oxygen that is driven by a gradient in oxygen tension from the capillaries into the intracellular compartment and that becomes a function of erythrocyte transit time in the capillaries. Within the cell, oxygen diffusion is facilitated by its reversible combination with myoglobin and the translational diffusion of oxymyoglobin. During acute increments in work, myoglobin content and mitochondrial oxygen tension remain unchanged while coronary flow increases. This increment in flow involves the redistribution of blood flow from nonexchanging to exchanging vessels, in a manner analogous to the concept of ventilation:perfusion ratios in the lungs, and the recruitment of perfused channels, or the density of open capillaries. Oxygen extraction will also increase with an augmented work load. Because oxygen extraction in the heart is already rather high (see Chapter 2), this response is less than the elevation in flow. In the chronically overloaded, hypertrophied heart, it is not clear whether a proliferation of the capillary bed occurs (thereby preserving the normal diffusion distance for oxygen between the hypertrophied myocyte and its capillary bed) or whether part of the adaptation process involves myoglobin or mitochondrial energetics. Nonetheless, the compensatory adjustments in both flow and oxygen extraction represent the metabolic reserve of the heart. Regrettably, however, the oxidative reserve of the myocardium has finite limits, as we will discuss later.

Capillary oxygen delivery is established by coronary blood flow and arterial oxygen content. The ratio of the amount of delivered oxygen (coronary flow × arterial oxygen content) to that which is consumed (coronary flow × coronary-arteriovenous oxygen difference) is represented by the oxygen extracted (ratio of coronary arteriovenous oxygen difference to the arterial oxygen content). These measurements, however, do not establish the adequacy of mitochondrial oxygen content. Rather, they only approximate the kinetics of intracellular molecular oxygen. However, the lactate-to-pyruvate ratio, or the ratio of reduced to oxidized nicotinamide adenine dinucleotide, reflects the proportion of reduced to oxidized substrate. These ratios provide a better description of the adequacy of oxygen availability. Measurements of coronary sinus lactate and pyruvate have been used clinically for this purpose. Normally, the myocardium extracts 30 to 40 per cent of the lactate in arterial blood. With myocardial ischemia and anaerobic conditions, the myocardium produces lactate so that coronary sinus lactate concentration exceeds that of arterial blood. Lactate production has been demonstrated in patients with myocardial ischemia and in those with aortic stenosis and marked myocardial hypertrophy but patent coronary arteries. For an excellent review of the advantages and disadvantages of measuring lactate extraction across the myocardium to reflect the state of oxygen availability, the reader is referred to a recent publication by Gertz and coworkers.[35]

The Oxidative Reserve of the Heart

Myocardial oxygen extraction ranges from 65 to 75 per cent under a wide variety of conditions,[36] including exercise, catecholamine infusion, hyperthyroidism, and various cardiac diseases associated with ventricular hypertrophy. This level of oxygen extraction, however, is not a physiologic limit. When coronary flow is restricted, oxygen extraction rises to 80 per cent or more (Fig. 4–15). The relevant issue to oxygen extraction is therefore the relation between the demand for oxygen and its availability. Even though a large fraction of the delivered oxygen is used by the heart under a variety of circumstances, oxygen extraction is not maximal unless the coronary vascular reserve or coronary vasodilation has been fully used or unless the oxygen-carrying capacity of blood is compromised.

The reserve in oxygen extraction represents a minor component of the heart's metabolic reserve to increments in aerobic work. It is only brought into play under conditions in which oxygen delivery is impaired. The coronary vascular reserve represents the major compensatory response to increased $M\dot{V}O_2$. The importance of increments in coronary flow has been amply demonstrated during the increased $M\dot{V}O_2$ attendant with exercise, atrial pacing, or when the oxygen-carrying capacity was purposely reduced. A substantial decline in coronary vascular resistance occurs during such increments in aerobic demand. This coronary vasodilation permits an increased delivery of oxygen. When

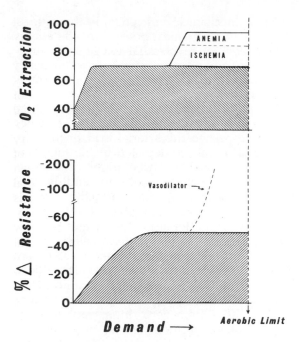

FIGURE 4–15. The metabolic reserve of the heart may be described by the changes in O_2 extraction (per cent) and the per cent decrease in coronary vascular resistance that occur in response to a progressive elevation in metabolic demand. Note that O_2 extraction reaches a plateau early and does not increase again until the coronary vascular reserve has reached its optimal level. Myocardial ischemia or anemia will promote a greater extraction of O_2. Coronary vasodilators, such as dipyridamole, may increase coronary flow beyond its optimal limits. Once O_2 extraction and coronary flow are maximal, additional increments in demand result in cell hypoxia, and thus the aerobic limit of the heart is exceeded. (From Weber KT, Janicki JS. The metabolic demand and oxygen supply of the heart: Physiologic and clinical considerations. Am J Cardiol 44:722–729, 1979.)

the metabolic reserve of the heart is fully utilized, oxygen extraction and coronary vasodilatation are maximal. Any further demand for oxidative metabolism cannot be satisfied. We have viewed this state as representing the *aerobic limit of the heart*.[16] Beyond the aerobic limit, additional increments in oxygen requirements create a situation in which metabolic demand exceeds the oxygen supply. Cellular hypoxia and intracellular anaerobic metabolism are the result. Lactate accumulates, as reflected by a reversal in the arterial-to-coronary sinus lactate difference and the calculation of lactate extraction. During myocardial anaerobiosis, ventricular performance falls quickly and pulsus alternans appears. Pulsus alternans refers to a normal contraction and development of force being followed in alternate beats by a weak contraction. Pulsus alternans is a characteristic of the severely failing heart.

Over the years, several schools of thought have developed regarding those events that initiate heart failure. One supported theory[37] emphasizes a feedback control of ventricular hypertrophy based on normalizing wall force per unit of muscle or wall stress. Hypertrophy, which may have served for many years to normalize the augmented wall force of the pressure- or volume-overloaded heart, eventually becomes incapable of compensating for the increased hemodynamic load. Hence, the heart is accompanied by progressive chamber enlargement. The explanation for this inappropriate response in wall thickness and, presumably, in protein synthesis, is unknown. It has also been theorized[38] that the metabolic demand of the mechanically overburdened heart eventually exceeds its oxygen availability, and, as a result, a defect in mechanical performance and protein synthesis ensues. It is these events that lead to progressive chamber dilation and an inappropriate elevation in wall stress without adequate concomitant hypertrophy.

Table 4–2. Ventricular Mass and Energetics in Aortic Stenosis

	Normal Heart	Compensated AS	Decompensated AS
Peak systolic wall force (grams)	2835	8160	13,060
End diastolic volume (cc)	100	125	250
LV pressure (mm Hg)	80	200	200
LV mass (grams)	125	450	600
Peak systolic wall stress	152	146	216
$M\dot{V}O_2$ (ml/min)	10	36	48
Coronary blood flow (ml/min)	100	360	480
O_2 extraction (%)	75	75	80
$M\dot{V}O_2$ (ml/min per 100g)	8	8	8
Coronary blood flow (ml/min per 100 grams)	80	80	80

AS, aortic valve stenosis; LV pressure, left ventricular pressure at aortic valve opening, which approximates the point of peak systolic wall force; $M\dot{V}O_2$, myocardial oxygen consumption; normal heart, trivial to nonexistent aortic valve gradient.

A common range for coronary flow and $M\dot{V}O_2$ when expressed per 100 g of ventricle (Table 4–2) has been observed in patients with cardiac disease.[36] This range corresponds to that observed in patients without significant cardiac disease. Because of the increased muscle mass with cardiac disease, total coronary flow and $M\dot{V}O_2$ in patients at rest with compensated and decompensated failure has also revealed no differences, even though wall stress was shown to be greater in patients with symptomatic failure. However, when $M\dot{V}O_2$ is raised in patients with heart failure, as may occur with atrial pacing or isoproterenol administration,[39–41] both simulating the response to exercise, evidence of cellular hypoxia may result with myocardial lactate production despite the absence of obstructive coronary disease. This response suggests that under these circumstances, metabolic demand exceeds the given metabolic supply. Considering that the total coronary flow (expressed in ml/min) may be increased three to four times above normal, commensurate with the increase in muscle mass, it is not surprising that the coronary vascular reserve may be fully used under these circumstances.

THE EFFICIENCY OF THE MUSCULAR PUMP

To this point in this chapter, we have considered the mechanics and energetics of ventricular contraction as separate entities. As a working muscular pump, however, the two entities are inseparable in that they are interactively determined by each other. One of the ways of simultaneously examining both the mechanical and metabolic behavior of the ventricle is the concept of mechanical efficiency. The following discussion briefly presents this concept and also its potential usefulness in assessing the coupling of the left ventricle to its external load.

The Concept of Efficiency

Under the conditions of aerobic metabolism, one can compute the energy equivalent of myocardial oxygen consumption by multiplying oxygen consumption by a conversion factor (20.3 joules/ml of oxygen for cardiac muscle). Part of the input energy (ie, energy equivalent of oxygen consumption) is used in performing mechanical work, while the remainder is lost as heat. Thus, one can define mechanical efficiency as the ratio of the mean mechanical power and the energy equivalent of myocardial oxygen consumption. In other words, mechanical efficiency represents the relative cost of performing useful work.

Intuitively, one would predict that there should be a maximum mechanical efficiency with respect to the arterial load of the ventricle. This can be depicted in the following manner. Consider three different contractions, each having a constant end-diastolic volume, heart rate, and contractile state but different arterial loads (Fig. 4–16); an extremely high arterial load such that the contraction is isovolumetric (ie, no ejection, *loop ADA*); an intermediate arterial load (*loop ACEHA*); and an extremely low arterial load (*loop ABFGA*). It is clear that mechanical work (ie, area enclosed by the pressure-volume loop) varies from zero (high load) to some finite value (intermediate load) and then back to a low value (low load). Even for the isovolumetric contraction, in which external power is equal to zero, there will be a finite amount of oxygen uptake by the myocardium, and therefore, the mechanical efficiency will equal zero. With a reduction in

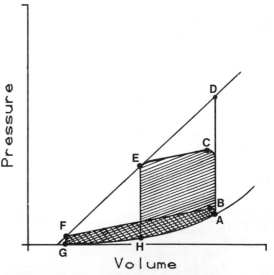

FIGURE 4–16. Three pressure-volume trajectories corresponding to different arterial loads: high (loop ADA), intermediate (loop ACEHA), and low (loop ABFGA). All three contractions have the same end-diastolic volume and contractile state. Lines GHA and FED represent the end-diastolic and end-systolic pressure-volume relations, respectively. It is evident that stroke work (i.e., the area enclosed by the pressure-volume loop) diminishes for extremely low or high arterial loads. Therefore, a maximum of stroke work with respect to arterial load can be expected.

load from its isovolumetric level, efficiency will gradually increase, reaching a maximum at a certain load. Further reductions in load may either have little effect on efficiency or reduce efficiency, depending on the relative rates of this decline in power and oxygen consumption.

The crucial point to note is that there is a load above which efficiency declines and below which efficiency either remains the same or declines. It should also be noted that one cannot reduce arterial load to any arbitrarily low value, as there are physiologic limits set by systemic perfusion. Using an isolated servocontrolled canine heart preparation,[42] we have observed that for the normal heart, there exists an arterial load such that mechanical efficiency is maximized. In addition, the same load produced maximum mechanical power and physiologic levels of mean arterial pressure. Thus, the natural design of the two systems, the left ventricle and its arterial load, is such that both the mechanical performance and energetics of the myocardium are simultaneously maximized. Finally, it should be recalled that in addition to arterial load, end-diastolic volume, contractile state, and heart rate will also affect myocardial oxygen consumption and hence mechanical efficiency.

In the diseased heart, it is conceivable that the equilibrium among arterial load, end-diastolic volume, contractile state, and heart rate has been altered such that mechanical power or mechanical efficiency or both are no longer near their maximum. For example, in the case of cardiomyopathy, with reduced cardiac output, the arterial load and end-diastolic volume are often markedly elevated with relatively normal heart rate and mean arterial pressure. The increased arterial load and end-diastolic volume will reduce efficiency, whereas the compromised contractile state of the myocardium will increase its efficiency. The overall or net effect of these alterations usually translates into a reduction in efficiency.[43] One can now manipulate arterial load with vasodilators; end-diastolic volume with vasodilators, inotropes, or diuretics; and contractile state with inotropic agents to shift the equilibrium point such that efficiency is improved and is closer to its maximum. At the same time, the salutory hemodynamic effects (ie, improved cardiac output, reduced arterial load, and end-diastolic volume) of these drugs can also be attained.

In closing, the assessment of the heart's mechanical efficiency may prove useful in deriving objective and rational manipulations of the cardiovascular system; the utility of this approach, however, requires careful evaluation. The advantage of the mechanical efficiency concept over that of power is that it considers both the mechanical and metabolic aspects of cardiac performance.

REFERENCES

1. Braunwald E, Ross J, Sonnenblick EH. Mechanisms of Contraction of the Normal and Failing Heart. Little, Brown and Co, Boston, 1976.
2. Mirsky I, Ghista DN, Sandler H. Cardiac Mechanics. Physiological, Clinical and Mathematical Considerations. John Wiley and Sons, New York, 1974.
3. Noble MUM. The Cardiac Cycle. Blackwell Scientific Publications, 1979.
4. Wiggers CJ. The interpretation of the intraventricular pressure curve on the basis of rapidly summated fractionate contractions. Am J Physiol 80:1–11, 1927.
5. Wiggers CJ. Pressure Pulses in the Cardiovascular System. New York, Longmans, Green, 1928, p 107.
6. Hefner LL, Sheffield LT, Cobbs GC, Klip W. Relation between mural force and pressure in the left ventricle of the dog. Circ Res 11:654–663, 1962.
7. Gould KL, Lipscomb K, Hamilton GW, Kennedy JW. Relation of left ventricular shape, function, and wall stress in man. Am J Cardiol 34:627–634, 1974.
8. Hood WP Jr, Rackley CE, Rolett EL. Wall stress in the normal and hypertrophied human left ventricles. Am J Cardiol 22:550–558, 1968.
9. Weber KT, Reichek N, Janicki JS, Shroff S. The pressure overloaded heart: physiological and clinical correlates, in Strauer B (ed). The Heart in Hypertension. Springer-Verlag, Berlin, 1981, pp 287–306.
10. Woods RH. A few applications of a physical theorem to membranes in the human body in a state of tension. J Anat Physiol 26:362–370, 1892.
11. Weber KT, Janicki JS, Reeves RC. Determinants of stroke volume in isolated canine heart. J Appl Physiol 37:742–747, 1974.
12. Weber KT, Janicki JS, Reeves RC, Hefner LL. Factors influencing left ventricular shortening in isolated canine heart. Am J Physiol 230:419–426, 1976.
13. Weber KT, Janicki JS, Hefner LL. Left ventricular force-length relations of isovolumic and ejecting contractions. Am J Physiol 231:337–343, 1976.
14. Weber KT, Janicki JS. Instantaneous force-velocity-length relations in isolated dog heart. Am J Physiol 232:H241–H249, 1977.
15. Weber KT, Janicki JS. The dynamics of ventricular contraction: force, length and shortening, in Weber KT, Janicki JS (eds): Symposium on Cardiac Mechanics. Fed Proc 39:188–195, 1980.
16. Weber KT, Janicki JS, Fishman AP. The aerobic limit of the heart perfused at constant pressure. Am J Physiol 238:118–125, 1980.
17. Weber KT, Janicki JS, Shroff SG, Fishman AP. Contractile mechanics and interaction of the right and left ventricles. Am J Cardiol 47:686–695, 1981.

18. Grossman W, Braunwald E, Mann T. Contractile state of the left ventricle in man as evaluated from end systolic pressure-volume relations. Circulation 56:845–852, 1977.
19. Borow KM, Green LH, Grossman W, Braunwald E. Left ventricular end-systolic stress-shortening and stress-length relations in humans. Am J Cardiol 50:1301–1308, 1982.
20. Borow KM, Neumann A, Wynne J. Sensitivity of end-systolic pressure-dimension and pressure-volume relations to the inotropic state in humans. Circulation 65:988–997, 1982.
21. Linzbach AJ. Heart failure from the point of view of quantitative anatomy. Am J Cardiol 5:370–383, 1960.
22. Burch GE, Ray CT, Cronvich JA. Certain mechanical peculiarities of the human cardiac pump in normal and diseased states. Circulation 5:504–513, 1952.
23. Sarnoff SJ, Berglund E. Ventricular function. I. Starling's law of the heart studied by means of simultaneous right and left ventricular function curves in the dog. Circulation 9:706–718, 1954.
24. Weber KT, Janicki JS. The metabolic demand and oxygen supply of the heart: physiologic and clinical considerations. Am J Cardiol 44:722–729, 1979.
25. Harden WR, Barlow CH, Simson MB, Harken AH. Myocardial ischemia and left ventricular failure in the isolated, perfused rabbit heart. Am J Cardiol 44:741–746, 1979.
26. Weber KT, Janicki JS. Myocardial oxygen consumption: the role of wall force and shortening. Am J Physiol 233:H421–H430, 1977.
27. Weber KT, Janicki JS. Interdependence of cardiac function, coronary flow and oxygen extraction. Am J Physiol 235:H784–H793, 1978.
28. Benotti JR, Grossman W, Braunwald E, Carabello BA. Effects of amrinone on myocardial energy metabolism and hemodynamics in patients with severe congestive heart failure due to coronary artery disease. Circulation 62:28–34, 1980.
29. Rude RE, Turi Z, Brown EJ, Lorell BH, Colucci WS, Mudge GH, Taylor CR, Grossman W. Acute effects of pirbuterol on myocardial oxygen metabolism and systemic hemodynamics in chronic congestive heart failure. Circulation 64:139–145, 1981.
30. Martin JL, Likoff MJ, Janicki JS, Laskey WK, Hirschfeld JW, Weber KT. Myocardial energetics and clinical response to the cardiotonic agent MDL 17,043 in advanced heart failure. JACC 4:875–881, 1983.
31. Bendersky R, Chatterjee K, Parmley WW, Brundage BH, Ports TA. Dobutamine in chronic ischemic heart failure: alterations in left ventricular function and coronary hemodynamics. Am J Cardiol 48:554–558, 1981.
32. Hoh JFY, McGrath MA, Hale PT. Electrophoretic analysis of multiple forms of rat cardiac myosin: effects of hypophysectomy and thyroxine replacement. J Mol Cell Cardiol 10:1053–1076, 1977.
33. Pagani ED, Julian FJ. Rabbit papillary muscle myosin isozymes and the velocity of muscle shortening. Circ Res 54:586–594, 1984.
34. Alpert NR, Mulieri RA. Increased myothermal economy of isometric force generation in compensated cardiac hypertrophy induced by pulmonary artery constriction in rabbit. A characterization of heat liberation in normal and hypertrophied right ventricular papillary muscles. Circ Res 50:491–500, 1982.
35. Gertz EW, Wisneski JA, Neese R, Bristow JD, Searle GL, Hanlon JT. Myocardial lactate metabolism: evidence of lactate release during net chemical extraction in man. Circulation 63:1273–1279, 1981.
36. Bing RJ, Hammond MM, Handelsman JC, Powers SR, Spencer FC, Eckenhoff JE, Goodale WT, Hafenschiel JH, Ketty SS. The measurement of coronary blood flow, oxygen consumption, and efficiency of the left ventricle in man. Am Heart J 38:1–24, 1949.
37. Sandler H, Dodge HT. Left ventricular tension and stress in man. Circ Res 13:91–98, 1963.
38. Badeer HS. Myocardial blood flow and oxygen uptake in clinical and experimental cardiomegaly. Am Heart J 82:105–119, 1971.
39. Rowe GG, Afonso S, Lugo JE, Castillo CA, Boake WC, Crumpton CW: Coronary blood flow and myocardial oxidative metabolism at rest and during exercise in subjects with severe aortic valve disease. Circulation 32:251–257, 1965.
40. Trenouth RS, Phelps NC, Neill WA. Determinants of left ventricular hypertrophy and oxygen supply in chronic aortic valve disease. Circulation 53:644–650, 1976.
41. Fallen EL, Elliott WC, Gorlin R. Mechanisms of angina in aortic stenosis. Circulation 36:480–488, 1967.
42. Shroff SG, Janicki JS, Weber KT. The relation between left ventricular efficiency and arterial load. Clin Res 31:463A, 1983.
43. Baxley WA, Dodge HT, Rackley CE, Sandler H, Pugh D. Left ventricular mechanical efficiency in man with heart disease. Circulation 55:564–568, 1977.

LARRY C. CASEY
KARL T. WEBER

5

Ventilatory System Mechanics and Gas Exchange

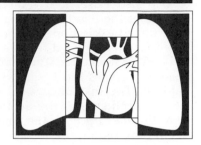

The process of respiratory gas exchange that exists between the atmosphere and alveolar capillary blood is termed *external respiration*. *Internal respiration* refers to the gas exchange process that occurs between the metabolizing cells and the capillaries of the systemic circulation. It is the lungs that allow humans to derive oxygen from the atmosphere while permitting the egress of the end-product of oxidative metabolism, carbon dioxide, into the atmosphere. The ventilatory system must maintain the most appropriate physiologic concentrations of oxygen and carbon dioxide in the alveoli. Of equal importance to gas exchange is the fact that, functionally, each of the 600 million alveoli has its own capillary to permit the ready diffusion of these repiratory gases into and out of the pulmonary circulation. Pulmonary blood flow averages 4 to 6 liters/min. It delivers, on the average, 200 ml of carbon dioxide each minute to the alveoli while taking up 250 ml of oxygen each minute from the alveoli.

The focus of this chapter is the dynamic behavior of the normal ventilatory system, its gas exchange function, and the complex system of controls that closely links these functions to the metabolic requirements of the tissues at rest and during exercise.

THE AERODYNAMIC BEHAVIOR AND MECHANICS OF THE LUNG

Ventilation is that process in which ambient air is brought into and exchanged with the air in the lungs. As we indicated in Chapter 1, ambient air passes through a conductance network composed of the nose, mouth, and pharynx, where it is warmed, humidified, and filtered on its passage to the trachea and the bronchi. Eventually, the air reaches the alveoli. Air is brought into the lungs by the respiratory effort, which consists of the contraction of the diaphragm. Diaphragmatic contraction increases the size of the thorax, lowers intrathoracic pressure, and draws air into the lungs. This sequence of events encompasses the mechanics of ventilation.

Ventilatory Volumes and Capacities

The amount of air that is moved into the lungs in 1 minute is termed the *minute ventilation* ($\dot{V}E$). It is determined by the *respiratory rate*, or the number of breaths taken in a minute, and the amount of air inhaled for each breath, the *tidal volume*. As we noted previously, an average $\dot{V}E$ equals 9 liters of air obtained by breathing 15 times per minute with a tidal volume of 600 ml. As the need to increase $\dot{V}E$ occurs with exercise, larger tidal volumes and higher respiratory rates are necessary. To understand how the lung is able to increase its tidal volume, it is first necessary to understand lung volume and the various reserves in lung volume that exist.[1]

The *total lung capacity* (TLC) averages 6 liters. An average tidal volume of 500 to 750 ml occupies only a small fraction, around 12 per cent of the total lung capacity. This ratio is similar to the ejection fraction of the heart (i.e., the stroke volume to filling volume ratio). Increments in tidal volume are derived from the inspiratory and expiratory reserve volumes. The *inspiratory reserve volume*, similar to the diastolic reserve of the heart, can be demonstrated when a subject inhales as deeply as possible above tidal volume; it averages 2.5 to 3.5 liters above the average tidal volume (Fig. 5–1). An *expiratory reserve volume* also exists that mimics the systolic reserve of the heart. It can be demonstrated by a forced expiration in which as much air as possible is expelled from the lungs below the end-tidal volume. The normal expiratory reserve averages 1 to 1.5 liters below the tidal volume. The inspiratory and expiratory reserves together with the tidal volume represent the *vital capacity* of the lungs. In practice, the thorax uses more of the inspiratory reserve than the expiratory reserve in raising tidal volume. Since the total lung capacity is approximately 6 liters and the vital capacity averages 5 liters, it is apparent that there must be an average *residual volume* of 1 liter that cannot be expelled no matter how forceful the expiration. This residual volume prevents the complete collapse of the lung while maintaining a certain degree of gas exchange at all times. Therefore, the normal tidal volume terminates at a lung volume, termed the *functional residual capacity*, that includes the expiratory reserve and residual volumes. The *inspiratory capacity* equals the tidal volume and inspiratory reserve volume.

A dynamic test of ventilatory capacity that can be obtained with a subject at rest is the *maximal voluntary ventilation* (MVV). It consists of the amount of air that can be moved during 15 seconds of deep, vigorous breathing. Because it is a short-lived period of maximal breathing effort, it normally is 25 per cent or more higher than the maximal VE that can be sustained during vigorous exercise. The MVV averages 140 to 160 liters/min.

Alveolar Ventilation

Each tidal volume averages 500 ml. At rest, approximately 30 per cent, or 150 ml, of each breath never reaches the alveoli and remains in the conductance network. This air is not available for gas exchange and is termed *anatomic dead space* ventilation. Thus, the true *alveolar ventilation* consists of 350 ml of fresh air, plus 150 ml of dead space air from the previous breath that reaches the alveoli and mixes with its existing air composition. The fraction of the tidal volume that represents dead space ventilation is not fixed. It may be increased during rapid shallow breathing, in which much of the inspired air only fluctuates in the trachea; or, as the tidal volume increases with a greater inspiratory effort, the anatomic dimensions of the conductance network are also increased. During exercise the ratio of dead space ventilation to tidal volume falls from its normal resting value of 30 per cent to less than 20 per cent, as a result of a larger tidal volume. Thus, alveolar ventilation increases from 70 per cent of minute ventilation at rest to over 80 per cent with exercise.

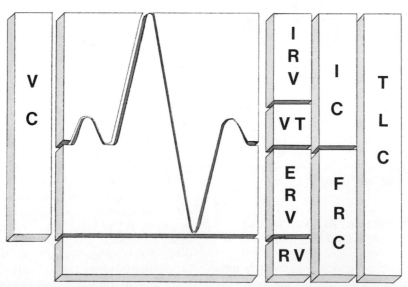

FIGURE 5–1. The volumes and capacities of the lung. The vital capacity (*VC*) includes the inspiratory (*IRV*) and expiratory (*ERV*) reserve volumes from which a given tidal volume (*VT*) is derived at rest or during exercise. *VC*, therefore, represents a ventilatory reserve from which the exercise response is obtained. For most workloads, tidal volume rarely exceeds 50 per cent of *VC*. The residual volume (*RV*) is never used for this purpose and sustains a steady state of gas exchange in the alveoli. Inspiratory capacity (*IC*) includes *VT* and *IRV*. The functional residual capacity (*FRC*) includes *RV* and *ERV*; total lung capacity (*TLC*) includes both *VC* and *RV*.

Alveolar ventilation determines the adequacy of respiratory gas exchange. However, it must be matched to alveolar capillary blood flow. At rest, the ratio of alveolar ventilation to alveolar blood flow, termed the *ventilation:perfusion ratio*, is 0.80. Thus, for each liter of blood flow 800 ml of alveolar ventilation is available for gas exchange. During exercise, alveolar ventilation and alveolar blood flow increase so that the ventilation:perfusion ratio approaches 5.0. Under certain circumstances, alveolar ventilation will fall. As a result, gas exchange is less efficient and there exists a *physiologic dead space* in contradistinction to the anatomic dead space. Alternatively, a reduction in alveolar capillary blood flow relative to alveolar ventilation is also a cause of physiologic dead space. Together, the anatomic and physiologic dead spaces equal the *total dead space*. If the total dead space of the lung exceeds 60 per cent of the total lung capacity, gas exchange will no longer be adequate.

Regional Distribution of Ventilation

The regional distribution of ventilation is partly a function of the resistance and compliance of regional lung units.[2] The product of resistance and compliance is termed the time constant. The normal resistance is 2 cm H_2O/liter/sec and the normal compliance is 0.3 liter/cm H_2O. Thus, the time constant is 0.6 sec. In one time constant, the lung unit is 63 per cent inflated; in two time constants, 95 per cent; and in three time constants, 100 per cent inflated. Therefore, in 0.6 sec the lung would receive 63 per cent of its ventilation, and in 1.2 sec, 95 per cent of its ventilation. If the resistance of a lung unit were to increase, then the time constant would increase and a longer period of time would be needed for that lung unit to receive all its normal ventilation. In patients with lung disease, regional differences in resistance or compliance or both might result in prolonged time constants. During exercise, the increased respiratory rate may not allow sufficient time for complete ventilation of lung units with abnormal time constants. As a result, areas of the lung may develop abnormal ventilation:perfusion ratios.

Ventilatory Mechanics

The thorax contains the heart and lungs. It is a closed chamber, separated from the atmosphere by the pleura. As a result, alterations in intrathoracic volume create changes in pleural pressure that are independent of atmospheric pressure.

Air flows into the lung because of pressure differences.[2] Four different pressures in the ventilatory system regulate airflow: (1) mouth pressure; (2) airway pressure; (3) alveolar pressure; and (4) pleural pressure. Because of the resistance to airflow imparted by the bronchi, as air flows from the mouth through the airways to the alveoli there is a continuous drop in pressure. The difference between the pressure at the mouth and the pleural pressure is called the *transpulmonary pressure* (P_{TP}), and the difference between the mouth pressure and alveolar pressure is called the *transairway pressure* (P_{TAW}). The transpulmonary pressure gradient depends on three mechanical properties of the lung: elastance (E), resistance (R), and inertance (I). The total pressure difference generated across the lung from the mouth to the pleural space (P_{TP}) is the sum of the pressures necessary to overcome each of these three elements, or $P_{TP} = P_R + P_E + P_I$. Resistance is defined as pressure/flow; elastance as pressure/volume; and inertance as pressure/acceleration. Usually, the inertance component is so small that it is ignored. However, during exercise it may become more important.

The mechanics of a breath thus can be characterized by determining the P_{TP} and the resulting flow that produces a change in volume. The interrelationship between tidal volume and intrapleural pressure, which reflects the time course of P_{TP}, is illustrated in Figure 5–2.[3]

Starting at the functional residual capacity (FRC) (the volume of the lung at end-exhalation), the forces of the chest wall that are acting to expand the chest and the forces of the lung that are trying to collapse the lung are exactly equal, and the pleural pressure at this time is approximately −3 cm H_2O. As inspiration begins, the diaphragm descends and the rib cage elevates; this combination produces a further decrease in the pleural pressure to −6 cm H_2O. This decrease in the pleural pressure is transmitted to the alveolus. Because alveolar pressure is lower than mouth pressure, air flows from the mouth into the alveoli, resulting in an increase in lung volume.

Lung expansion ceases when the inspiratory motion of the diaphragm is completed. At rest, this ventilatory process causes 7 to 12 liters/min of air to enter the lungs during inspiration—on an average, 14 to 16 breaths per minute, each having a tidal volume of

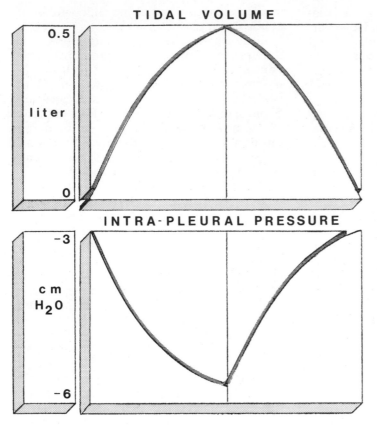

TIDAL VOLUME

INTRA-PLEURAL PRESSURE

FIGURE 5–2. The response of intrapleural pressure during the course of a simplified tidal volume response. With inspiration there is a fall in pleural pressure, which then reverses during expiration. Because of tissue and airway resistances the changes in pleural pressure are not linear.

500 to 750 ml. Inasmuch as the lung has no muscle of its own, its expansion depends on the thoracic pump and its muscular elements (see Chapter 1). The diaphragm and its contraction are adequate to move a sufficient amount of ambient air into and out of the lungs at rest. During exercise, when minute ventilation must increase, additional muscle elements like the scalenes and intercostals are required to move large volumes of air. These muscle groups are also brought into play when airway resistance or interstitial compliance of the lungs is altered by a disease process. The specific actions of the various muscle groups that alter thoracic volume and thereby aid in inspiratory motion during exercise or in disease are discussed in Chapter 1 and will not be recounted here.

Expiration occurs as the various muscular elements of the thorax relax, reducing thoracic size, and the elastic recoil of the lungs compresses the alveoli, permitting air to escape into the atmosphere. Expiration is therefore a passive process. Only during a forced expiration do various muscle groups of the abdomen participate to forcibly express air from the lungs. Transpulmonary pressure falls slowly during a normal expiration down to approximately atmospheric pressure; with exercise, the contraction of various muscle groups may aid in returning transpulmonary pressure to zero more quickly.

The major part of the pleural pressure generated during quiet breathing is used to overcome the elastic characteristics of the lung; however, the resistance of the lung parenchyma and airways also contributes.[4] During exercise, because of the increased respiratory rate and attendant high flow rates, more of the pressure must be used to overcome the resistive elements to airflow.

Airway resistance is created by friction between molecules of the flowing gas and between molecules of residual gas and the wall of the bronchial tubes.[1] As gas flows slowly through a straight, smooth, rigid large caliber tube, a laminar flow pattern develops. Friction between the gas molecules and the wall of the tube retards the outer layer of gas; this layer, in turn, retards the next closest gas layer in the lumen. As a result, multiple concentric layers of gas are generated, which flow parallel to the walls of the bronchi. The friction is greatest between the wall of the tube and the first layer of gas, decreases for layers of gas flow that are removed from the wall of the tube, and is least at the center of the tube. The laminar flow pattern thus has a parabolic velocity profile (Fig. 5–3). For laminar blood flow, airway resistance varies directly with the viscosity of the gas and the length of the tube and inversely with the fourth power of the radius of the lumen of the tube. If the resistance is small (short or wide tube) and the flow is small, only a small driving pressure is required. If the resistance is increased (long or narrow tube), more pressure is required to produce the same flow. If a greater flow is required through the same resistance, then more driving pressure is required.

When the molecules of gas flowing through a tube reach a critical linear velocity, the character of the flow changes. The concentric layers of gas no longer flow smoothly over adjacent layers but instead form eddy currents and turbulence. With turbulent gas flow, the gas tends to advance along the tube at the same velocity at the center as it does adjacent to the wall, thus abolishing the parabolic velocity profile that is characteristic of laminar flow.

In smooth, straight tubes, turbulent flow occurs only at high velocities. However, the tracheobronchial tree has hundreds of thousands of branchings, and these tend to cause

eddy formation and turbulent flow. Turbulent flow is also apt to occur at low flow rates if there are irregularities in the bronchus caused by mucus, exudate, or tumors. As Figure 5–3 illustrates, flow in the tracheobronchial tree is likely to consist of a combination of both laminar and turbulent flow. Also, as gas flows toward the periphery of the bronchial tree into smaller bronchi, the velocity of gas flow greatly diminishes. Thus, airflow tends to be laminar in the bronchioles but turbulent in the large airways.

With exercise, the increase in respiratory rate and tidal volume dictates that the velocity of gas flow must also increase. Therefore, during exercise, flow is likely to be more turbulent, and a greater transpulmonary pressure will be required to generate air flow. In addition, it is obvious that patients with lung disease who have airflow obstruction and increased airway resistance will be prone to the development of turbulent flow and thus require the generation of larger transpulmonary pressures to maintain adequate ventilation. The pattern of airflow has an important influence on the level of transpulmonary pressure required to sustain alveolar ventilation and, by inference, the work load that will be placed on the respiratory muscles and their corresponding VO_2.

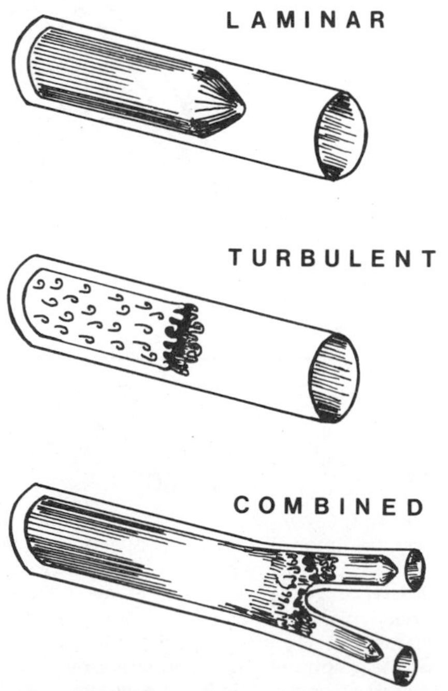

LAMINAR

TURBULENT

COMBINED

FIGURE 5–3. Airflow through the tracheobronchial tree may follow several patterns, including laminar or turbulent flow. At points of bifurcation, turbulence will disrupt laminar flow. See text for additional discussion.

Maximal Expiratory Flow

In addition to the movement of an absolute volume of air into the lungs, the rate of airflow is important to ensure proper gas exchange. The conductive network and the lungs normally offer only a modest resistance to the velocity of airflow. A standard expression of this resistance is derived by having a subject expel his or her vital capacity as quickly as possible. The volume expelled in 1 second is termed the *forced expiratory volume* (FEV_1). Normally, 80 per cent of the vital capacity can be exhaled in 1 second, and nearly 95 per cent is expelled in 3 seconds. FEV_1 can be used to calculate maximal voluntary ventilation (MVV)—that is, $FEV_1 \cdot 35$ = MVV.

The maximal flow ($\dot{V}max$) that a patient can forcibly generate is the net result of the forces acting to drive air out of the lungs (muscular contraction of diaphragm and abdominal muscles and elastic recoil of the lung) and the opposing airway resistance.[2]

Muscular pressure is the major determinant of the effort-dependent portion of the flow volume curve.[2, 3] It can be measured by

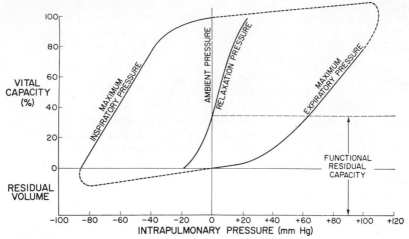

FIGURE 5–4. The relationship between lung volume expressed as per cent of vital capacity (*VC*) and the maximal pressure (*P*) that can be generated. See text for discussion. (From Tisi GM. Pulmonary Physiology in Clinical Medicine. Williams and Wilkins, Baltimore, 1983.)

determining the positive pressure generated during exhalation from TLC down to RV and the negative pressure generated during inspiration from RV to TLC (Fig. 5–4). The assessment of respiratory muscle strength is done clinically by measuring the maximal inspiratory pressure at FRC and the maximal expiratory pressure at TLC.

The elastic recoil of the lung is also a function of lung volume, being highest at total lung capacity and lowest at functional residual capacity (Fig. 5–5).[2] Airway resistance is also a function of lung volume, being greatest at residual volume and least at total lung capacity. This behavior may be accounted for by the fact that airway resistance depends on the diameter of the airway, which in turn depends on the pressure difference across the wall of the bronchus. Because pleural pressure is lower at increasing lung volume, more pressure acts to pull the lumen of the bronchus to a larger diameter (Fig. 5–6).

Since all the forces that tend to regulate air flow (pleural pressure, elastic recoil, and airway resistance) depend on lung volume, a common pulmonary function test is based on the relationship between flow and volume obtained during a maximal expiratory effort.[4] The results of such tests are depicted in Figure 5–7. Note the similarity of this relationship to the velocity-length relationship of cardiac muscle. The peak flow generated depends on the patient's effort. If the same maximal inspiration is achieved but a poor expiratory effort is made (see *a*, Fig. 5–7), then peak flow will be less but, as the lung

volume decreases, it will reach the point where it joins the curve generated during a maximal effort, and thereafter the curves are identical. On the other hand, if the patient fails to take in a maximal inspiration (to less than total lung capacity) and then performs a maximal exhalation, the peak flow tran-

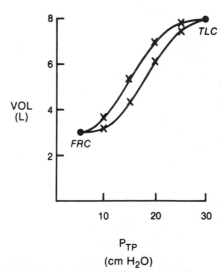

FIGURE 5–5. The compliance of the lung can be described by the interrelationship between lung volume (*Vol*) and transpulmonary pressure (P_{TP}). Compliance = $\Delta V/\Delta P$. Elastance = $\Delta P/\Delta V$. Points along the pressure-volume relation that correspond to total lung capacity (*TLC*) and functional residual capacity (*FRC*) are identified. Note that the graph depicts a loop rather than a line. The lung volumes during exhalation are higher than during inspiration at similar pressure points. This phenomenon is called hysteresis. (From Tisi GM. Pulmonary Physiology in Clinical Medicine. Williams and Wilkins, Baltimore, 1983.)

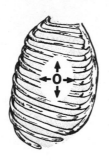

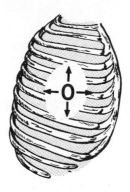

FIGURE 5–6. Bronchial lumen size and intrapleural pressure. The influence of intrapleural pressure on the wall and lumen size of a bronchus (open ellipse) is depicted by the arrows. At total lung capacity, in which elastic recoil pressure is increased, the lumen will be larger than that at the residual volume of the lung.

RESIDUAL VOLUME   TOTAL LUNG CAPACITY

siently increases above the flow expected for that lung volume (see *b*, Fig. 5–7) but then immediately decreases and follows the curve generated by a maximal exhalation from TLC. The portion of these curves that are all the same is the effort independent portion and is the most useful portion of the curve for diagnosing airway obstruction.

Several flow-volume curves are shown in Figure 5–8: one for a normal patient; one for a patient with airway disease; and one for a patient with restrictive lung disease (*B*). The effort-independent portion of the curve is indicated (*A*) and is analogous to that shown in Figure 5–7.

Mead and colleagues developed a model

FIGURE 5–7. Instantaneous airflow rates are shown as a function of lung volume. In (*a*), several expirations are depicted from total lung capacity; each expiration used a different level of effort. The early disparity seen in the course of these curves is due to differences in effort. Later on, however, these curves converge to a common flow rate curve that is effort independent. Note the similarity in these relations to the velocity-length regulation of the heart. In (*b*) are seen several forced expirations from different lung volumes. See text. (From Nunn JF. Applied Respiratory Physiology. Butterworth and Co., London, 1977.)

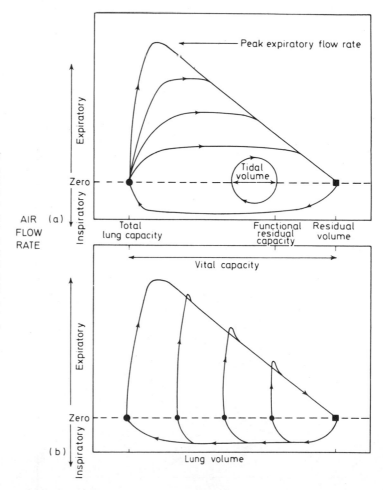

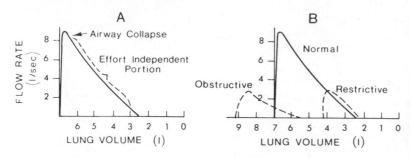

FIGURE 5–8. A series of forced expiratory flow-volume curves are shown. Each is obtained at total lung capacity. *A* shows the effort-independent portion of a normal flow-volume curve. Abnormalities in the curves are produced by obstructive or restrictive lung disease (*B*). (From West J. Respiratory Physiology—The Essentials. Williams and Wilkins, Baltimore, 1974.)

to explain airflow limitation that is based upon airway compression.[5] In this model, during forced exhalation, pleural pressure increases and is transmitted to the alveoli. The pressure in the alveolus is then composed of the pressure generated by the natural elastic properties of the lung that are acting to collapse the lung (Fig. 5–9) plus the transmitted pleural pressure.[2] Since mouth pressure is zero, it stands to reason that there is a decreasing pressure gradient from the alveolus to the mouth. Likewise, it is apparent that at some location in the tracheobronchial tree, there is a point at which the pressure inside the airway is equal to the pressure outside the airway. This point is called the *equal pressure point* (EPP).

The significance of the equal pressure point is that the portion of the tracheobronchial tree that is downstream (from the site of this point in the trachea) is subject to the development of airway compression and closure. Whether or not compression and closure will occur depends on the magnitude of the transmural pressure and the rigidity of the bronchial wall. This concept is extremely important during exercise since exhalation is forced and intrapleural pressures are high, thus allowing the equal pressure point to be reached at a higher lung volume. This problem is especially important in patients with obstructive lung disease whose bronchial

walls have decreased rigidity and who try to force their exhalations during exercise.

Work of Breathing

Breathing involves muscular work.[6] Work is defined as a force applied over a distance. As in the heart, the work of the respiratory pump can be expressed in the pressure and volume domain. The work of a single inspiration can be divided into the work required to overcome the elasticity of the lung and that required to overcome friction. Nearly 80 per cent of the nonelastic work is used to overcome airway resistance. Figure 5–10 depicts the force-distance and pressure-volume relations for a single breath. If there were no friction, the relation between force and distance would be the line in *B*. The work involved in overcoming the elastic resistance would be represented by the cross-hatched area between the ordinate and the line. If nonelastic forces (frictional) are present, the relationship between pressure and volume becomes curvilinear (*C*), and the work required to overcome the nonelastic forces and airways resistance is the stippled area between the line and the curved line.

Normally, during quiet spontaneous breathing expiration is passive, and hence the work of breathing is derived mostly during inspiration. The work required for exhal-

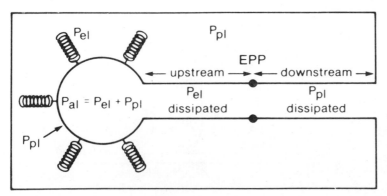

FIGURE 5–9. A model of the equal pressure point (*EPP*) concept. P_{pl}, pleural pressure, P_{al}, alveolar pressure; P_{el}, elastic pressure. (From Tisi GM. Pulmonary Physiology in Clinical Medicine. Williams and Wilkins, Baltimore, 1983.)

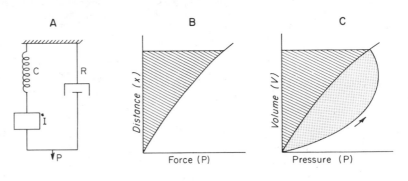

FIGURE 5–10. A simplified mechanical analog of the respiratory system. A three-element model is shown. *A* depicts the elastance (*C*), resistance (*R*), and inertance (*I*) of the lung. In *B*, the work performed in stretching an elastic element, such as a spring, is shown. *C* shows the work needed to inflate a balloon, which has a resistance opposing inflation (denoted by the stippled area), as well as the elastic work. (From Ruch TC, Patton HD (eds). Physiology and Biophysics. II. Circulation, Respiration and Fluid Balance. WB Saunders, Philadelphia, 1974.)

ation is derived from energy stored in the lung-thorax system during the preceding inspiration. The remainder of the stored energy is transformed into heat. When expiration is active, as it is during exercise, more work is done per breath. When lung compliance decreases or airway resistance increases, the work of breathing must increase.

Like skeletal muscle work, the work of breathing also can be expressed in metabolic terms.[3] The metabolic cost of breathing is low during quiet breathing, representing approximately 5 per cent of the total oxygen consumption; it increases with increasing minute ventilation (Fig. 5–11). In patients with emphysema, the $\dot{V}O_2$ and, in fact, the oxygen cost of additional ventilation may exceed the additional oxygen provided by the increase in $\dot{V}_E$. Furthermore, the increased work of breathing may generate extra carbon dioxide at a rate in excess of the augmentation in alveolar ventilation, thus leading to carbon dioxide retention.

The concept of efficiency is described in Chapter 4. For the respiratory apparatus, the optimal (from the efficiency standpoint, or work-performed-to-energy-consumed ratio) rate and depth of breathing should be those that produce the required alveolar ventilation with the minimal amount of work required by the respiratory muscles. If a constant minute volume is maintained, the work necessary to overcome elastic recoil is increased when breathing is deep and slow. On the other hand, the work expended to overcome airway resistance is increased when breathing is rapid and shallow. Figure 5–12 presents the relationship between work and respiratory rate.[4] The optimal respiratory rate is at the lowest total work of breathing. Normally, the respiratory rate under resting conditions is 15 bpm or less. In disease states in which there is decreased compliance of the lung (e.g., restrictive lung disease), respiratory rate increases and tidal volume decreases. If airway resistance is increased (e.g., asthma or emphysema), the respiratory rate is decreased and the tidal volume is increased. These breathing patterns serve to minimize the work of breathing.

RESPIRATORY GAS EXCHANGE

The atmosphere contains the oxygen required by the metabolizing cells. The amount of oxygen in the atmosphere depends on its concentration and pressure. Normally, 20.9 per cent of ambient air is oxygen. Carbon dioxide is produced by the cells and exchanged into the atmosphere; it normally occupies only 0.03 per cent of the air we breathe. Hence, the partial pressure that oxygen exerts in the atmosphere is equal to the product of 760 mm Hg, the atmospheric

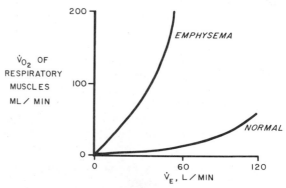

FIGURE 5–11. The work of breathing, which is performed by the muscles of the respiratory pump, utilizes O_2. The relationship between the $\dot{V}O_2$ of the respiratory muscles and minute ventilation ($\dot{V}_E$) is given for both a normal subject and one with emphysema. Restrictive lung disease also raises the work of breathing and the $\dot{V}O_2$ of the respiratory muscles. (From Slonim NB, Hamilton LH. Respiratory Physiology. CV Mosby, St. Louis, 1971.)

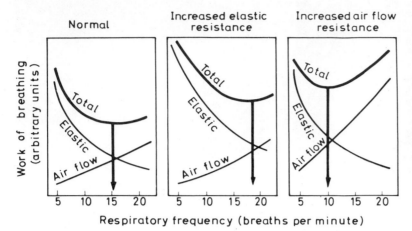

FIGURE 5—12. The work of breathing includes elastic and resistive elements, as depicted in Figure 5—10. The total work of breathing is at its minimum in the normal subject at 15 bpm. With interstitial lung disease and increased elastic resistance, a higher respiratory rate (18 bpm) is chosen to minimize work, whereas with increased airflow resistance a slower respiratory frequency (10 bpm) is more efficient for respiratory work. (From Nunn JF. Applied Respiratory Physiology. Butterworth & Co., London, 1977.)

pressure, and its 20.9 per cent concentration, or 159 mm Hg. Carbon dioxide has a much smaller partial pressure of only 0.2 mm Hg, or 0.0003 · 760 mm Hg. As air enters the nose, mouth, and trachea, it is humidified. The addition of water vapor lowers the pressure exerted by inspired gases. For example, from the atmospheric pressure of 760 mm Hg, 47 mm Hg of water vapor pressure are subtracted, leaving 713 mm Hg of pressure. This lowers the oxygen pressure in the trachea to 149 mm Hg—that is, 713 · 0.209. We can ignore the influence of water vapor on carbon dioxide because its concentration in ambient air is so low.

The partial pressure of oxygen in alveolar air is also less than that in the trachea or at the mouth. This is because the gas composition of alveolar air is a mixture of inspired and expired air. Alveolar air typically contains 14.5 per cent oxygen and 5.5 per cent carbon dioxide; thus, the partial pressure of oxygen is 103 mm Hg (0.145 · 713 mm Hg) and of carbon dioxide is 40 mm Hg (0.055 · 713 mm Hg). This pressure will drive oxygen from the alveolus into the capillary blood. Variations in these gas pressures are modest throughout the respiratory cycle. This "steady state" gas composition of the alveoli is mediated by the large functional residual capacity of air that remains in the lung at the end of each respiratory cycle.

Respiratory Gas Exchange in the Alveoli

Oxygen and carbon dioxide exchange from their gaseous phase in the alveoli into the liquid phase of the alveolar capillaries is through a passive process of diffusion determined by their partial pressures in the alveoli and blood and their solubility in blood.[7] We have already established that oxygen and carbon dioxide are under 103 and 40 mm Hg of pressure, respectively, in the alveoli; their respective pressures in the venous blood entering the alveolar capillary are 40 and 46 mm Hg. Thus, oxygen will be driven from the alveoli into the capillary blood while carbon dioxide will be driven out of the blood into the alveoli. A state of equilibrium exists for each respiratory gas when its transfer between the liquid and gas phases is balanced. At equilibrium there is no transfer of gas. Oxygen and carbon dioxide transfer between the alveoli and alveolar capillary blood is in equilibrium in less than 1 second. Conceptually, this occurs during the midpoint of the blood's transit through the lungs. As a result of this highly efficient process, the partial pressure of oxygen and carbon dioxide leaving the lungs is 100 and 40 mm Hg, respectively.

From its residence in the alveoli, oxygen is taken up by hemoglobin of the red blood cells that are present in the alveolar capillary blood, while a smaller quantity is dissolved directly in blood. The amount dissolved in plasma is only 0.003 ml per dl of blood and can be ignored. The iron composition of hemoglobin has a high affinity for oxygen. Each of the four iron atoms combines reversibly with oxygen to form oxyhemoglobin in accordance with the oxyhemoglobin dissociation relation, which describes the affinity of hemoglobin for oxygen. This means that 20 ml of oxygen are carried in every deciliter of blood. However, hemoglobin is never 100 per cent saturated, and therefore its per cent saturation, plus the oxygen-combining capacity, determines the arterial oxygen content. For an alveolar oxygen tension of 100 mm Hg, hemoglobin will be 98 per cent saturated. Consequently, the arterial oxygen content is

19 ml/dl of blood or 15 grams of hemoglobin 1.34 ml O_2/gram hemoglobin · 98 per cent saturation. The extent to which the hemoglobin molecule and its iron atoms are saturated is also a function of the acidity of the erythrocyte, its concentration of 2,3-diphosphoglycerate, and temperature.

Oxygen is avidly taken up by the metabolizing tissues. The partial pressure of oxygen outside and that within the cells is substantially lower than the 100 mm Hg of oxygen tension in arterial blood. As a result of this difference in oxygen pressure, oxygen is driven by diffusion from the blood of the capillaries into the tissue compartment. The oxygen tension outside the cell may be 40 mm Hg or more; within the cell it will be substantially lower and depend on the degree of oxidative metabolism. With heavy muscular work, it may fall to 3 mm Hg. By giving up a portion of its oxygen, hemoglobin in the capillaries is less saturated. The degree of oxygen saturation will depend on the amount of oxygen extracted by the tissues. In Chapter 2, Table 2–3, typical values of venous oxygen saturation are given for various organs. In the mixed venous blood of the pulmonary artery, representing the admixture of the various regional venous drainage sites, hemoglobin is 69 to 82 per cent saturated. This is a substantial quantity of oxyhemoglobin and suggests that overall oxygen extraction is only 25 per cent. The remaining oxyhemoglobin can serve as a reserve during heightened oxygen requirements by the tissues, when oxygen extraction can rise to 75 per cent or more. Thus, as oxygen requirements increase, tissue oxygen tension falls, favoring the passive diffusion gradient for oxygen from the capillary to the tissues.

Carbon dioxide is the end-product of oxidative metabolism. Inside the cell the partial pressure of carbon dioxide averages 46 mm Hg. Once again by passive diffusion, carbon dioxide moves along the gradient in carbon dioxide pressure into capillary blood where its tension is 45 mm Hg. As oxidative metabolism increases with exercise, for example, carbon dioxide tension in venous blood increases and may reach 90 mm Hg. The venous return to the lung carries the carbon dioxide for elimination into the alveoli and subsequently the atmosphere. Not all of the carbon dioxide of venous blood is eliminated, however. Recall that the average tension of carbon dioxide leaving the alveolar capillaries is 40 mm Hg. Carbon dioxide of arterial blood

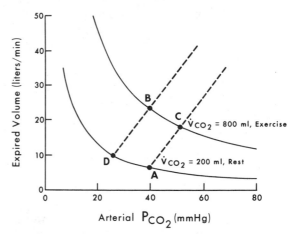

FIGURE 5–13. The relationship between expired volume and arterial CO_2 tension (pCO_2) is shown for two different isopleths of CO_2 production (VCO_2); one at rest with 200 ml/min and the other with exercise or 800 ml/min. Expired volume has to be increased more than twofold (from point A to B instead of A to C) to maintain eucapnia during exercise. Point D shows the increase in expired volume that occurs in order to decrease the PaCO_2. The dashed lines represent "normal" CO_2 response curves. (From Murray JF. The Normal Lung. The Basis for Diagnosis and Treatment of Pulmonary Disease. WB Saunders, Philadelphia, 1976.)

is a potent chemical stimulus to the control of breathing, as we will discuss later. The body's ventilatory response is designed for variations in carbon dioxide production and thereby metabolic demand, by maintaining a eucapnic state with minimal fluctuations in alveolar respiratory gas composition (Fig. 5–13).

Carbon dioxide can react with the free amino groups of hemoglobin and other proteins; however, the majority of carbon dioxide (i.e., 60 to 80 per cent) that leaves the cell is delivered to the lung in the form of bicarbonate. The carbon dioxide produced by the cells combines with water to form carbonic acid, a process mediated by carbonic anhydrase in the red blood cells. The carbonic acid ionizes to hydrogen and bicarbonate. The hemoglobin protein buffers the hydrogen to maintain a constant pH of blood. The bicarbonate formed within the erythrocyte is quite soluble and enters into the plasma in exchange for chloride.

VENTILATORY CONTROL

A complex control system is responsible for the coordination and synchronization of respiration with the metabolic requirements of the tissues. As a result of this control system, the oxygen requirements of the tissues can be met and the carbon dioxide produced can be eliminated according to physiologic priorities that vary on a moment-to-moment basis. Moreover, despite variations in $\dot{V}O_2$, arterial oxygen tension, hemoglobin oxygen saturation, and arterial carbon dioxide tension remain constant. Even more remarkable may be the fact that the control system logic integrates both respiratory and cardiocirculatory performance relative to internal respiration.

The control system has several key components, including peripheral and central receptors, neural pathways, and integrating centers within the brain and spinal cord. A detailed description of the control of breathing is beyond the scope of this text but may be found in references 8 and 9. In the following discussion, we will highlight several key elements of the system that are important to the integrated function of the cardiopulmonary unit, particularly during the physiologic stress of exercise.

Metabolic Factors That Regulate Ventilation

The mechanisms that regulate ventilation relative to $\dot{V}O_2$ and $\dot{V}CO_2$ are not well understood. That arterial oxygen and carbon dioxide tension will remain unchanged during exercise as $\dot{V}O_2$ and $\dot{V}CO_2$ each rise considerably is a remarkable fact that has attracted many investigators. Perhaps no one mechanism is responsible but rather an integrated system of multiple controls. Carbon dioxide appears to be an important factor that regulates the ventilatory response.

Arterial carbon dioxide tension is a direct function of the $\dot{V}CO_2$ found during exercise; it is inversely determined by alveolar ventilation. The inverse relationship between carbon dioxide tension and $\dot{V}E$ (used to reflect alveolar ventilation) is depicted in Figure 5–13 for both the resting state and for exercise when $\dot{V}CO_2$ is increased. The rise in $\dot{V}CO_2$ with exercise would lead to an increase in carbon dioxide tension if alveolar ventilation did not increase.

Receptor cells situated in the aortic arch and carotid body respond to changes in carbon dioxide tension, as well as to the acidity of arterial blood and its oxygen tension. Signals from these chemoreceptors travel to the brain via the vagus and glossopharyngeal nerves, respectively. These receptors may play a central role in maintaining eucapnia

during exercise. Recall that the heart's venous return is also the carbon dioxide delivery (CO_2 content · venous return) to the lung. Changes in venous return and thereby carbon dioxide delivery may stimulate respiration via these peripheral chemoreceptors. Studies on ventilatory control during exercise that were conducted in patients with carotid body resection suggest that the carotid bodies are the most important of these chemoreceptors in mediating the ventilatory response to exercise.[10] The nature of the integration between these peripheral chemoreceptors and the central chemoreceptors of the brain requires further investigation.

Receptors in the Musculoskeletal System and Other Factors

Nonmetabolic factors may also stimulate ventilation during exercise. A reflex mechanism arising from within proprioreceptors or muscle spindles of contracting skeletal muscle or a moving joint, and mediated via the anterior horn cells of the spinal cord, may be responsible. For example, passive movement of the limbs will raise ventilation even when the blood supply to the limb is occluded.[9] Controversy exists, however, about the true role played by a neuronally mediated increase in exercise ventilation, mediated from the working limb.

During vigorous, prolonged exercise the body's heat production rises considerably. As a result, there is a need to avoid hyperthermia and to dissipate this heat. This may be accomplished not only by sweating but also by increased ventilation. An elevated body temperature increases $\dot{V}CO_2$ and carbon dioxide sensitivity, each of which is known to increase $\dot{V}E$.[9]

Finally, psychogenic influences may participate in determining the ventilatory response to exercise, as can be seen by the hyperventilation that accompanies the anticipation of exercise. The type of exercise also appears to determine the pattern of ventilation.

Ventilatory Response to Exercise

During incremental exercise, $\dot{V}O_2$ and $\dot{V}E$ increase in proportion to one another in a nearly linear fashion until approximately 60 per cent of the maximal work capacity is reached (Fig. 5–14).[11] Above this level of work, $\dot{V}E$ continues to rise, but in a manner disproportionate to $\dot{V}O_2$ though more closely proportional to $\dot{V}CO_2$. This phenomenon is

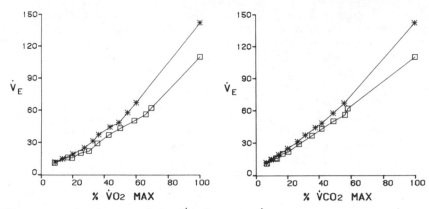

FIGURE 5–14. The response in minute ventilation ($\dot{V}_E$), O_2 uptake ($\dot{V}O_2$), and CO_2 production ($\dot{V}CO_2$) to incremental treadmill exercise in two normal subjects.

the result of two additional factors that stimulate ventilation, both of which are related to increased lactic acid production at higher work loads: (1) the added amount of carbon dioxide produced from the buffering of lactic acid by bicarbonate; and (2) increased hydrogen ion concentration caused by the reduction in bicarbonate concentration.[11]

The increase in $\dot{V}E$ that occurs with exercise is achieved by an increase in both respiratory rate and tidal volume. The rise in respiratory rate and tidal volume occurs in proportion to the increment in $\dot{V}O_2$ for light to moderately heavy work loads. At maximal loads the frequency of breathing has risen to a level that is approximately threefold greater than

its resting value. At a $\dot{V}O_2$ max of 30 to 40 ml/min/kg, for example, the respiratory rate of a normal individual will range between 40 and 45 breaths per minute. Tidal volume increases to values that are roughly three to four times its resting value, reaching levels of 2200 to 2600 ml per breath for this aerobic capacity. At a higher $\dot{V}O_2$ max of 50 to 60 ml/min/kg, the respiratory rate rises to the same level as noted for the lesser aerobic capacity; tidal volume, on the other hand, may reach values of 3 liters or more. The pattern of response in tidal volume and respiratory rate during exercise, however, appears to vary among individuals (Fig. 5–15), which may be related to differences in the ventilatory response to carbon dioxide.

The ventilatory response to exercise also depends upon the type of exercise test employed. Figure 5–14 depicts the ventilatory response to our 2 minute incremental tread-

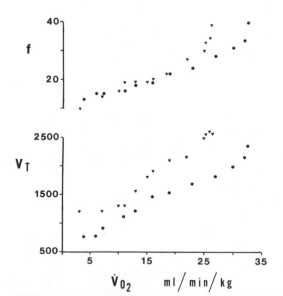

FIGURE 5–15. The response in respiratory rate (*f*) and tidal volume (V_T) to incremental treadmill exercise for two normal subjects. Note the differences in the tidal volume response.

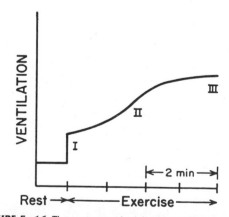

FIGURE 5–16. The response in minute ventilation during constant work rate exercise can be broken down into three phases (I, II, and III). See text. (From Wasserman K. Breathing during exercise. N Engl J Med *298*:780–785, 1978.)

mill test, whereas Figure 5–16 shows the ventilatory response to constant work-rate exercise. The ventilatory response to constant work-rate exercise has three phases: (a) an immediate increase in ventilation at the start of exercise; (b) a slower increase in ventilation to a steady state level; and (c) the steady state level.[11] This pattern holds true for aerobic and anaerobic steady state work loads, except that for anaerobic work the second phase is significantly delayed, thus prolonging the time required to attain the steady state.

Integrated Cardiopulmonary Response to Exercise

The ability to reach a maximum predicted work load for any individual depends upon the integrated performance of the cardiopulmonary unit. Figure 5–17 illustrates the cardiac and the ventilatory responses to incremental treadmill exercise and increasing $\dot{V}O_2$ for a normal subject studied in our laboratory. Each response demonstrates that with

the increase in $\dot{V}O_2$ there must be a corresponding increase in both ventilation and cardiac output. The increases in $\dot{V}E$ and cardiac output are achieved by an increase in both the rate and the volume of air and blood that enter and leave the thorax. During maximal exercise, a normal untrained individual will raise his or her tidal volume three to five times and the respiratory rate three to four times. Thus, it is possible for maximum exercise $\dot{V}E$ to reach a value that exceeds resting $\dot{V}E$ by eight- to tenfold. The heart's ability to raise blood flow during maximal exercise, on the other hand, is more limited than the ability of the lungs to increase airflow. Stroke volume will increase only twofold whereas heart rate can increase threefold with maximal exercise. Hence, cardiac output will not rise more than four to five times above its resting value.

In the process of increasing cardiac output and $\dot{V}E$ during exercise, there are metabolic costs to the myocardium and respiratory muscles. For the heart, a 300 gram organ, myocardial oxygen consumption can double

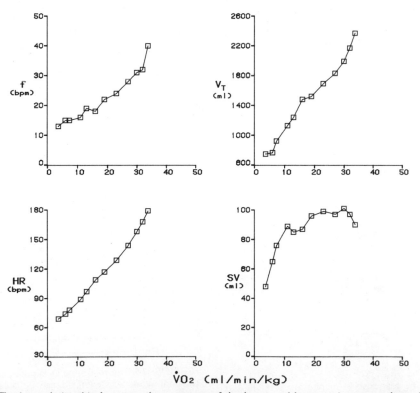

FIGURE 5–17. The interrelationship between the response of the heart and lungs to incremental treadmill exercise is shown for a normal subject. Given are the frequency and amount of air and blood that enter and leave the cardiopulmonary unit. HR, heart rate; f, respiratory rate; SV, stroke volume; and V_T, tidal volume.

with moderate level exercise.[13] In terms of the milliliters of oxygen consumed by the myocardium/min/kg of body weight, however, this is an inconsequential elevation in $\dot{V}O_2$. Respiratory muscle work, on the other hand, has a more significant impact on $\dot{V}O_2$. This larger muscle mass can raise $\dot{V}O_2$ by 300 to 400 ml/min[14] or by 4.0 to 5.0 ml/min/kg in a 75 kg individual with an average body surface area of 1.75 m². Normally, the heart provides 600 ml/min/m² of blood flow for each 100 ml/min/m² increment in $\dot{V}O_2$ (see Chapter 14). Thus, the elevation in $\dot{V}O_2$ of 200 ml/min/m² that accompanies the work of maximal ventilation requires an increase in systemic blood flow of 1200 ml/min/m².

REFERENCES

1. Comroe JH. The Lung. Clinical Physiology and Pulmonary Function Tests. Year Book Medical Publishers, Chicago, 1970.
2. Tisi M. Pulmonary Physiology in Clinical Medicine. Williams & Wilkins, Baltimore, 1983.
3. Slonim NB, Hamilton LH. Respiratory Physiology. C. V. Mosby, St. Louis, 1981.
4. Nunn JF. Applied Respiratory Physiology. Butterworth & Co, London, 1977.
5. Mead J, Turner JM, Macklem PT, et al. Significance of the relationship between lung recoil and maximum expiratory flow. J Appl Physiol 22:95–108, 1967.
6. Ruch TC, Patton HD (eds). Physiology and Biophysics. II. Circulation, Respiration and Fluid Balance. W. B. Saunders, Philadelphia, 1974.
7. Comroe J. Physiology of Respiration. Year Book Medical Publishers, Chicago, 1971.
8. Murray JF. The Normal Lung. The Basis for Diagnosis and Treatment of Pulmonary Disease. WB Saunders, Philadelphia, 1976.
9. Cherniack RM, Cherniack L. Respiration in Health and Disease. Philadelphia, WB Saunders, 1983.
10. Wasserman K, Whipp BJ, Casaburi R, Golden M, Beaver WL. Ventilatory control during exercise in man. Bull Eur Physiopathol Resp 15:27, 1979.
11. Wasserman K. Breathing during exercise. N Engl J Med 298:780–785, 1978.
12. West J. Respiratory Physiology—The Essentials. Williams & Wilkins, Baltimore, 1974.
13. Ferguson RJ, Cote P, Gauthier P, Bourass M. Changes in exercise coronary sinus blood flow with training in patients with angina pectoris. Circulation 58:41–47, 1978.
14. Bradley ME, Leith DE. Ventilatory muscle training and the oxygen cost of sustained hyperpnea. J Appl Physiol 45:885–892, 1978.

6

KARL T. WEBER
JOSEPH S. JANICKI

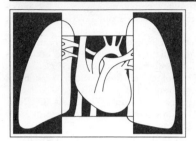

Acute Cardiac Failure

We will conclude the section on physiologic principles with a discussion of acute cardiac failure. The evaluation and management of cardiac failure, whether it be acute in onset or of long-term duration, requires a knowledge of the fundamental concepts of oxygen transport. In acute cardiac failure, the defect in oxygen delivery, relative to oxygen consumption ($\dot{V}O_2$), elicits many of the responses seen during exercise, when $\dot{V}O_2$ is increased relative to oxygen delivery. Because the deficit in oxygen delivery is severe in patients with acute cardiac failure, exercise testing is neither required nor advisable.

The past decade has seen a dramatic increase in the annual incidence of patients discharged from the hospital with the diagnosis of congestive heart failure (unpublished data, National Center for Health Statistics). A recent report[1] suggests that heart failure currently represents the most prevalent cause of death in hospitalized patients. Thus, the evaluation and treatment of patients with heart failure represents a major challenge to the practicing cardiologist. In this connection, knowledge of the concepts of oxygen delivery and oxygen availability will prove invaluable.

Regardless of the etiologic basis of heart disease, invasive hemodynamic monitoring in an intensive care setting is required to characterize the hemodynamic status and oxygen delivery of the patient with acute cardiac failure, as well as to determine the response to various therapeutic interventions. The principles governing the treatment of acute cardiac failure include an understanding of the following major issues: the nature and severity of the underlying disease; the role of associated conditions, such as infection, anemia, or hyperthyroidism, which may precipitate heart failure; the pathophysiology of acute cardiac failure; and the pharmacologic basis of medical therapy. A discussion of each issue is beyond the scope of this text. The purpose of this chapter will be to review the pathophysiology of acute cardiac failure and to develop broad guidelines for its treatment.

PATHOPHYSIOLOGY OF CARDIAC FAILURE

As we have indicated in Chapter 2, the oxidation of carbohydrates and fats is the major source of chemical energy from which cells sustain their many biologic functions. Oxidative metabolism cannot take place in the absence of oxygen. The consumption of oxygen during oxidative metabolism leads to the production of carbon dioxide ($\dot{V}CO_2$). $\dot{V}O_2$ and $\dot{V}CO_2$, and the resultant exchange of these repiratory gases with the capillary blood of the systemic circulation, form the process that is termed *internal respiration* (Fig. 6–1). Internal respiration mandates that the tissues be linked to the atmosphere for its supply of oxygen and for the elimination of the metabolic end-product carbon dioxide. The process whereby these two respiratory gases are exchanged between the atmosphere and the alveolar capillary blood is termed *external respiration*. The heart and lungs, together with hemoglobin, are responsible for the transport and exchange of oxygen and carbon dioxide. The lungs provide the exchange surface for the body's supply of oxygen and its expulsion of carbon dioxide, whereas the heart is responsible for the delivery of these gases to and from the tissues

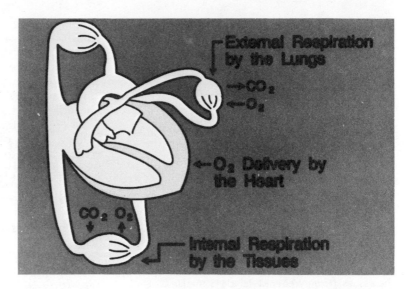

FIGURE 6–1. The body's exchange and transport of the respiratory gases O_2 and CO_2. The heart and lungs, together with hemoglobin, link the metabolizing tissues with the atmosphere. (From Weber KT, Janicki JS, Maskin CS. Pathophysiology of cardiac failure. Am J Cardiol 56:3B–7B, 1985.)

and the lungs. *Heart failure* may be defined in physiologic terms as that circumstance in which oxygen delivery to the tissues is inadequate, relative to their aerobic requirements. The term *acute heart failure* indicates that the appearance of this defect in oxygen supply and demand has been relatively sudden.

The heart's ability to deliver oxygen to the tissues may be compromised by a host of cardiovascular diseases or conditions. The late Louis N. Katz[2] suggested that conditions that do not affect the myocardium (eg, hypovolemia or acute valvular incompetence) are causes of *circulatory failure*. Acute myocardial infarction, severe myopathic heart disease, or an exacerbation of chronic cardiac failure, on the other hand, are causes of acute *cardiac* (or *myocardial*) *failure*. The sole focus of this chapter will be on acute cardiac failure.

Oxygen Availability

In accordance with our physiologic definition of heart failure, the delivery and availability of oxygen to the tissues is central to the pathophysiology of acute cardiac failure. The concepts of oxygen availability, delivery, and utilization have been reviewed in Chapter 2. In brief, *oxygen availability* to the metabolizing cells is a function of oxygen delivery to the tissues and oxygen that is extracted from the systemic capillaries by the cells. Cardiac output, which normally averages 5000 ml/min, is a function of the heart's frequency of contraction and the volume of blood ejected per contraction. The rate with which oxygen is transported to the tissues is

termed *oxygen delivery*; it is equal to the product of cardiac output and the arterial oxygen content and averages 950 ml/min. From the oxygen delivered to the capillaries, a certain amount of oxygen is extracted. Systemic *oxygen extraction* may be estimated from the ratio of the difference in oxygen content between an artery and the mixed venous blood of the pulmonary artery to the arterial oxygen content. Arterial oxygen content averages 19 ml/dl and is determined by the hemoglobin concentration of blood, its degree of oxygen saturation, and oxygen-combining capacity.

In patients with acute cardiac failure, in whom a low cardiac output is a hallmark, it is necessary to monitor tissue oxygen availability. In the intensive care setting, this can be accomplished by measuring the *cardiac output* directly to reflect oxygen delivery, or by monitoring the *oxygen saturation of mixed venous blood* in the pulmonary artery to reflect indirectly oxygen delivery and the level of oxygen extraction, or by both methods. Because the amount of hemoglobin in venous and arterial blood is essentially the same, the amount of oxygen leaving the capillaries is reflected by the oxygen saturation of venous blood.

The oxygen saturation of the mixed venous blood observed in the pulmonary artery is therefore an estimate of systemic blood flow and the body's overall extraction of oxygen. In Figures 6–2 and 6–3, the relationship between mixed venous oxygen saturation, or SvO_2, is given as a function of the resting cardiac output and arteriovenous oxygen difference, respectively.[3] It can be seen that as

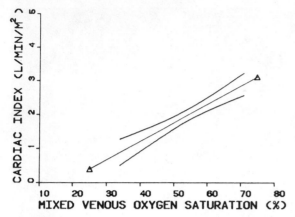

FIGURE 6–2. The relationship between resting cardiac output and mixed venous O₂ saturation. It can be seen that as cardiac output falls, O₂ saturation declines commensurate with an augmented level of O₂ extraction by the tissues. (From Weber KT, Janicki JS, Maskin CS. Pathophysiology of cardiac failure. Am J Cardiol, *56*:3B–7B, 1985.)

resting cardiac output falls, SvO_2 declines commensurate with the greater extraction of oxygen by the tissues. As SvO_2 declines, there is a resultant increase in the arteriovenous oxygen difference. As long as oxygen extraction rises appropriately, oxygen availability relative to oxygen uptake will be assured and oxidative metabolism will be sustained.

The normal resting $\dot{V}O_2$ averages 3.5 ml/min/kg; it is termed one *metabolic equivalent*. For an average-sized 70-kg adult, $\dot{V}O_2$ therefore averages 245 ml/min. The ability to

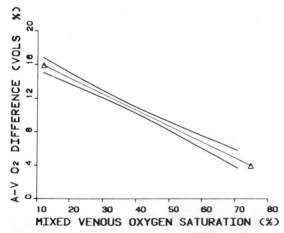

FIGURE 6–3. The relationship between the arteriovenous O₂ difference across the systemic circulation and the O₂ saturation of mixed venous blood. O₂ saturation falls as tissue O₂ extraction increases and the arteriovenous O₂ difference becomes greater. (From Weber KT, Janicki JS, Maskin CS. Pathophysiology of cardiac failure. Am J Cardiol, *56*:3B–7B, 1985.)

increase oxygen extraction serves as the primary reserve whereby cellular aerobic metabolism is maintained in patients with acute cardiac failure. We might develop a theoretical example to describe this circumstance more adequately. Actual clinical findings are described in the following discussion.

Oxygen extraction appears to have a physiologic limit of 75 to 80 per cent, which corresponds to an arteriovenous oxygen difference of approximately 15 ml/dl and an SvO_2 of 35 per cent or less. Therefore, cardiac output can decline to 1.75 liters/min, which corresponds to an oxygen delivery of roughly 330 ml/min (1.75 liters/min × 19 ml/dl), and oxygen availability relative to oxygen demand will still be preserved. Below this level of systemic blood flow, oxygen uptake exceeds oxygen delivery. Table 6–1 depicts this reserve in oxygen availability as oxygen extraction rises in the face of a declining cardiac output that characterizes acute cardiac failure.

In this theoretical case of acute cardiac failure, we have considered the whole body to be a homogeneous organ extracting oxygen uniformly across its various circulations. This is clearly an oversimplification. Conditions for oxygen extraction are different in each organ (see Chapter 2). Differences between this theoretic case and clinical practice are therefore based on the lack of homogeneity in oxygen extraction that exists between organs. Hence, one tissue may become anaerobic before another does.

When oxygen availability relative to tissue oxygen uptake is inadequate, less efficient anaerobic sources of energy are utilized by the tissues. Anaerobic cells actively produce lactate, which appears in the venous blood draining these tissues. If lactate production is of sufficient quantity to exceed the buffer-

Table 6–1. *Theoretical Example of the Reserve in O₂ Availability as Cardiac Output Falls and O₂ Extraction Increases*

CO (l/min)	AV̇O₂ (ml/dl)	O₂ Ext* (%)	O₂ Delivery (ml/min)	V̇O₂ (ml/min)
5	5.00	26	950	250
4	6.25	33	760	250
3	8.33	44	570	250
2	12.50	66	380	250
1.75	14.25	75	333	250

*Based on arterial O₂ content of 19 ml/dl.

CO, cardiac output; AV̇O₂, arteriovenous O₂ difference; O₂ Ext, O₂ extraction; V̇O₂, O₂ uptake.

ing capacity of bicarbonate, the lactate concentration of mixed venous blood will rise and lead to the appearance of *metabolic acidosis*. This acidosis further complicates the low cardiac output state. In Figure 6–4, it can be seen clinically that when the oxygen saturation of mixed venous blood falls below 35 per cent, the lactate concentration of mixed venous blood rises above 12 mg% (i.e., the upper limit of normal in our laboratory); this is the level above which a metabolic acidosis will occur. An SvO_2 below 35 per cent corresponds to a resting cardiac output of less than 1.5 liter/min/m² and an arteriovenous oxygen difference of more than 12 ml/dl (i.e., a level of systemic oxygen extraction in excess of 60 percent. Systemic oxygen extraction does not appear to be at its physiologic limit of 80 per cent, but this is secondary to the admixture of mixed venous blood with venous blood of all tissues that are extracting variable quantities of oxygen.

Hypotension may complicate acute cardiac failure. Arterial blood pressure is a function of cardiac output and the vascular resistance of the systemic circulation. Normally, mean arterial pressure averages 80 mm Hg, because the resting cardiac output is 5 liters/min and the vascular resistance is 1200 dynes · sec · cm⁻⁵. Even when cardiac output falls to one half of its normal value in patients with acute cardiac failure, mean arterial pressure is preserved because systemic arterioles vasoconstrict and vascular resistance will increase

twofold. Systemic hypotension, or shock, generally appears when cardiac output falls below 2 liters/min/m² or when vascular resistance fails to rise appropriately, or both.

The rise in vascular resistance occurs as an ordered process. Several regional (e.g., cutaneous) circulations demonstrate a preferential vasoconstriction relative to other (e.g., coronary and cerebral) circulations. This reapportionment and redistribution of systemic blood flow follows in accordance with the oxygen requirements and oxygen availability of the tissues. In all likelihood, it is mediated largely by a varying population, or sensitivity of alpha receptors within each regional circulation, or both. The skin and kidneys, for example, which extract only a small amount of their arterial oxygen supply (i.e., 6 to 7 per cent, respectively), are quite sensitive to circulating catecholamines. They are able to have their blood flow reduced through vasoconstriction without compromising their oxygen availability and oxidative metabolism. An enhanced extraction of oxygen by the kidneys or skin, in the face of reduced oxygen delivery, sustains their oxidative metabolism and preserves their viability.

Thus, the pathophysiologic cycle of acute cardiac failure is initiated by myocardial failure and reduced cardiac output, which accompanies a reduction in myocardial contractility secondary to ischemic or myopathic heart disease. The reduction in cardiac output and tissue oxygen delivery is followed by an ordered process of vasoconstriction similar to that seen with hemorrhagic shock. The vasoconstriction raises systemic vascular resistance and preserves systemic arterial pressure while maintaining regional oxygen availability. As a consequence of this increased vascular resistance, the impedance to left ventricular ejection is increased. This represents an additititional hemodynamic burden for the failing heart (see Chapter 3). A vicious cycle ensues with both the reduction in myocardial contractility and the elevation in vascular impedance each fostering the low cardiac output state.

Hemodynamic Monitoring

The advent of the flotation catheter, designed by Drs. H. J. C. Swan and W. Ganz, has aided in the bedside monitoring of the patient's hemodynamic status. An overview of the flotation catheter and its use in obtaining the hemodynamic profile of the patient with acute cardiac failure follows.

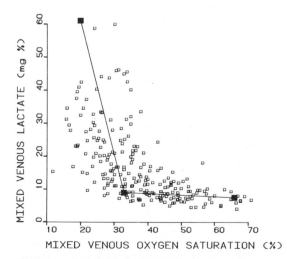

FIGURE 6–4. The relationship between the lactate concentration of mixed venous blood and the mixed venous O_2 saturation. Lactate production and a metabolic acidosis occur when O_2 saturation falls below 35 per cent. See text for further details. (From Weber KT, Janicki JS, Maskin CS. Pathophysiology of cardiac failure. Am J Cardiol, 56:3B–7B, 1985.)

The catheter itself represents a major advance in our ability to evaluate and manage critically ill patients by providing hemodynamic data from which to assess the nature and severity of acute cardiac failure. Moreover, these data can be monitored continuously over days and the response to therapeutic intervention evaluated objectively. In experienced hands, the insertion of the catheter is straightforward. In most cases, it can be inserted into the pulmonary artery without fluoroscopy; bedside pressure monitoring alone will suffice for monitoring catheter position during insertion, as we will review subsequently. The requisite instrumentation that is part of bedside hemodynamic monitoring will be reviewed in Chapter 8 and therefore will not be recounted here.

The catheter itself is quite flexible. Every 10 cm of the catheter's external length is scored with a thin black circle; every 50 cm has a heavy circle. This scoring of length aids in monitoring catheter position during insertion (vide infra). The triple-lumen 7F catheter that we prefer houses three lumina: (1) a lumen for the monitoring of central venous or right atrial pressure that terminates in an ostia located 30 cm from the tip of the catheter; (2) a lumen that traverses the entire length of the catheter and whose opening is at the end of the catheter through which pulmonary artery and occlusive wedge pressures can be monitored; and (3) a lumen for inflating the balloon that is situated at the distal end of the catheter. The catheter also contains a thermistor. The termistor exits near the catheter tip and is used to monitor cardiac output by thermodilution technique (see Chapter 8). Blood samples can be withdrawn from the proximal (right atrium) and distal (pulmonary artery) ports.

Every cardiologist has his or her own preference as to the site and manner of catheter insertion. The antecubital or femoral vein or internal jugular vein can be used for the catheter's insertion to the right heart. Herein we will describe an approach we have found quite useful over the years, particularly in patients receiving anticoagulant agents. Figure 6–5 depicts several phases of the catheter insertion procedure. We begin by placing a tourniquet around either upper arm (1). The tourniquet causes the distension of the vessels of the arm; we are particularly interested in the vessels lying in the medial aspect of the antecubital fossa. Lateral vessels are less preferable, because the catheter will have to cross over the shoulder to enter the thorax and may be more difficult to accomplish. The arm is prepared with a bacteriocidal-bacteriostatic iodine solution, draped, and the subcutaneous tissue overlying the chosen vein injected with lidocaine. Thereafter, a small (0.5 to 0.75 inch) skin incision is made and the vein isolated (2, 3). Chromic suture is used to encircle both ends of the visible vessel. The sutures are tethered under tension to the drapes above and below the incision by hemostats (4). This arrangement will assist in maintaining hemostasis when the vessel is incised. Fine ocular scissors are used to create an incision perpendicular to the long axis of the vein. With the hypothenar surface of the right hand, a downward traction is applied to the distal chromic suture, while the catheter is held with the thumb and forefinger of the right hand. The left hand is used to place traction on the proximal suture and hold the introducer, which opens the incision to permit the insertion of the catheter (5, 6). The tourniquet can then be loosened through the sterile drape to permit catheter advancement. The catheter itself should have been previously fluid-filled with saline, closed stopcocks should have been inserted into each of its ports, and the balloon should have been inflated under sterile saline or dextrose to check for defects; finally, the catheter should have been attached to a pressure transducer.

Each catheter port should be connected directly via stopcocks to the pressure transducer and to a container of 5 per cent dextrose in water that can be pressurized and used to continuously flush the proximal and distal lumina of the catheter. This will ensure catheter patency.

The pressure transducer to which the catheter is attached should be placed at heart level; this corresponds to the midaxillary line. If additional tubing is necessary to connect the two pressure ports of the catheter to the transducer, its length should be kept at a minimum and it should be stiff-walled to reduce damping of the pressure wave form. The connector tubing can be connected via stopcocks to the transducer. Simple opening of one stopcock and closure of the other permits periodic examination of the right atrial or central venous pressure, as well as the more continuous read-out of pulmonary artery pressure.

A pressure monitor can be used to follow catheter position during insertion. Respira-

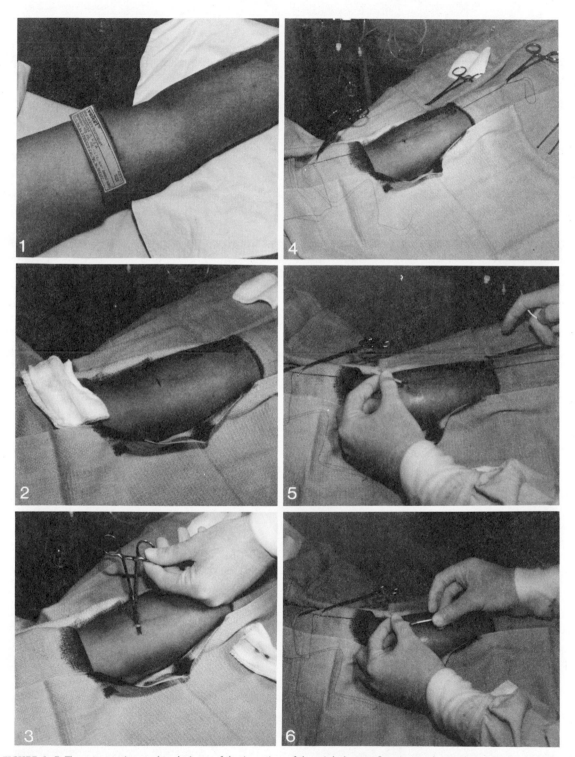

FIGURE 6–5. The preparation and technique of the insertion of the triple lumen flotation catheter through an antecubital vein. See text for explanation.

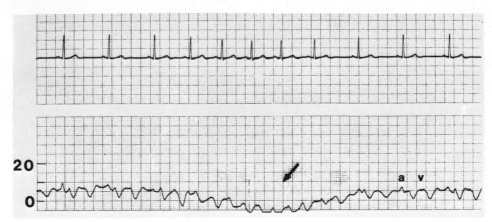

FIGURE 6–6. A recording of intrathoracic venous pressure. A drop in pressure can be seen during an inspiratory effort (arrow). The *a* and *v* waves of right atrial pressure tracing are identified.

tory variations in intravascular pressure become apparent once the catheter has entered the thorax; a deep inspiration can verify this fact should there be any question (Fig. 6–6). From the right antecubital fossa, 30 to 40 cm of the catheter will have to be advanced to enter the chest and to be positioned in the central venous system; an additional 10 cm

is required to reach the vena cava from the left arm. Figure 6–6 also depicts a typical right atrial pressure trace with its *a* and *v* wave components. Once in the right atrium, the balloon is inflated and the catheter advanced. The flow of venous return will transport the flotation (balloon) catheter across the tricuspid valve into the right ventricle,

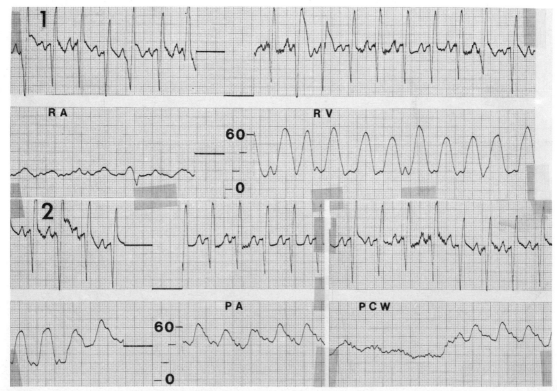

FIGURE 6–7. Monitoring right heart pressures to guide the insertion of the flotation catheter into the pulmonary artery. In panel *1*, right atrial (*RA*) and right ventricular (*RV*) pressures are shown, together with a chest lead electrocardiogram. In panel *2*, the transition from RV to pulmonary artery (*PA*) pressures is seen on the extreme left; pulmonary capillary wedge pressure (*PCW*) is given on the far right, as well as the return to PA pressure. The elevation in right heart and PCW pressures is apparent for this patient with acute cardiac failure secondary to a dilated cardiomyopathy.

where a typical ventricular pressure tracing becomes apparent (Fig. 6–7). The catheter is generally at 50 to 60 cm of its length at this point. Further advancement will bring the catheter into the pulmonary artery, where the pressure wave form is also distinguishable from that of the right ventricle. We prefer to continue catheter advancement with the balloon inflated until the catheter becomes wedged in a terminal portion of the pulmonary arterial circulation. Here the pressure wave form once again resembles an atrial pressure (left atrium) tracing.

The occlusive wedge pressure reflects the pressure within the pulmonary venous system and the left atrium. In the absence of mitral stenosis, the wedge pressure tracing will also be representative of mean left ventricular filling pressure. Thus, the pressures within the right heart and the diastolic pressure of the left heart can be easily and safely monitored with the flotation catheter. The systolic pressure of the left ventricle, which is equivalent to the arterial systolic blood pressure, can be monitored with an inflatable cuff around the opposite arm. In the presence of shock, an intra-arterial catheter should be inserted. This can be accomplished percutaneously after lidocaine infiltration over the radial or brachial artery.

Once the flotation catheter has been wedged and the pressure tracing obtained, the balloon is deflated and the wave form observed. At this time, pulsatile pulmonary artery pressure should be present. If the catheter remains wedged with the balloon deflated, the catheter should be withdrawn gradually until pulmonary artery pressure is again obtained. Here, the balloon should be reinflated to determine if the wedge pressure can be obtained from this catheter position. If not, the catheter should be advanced until a position is found where both pulsatile pulmonary artery and wedge pressures can be obtained reproducibly (Fig. 6–8). Once this position is established the distal chromic suture is used to ligate the vein, while the proximal suture is loosely tied over the catheter to secure its position within the vein and to maintain hemostasis. Generally 80 to 90 cm of catheter length will have been used in reaching this position in an average-sized adult. Whenever the right heart is markedly enlarged, it may be necessary to insert the full 100 cm length of the catheter.

The skin incision is closed with silk suture; only three or four sutures are required, and the catheter should be positioned between sutures and not to one end of the incision. This will promote better tissue healing and reduce the risk of infection. A bacteriocidal solution is applied over the incision, the area draped with gauze, and the catheter taped to the arm. An arm board can be used and taped to the arm to prevent flexion of the elbow and kinking of the catheter. The patient should be informed, however, that it is not necessary to maintain the arm immobile;

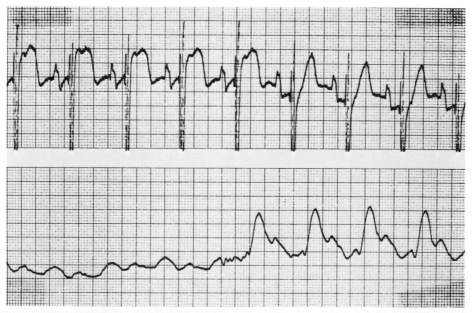

FIGURE 6–8. A chest lead electrocardiogram and tracing of wedge pressure (left half) and pulmonary artery pressure (right half) obtained with the flotation catheter at its optimal insertion length.

rotation and extension are encouraged to minimize discomfort at the elbow, shoulder, and wrist. Also, the patient should be instructed to open and close the hand periodically.

The importance of a compulsive attitude toward the calibration of the transducer and the maintenance of catheter patency cannot be overemphasized. The calibration procedure is described in detail in Chapter 8.

Artifacts and issues that may obscure or confuse the recording of right heart and wedge pressures, and examples of the typical pressure wave forms that can be expected in patients with acute cardiac failure, are shown in Figures 6–9 through 6–15.

First and foremost, it is important to recognize the inter-relationship between the electrocardiogram and the pressure pulses. The timing of pressure events bears a close relationship to the electrical activity of the heart (Fig. 6–9). The QRS complex heralds myocardial depolarization; ventricular contraction and the subsequent opening of the pulmonic valve follow soon thereafter. In patients with mitral regurgitation, a large regurgitant *v* wave (Fig. 6–10) can be confused with pulsatile pulmonary artery pressure.

In timing pressure events relative to the electrocardiogram, one must also be mindful of the delay within the pressure tracings that is a function of the length of the connecting tube system. The length of the connecting tubing between the catheter and transducer must be minimized.

Also note in Figure 6–9 that the wedge and diastolic pressures of the pulmonary artery are nearly equal. As a result, pulmonary artery diastolic pressure can be used to indicate wedge pressure. This may prove valuable under various circumstances when wedge pressure can no longer be obtained. The agreement between these pressures should be verified at the time of catheter insertion.

On a separate note, it should be appreciated that an inflated balloon, if left unattended, will create ischemia with possible pulmonary infarction and consequent hemoptysis.

Other factors can affect the pulmonary artery pressure tracing. In Figure 6–11, the influence of several premature ventricular contractions are shown. Note that, coincident with these contractions, there is no effective ejection of blood and pulsatile pulmonary artery diastolic pressure falls. This reduction in pulmonary artery diastolic pressure should not be considered the true diastolic pressure.

Variations in intrapleural pressure with respiration will also influence right heart pressure, as we have previously indicated. Figure 6–12 shows the decline in pulmonary artery and wedge pressures that occur during inspiration. Therefore, one should not use an electronic averaging of pulsatile pressures to determine the absolute level of these pressures. Instead, end-expiratory pressures should be determined manually to avoid significant underestimation of the pressures by signal averaging. End expiration is chosen because it represents the point (i.e., functional residual capacity) when pulmonary vascular resistance is minimal and when intrathoracic pressure comes closest to atmospheric pressure.

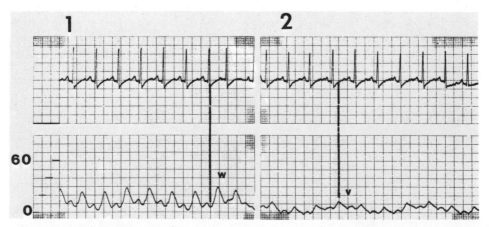

FIGURE 6–9. Panel *1* shows a pulmonary artery pressure tracing. The timing of the upstroke relative to the QRS of the electrocardiogram is indicated by line *w*. Panel *2* shows the wedge pressure tracing. The patient has mild mitral regurgitation by examination and clinical history, with a small v wave in wedge pressure. The relationship of the v wave to the electrocardiogram is identified by line *v*.

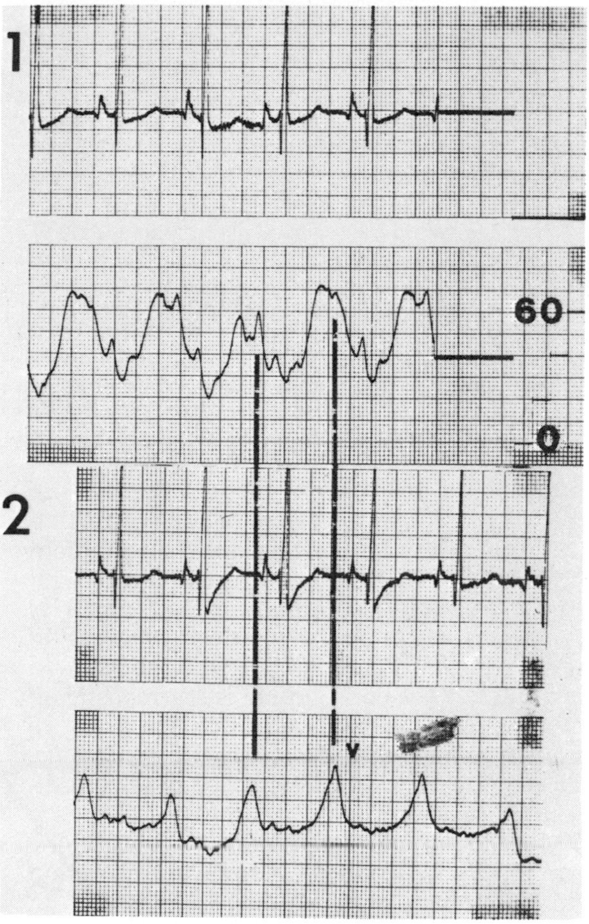

FIGURE 6–10. The superimposition of pulsatile pulmonary artery (panel *1*) and wedge (panel *2*) pressures is shown for a patient with significant mitral regurgitation and acute cardiac failure. The broken vertical lines demarcate the timing of the v wave relative to pulsatile pulmonary artery pressure and the electrocardiogram. It can be seen that the v wave in the left atrium is transmitted back to the pulmonary artery, where it causes an elevation in diastolic pulmonary artery pressure. The peak of the v wave occurs after the T wave of the electrocardiogram, whereas systolic pressure follows soon after the QRS complex during the ST segment.

During balloon inflation to determine wedge pressure, the balloon may interfere with the pressure sensing of the distal lumen. As a result, an "over-wedged" recording is obtained that is falsely higher than the true wedge pressure. This artifact is shown in Figure 6–13; an "over-wedge" pressure recording is given in *panel 2*. When uncertainty exists as to whether or not the wedge recording is true, it should be recalled that pulmo-

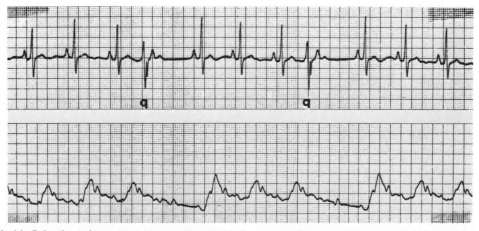

FIGURE 6–11. Pulsatile pulmonary artery pressure and the chest electrocardiogram. Two premature ventricular contractions (q beats) in which there is no right ventricular ejection are shown with their influence on pulmonary artery diastolic pressure.

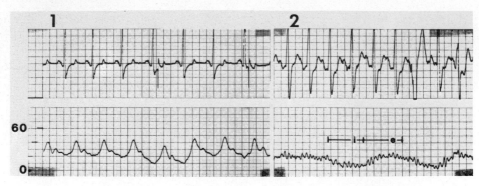

FIGURE 6–12. The influence of respiration on the pulmonary artery (panel *1*) and wedge pressures (panel *2*) is shown. During inspiration (*i*), a decline in these pressures accompanies the fall in intrapleural pressure. During expiration (*e*), these pressures once again rise. The "true" pressures should be measured at end-expiration.

nary blood flow cannot occur in the absence of a gradient in pressure between the pulmonary artery and left atrium. This gradient normally averages 8 mm Hg. In Figure 6–13, the "over-wedged" pressure is 47 mm Hg, while mean pulmonary artery pressure at end expiration is 50 mm Hg (not shown)—a small gradient of 3 mm Hg is not realistic on a physiologic basis. The true wedge pressure in this patient was 34 mm Hg and could have been inferred from the pulmonary artery diastolic pressure.

Motion of the exteriorized portion of the catheter will produce an artifactual variation in pulmonary artery pressure, as shown in Figure 6–14. This should not be confused with the aberration in pressure that can be seen during cardiac arrhythmia or mitral regurgitation. A whipping motion of the implanted portion of the catheter can also give

an erroneous pressure signal during systole or diastole, as indicated by the arrows in Figure 6–15.

Finally, it should be noted that the estimation of cardiac output by thermodilution technique may prove difficult in the presence of markedly reduced cardiac output or tricuspid regurgitation, when the cold dextrose-blood mixture flows forward and backward between the right atrium and ventricle. In either of these circumstances, mixed venous oxygen saturation may be more reliable. SvO_2 can be obtained by direct blood sampling of the pulmonary artery or through fiberoptic recording.

Hemodynamic Profile

The hemodynamic features of acute cardiac failure are outlined in Table 6–2. Generally

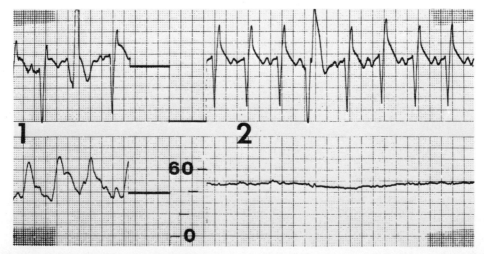

FIGURE 6–13. An "overwedged" pressure recording is shown in *2*. It bears little physiologic relationship to end-expiratory mean (not shown) or diastolic pulmonary artery pressure (panel *1*) and the expected gradient in pressure across the lung that sustains pulmonary blood flow.

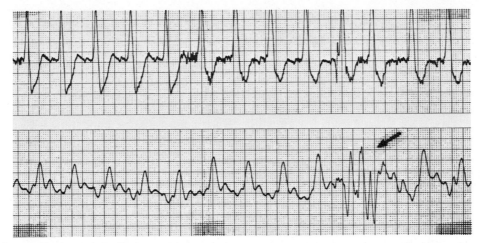

FIGURE 6–14. Motion of the exteriorized portion of the flotation catheter or the connecting tubing will produce an artifactual variation in pulmonary artery pressure, as shown by the arrow. This is not the type of variation that can be seen in pressure with an arrhythmia or mitral regurgitation.

speaking, cardiac index will be reduced to 2.0 to 2.4 liters/min/m². Accordingly, systemic oxygen extraction must increase, to preserve oxygen availability; SvO₂ will typically fall to 55 per cent or less, from its normal value of 70 to 75 per cent. Because of the impairment in systolic ventricular function, and occasionally because of the diastolic function of the ventricle secondary to myocardial ischemia or an infiltrative cardiomyopathy (e.g., amyloid), left ventricular filling pressure typically exceeds 15 mm Hg. With

the fall in cardiac output, systemic vascular resistance rises to values in excess of 1600 dynes · sec · cm⁻⁵. In patients with advanced cardiac failure, pulsus alternans may appear in the pulmonary artery pressure tracing, as in Figure 6–16 for a 62-year-old man with a dilated cardiomyopathy.

Hypotension complicates the clinical picture if the cardiac index is markedly reduced (ie, 1.5 to 2.0 liters/min/m² or less) or if vascular resistance fails to rise appropriately. The latter may occur when sepsis complicates the

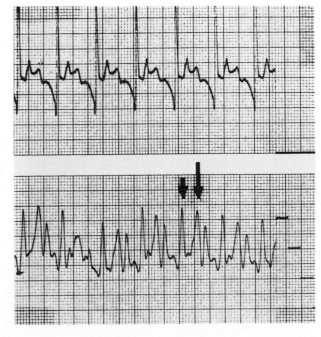

FIGURE 6–15. Catheter whip can occur in patients with acute cardiac failure, particularly when there is tricuspid regurgitation. The long and short arrows indicate the artifact in systolic and diastolic pulmonary artery pressures, respectively.

Table 6–2. *Hemodynamic Features of Acute Cardiac Failure*

Cardiac Failure Alone

Reduced cardiac output (2.0–2.4 l/min/m²)
Reduced SvO₂ (<55%)
Elevated LV filling pressure (>15 mm Hg)
Elevated systemic resistance (>1600 dynes · sec · cm⁻⁵)

Hypotension and Cardiac Failure

Markedly reduced cardiac output (1.5–2.0 l/min/m²)
Lack of appropriate rise in systemic resistance

Acidosis, Hypotension, and Cardiac Failure

Severely reduced cardiac output (<1.5 l/min/m²)
Elevation in lactic acid

SvO₂, mixed venous O₂ saturation; LV, left ventricle

clinical picture or when certain drugs with vasodilator properties are being administered. Finally, *lactic acidosis* will accompany acute cardiac failure if the cardiac index is severely reduced to 1.5 liters/min/m² or less.

Patients with acute myocardial infarction and cardiogenic shock typify acute cardiac failure. In Figure 6–17 the hemodynamic response to an acute reduction in coronary blood flow is depicted for an instrumented animal.[4] Typical clinical data[5] obtained in a large group of patients with either an acute anterior or an inferior infarction and a systolic arterial pressure of less than 90 mm Hg are shown in Figure 6–18. The hemodynamic features that are characteristic of cardiogenic shock are demonstrated by those patients with a cardiac index of less than 2 liters/min/m² and a left ventricular filling pressure of greater than 15 mm Hg; their survival rate is poor, as one might expect from such a com-

promise in ventricular function. Similar observations have been reported by Parr and associates[6] for children following open heart surgery, in whom cardiac output was significantly reduced (Fig. 6–19).

The interrelationship between ventricular performance and survival can be further demonstrated from the analysis of stroke work, left ventricular filling pressure, and cardiac output. The stroke work to filling pressure relation describes the ventricular function curve (Fig. 6–20A). If this relationship is derived from grouped patient data over a range of cardiac outputs, it is apparent that there is a progressive decline in ventricular function as cardiac output falls below normal levels. When this three-dimensional relationship was derived from a large body of data generated from the nine Myocardial Infarction Research Units around the country,[5] similar findings were demonstrated (Fig. 6–20B). Of interest is the fact that once stroke work fell below 20 gm-m/m², survival was only 4 per cent following either an acute anterior or an inferior myocardial infarction.

It should be noted that some patients with an acute myocardial infarction and a reduction in cardiac index may have a low filling pressure. This is the subset of patients shown in the lower left quadrant of Figure 6–18. These patients will respond to volume expansion, and their survival is much more favorable. Thus, there is a real need for hemodynamic monitoring in patients with acute cardiac failure following an acute myocardial infarction or open heart surgery. Table 6–3 identifies the major advantages of such monitoring in the evaluation and management of these patients. The institution of optimal

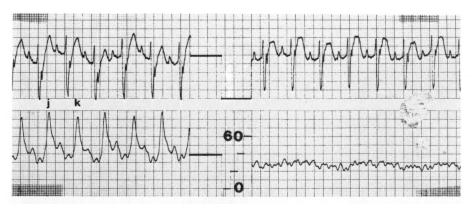

FIGURE 6–16. Pulsus alternans is typical of advanced cardiac failure. It is characterized by strong (*j*) and weak (*k*) contractions that appear in an alternating sequence. Pulsus alternans is seen in the pulmonary artery pressure tracing shown on the left. This patient also had an elevation in pulmonary artery systolic and diastolic pressures and the occlusive wedge pressure as well (shown on the right).

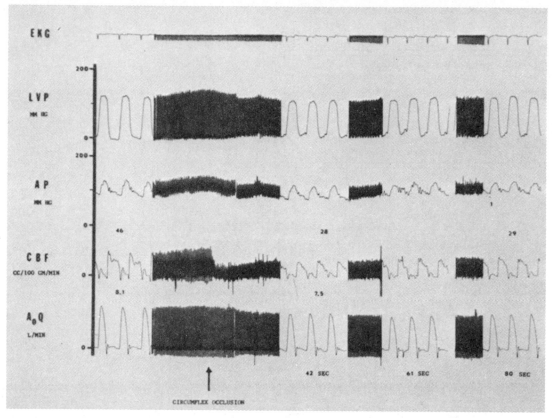

FIGURE 6–17. Recording of left ventricular and aortic pressures, left main coronary artery blood flow, aortic flow, and the electrocardiogram are given for an instrumented, unsedated calf. With the occlusion of the left circumflex coronary artery (by implanted cuff), left main coronary artery flow declines. There is a prompt fall in left ventricular and arterial systolic pressure as stroke volume declines. There also is a rapid elevation in left ventricular end-diastolic pressure following coronary occlusion. (From Weber KT, Malinin TI, Heck FJ, Dennison BH, Hastings FW. Experimental production of vascular and microvascular myocardial ischemia and infarction: the effects of different rates and degrees of coronary flow reduction in calves, *in* Malinin TI, Zeppa R, Gollan F, Callahan AB (eds). Reversibility of Cellular Injury Due to Inadequate Perfusion. CC Thomas, Springfield, IL, 1972, pp 266–287.)

FIGURE 6–18. The hemodynamic profile for patients with cardiogenic shock following an acute anterior or inferior myocardial infarction. Subsets of patients at high and lesser risk can be identified. See text. (From Weber KT, Janicki JS, Russell RO, Rackley CE. Identification of high risk subsets of acute myocardial infarction. Am J Cardiol *41*:197–203, 1978.)

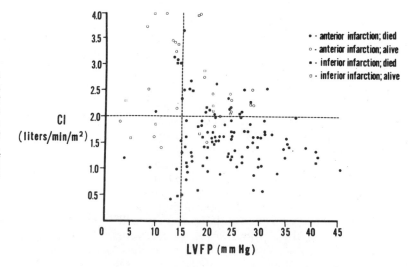

Table 6–3. *Information Derived from Hemodynamic Monitoring in Acute Myocardial Infarction*

Identification of the severity of left ventricular dysfunction that can be monitored serially

Identification of the high-risk patient, as well as those at lesser risk

Identification of the requisite information to select therapy

Identification of the response to therapy

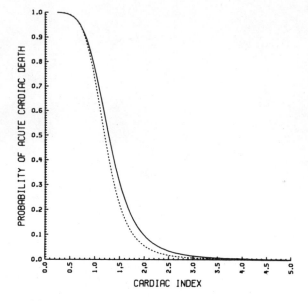

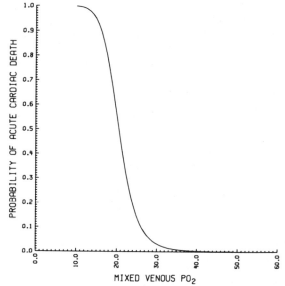

therapeutic intervention and the determination of therapeutic response can be gauged from monitoring oxygen delivery and ventricular and intravascular hemodynamics.

MANAGEMENT GUIDELINES FOR CARDIAC FAILURE

Acute Cardiac Failure Without Shock

From the foregoing discussion it can be concluded that in most cases acute cardiac failure is characterized by systolic dysfunction of the left ventricle with a reduced cardiac output and an elevated filling pressure. Therefore, an over-riding objective of medical therapy should be to enhance left ventricular emptying. As a result, cardiac output and oxygen delivery will increase, whereas ventricular filling pressure and pulmonary venous pressure will decrease. Based on relationships shown earlier for oxygen delivery and extraction, cardiac index should be raised to more than 2 liters/min/m^2 and SvO_2 to greater than 50 per cent, whereas filling pressure should be reduced to 20 mm Hg or less. The optimal level of pump function for each patient, however, must be based on monitoring that patient's hemodynamic and clinical status and response to therapy. The relative chronicity of cardiac failure will influence the nature of these responses. A reduction in calculated vascular resistance will accompany the increased cardiac output. A calculated vascular resistance of approximately 1900 dynes · sec · cm^{-5} represents a targeted end point as long as mean arterial pressure remains between 70 and 80 mm Hg in previously normotensive individuals. In patients with a history of systemic hypertension, higher levels of arterial pressure will be necessary; the optimal level of pressure

FIGURE 6–19. The probability of acute cardiac death for children following open heart surgery. Mortality escalates significantly once the cardiac index falls below 2 liters/min/m^2 or mixed venous O_2 tension falls below 30 mm Hg. The broken line indicates data derived from the measurement of mixed venous O_2 tension. (From Parr GVS, Blackstone EH, Kirklin JW. Cardiac performance and mortality early after intracardiac surgery in infants and young children. Circulation *51*:867–874, 1975.)

must be based on clinical response and systemic perfusion, particularly of the heart, brain, and kidneys. Generally speaking, mean arterial pressure should approximate 90 mm Hg or more in these patients with systemic hypertension.

The aforementioned hemodynamic objec-

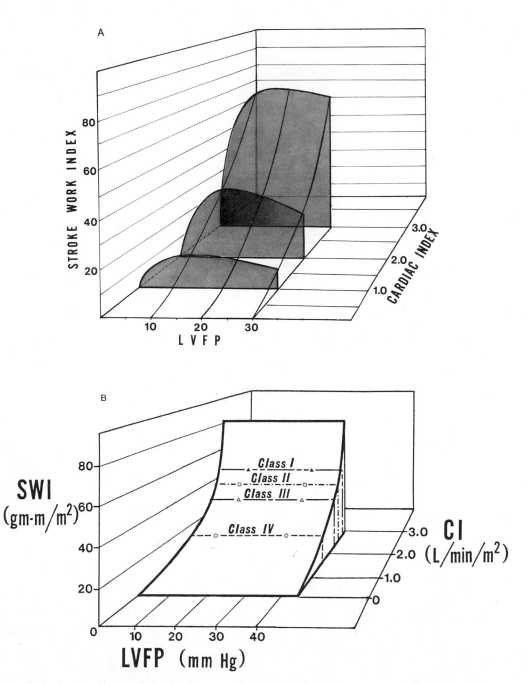

FIGURE 6–20. *A*, The theoretic family of ventricular function curves for patients with acute myocardial infarction. *B*, The actual clinical data for patients with acute myocardial infarction and left ventricular dysfunction of varying severity on clinical examination (class I, no failure; class II, rales or S₃ gallop; class III, pulmonary edema; class IV, shock). (From Weber KT, Janicki JS, Russell RO, Rackley CE. Identification of high risk subsets of acute myocardial infarction. Am J Cardiol *41*:197–203, 1978.)

Table 6—4. *Pharmacologic Agents for the Treatment of Acute Cardiac Failure*

Drug	Cardiocirculatory Effect	Average IV Dosage	Comments
Amrinone	Inotropy and vasodilation	0.75–1.5 mg/kg 5–20 µg/kg/min	Loading dose sustaining infusion
Dobutamine	Inotropy and vasodilation	5–15 µg/kg/min	Begin with 2.5 µg/kg/min and titrate upward
Dopamine	Inotropy and vasoconstriction	2–15 µg/min	Dopaminergic activity at 2–4 µg/min
Isoproterenol	Inotropy and vasodilation	0.5–5 µg/min	Chronotropic response and arrhythmia
Norepinephrine	Inotropy and vasoconstriction	1–8 µg/min	Decreased renal perfusion and arrhythmia
Nitroprusside	Vasodilation	0.5–10 µg/kg/min	Hypotension
Furosemide	Vasodilation	40–120 mg	Diuresis

tives can be attained with various pharmacologic agents, including those with positive inotropic effects on the myocardium. Agents such as amrinone and dobutamine, for example, have been shown to increase ventricular emptying in these patients.[7, 8] Moreover amrinone, a noncatecholamine- and non-digitalis-type drug, improves pump performance without adversely raising myocardial oxygen consumption.[9, 10] Another advantage to amrinone is the fact that tolerance to the drug has not been demonstrated. On the other hand, the dose-response curve for dobutamine and its effectivensss may decline after several days of administration.[11] Average doses of these and other drugs that are commonly used in these patients are presented in Table 6–4. Illustrative cases of acute cardiac failure and their initial response to various inotropic agents are given in Figures 6–21 to 6–23.

Intravenous nitroprusside, a potent vasodilator with balanced effects on the arterial and venous circulation, is also a useful agent for improving cardiac performance in patients with acute cardiac failure. It, however, may create a ventilation/perfusion mismatch with hypoxemia and may lead to thiocyanate poisoning if given over protracted periods of time. For a more detailed discussion of this and other vasodilator agents, the interested reader is referred elsewhere.[12] The potent loop diuretics, such as furosemide, when administered intravenously will promote sodium and water clearance and thereby aid in reducing left ventricular filling pressure in these patients. The potential to induce hypokalemia and cardiac arrhythmias must be recognized when using loop diuretics.

Acute Cardiac Failure with Shock

In patients with cardiac failure and shock, it is necessary to preserve mean arterial pressure and hence systemic perfusion. Thus, enhanced ventricular emptying plus vaso-

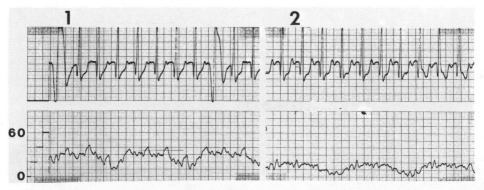

FIGURE 6—21. A wedge pressure tracing is shown in panel *1* for a 52 year old man with a dilated cardiomyopathy and acute cardiac failure. A murmur of mitral regurgitation was present, and small v waves were apparent in the wedge pressure tracing; wedge pressure at end-expiration averaged 34 mm Hg, and the patient was tachypneic and orthopneic. Intravenous dobutamine, a synthetic catecholamine, was started at 5 µg/kg/min, with a prompt reduction in wedge pressure to 18 mm Hg (panel *2*) and attenuation of the mitral regurgitation murmur. Cardiac output was increased from 2.1 liters/min/m² at baseline to 3.2 liter/min/m² after dobutamine.

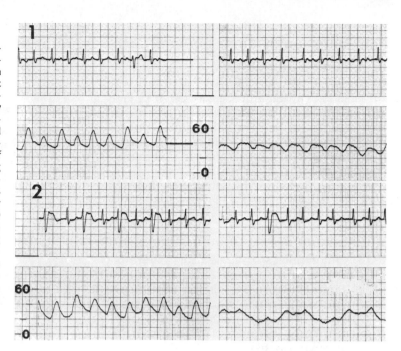

FIGURE 6–22. Panel *1* shows the pulmonary artery and wedge pressure recordings for a 62 year old woman with ischemic heart disease, acute cardiac failure, and atrial fibrillation. Pulsus alternans can be seen in the pulmonary artery tracing. Wedge pressure averaged 38 mm Hg, and the patient had clinical evidence of pulmonary congestion. Following the administration of intravenous amrinone (a 1.5 mg/kg loading dose and a 20 μg/min/kg sustaining infusion), the pulsus alternans disappeared and the end-expiratory wedge pressure was reduced to 30 mm Hg (panel *2*). Cardiac output rose from 1.8 liters/min/m² prior to the drug to 3.3 liters/min/m² after amrinone. Although the lower tracing indicates the presence of ventricular premature depolarizations, these were present before amrinone administration and did not increase in frequency afterward.

constriction of systemic arterioles is required. Because of their vasoconstrictor properties, dopamine or norepinephrine may be better suited for this purpose than amrinone or dobutamine. Dopamine, however, has less inotropic potency than the other positive inotropic agents, and therefore, in selected cases, dopamine together with agents such as dobutamine or amrinone may prove useful. Dopamine may also adversely raise ventricular filling pressure,[13] while dopamine and norepinephrine may cause ventricular arrhythmias. Finally, intra-aortic balloon counterpulsation may be required in patients with advanced cases of acute cardiac failure and shock who are poorly responsive to medical therapy.[14]

It should be recalled that the measurement of occlusive wedge pressure will identify those patients with relatively volume-contracted acute cardiac failure. These patients require intravenous fluids to raise their ventricular filling pressure and cardiac output. The optimal level of filling pressure is generally 15 to 18 mm Hg,[15] but this level must again be individualized for each patient based on the patient's intravascular volume and left ventricular compliance.

The ultimate selection of any drug or combination of drugs should be based on the relevant hemodynamic profile of each patient. As noted earlier, the measurement of SvO_2 adds much valuable information to the evaluation and management of oxygen deliv-

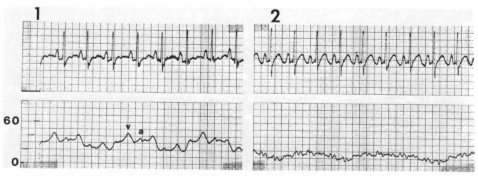

FIGURE 6–23. A 60 year old women with ischemic heart disease, mitral regurgitation on examination and by wedge pressure data (elevated v wave in panel *1*), and acute cardiac failure. She was marginally responsive to dobutamine. Following the intravenous administration of an experimental phosphodiesterase inhibitor, MDL 17,043 (panel *2*), there was a dramatic reduction in wedge pressure and her mitral regurgitation murmur disappeared. Cardiac output rose from 1.9 liters/min/m² before MDL 17,043 to 3.4 liters/min/m² after its administration.

ery and extraction. This parameter[16] can now be obtained at the bedside from a fiberoptic bundle that has been incorporated into the triple-lumen flotation catheter (see Chapter 8). The relationship between resting SvO_2 and resting cardiac output was given in Figure 6–2. In addition to providing a continuous read-out of SvO_2 and, by inference, cardiac output and oxygen delivery, the system eliminates the need for multiple determinations of cardiac output by the thermodilution technique. In turn, this minimizes the volume of fluid that must be given to a patient who already has pulmonary congestion, and also saves nursing time for other tasks related to the care of critically ill patients. In sensing SvO_2, other causes of acute heart failure or shock or both can be assessed as well, such as a ventricular septal rupture following acute myocardial infarction. In this instance, SvO_2 would be inappropriately high (e.g., 70 to 80 per cent), because of the left-to-right shunt in such a patient.

REFERENCES

1. Frommer PL. Workshop on congestive heart failure: introduction and overview, *in* Braunwald E, Mock MB, Watson JT (eds). Congestive Heart Failure: Current Research and Clinical Applications. New York, Grune and Stratton, 1982, pp 1–2.
2. Katz LN, Feinberg H, Shaffer AB. Hemodynamic aspects of congestive heart failure. Circulation *21*:95–111, 1960.
3. Weber KT, Janicki JS, Maskin CS. Pathophysiology of cardiac failure. Am J Cardiol *56*:3B–7B, 1985.
4. Weber KT, Malinin TI, Heck FJ, Dennison BH, Hastings FW. Experimental production of vascular and microvascular myocardial ischemia and infarction: the effects of different rates and degrees of coronary flow reduction in calves, *in* Malinin TI, Zeppa R, Gollan F, Callahan AB (eds). Reversibility of Cellular Injury Due to Inadequate Perfusion. Charles C Thomas, Springfield, 1972, pp. 266–287.
5. Weber KT, Janicki JS, Russell RO, Rackley CE. Identification of high risk subsets of acute myocardial infarction. Am J Cardiol *41*:197–203, 1978.
6. Parr GVS, Blackstone EH, Kirklin JW. Cardiac performance and mortality early after intracardiac surgery in infants and young children. Circulation *51*:867–874, 1975.
7. Weber KT, Andrews V, Janicki JS. Cardiotonic agents in the management of chronic cardiac failure. Am Heart J *103*:639–649, 1982.
8. Leier CV, Unverferth DV. Dobutamine. Ann Intern Med *99*:490–496, 1983.
9. Bennotti JR, Grossman W, Braunwald E, Carabello BA. Effects of amrinone on myocardial energy metabolism and hemodynamics in patients with severe congestive heart failure due to coronary artery disease. Circulation *62*:28–34, 1980.
10. Bendersky R, Chatterjee K, Parmley WW, Brundage BH, Ports TA. Dobutamine in chronic ischemic heart failure: Alterations in left ventricular function and coronary hemodynamics. Am J Cardiol *48*:554–558, 1981.
11. Unverferth DV, Blanford M, Kates RE, Leier CV. Tolerance to dobutamine after a 72 hour continuous infusion. Am J Med *69*:262–266, 1980.
12. Chatterjee K, Parmley WW. The role of vasodilator therapy in heart failure. Prog Cardiovasc Dis *19*:301–325, 1977.
13. Leier CV, Heban PT, Huss P, Bush CA, Lewis RP. Comparative systemic and regional hemodynamic effects of dopamine and dobutamine in patients with cardiomyopathic heart failure. Circulation *58*:466–475, 1978.
14. Weber KT, Janicki JS. Intra-aortic balloon counterpulsation: a review of physiologic principles, clinical results and device safety. Ann Thorac Surg *17*:602–636, 1974.
15. Russell RO, Rackley CE, Pombo JH, Hunt D, Potanin C, Dodge HT. Effects of increasing left ventricular filling pressure in patients with acute myocardial infarction. J Clin Invest *49*:1539–1559, 1970.
16. Divertie MB, McMichan JC. Continuous monitoring of mixed venous oxygen saturation. Chest *85*:423–428, 1984.

SECTION II

CARDIOPULMONARY EXERCISE (CPX) TESTING IN HEART AND LUNG DISEASE

JOSEPH S. JANICKI
SANJEEV G. SHROFF
KARL T. WEBER

7

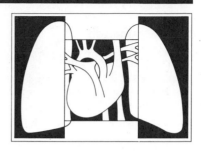

Instrumentation for Monitoring Respiratory Gas Exchange

To this point in the text we have focused on the anatomic and physiologic characteristics of the cardiopulmonary unit, a unit whose integrated metabolic function is responsible for the exchange and transport of the respiratory gases oxygen and carbon dioxide. The monitoring of oxygen and carbon dioxide exchange is therefore central to the evaluation of cardiopulmonary function, whether performed in the resting or in the exercising patient. In the past, these techniques were complicated, cumbersome, and time consuming. The advent of rapidly responding gas analyzers has simplified the technique considerably. Consequently, determination of the respiratory gas exchange process on a breath-by-breath basis is now possible. With proper training, these techniques can be used by practicing physicians and their paramedic personnel; they no longer need to be confined to select academic facilities. However, this cannot be accomplished without proper attention to detail and a working knowledge of the instrumentation, including its maintenance and calibration.

This chapter is designed to provide the reader with an understanding of the theory underlying the calculation of oxygen uptake ($\dot{V}O_2$) and carbon dioxide production ($\dot{V}CO_2$). From this background it will become apparent that in order to calculate $\dot{V}O_2$ and $\dot{V}CO_2$, one must be able to measure three variables in expired air: (1) the fractional amount of oxygen; (2) the fractional amount of carbon dioxide; and (3) the volume. Accordingly, this chapter will familiarize the reader with the methods and instrumentation used at present for calculating $\dot{V}O_2$ and $\dot{V}CO_2$ at rest and during exercise.

Oxygen Uptake Equation

When we breathe, a portion of the oxygen contained in atmospheric air diffuses across the alveolar capillary wall to bind with hemoglobin. Consequently, the air we expire contains a lesser amount of oxygen than the 20.9 per cent in the atmospheric air that was inspired. In order to calculate the amount of oxygen removed from the alveoli per breath, one needs to know the amount, or the volume, of oxygen present in inspired and expired air. The difference between the volume of oxygen inspired and that expired represents the oxygen that is taken up by the body for each breath:

$$O_2 \text{ Uptake per Breath} = \text{Inspired } O_2 \text{ Volume} - \text{Expired } O_2 \text{ Volume} \qquad (1)$$

It should be noted that, by convention, the volume of gas exchanged is expressed as the volume the gas would occupy as a dry gas at standard temperature (0°C) and pressure (760 mm Hg) (*Standard Temperature Pressure Dry*, or STPD). The equations for this conversion are presented in the appendix to this chapter. Inspired and expired oxygen volumes can be obtained from the inspired and expired volumes of air and their respective fractional amounts of oxygen (see Equation 2).

$$O_2 \text{ Volume} = \text{Volume of Air} \cdot \text{Fractional Amount of } O_2 \qquad (2)$$

From Equations 1 and 2, the following equation for oxygen uptake per breath ($\dot{V}O_2$) is obtained.

113

$$VO_2 = (V_I \cdot F_IO_2) - (V_E \cdot F_EO_2) \qquad (3)$$

where V_I and V_E are the inspiratory and expiratory volumes, and F_IO_2 and F_EO_2 are the fractional amounts of oxygen in the inspired and expired air, respectively. The oxygen uptake per *minute* ($\dot{V}O_2$) is obtained by multiplying equation 3 by the respiratory rate (f). If we set $\dot{V}O_2 = VO_2 \cdot f$, $\dot{V}_I = V_I \cdot f$, and $\dot{V}_E = V_E \cdot f$, then the equation for average oxygen uptake per *minute* can be written as

$$\dot{V}O_2 = (\dot{V}_I \cdot F_IO_2) - (\dot{V}_E \cdot F_EO_2) \qquad (4)$$

From Equation 4, it can be seen that the volume of air inspired and expired per minute, along with the fractional amounts of oxygen in inspired and expired air, must be known for the determination of $\dot{V}O_2$.

Instead of directly measuring both inspired and expired air volumes, however, a simpler procedure is to measure only the expired air volume, and to calculate the inspired air volume from the expired air volume and the fractional amounts of oxygen and carbon dioxide. This simplification is possible because the quantities of nitrogen and other inert gases in the atmosphere are not involved nor altered in the gas exchange process. Thus, for the inert gases we have

$$F_I \text{ (inert)} \cdot \dot{V}_I = F_E \text{ (inert)} \cdot \dot{V}_E \qquad (5)$$

where F_I (inert) and F_E (inert) represent the fractional amount of inert gases in inspired and expired air, respectively. The fractional composition of dry inspired or room air is constant and the values are as follows:

$$
\begin{aligned}
F_I \text{ (inert)} &= 0.7903 \\
F_IO_2 &= 0.2094 \qquad (6)\\
F_ICO_2 &= 0.0003
\end{aligned}
$$

For expired air, F_E (inert) can be obtained from the measured variables F_EO_2 and F_ECO_2.

$$F_E \text{ (inert)} = 1 - F_EO_2 - F_ECO_2 \qquad (7)$$

If Equations 6 and 7 are substituted into Equation 5, and Equation 5 is solved for $\dot{V}_I$, then $\dot{V}_I$ can be expressed in terms of the easily measurable quantities F_EO_2, F_ECO_2 and $\dot{V}_E$. That is,

$$\dot{V}_I = \frac{[\dot{V}_E \cdot (1 - F_EO_2 - F_ECO_2)]}{0.7903} \qquad (8)$$

Equation 4 can also be expressed in terms of these measurable quantities, by substituting Equation 8 for $\dot{V}_I$. Accordingly,

$$\dot{V}O_2 = \frac{[\dot{V}_E \cdot (1 - F_EO_2 - F_ECO_2) \cdot 0.2094]}{0.7903} - (\dot{V}_E \cdot F_EO_2) \qquad (9)$$

or

$$\dot{V}O_2 = \dot{V}_E [0.265 (1 - F_ECO_2) - 1.265\, F_EO_2] \qquad (10)$$

Both these methods (i.e., Equations 4 and 10) for obtaining $\dot{V}O_2$ are depicted in Figure 7–1. Method 1 requires the measurement of inspiratory and expiratory volumes and the fractional amount of oxygen in the expired air (see Equation 4). In method 2, the measurement of expiratory volume and the fractional amounts of oxygen and carbon dioxide in the expired air are needed (see Equation 10).

Carbon Dioxide Production Equation

The equation for carbon dioxide production per minute ($\dot{V}CO_2$) is derived in a similar fashion to that for $\dot{V}O_2$:

$$\dot{V}CO_2 = (\dot{V}_E \cdot F_ECO_2) - (\dot{V}_I \cdot F_ICO_2) \qquad (11)$$

As noted earlier, the fractional amount of inspired carbon dioxide is very small (see Equation 6) and therefore can be neglected. Accordingly, Equation 11 reduces to

$$\dot{V}CO_2 = \dot{V}_E \cdot F_ECO_2 \qquad (12)$$

Thus, $\dot{V}CO_2$ is calculated from a subset of the measurements required for the calculation of $\dot{V}O_2$.

Methods to Obtain $\dot{V}O_2$ and $\dot{V}CO_2$

Three data acquisition techniques can be used to obtain the requisite information for calculating $\dot{V}O_2$ and $\dot{V}CO_2$. These include the timed collection of expired air, a mixing chamber method, and the breath-by-breath determination of the respiratory gases. These techniques are similar in that they each require the patient to exhale through a tube so that the volume, F_EO_2 and F_ECO_2 of the expired air can be measured. This is usually accomplished by clamping the nose and having the patient breathe through a mouthpiece attached to a nonrebreathing valve (Fig. 7–2).

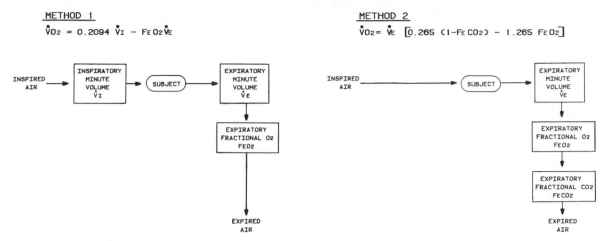

METHOD 1

$$\dot{V}O_2 = 0.2094\ \dot{V}_I - F_EO_2\dot{V}_E$$

METHOD 2

$$\dot{V}O_2 = \dot{V}_E\ [0.265\ (1 - F_ECO_2) - 1.265\ F_EO_2]$$

FIGURE 7–1. Two methods of obtaining O₂ uptake. Method 1 requires the measurements of inspiratory and expiratory minute volumes and the expiratory fractional amount of O₂; method 2 requires the measurement of expiratory minute volume and the fractional amounts of O₂ and CO₂.

As shown in Figure 7–3, the nonrebreathing valve consists of three ports, one for inspired air, one for expired air, and one for the patient. During inspiration, valve A is open and valve B is closed, allowing air to be drawn into the lungs solely through port A. During expiration the opposite occurs; valve A is closed and valve B is opened, so that all of the expired air exits through port B.

A wide selection of nonrebreathing valves is available. However, their sole function is to prevent the mixing of expired and inspired air. The choice of a particular valve should consider the trade-off between the dead-space volume of the valve and its resistance to airflow. In general, the smaller valves (ie, minimum dead-space volume) have the highest resistance. For adults, we use a Hans Rudolph valve that has a dead-space volume of 90 ml. It is possible to account for this dead space by adding a correction factor to Equations 10 and 12.[1] When this is done, Equation 10 becomes

$$\dot{V}O_2 = \dot{V}_E\ [0.265\ (1 - F_ECO_2) - 1.265\ F_EO_2] - (0.2094 - F_{ET}O_2)\ VBV \qquad (13)$$

and Equation 12 becomes

$$\dot{V}CO_2 = \dot{V}_E \cdot F_ECO_2 - F_{ET}CO_2 \cdot VBV \qquad (14)$$

Here $F_{ET}O_2$ and $F_{ET}CO_2$ are the fractional amounts of oxygen and carbon dioxide at end expiration (end-tidal), and VBV, the dead-space volume of the valve.

To obtain $\dot{V}O_2$ and $\dot{V}CO_2$ by the first method, expired air from the nonrebreathing valve passes through a large bore, low resistance tube, typically 30 mm in diameter, to one of the ports of a manual three-port valve. A meteorologic or Douglas type of bag is attached to another port, as depicted in Figure 7–4. Prior to gas collection, the bag is voided of all air and hung vertically to reduce resistance. At this point, the patient's expired air is being vented to the atmosphere via the third port. Once a steady state is achieved, the manual valve is turned so that all expired air flows into the bag. The timed collection period should last a minute or more and include a series of complete respiratory cycles, beginning and ending the collection

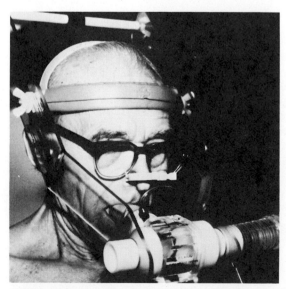

FIGURE 7–2. A patient with mouthpiece in place and nose clamped. The weight of the nonrebreathing valve and tubing is borne by the head by means of the headpiece.

FIGURE 7–3. Diagram of a non-rebreathing valve, showing the position of valves *A* and *B* during inspiration (*A* opened and *B* closed) and expiration (*A* closed and *B* opened). With inspiration, all air flows through the inspiratory port to the subject; with expiration, all air flows from the subject through the expiratory port.

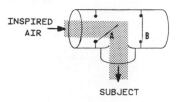

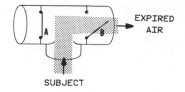

INSPIRATION   EXPIRATION

STEP 1

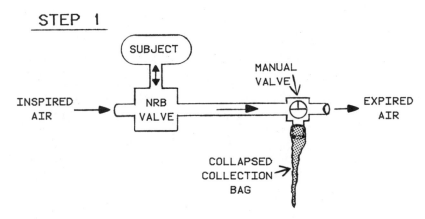

STEP 2

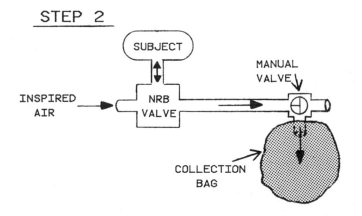

FIGURE 7–4. The three steps of the timed collection method to obtain the requisite information for calculating $\dot{V}O_2$ and $\dot{V}CO_2$. In step 1, all expired air that flows from the nonrebreathing (*NRB*) valve is exhausted to the atmosphere. In step 2, the manual valve is rotated so that all expired air flows into the bag. Finally, in step 3, the volume, O_2, and CO_2 of the collected gas are measured.

STEP 3

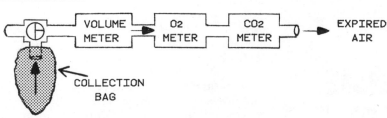

period at the same point in the respiratory cycle, preferably during inspiration. After the sample has been collected, the bag should be squeezed to ensure good mixing of the gas. The fractional amounts of oxygen and carbon dioxide are then measured along with the volume of collected gas. When the volume is being measured, it is important to record the temperature of the gas and then to calculate the volume at body temperature. The volume of gas in the lungs is, by convention, reported at body temperature (BT) and pressure (P) and saturated with water vapor (S) or *Body Temperature Pressure Saturated* (BTPS), even though it is measured at ambient temperature (AT) and pressure and saturated with water vapor (*Ambient Temperature Pressure Saturated*, or ATPS). The procedure for converting volume from ATPS to BTPS is presented in the appendix to this chapter.

From the above method, the average $\dot{V}O_2$ and $\dot{V}CO_2$ for the time period of gas collection are obtained. It is possible to use this technique during progressive exercise, provided the time interval of each work level is sufficiently long to ensure adequate time for the attainment of a steady state and for the subsequent collection of a number of expired volumes. If the change in the level of work is not too large (eg, <25 watts) then 2-minute work intervals should suffice. To use this method during progressive exercise, one obviously needs to have on hand a number of deflated bags that could be quickly incorporated into the system following completion of each gas collection. Measurements of volume and the fractional amounts of oxygen and carbon dioxide are then made following the completion of the exercise protocol.

While the above technique is relatively inexpensive and uncomplicated, there are several inherent disadvantages. Shorter "non–steady-state" testing protocols cannot be used.[2] End-tidal measurements of oxygen and carbon dioxide cannot be obtained, and, as a result, it is not possible to correct for the dead space of the nonrebreathing valve

(Equations 13 and 14). Moreover, it will not be known during the exercise test whether the subjects crossed their anaerobic threshold or achieved their maximum $\dot{V}O_2$. Instead, one must wait for the completion of the protocol before analyzing the collected gases. In addition, because of the paucity of gas-exchange data (ie, one set of data per work level), the determination of the anaerobic threshold and maximum $\dot{V}O_2$ may not be possible. The criteria for determining the anaerobic threshold and maximum $\dot{V}O_2$ are given in Chapter 10.

The second method of obtaining $\dot{V}O_2$ and $\dot{V}CO_2$ makes use of a mixing chamber, so that mixed expired air can be continuously analyzed. A schematic representation of this technique is presented in Figure 7–5. Expired air from the nonrebreathing valve flows through a tube into the mixing chamber. Typically, the volume of the mixing chamber is between 5 and 10 liters. The required size of the chamber depends on the intended application. In general, the larger the chamber, the more complete the mixing of expired gases. However, the responsiveness to variations in gas composition is greatly reduced because of the increased "wash-out" time. Gas mixing is facilitated by including a number of strategically placed baffles within the chamber, which the expired air encounters en route from the input to the output port (Fig. 7–6).

Volume, temperature, and the fractional amounts of oxygen and carbon dioxide in the expired gas are measured distal to the output port of the chamber. An absence of respiratory variations in the fractional amounts of oxygen and carbon dioxide is indicative of adequate mixing. Expired gas volume can be measured either directly (eg, via Tissot spirometer) or indirectly by integrating the measured flow of expired gas. The SensorMedics Horizon System is an example of a commercially available integrated system that uses a mixing chamber. A diagram depicting the flow of expired gas through this system is presented in Figure 7–7.

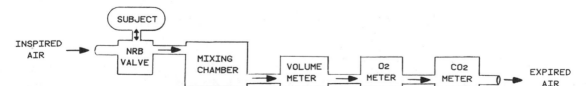

FIGURE 7–5. The mixing chamber technique to obtain $\dot{V}O_2$ and $\dot{V}CO_2$. All expired air flows from the nonrebreathing (*NRB*) valve to the mixing chamber where it is thoroughly mixed. From there the mixed air is continuously sampled for its O_2 and CO_2 content, and the minute ventilation is measured.

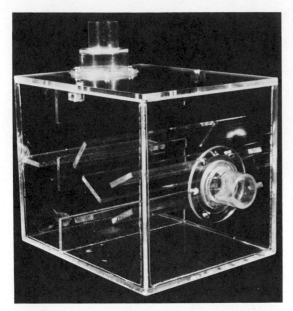

FIGURE 7–6. A mixing chamber. The internal arrangement of baffles ensures complete mixing of the expired air. The top port is the input to and the side port is the output of the mixing chamber.

The advantages of the mixing chamber method over the timed gas collection technique are the ability to acquire more data for a given workload and to have some of the results displayed during the exercise test. For example, the Horizon System provides a graphic display of $\dot{V}O_2$, $\dot{V}CO_2$, and $\dot{V}_E$ during the exercise test. Consequently, the anaerobic threshold and maximal $\dot{V}O_2$ are easier to discern. Moreover, the cumbersome task of replacing bags following each timed collection is eliminated, thereby allowing the technician to perform other duties during the exercise test. These advantages are not without cost, because a recording device for the continuously measured data is needed. As is the case with timed collections, it is not possible with the mixing-chamber method to acquire end-tidal measurements of oxygen and carbon dioxide and to use shorter "non-steady-state" testing protocols. Also, with intense workloads, the data may become inaccurate because of inadequate mixing at higher $\dot{V}_E$.

The breath-by-breath method provides the most comprehensive representation of the gas exchange response during exercise. As depicted in Figure 7–8, air is removed from the nonrebreathing valve at a constant rate of 200 to 500 ml/min and delivered to the oxygen and carbon dioxide analyzers for a continuous determination of the percentages of these two gases in expired air. Expiratory flow, $\dot{V}(t)$, is also continuously measured.

An example of typical breath-by-breath $O_2(t)$, $CO_2(t)$ and $\dot{V}(t)$ data is given in Figure

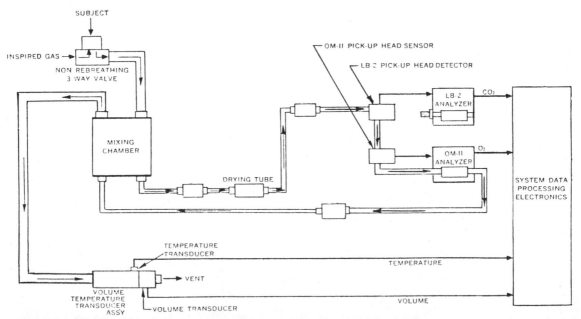

FIGURE 7–7. Gas flow diagram for a SensorMedics Horizon System. Expired air flows to the mixing chamber and then to the volume, temperature transducer assembly. In addition, air from the mixing chamber is pumped to the OM-11 and LB-2 analyzers for measurement of O_2 and CO_2, respectively. The volume, O_2, and CO_2 data are then supplied to the system computer for the calculation of $\dot{V}O_2$ and $\dot{V}CO_2$.

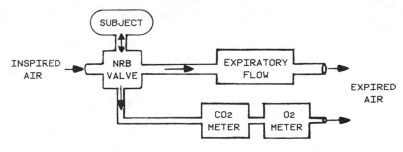

FIGURE 7–8. The breath-by-breath method of measuring volume, O_2, and CO_2 for the subsequent calculation of $\dot{V}O_2$ and $\dot{V}CO_2$. The flow of expired air is continuously measured. In addition, air is continuously removed from the nonrebreathing (NRB) valve at a rate of 200 to 500 ml/min and pumped through the CO_2 and O_2 analyzers.

7–9. As can be seen, there are inherent time delays in the measurement of $O_2(t)$ and $CO_2(t)$ with respect to $\dot{V}(t)$. Consequently, $O_2(t)$ and $CO_2(t)$ have to be shifted by their respective delays before expiratory volume (V_E) and the fractional amounts of expired O_2 (F_EO_2) and CO_2 (F_ECO_2) can be computed as follows:

$$V_E = \int \dot{V}(t) \cdot dt \qquad (15)$$

$$F_EO_2 = \int \dot{V}(t) \cdot O_2(t) \cdot dt \qquad (16)$$

$$F_ECO_2 = \int \dot{V}(t) \cdot CO_2(t) \cdot dt \qquad (17)$$

Here the integrations are evaluated from the onset to the end of expiration. Average minute ventilation, $\dot{V}_E$, is obtained by multiplying V_E by the respiratory rate, which is the reciprocal of the respiratory cycle time in seconds multiplied by 60 sec/min. These calculated values are then substituted into Equations 13 and 14 to yield $\dot{V}O_2$ and $\dot{V}CO_2$.

Owing to the large amount of measured data and subsequent calculations, a computer and a rather sophisticated computer program are required for the breath-by-breath method. The associated costs are therefore much greater than are those of the other two methods. On the other hand, for this additional cost the limitations of the other two methods no longer exist. That is, nonsteady-state exercise tests can be performed, end-tidal data are readily available, and the anaerobic threshold and $\dot{V}O_2$ max are clearly delineated during testing (see Chapter 10).

From the foregoing discussion it is clear that in order to measure $\dot{V}O_2$ and $\dot{V}CO_2$ one must be able to measure the fractional amounts of oxygen and carbon dioxide in expired air as well as the volume of expired air. Rather than an extensive review of the available instrumentation for the measurement of these variables, a brief discussion of the instruments that we currently use will be presented. For a more complete listing of pulmonary and respiratory equipment and manufacturers, the reader is referred to the annual review that appears in *Medical Electronics*.[3]

Oxygen Analyzer

The acquisition of breath-by-breath gas exchange data during exercise has been possible only within the past 15 years following

FIGURE 7–9. Typical breath-by-breath data of per cent O_2, per cent CO_2, and flow ($\dot{V}$). During inspiration, $\dot{V}$ is zero because the expiratory valve of the nonrebreathing valve is closed. *a* and *b* represent the delay times for per cent CO_2 and O_2, respectively. These delays are due to the transport time of the gas and the inherent response time of the analyzer. The delay for per cent O_2 is greater because the two analyzers were coupled in series with the CO_2 analyzer first receiving the gas.

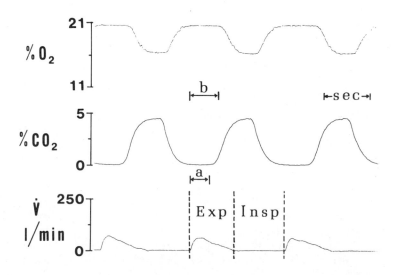

the development of a relatively inexpensive, rapidly responding, oxygen analyzer. Prior to that, only manometric (eg, Scholander or Haldane) methods that require careful technique and are subject to error from many sources, the slow responding oxygen analyzer (eg, paramagnetic oxygen meter), and the mass spectrometer were available. Although the mass spectrometer has an extremely fast response, a low sampling flow, and a freedom from interference by other gases, it is expensive, bulky, and complex to use. Also, it is sensitive to water vapor, thus requiring the drying of the expired gas prior to analysis. For these reasons, the mass spectrometer, despite its fast response time, is not commonly used to measure the composition of expired air.

With the timed collection technique there is no need for a rapidly responding system, and one need only be concerned with the accuracy of the oxygen measuring device. As mentioned earlier, the manometric methods require careful technique and a great deal of time. When using electronic oxygen analyzers, care must be taken either to dry the gas or to correct for the water vapor pressure. In addition, the accuracy of all electronic analyzers is only as good as the calibration techniques and the quality of the calibration gas. The oxygen concentration of the calibration gas should be known to within ± 0.03 per cent. In this respect, the manometric techniques remain the "gold standard," because gas supply firms use these techniques to analyze the composition of the calibration gases they market.

Both the mixing chamber and breath-by-breath methods require an electronic oxygen analyzer with a linear output. Although accuracy and linearity are important to both techniques, a fast response time is much more critical to the breath-by-breath method.

Several types of oxygen analyzers have sufficiently rapid response times for breath-by-breath analysis. These include the mass spectrometer, the polarographic electrode, the fuel cell oxygen analyzer, and the rapid paramagnetic analyzer. We have had the opportunity to use the OM-11 oxygen analyzer in a custom-built system. It is also incorporated in the SensorMedics Horizon System. We currently use the Medical Graphics System 2000, which uses the Applied Electrochemistry, Incorporated, oxygen analyzer (model S-3A).

The OM-11 uses the polarographic oxygen sensor, which consists of a gold cathode and a silver anode. These two electrodes are mounted behind a thin Teflon membrane that is permeable to oxygen, and are immersed in a buffered potassium chloride gel. In operation, a polarizing voltage is applied across the electrodes, and the resultant current flow is directly proportional to the partial pressure of oxygen. The sensor is insensitive to temperature, to all other gases normally associated with respiration, and to water vapor. Its output is linear over the entire range (ie, 0 to 100 per cent oxygen), and the response time (ie, the time required for the output of the instrument to reach 90 per cent of the final value, following a step change in the input) is short, typically 100 msec. This response time implies that for a respiratory rate in excess of 130 breaths per minute, the measured value of end-tidal oxygen is in error by approximately 0.2 per cent.

The S-3A oxygen analyzer has characteristics similar to the OM-11, but the principle of operation is different. Its sensor contains a zirconium oxide high-temperature electrochemical cell. The cell is heated to 750°C, and whenever the oxygen partial pressures on the inside and outside (ie, room air) of the sensor are different, a voltage proportional to the difference is generated.

It should be noted that, although the output of these oxygen analyzers is a percentage, they are in the strictest sense partial pressure–sensing devices. However, for a given barometric pressure, the percentage of oxygen is simply the ratio of the partial pressure of oxygen to the barometric pressure. The factor for the conversion from partial pressure to pecentage is adjusted by the instrument gain at the time of calibration. That is, the gain is adjusted so that the instrument displays the correct percentage of oxygen in the calibration gas, thereby taking into account the existing barometric pressure. Accordingly, the analyzer should be recalibrated if there is a sudden change in barometric pressure (ie, the passing of a weather front).

In an integrated gas-exchange system, the design of the interconnections to the gas-sensing units is already optimized by the manufacturer of the system. However, if one were to assemble one's own system, then the type, diameter, and length of interconnecting tubing and the rate of air flow through the sensors are important considerations. The major portions of the oxygen and carbon dioxide delays in Figure 7–9 are due to the time required to transport the sample

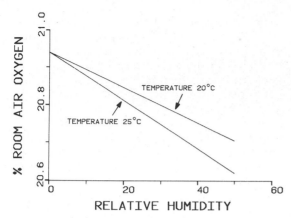

FIGURE 7–10. Per cent room air oxygen plotted versus relative humidity for two temperatures.

of gas from the nonrebreathing valve to the oxygen and carbon dioxide sensors.

Since the two oxygen analyzers just described actually are measuring the partial pressure of oxygen, one need not be concerned with correcting for water vapor. For example, if the room temperature was 25°C and the relative humidity 38 per cent, then the percentage of room air oxygen displayed by the analyzer would be 20.7 per cent. The linear, inverse relations between per cent oxygen in room air and relative humidity for two ambient temperatures, 20°C and 25°C, are given in Figure 7–10.

Carbon Dioxide Analyzer

Carbon dioxide is usually measured with an infrared analyzer, although it also can be measured with a mass spectrometer. As mentioned earlier, however, the mass spectrometer is not commonly used to measure the composition of expired air. With respect to the two integrated systems mentioned previously, the SensorMedics Horizon System incorporates the LB-2 Medical Gas CO_2 Analyzer, and the Medical Graphics System 2000 uses the Datex Instrumentation CD102 Normocap CO_2 monitor, both of which are infrared analyzers.

The infrared technique of measuring carbon dioxide is based on the fact that carbon dioxide absorbs energy from a specific portion of the infrared spectrum. The radiation from the gas in the measuring chamber is then compared with the radiation from a known gas mixture in a reference chamber. The difference, which is measured electronically, is proportional to the partial pressure of carbon dioxide in the gas being sampled.

The reference and the manner by which the difference in radiation is converted to an electric signal varies from manufacturer to manufacturer. Most manufacturers, however, report a rapid response time. For example, the typical time required for the LB-2 to reach 90 per cent of the final value, following a step change in carbon dioxide, is 100 msec. The carbon dioxide analyzers are linear over the 0 to 10 per cent carbon dioxide range, with the accuracy ranging from ±0.2 per cent (CD102) to ±2.0 per cent (LB-2).

Even though the infrared analyzer is specifically sensitive to carbon dioxide, other organic compounds have overlapping bands of infrared absorption that will interfere with their measurement. The anesthetic gas nitrous oxide, for example, produces infrared absorption peaks on both sides of the carbon dioxide peak and will interfere with the measurement of carbon dioxide. Although this is not normally a problem with room air, one should be aware of it, particularly if special gas mixtures are used. If there is any doubt, the reference manual or the manufacturer should be consulted.

Measurement of Volume

There are numerous techniques for measuring gas volume, consisting of those that directly measure displacement of volume (eg, the water-seal metal bell spirometer) and those that derive volume by integrating a flow signal (eg, the pneumotachygraph). Regardless of its application, the measuring device should be stable for the testing period, and in the case of exercise testing, it should be accurate over the wide range of volumes and flow rates encountered during light, moderate, and heavy exercise (Chapter 10). Moreover, because the mixing chamber and breath-by-breath methods require the continuous measurement of volume, the device should have a low resistance, a low inertia, and a sufficiently rapid response time.

In 1979, the American Thoracic Society recommended the following minimum requirements for the measurement of the forced expiratory volume in 1 second (FEV_1): the volume measuring device should have a range of 7 liters and an accuracy of ±3 per cent of the measured value, or 50 ml, whichever is greater for flows of 0 to 12 liters/sec; and a resistance of less than 1.5 cm H_2O/liter/sec at a flow of 12 liters/sec.[4]

Regardless of the type of volume-measuring device, spirometers can be used to measure respiratory volume in conjunction with the timed collection and mixing chamber methods for measuring $\dot{V}O_2$ and $\dot{V}CO_2$. However, only the spirometers that directly measure displacement of volume are used for this purpose; the other types are used exclusively for pulmonary function testing. Those that directly measure volume are limited by their maximum volume capacity. For example, the Stead Wells (Warren E. Collins, Inc.) has a 10-liter capacity; the Jones Pulmonor, a 7-liter capacity; and the Tissot (Warren E. Collins, Inc.) a 50- to 600-liter capacity. Consequently, the ventilation record must be interrupted whenever the maximum capacity is reached, in order to vent and reset the spirometer. Obviously, the smaller the capacity of the spirometer, the less suitable it is for the measurement of respiratory volume during exercise.

The indirect method of obtaining volume from an integrated flow signal is best suited for continuously monitoring ventilation and can be used with either the mixing chamber or the breath-by-breath method. The most popular techniques for measuring respiratory flow are based on thermal dissipation (hot-wire anemometer), pressure drop (pneumotachygraph), and the rotating vane (turbine).

The thermal dissipation technique uses a thermistor that is maintained at a constant temperature (200 to 220°C) by the associated electronic circuitry. Airflow across the thermistor reduces temperature. This reduction is electronically sensed and the heating current to the thermistor is increased to compensate for the loss. Thus, airflow is proportional to the thermistor current. The relation between airflow and thermistor current, however, is nonlinear, necessitating the use of linearizing circuits. Advantages of this technique include its insensitivity to changes in ambient and gas temperatures, barometric pressure, and water vapor. On the other hand, stability can be a problem, and frequent calibration is necessary to maintain consistent performance. In addition, this device cannot distinguish between forward and backward airflow.

The pneumotachygraph is a device that creates a small resistance to the flow of gas so as to create a measurable pressure drop. Resistance is produced either by a fine mesh screen or by a bundle of small diameter tubes. As long as flow is laminar, the pressure difference across the resistance is linearly related to the flow. The differential pressures that are induced, however, are not large; and a sensitive pressure transducer, such as the Validyne model MP 45-1 with a minimum operating range of ± 2 cm H_2O, is needed. Most pneumotachygraphs can be heated to body temperature in order to prevent condensation at the resistance site and to eliminate the need to measure temperature. We have found this device to be extremely stable with virtually no day-to-day variation in the calibration, and, unlike the hot-wire anemometer, it can distinguish the direction of flow.

The rotating vane flowmeter is a unidirectional flow-sensing device, consisting of a delicately balanced turbine that is caused to rotate by the flow of gas. The rotational speed of the turbine is directly proportional to the volumetric flow rate. The manner by which the number of revolutions are counted varies among the various rotating vane flowmeters. The SensorMedics Horizon System, for example, uses a light-sensing technique to count revolutions. As the turbine blade rotates, it interrupts a light beam that falls on a phototransistor. The result is a train of pulses, the number of pulses being proportional to the number of revolutions. These pulses are integrated to yield an accumulating volume. Other designs use a magnet mounted in the rotor, which induces a pulsating current in a pick-up coil mounted in the housing. The resulting pulses are then amplified and integrated. When tested for its ability to measure volume, this type of flowmeter was found to be accurate to within 2 per cent of the actual volume as measured by the Tissot spirometer. It is as stable as the pneumotachygraph, and its output is linear in the range of 3 to 600 liters/minute.

The application of the ultrasonic flowmeter to the measurement of respiratory gas flow has been achieved.[5] This type of flowmeter consists of two ultrasound transducers; each transducer acts alternately as transmitter and receiver. The velocity of the gas is detected by sending an ultrasonic or high-frequency (100 KHz) wave back and forth between the transducers and measuring the phase shift between the transmitted and received waves. The advantages are many and include a fast response time, no moving parts, little obstruction to flow, insensitivity to gas composition, a linear output in the range 0 to 200 liters/min, and an ability to measure flow in both directions.

Calibration of these direct and indirect volume-measuring devices consists of varying volume or flow by known amounts and of recording and adjusting the output of the volume-sensing device. Calibration syringes up to 3 liters are available (eg, Hans-Rudolph) for varying volumes by a known amount. To obtain a calibration curve, the output of the syringe can be adjusted to within ±50 ml for any amount between 0 and 3 liters. Flowmeters can also be calibrated using this syringe. That is, known syringe volumes can be imposed at different flow rates (ie, average flow rate equals volume infused divided by infusion time). The flowmeter output is then integrated to obtain the average output that is equated to the average flow rate. It can also be directly calibrated if a constant, known flow source is available. Many laboratories use a homemade flow-calibrating system consisting of a rotameter flowmeter and a vacuum cleaner, as depicted in Figure 7–11. Flow rate to the device is adjusted by varying the position of the flow regulatory valve. The rotameter is a tapered glass tube with a calibrated float having a constant cross-sectional area. As the flow rate varies, the float moves up or down in the tube to maintain a constant pressure drop across the anular orifice. With proper calibration of the float position, the tube can be marked to give flow readings directly.

Metabolic Rate ($\dot{V}O_2$) Monitor

The Waters Instrument Company manufactures a portable device for the direct and continuous measurement of $\dot{V}O_2$. This instrument was referred to as the metabolic rate monitor (MRM) by its developers Webb and Troutman.[6] As shown in Figure 7–12, the blower draws ambient air through the face mask to a polarographic oxygen sensor. The flow of air is servocontrolled so as to keep the partial pressure of oxygen (pO_2) at the sensor constant. For example, if $\dot{V}O_2$ suddenly increased, there would be a drop in pO_2 at the sensor and an increase in the error signal (i.e., the difference between pO_2 of ambient air and pO_2 of the sensor). This error signal increases the speed of the blower, thereby drawing in more room air via the air mask and raising the sensor pO_2. This process continues until the error signal is zero. If the respiratory gas exchange ratio (R) is assumed to be 1, then it can be shown that $\dot{V}O_2$ is equal to 0.01 times the volume flow through the blower.[6] The error associated with this assumption, ranges from +3.2 per cent to −3.2 per cent, as R varies between 0.8 and 1.2. When tested against the timed gas collection method, the calculated values for $\dot{V}O_2$ were within ±0.1 liter/min for values up to 3 liters/min.

The advantages of this instrument are its portability and its ease of operation. Accordingly, it can be used to measure $\dot{V}O_2$ of patients during actual or simulated activities (eg, household chores). The fact that only $\dot{V}O_2$ is measured can be considered a possible disadvantage, unless the aerobic capacity of the subject or patient was determined previously. In addition, it typically takes more than a minute to ascertain whether a steady state has been reached following an increase in $\dot{V}O_2$.

APPENDIX

Converting Gas Volumes to Standard Conditions

In calculating $\dot{V}O_2$ and $\dot{V}CO_2$, the gas volumes must be converted to standard condi-

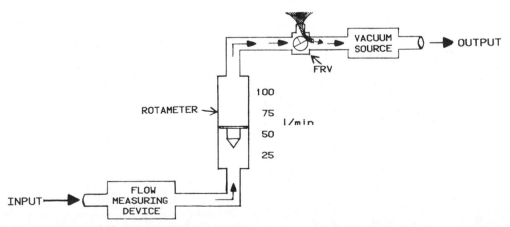

FIGURE 7–11. Apparatus for calibrating flow-measuring devices. Flow through the device is varied by means of a flow regulatory valve (*FRV*). Flow is measured by a rotameter and plotted versus the output of the device.

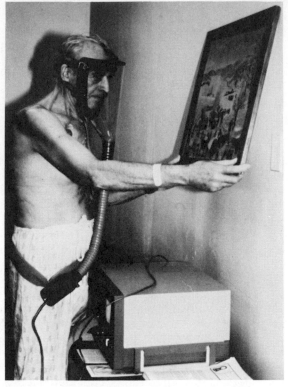
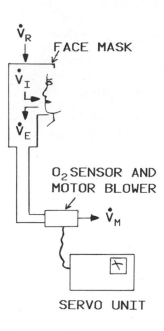

FIGURE 7–12. The metabolic rate monitor. Room air enters the face mask at a rate $\dot{V}_R$. $\dot{V}_I$ is the inspiratory air flow; $\dot{V}_E$, the expiratory air flow; and $\dot{V}_M$, the flow of air through the blower (see text).

tions in order to be proportional to grams or moles of gas exchanged. The conventional standard conditions are a temperature of 0°C, or 273°K; a pressure of 760 mmHg, and a perfectly dry gas. These conditions are commonly abbreviated as STPD (Standard Temperature Pressure Dry.)

When obtaining the gas-exchange response, volume is usually measured on wet expired air under variable room (ambient) conditions, where the pressure is the barometric pressure (P_A) and the temperature is that at the site of measurement (T_A). These conditions are abbreviated ATPS (Ambient Temperature Pressure Saturated). To convert volume from ATPS to STPD, we make use of the general gas law, which states that gas pressure (P) multiplied by gas volume (V) and divided by gas temperature (T) is equal to the gas constant R, or

$$\frac{P \cdot V}{T} = R \qquad \text{(A-1)}$$

Accordingly, for *ambient* conditions we have

$$\frac{P_A \cdot V_A}{T_A} = R \qquad \text{(A-2)}$$

and for *standard* condition we have

$$\frac{P_S \cdot V_S}{T_S} = R \qquad \text{(A-3)}$$

Combining Equations A-2 and A-3 yields

$$\frac{P_S \cdot V_S}{T_S} = \frac{P_A \cdot V_A}{T_A} \qquad \text{(A-4)}$$

Because the number of water molecules in a wet gas varies with temperature and total pressure, the ambient or barometric pressure must be corrected for water vapor pressure $P_{A(H_2O)}$

$$\frac{P_S \cdot V_S}{T_S} = (P_A - P_{A(H_2O)}) \cdot \frac{V_A}{T_A} \qquad \text{(A-5)}$$

Since standard conditions are those obtained with a dry gas, a similar correction to P_S is not necessary. In addition, we can substitute 760 mmHg for P_S and 273°K for T_S. Solving for V_S then results in the derived equation for correcting a volume measured at ATPS to one measured at STPD:

Volume at STPD = Volume at ATPS ·

$$\left[\frac{P_A - P_{A(H_2O)}}{760 \text{ mmHg}}\right] \cdot \left[\frac{273}{273 + T_A}\right] \quad \text{(A-6)}$$

where P_A is barometric pressure, and $P_{A(H_2O)}$ is the water vapor pressure of saturated air at temperature T_A measured in degrees centigrade.

In reporting tidal volume or minute ventilation, it is conventional to calculate the conditions existing within the lung. The conventional body conditions are body temperature (37°C), the barometric pressure (P_A), and saturation with water vapor. These conditions are abbreviated BTPS (*Body Temperature Pressure Saturated*).

The conversion equation for changing volumes measured at ATPS to equivalent volumes at BTPS is derived in a similar fashion as in Equation A-6. This equation can be written as

Volume at BTPS = Volume at ATPS ·

$$\left[\frac{P_A - P_{A(H_2O)}}{P_A - P_{B(H_2O)}}\right] \cdot \left[\frac{273 + 37°C}{273 + T_A}\right] \quad \text{(A-7)}$$

Here, $P_{B(H_2O)}$ is the water vapor pressure of fully saturated gas at 37°C, which is equal to 47 mm Hg. Therefore, Equation A-7 becomes

Volume at BTPS = Volume at ATPS ·

$$\left[\frac{P_A - P_{A(H_2O)}}{P_A - 47 \text{ mmHg}}\right] \cdot \left[\frac{310}{273 + T_A}\right] \quad \text{(A-8)}$$

MANUFACTURERS CITED

1. Applied Electrochemistry, Incorporated
   735 North Pastoria Avenue
   Sunnyvale, California 94086

2. Warren E. Collins, Incorporated
   220 Wood Road
   Braintree Massachusettes 02184

3. Datex Instrumentation OY
   P.O. Box 357 00101
   Helsinki 10 Finland

4. Medical Graphics Corporation
   501 West Country Road E
   St. Paul, Minnesota 55112

5. Hans Rudolph
   7200 Wyandotte
   Kansas City, Missouri 64114

6. SensorMedics Corporation
   1630 South State College Boulevard
   Anaheim, California 92806

7. Validyne Engineering Corporation
   19414 Londelius Street
   Northridge, California 91324

8. Waters Instruments, Incorporated
   2411 Seventh Street, N.W.
   Rochester, Minnesota 55901

REFERENCES

1. Beaver WL, Wasserman K, Whipp BJ: On-line computer analysis and breath-by-breath graphical display of exercise function tests. J Appl Physiol 34:128 132, 1973.
2. Whipp BJ, Davis JA, Torres F, Wasserman K: A test to determine parameters of aerobic function during exercise. J Appl Physiol 50:217–221, 1981.
3. Aronson MH (ed). Pulmonary-Respiratory. Med Electronics 84:162–179, 1983.
4. Gardner RM (Chmn). ATS statement—Snowbird workshop on standardization of spirometry. Am Rev Respir Dis 119:831–838, 1979.
5. Kou AH, Peickert WR, Polenske EE, Busby MG: A pulsed phase measurement ultrasonic flowmeter for medical gases. Ann Biomed Eng 12:263–280, 1984.
6. Webb P, Troutman SJ Jr: An instrument for continuous measurement of oxygen consumption. J Appl Physiol 28:867–871, 1970.

8

JOSEPH S. JANICKI
SANJEEV G. SHROFF
KARL T. WEBER

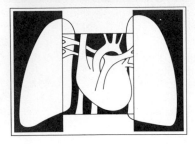

Instrumentation for Monitoring Respiratory Gas Transport

In addition to the gas exchange process in the lung, oxygen must be transported throughout the body, and the carbon dioxide produced by the metabolizing tissues must be returned to the lung. Thus, the heart and circulatory system can be viewed as part of the body's gas transport system. To assess the status of the system and its response during exercise, the following measurements are possible with present technology: intrathoracic (ie, esophageal pressure), intravascular, and intracardiac pressures; cardiac output; regional blood flow; arterial and venous blood oxygen saturations; and arterial and venous blood lactate concentrations. Note that the measurement of instantaneous cardiac chamber volumes, which is essential for a complete evaluation of the gas transport system, presently cannot be made during upright, progressive exercise. This chapter is devoted to a discussion of the techniques and equipment used to characterize the response of the gas transport system during progressive exercise.

PRESSURE

To measure pressure at a particular point in the cardiovascular system, a catheter capable of transmitting this pressure to a transducer or one with the transducer mounted on its tip must be positioned at the site of interest.[1] The transducers then convert the pressure into an electrical signal for amplification, recording, and display (Fig. 8–1). Figure 8–1 shows the three types of pressure catheters available for human use.

Regardless of which catheter system is used, however, a means of calibration must be available. Typically, the mercury manometer is used for this purpose, as depicted in Figure 8–2. The calibration procedure consists of exposing the transducer to a known (manometrically measured) pressure and adjusting the gain of the electronics to give the desired deflection on the recording system. Finally, the linearity of the system over the range of pressures to be measured is checked

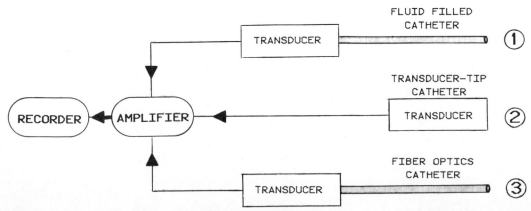

FIGURE 8–1. The three types of catheters available for measuring pressure in humans. Once the pressure is transduced into an electrical signal, the signal is amplified and then recorded.

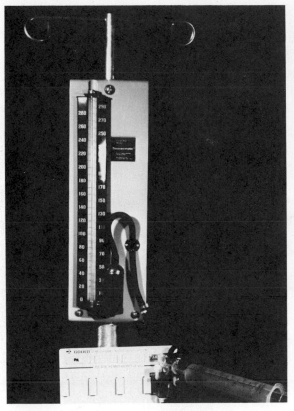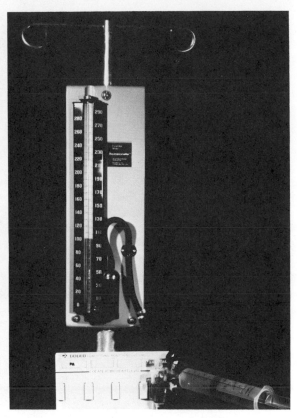

FIGURE 8–2. The apparatus used for calibrating a pressure transducer. Pressure in the system is varied by means of the syringe. The output of the transducer is then compared with the level of the mercury column. Left picture, 0 mm Hg; right, 100 mm Hg.

by exposing the transducer to several other known pressures within this range.

Fluid-Filled Catheter

All our exercise hemodynamic studies have been performed using the fluid-filled catheter; in particular, a 5 or 7 French (each French unit is equal to 0.33 millimeter; Table 8–1) triple lumen, thermodilution, flotation catheter (Fig. 8–3). This catheter is designed to allow measurement of pulmonary arterial pressure via the distal port, right atrial pressure via the proximal port, and thermodilution cardiac output via a thermistor mounted between the ports when its tip is positioned in the pulmonary artery. In addition, when the balloon at the tip of the catheter (Fig. 8–3) is inflated, it wedges the catheter in a smaller pulmonary artery. Fluoroscopically, the tip of the catheter appears to have little motion when it is in the wedged position. Once wedged, the pulmonary capillary wedge pressure, which reflects left atrial pressure, is measured via the distal port. Details regarding the insertion and position-

ing of the catheter and examples of pressure recordings are presented in Chapter 6. In addition to these pressures, we have also measured radial artery pressure during exercise, using a 20 gauge (Table 8–2), over-the-needle Teflon catheter.

Also apparent in the examples of pressure recordings given in Chapter 6 are the respiratory variations; with each inspiration the pressures shift downward by 5 to 10 mm Hg, reflecting the decrease in intrathoracic pres-

Table 8–1. Catheter Dimensions

French Size	Outside Diameter (mm)	Inside Diameter (mm)	Lumen Area (mm²)
2	0.66	—	—
3	1.00	—	—
4	1.33	0.78	0.48
5	1.67	0.97	0.74
6	2.00	1.19	1.11
7	2.33	1.42	1.58
8	2.67	1.65	2.14
9	3.00	1.88	2.78
10	3.33	2.11	3.50

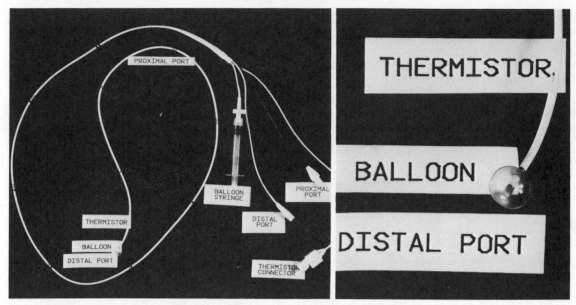

FIGURE 8–3. Left, a triple lumen, flotation thermodilution catheter. Right, a close-up of the catheter tip.

sure. In analyzing the data, the pressure values should be obtained at or near the end of expiration since the difference between intrathoracic and atmospheric pressure at this point in the respiratory cycle is at a minimum and the vascular resistance of the pulmonary circulation is at its nadir. Accordingly, intravascular pressures at the end of expiration are reasonable approximations of transmural pressures (that is, with respect to intrathoracic pressure).

Intrathoracic pressure during exercise can be determined indirectly from measurements of pressure within the lower esophagus. These measurements can be made without surgical intervention and have been shown

to be a reliable estimate of intrathoracic pressure.[2] The most common method for obtaining esophageal pressure utilizes an air-filled latex balloon (Hyatt Esophageal Balloon) sealed over a catheter that transmits balloon pressure to a pressure transducer. Traditionally, air has been used as the medium for transmitting pressure to the transducer when measuring esophageal pressure. However, the principles of measurement are the same as with the fluid-filled catheter system. Typically, the balloon is about 10 cm in length and 1 to 2 cm in diameter. It is introduced through the nose into the esophagus and, in adults, placed so that the balloon tip is about 45 cm from the nares. The balloon is then inflated with 5 to 10 ml of air to distend its walls evenly. Following this, the air is withdrawn until only 0.2 ml remains. For this size of balloon and balloon volume, esophageal pressure has been found to reflect closely the local absolute pleural pressure.[2]

A strain gauge transducer is used in conjunction with the fluid-filled catheter system. We routinely use the Gould Model T4812-AD disposable pressure transducer, although there are numerous transducers of similar quality.[3] The transducer consists of three parts: a fluid-filled dome, a diaphragm, and a strain gauge. The dome has two ports, one for the catheter and the other for debubbling and zero reference. For accurate pressure recordings, one should visually inspect the transducer to ensure that all air bubbles have been removed. The strain gauge or resistance

Table 8–2. Needle Dimensions

Gauge	Outside Diameter (mm)	Inside Diameter (mm)*	Lumen Area (mm²)
24	0.56	0.30	0.07
23	0.64	0.33	0.09
22	0.71	0.41	0.13
21	0.81	0.51	0.20
20	0.89	0.58	0.27
19	1.07	0.69	0.37
18	1.27	0.81	0.52
17	1.47	1.04	0.85
16	1.65	1.19	1.12
15	1.82	1.37	1.48
14	2.11	1.60	2.01
13	2.41	1.80	2.55
12	2.77	2.16	3.39
11	3.05	2.39	4.48

*Regular wall thickness.

wire is bonded to the nonfluid side of the diaphragm. The resistance wire forms one arm of an electronic bridge circuit. When the diaphragm is deformed by a change in pressure on its fluid side, the resistance of the strain gauge is changed and the bridge circuit becomes unbalanced. The amount of current required to rebalance the bridge circuit is proportional to the change in pressure. This change in bridge current is then amplified to a level suitable for recording.

When a triple lumen catheter is used, it is possible to obtain right atrial and pulmonary arterial pressures with only one transducer, as shown in Figure 8–4. The advantage of this arrangement is reduced cost and simplicity. The disadvantage is a disruption of one pressure recording to record the other. This, however, is not a serious problem if the stage of exercise is sufficiently long to permit the attainment of a steady state. For example, using the 2 minute stages of our incremental treadmill protocol (Chapter 9), we have found pulmonary artery pressure to reach a steady state within the first minute of each stage. Accordingly, during the second minute we are able to measure sequentially mean and pulsatile pulmonary artery pressures, pulmonary capillary wedge pressure, and mean and pulsatile right atrial pressures. Each pressure is recorded for several respiratory cycles.

The measurement of pressure with a fluid-filled system requires a reference zero pressure level that depends on the location of the distal end of the catheter. Generally, the procedure for obtaining a reference zero is to place the transducer at the same level as the tip or distal port of the catheter. In doing this, the possibility of an error caused by the hydrostatic pressure in the fluid-filled catheter is avoided. It is easy to demonstrate this type of error. For example, if the reference zero is obtained with a subject sitting, one would note an upward shift of the pressure as the subject stands up. That is, the tip of the catheter becomes higher than the transducer, and a hydrostatic pressure is gener-

ated because of the catheter fluid column that now lies above the transducer. The addition of this hydrostatic pressure causes the pressure recording to shift upward. The hydrostatic pressure can be seen to disappear as the transducer is raised to the same level as the distal pressure port. Although the location of the distal port is not known exactly with respect to an external reference, it is common practice to adjust the height of the transducer to the midheart level. When the subject is sitting or standing, the midheart level is taken to be midway between the sternal angle and the xiphoid process.

The major disadvantages of the fluid-filled catheter transducer system are its limited frequency response (10 Hz) and the motion artifact that is superimposed on the pressure waveform. At high work loads, motion artifact could be significant. Such problems are not encountered with the other types of catheters.

Transducer-Mounted Catheter

As mentioned earlier, two other types of pressure catheters are available for clinical use (see Fig. 8–1). Since we have not used either of these catheters during upright exercise, they will be described here briefly. The catheter with the transducer mounted at its tip was developed to overcome the limited frequency response and the motion artifacts associated with the fluid-filled catheter system. In addition, reference zero is automatically obtained since there is no fluid-filled catheter hydrostatic column. The Mikro-Tip Pressure Transducer manufactured by Millar Instruments, Inc., is an example of such a catheter that is presently used for measuring human pressures. The pressure sensor is an ultraminiature semiconductor strain gauge designed for catheter transducer applications. It is reported to have exceptional thermal stability and linearity, negligible hysteresis, and a flat frequency response to 20 KHz. Catheters are available in sizes from 3 to 9

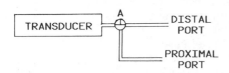

PULMONARY ARTERIAL PRESSURE

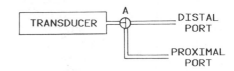

RIGHT ATRIAL PRESSURE

FIGURE 8–4. The tubing and stopcock (A) arrangement for measuring two pressures with one transducer. The position of the stopcock determines whether pulmonary arterial pressure or right atrial pressure is transmitted to the transducer.

French (see Table 8–1); custom-designed catheters can also be purchased.

While this type of pressure catheter has many advantages over the fluid-filled system, it is usually stiffer. Consequently, it is more difficult to position it in the pulmonary artery. To date, this catheter has been used primarily to measure left ventricular and aortic pressures. Its use during exercise has been limited to supine exercise in which the upper part of the body is relatively motionless.[4]

Fiberoptic Catheter

The other type of nonfluid-filled pressure catheter available for human use is constructed with fiberoptics (see Fig. 8–1); it has only recently become commercially available. It has similar advantages to the transducer-mounted pressure catheter, although the manufacturer (Camino Laboratories) reports a flat frequency response to only 20 Hz. This system consists of several fiberoptic bundles mounted within a catheter for the transmission and reception of light. At the tip of the catheter is a deformable membrane, the shape of which is sensitive to external pressure. As the shape of the membrane changes, so does the amount of reflected light. This reflected light is returned via the fiberoptic bundle to light-sensitive electronics where it is transduced into a signal for recording. Hence, reflected light is a function of intravascular pressure.

Camino Laboratories has incorporated the fiberoptics into the distal port of a triple lumen flotation catheter. Thus, it is possible to use this new technology with the versatile multipurpose flotation catheter system. Because of the limited experience with this product, however, there have been no reports of its utility in assessing the exercise response.

CARDIAC OUTPUT

Cardiac output (liters/min) can be measured during exercise by thermodilution, the Fick principle, carbon dioxide rebreathing, or directly measured flow.[5] Often, cardiac output is normalized using the body surface area (BSA) and reported as cardiac index (cardiac output/BSA; liters/min/m²). One can obtain the BSA from the height and weight of the subject and a nomogram such as the one presented in Figure 8–5.

Thermodilution Technique

To measure cardiac output by the thermodilution method, a triple lumen flotation catheter (as described previously) must be inserted into the pulmonary artery. The thermistor, located 4 cm from the tip of the catheter, allows measurement of blood temperature changes that are directly related to blood flow.[6] The rapid injection of 5 or 10 ml of cold solution, usually 5 per cent dextrose in water (D5W) at 0 to 4°C, into the right atrium via the proximal port of the catheter lowers the temperature of the blood with which it mixes. The change in temperature versus time relation as the cooled blood clears the right ventricle is then measured by the thermistor. From the thermodilution curve and the following equation, cardiac output (CO; liters/min) is calculated.

$$CO = \frac{(1.08)\ (K)\ VI\ (TB - TI)\ (60\ sec/min)}{\int_0^\infty \Delta T(t)dt} \quad (1)$$

Here 1.08 is the product of the density and specific heat of D5W, divided by the density-specific heat product of blood; K is the thermal transfer and lumen volume correction constant (see subsequently); VI is the injectate volume in liters; TB − TI is the difference between the preinjection blood and injectate temperature measured in degrees centigrade;

and $\int_0^\infty \Delta(t)dt$ is the integral of, or the area under, the thermodilution curve (units = degrees centigrade · seconds).

Several thermodilution computing devices are manufactured.[7] They automatically record and integrate the temperature-time curve associated with an injection of chilled D5W to derive cardiac output. We currently use one such device manufactured by American Edwards Laboratories. A distinct advantage of this instrument is the availability of an optional temperature probe that continually senses the temperature of the injectate. This probe connects to a specially designed syringe, which is also supplied by American Edwards as part of a complete, closed injectate delivery system (CO-Set Model 93-500). The CO-Set is depicted in Figure 8–6. The ability to measure injectate temperature directly increases the accuracy of the cardiac output determination. In addition, the CO-Set eliminates the need of using many syr-

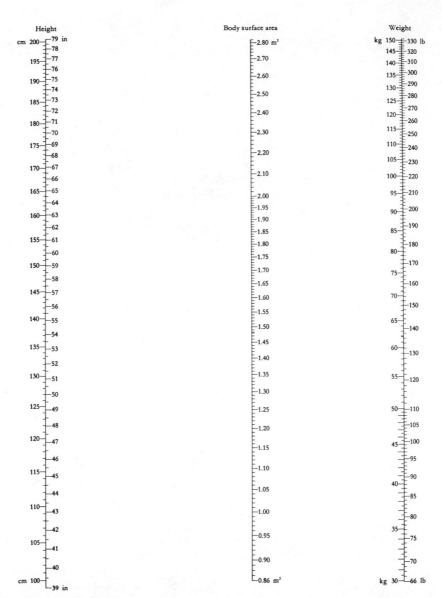

FIGURE 8–5. Nomogram for determining body surface area (BSA) from the height and weight of adults. (The nomogram is constructed from the formula of DuBois and DuBois: Arch Intern Med *17*:863, 1916.) For example, an individual with a height of 170 cm and a weight of 80 kg has a predicted BSA of 1.92 m². This is obtained by connecting the height and weight with a straight line and reading the BSA value where the line intersects the body surface area scale.

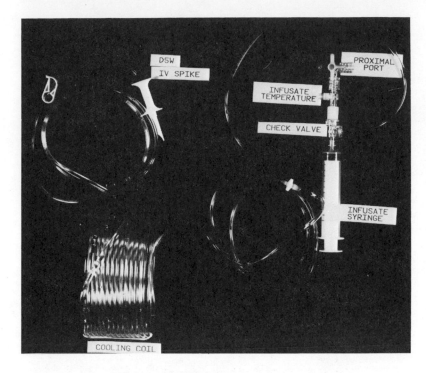

FIGURE 8–6. The CO-Set, closed injectate delivery system. As 5 per cent dextrose in water is drawn into the 10 ml infusate syringe, it is chilled by passing through the cooling coil of tubing that is surrounded by ice. It is then quickly injected through the proximal port of the catheter; a check valve prevents retrograde flow to the coil. An infusate temperature probe continuously measures the temperature of the injectate and transmits it to the output computer.

inges containing chilled D5W, thereby reducing the chance of infection. Most of the thermodilution computing devices provide an external adjustment for setting the proper correction factor or K value (equation 1). In addition, a chart or table is included in the operations manual, which lists the K value corresponding to the amount and temperature of the injectate and the type of catheter being used.

Typically, from 15 to 30 seconds following the injection of a 10 ml bolus are needed for the cardiac output to be calculated. The lower the output, the longer the wash-out time for the injectate. Thus, it is possible to obtain two thermodilution cardiac outputs per 2 minute exercise stage. As part of our protocol we measure cardiac output at the 1 minute point and then again 15 seconds before the end of the stage.

Fick Principle

Although the theorem of Adolf Fick was presented in 1870, the Fick principle was not used clinically until the early 1940s. It is based on the conservation of mass in a three port system (ie, input, output, and extraction ports) and can be used for obtaining cardiac output as well as organ blood flow, such as kidney or liver. The principle states that the flow rate through a system is equal to the extraction rate at the extraction port divided by the input-output difference in concentra-

tion of the material being extracted. For cardiac output estimations, oxygen is usually the indicator or material being extracted. Therefore, the extraction rate is $\dot{V}O_2$ and the input-output difference is the arteriovenous difference in blood oxygen content. We can write:

$$\text{Cardiac output} = \dot{V}O_2/(\text{arteriovenous } O_2 \text{ content difference}) \quad (2)$$

Note that the venous oxygen content measurement must be made·on blood obtained from the pulmonary artery, or what is commonly referred to as mixed venous blood. Clearly, a blood sample from a peripheral vein is not acceptable for cardiac output determinations since it only reflects the balance between oxygen uptake and blood flow in the tissue that is drained by that vein. Therefore, to obtain cardiac outputs using the Fick principle, a catheter must be positioned in the pulmonary artery.

Another requirement for this principle to be valid is a steady state. As discussed in Chapter 7, a steady state is achieved within the first minute of each stage of our exercise protocol (Chapter 9). Therefore, our procedure is to obtain a mixed venous sample of blood from the distal port of the catheter during the second minute of each stage, and in particular during the time when right atrial pressure is being recorded. If the subject has an arterial catheter, arterial blood samples would also be drawn at this time. Noninvasive techniques for measuring arterial oxygen saturation are presented subsequently (Arterial and Venous Oxygen Content section). Usually, 3 to 5 milliliters are obtained in preheparinized syringes and then stored on ice for subsequent analysis. Techniques for measuring $\dot{V}O_2$ have been discussed in Chapter 7 and methods for determining oxygen content will be discussed later.

Although it is our policy to obtain one or two thermodilution cardiac outputs and a Fick cardiac output at each stage of exercise (see Chapter 10), only the Fick cardiac outputs are used in analyzing and reporting the exercise results. Thermodilution cardiac outputs are obtained to provide us with immediate cardiac output information during the test and to serve as back-up data if needed. Nevertheless, we have found reasonable correlation between the two methods (r = 0.82) throughout the exercise test, with a tendency for the thermodilution method to slightly overestimate (5 per cent) Fick-determined cardiac output at the higher levels of work. The slope and intercept of the regression line equation were 1.05 and 0.04 (liters/min), respectively, and the regression line was statistically not different from the line of identity.

Carbon Dioxide Rebreathing Method

The carbon dioxide rebreathing method for calculating cardiac output is also based on the Fick principle. The equation is:

Cardiac output =
$\dot{V}CO_2$/(venoarterial CO_2 content difference) (3)

This technique was developed in an attempt to assess cardiac output noninvasively. To use it, one must be able to measure tidal volume and breath-by-breath carbon dioxide. From these measurements, $\dot{V}CO_2$ can be calculated (Chapter 7). The total carbon dioxide concentration or content of the arterial blood is then estimated by first obtaining the partial pressure of carbon dioxide at the end of expiration, commonly referred to as end-tidal carbon dioxide. This parameter, represented as $PetCO_2$, approximates the alveolar partial pressure of carbon dioxide. Jones et al[8] have shown that $PetCO_2$ reflects the partial pressure of carbon dioxide in arterial blood ($PaCO_2$), and they derived the following empiric relation for calculating $PaCO_2$ from $PetCO_2$ and tidal volume:

$PaCO_2$ =
5.5 + 0.09 ($PetCO_2$) − 0.0021 (tidal volume) (4)

Arterial blood carbon dioxide content is then obtained from $PaCO_2$ by means of the carbon dioxide dissociation curve.[9]

The noninvasive measurement of the partial pressure of carbon dioxide in mixed venous blood requires breathing in and out of a 5 liter bag, with breath-by-breath analysis of the carbon dioxide content in the bag. The closed lung-bag system functions as a tonometer in which the carbon dioxide content in the bag equilibrates with the carbon dioxide of the mixed venous blood.[10] The equilibrium partial pressure of carbon dioxide, however, has been found to overestimate that of mixed venous blood ($P\bar{v}CO_2$). Consequently, the following empiric relation[11] is used to correct the equilibrium value:

$P\bar{v}CO_2$ =
0.76 (equilibrium partial pressure of CO_2) + 11 (5)

This corrected value is then converted to mixed venous carbon dioxide content using the standard dissociation curve.

There are two rebreathing methods for estimating the partial pressure of carbon dioxide in mixed venous blood: the exponential and the equilibrium methods. The exponential method consists of rebreathing from a bag containing 96 to 100 per cent oxygen. As rebreathing takes place, the partial pressure of carbon dioxide in the bag increases until it equilibrates with the $P\bar{v}CO_2$. The equilibrium method involves the use of a bag containing 10 per cent or more carbon dioxide (that is, slightly higher than the expected mixed venous carbon dioxide content). As the subject rebreathes, the gas within the bag and the $P\bar{v}CO_2$ rapidly equilibrate, usually within 3 to 4 breaths, provided the carbon dioxide content of the bag gas was only slightly greater than that in the mixed venous blood. Of the two methods, the equilibrium method has been found to be more accurate.[12]

It is also possible to use foreign gases together with the Fick principle for determining cardiac output. However, the accuracy associated with the use of these gases is not as good as with carbon dioxide rebreathing. The gas has to be highly diffusible across the alveolar capillary wall so that the gas pressure in pulmonary capillary blood rapidly equilibrates with that in the alveoli during the time the blood is in the lungs. The foreign gases that have been used for this purpose include nitrous oxide, ethylene, ethyl iodide, and acetylene.[5] Of these, acetylene has been the most widely used.

There are two major difficulties with the

use of all foreign gases. First, precise measurements of alveolar gas concentrations and rate of gas absorption cannot be made, and second, to avoid errors associated with recirculation, the entire measurement must be made within the 8 to 12 seconds before the blood begins to recirculate through the lungs. In spite of many modifications to the methods of using foreign gases, no one has been able to devise a method whereby the gas can be brought to equilibrium and two successive samples of alveolar air removed in 10 seconds. Accordingly, all foreign gas methods require more than 10 seconds, resulting in a 30 to 40 per cent underestimation of cardiac output.[5]

Flow Velocity Technique

The Millar Instruments Company has developed a catheter, which, in addition to the pressure transducer at the distal end, has a velocity sensor mounted near the pressure transducer. There are two platinum electrodes on opposite sides of the probe and two electromagnets to generate magnetic fields, with their magnetic fluxes concentrated at the electrodes. When an ionic solution, such as blood, passes through each zone of magnetic flux, a potential is generated that is sensed at the electrodes. The magnitude and polarity of these potentials are directly proportional to the fluid velocity and direction of flow, respectively. With certain assumptions, such as a blunt velocity profile and a constant cross-sectional area (cross-sectional area is obtained from aortic angiograms or echocardiograms), the velocity measurement can be converted to blood flow (Fig. 8–7). If the velocity sensor is positioned in the ascending aorta, the blood flow signal can then be integrated and stroke volume

calculated. In this manner cardiac output can be calculated on a beat-by-beat basis. As discussed earlier, this rather stiff catheter, with or without the velocity sensor, has been used only during supine exercise.[4]

REGIONAL BLOOD FLOW

The [133]xenon clearance method has been used to determine muscle blood flow during exercise.[13] With the patient at rest, a bolus of ^{133}Xe-labelled saline is injected into the muscle and a small radiation detector is taped directly over the injection site. This element passes from tissue to blood, and its elimination is in most cases governed only by local blood flow. Moreover, it is almost totally eliminated in the lungs during its first pass so that recirculation does not exist. Ideally, the decrease in activity at the site of injection is a monoexponential function of time, so that a straight line is obtained when clearance versus time is plotted on semilog paper.

In a constantly and uniformly perfused tissue, the elimination of the tracer is described by the equation

$$C_t = Co \cdot e^{-kt} \qquad (6)$$

where Co and C_t are tissue concentrations initially and at time t, respectively, and k is the clearance constant, which can be derived from equation 7:

$$k = \ln 2/t_{1/2} \qquad (7)$$

Here $t_{1/2}$ is the half time of decay or the time required for half of the material to lose its radioactivity and is calculated from the straight line semilog plot of equation 6. Finally, flow is obtained from the formula

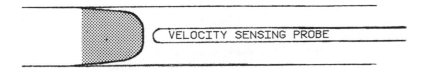

FIGURE 8–7. To calculate flow from velocity the velocity profile must be blunt and the cross-sectional area constant.

VELOCITY SENSING PROBE

ASSUMPTIONS: 1) BLUNT VELOCITY PROFILE

2) CONSTANT CROSS–SECTIONAL AREA

FLOW =   VELOCITY ● CROSS–SECTIONAL AREA

$$Q = k \cdot s \cdot 100 \qquad (8)$$

where s is the tissue blood partition coefficient of Xe divided by the specific weight of the tissue. At each work load, there is a change in the clearance rate that can be related to the change in muscle flow. Accordingly, all flow determinations can be performed with a single injection of ^{133}Xe.

ARTERIAL AND VENOUS OXYGEN CONTENT

The oxygen content of arterial and mixed venous blood samples must be determined to calculate cardiac output by the Fick principle. In addition, a knowledge of the amount of oxygen extracted by the tissues, which is a function of work load and flow, is useful in assessing whether there are abnormalities in the ability of the tissue to extract oxygen (Chapter 2).

The classic method for accurately measuring oxygen content in blood has been the van Slyke vacuum extraction and manometric procedure. However, it is very time consuming and requires considerable skill. Oxygen content can also be measured directly using the Lex-O$_2$-CON oxygen galvanic cell (Lexington/Evans Instruments), but it too requires careful technique and operator skill. Because of the time and skill required by these two methods, most laboratories calculate oxygen content from measurements of oxygen saturation and hemoglobin. With today's technology these measurements are easily made using analyzers that require only 25 microliter blood samples (e.g., OSM2 Hemoximeter, Radiometer, and Instrument Laboratory CO-Oximeter 282).

Oxygen saturation can be defined by the ratio: O$_2$ content · 100%/O$_2$ capacity. This refers to the amount of oxyhemoglobin in the sample. Total oxygen capacity of the blood sample is simply the product of total hemoglobin and the oxygen-carrying capacity of human hemoglobin (that is, 1.34 ml of oxygen per gram of hemoglobin). Hemoglobin can be present in several forms—for example, oxyhemoglobin, carboxyhemoglobin, methemoglobin, and reduced hemoglobin. Ideally, all forms should be directly measured. However, carboxyhemoglobin and methemoglmobin normally are present in negligible amounts. Consequently many instruments measure oxyhemoglobin and reduced hemoglobin only. It is also possible to estimate the per cent oxygen saturation of hemoglobin from the normal dissociation curve if the partial pressure of oxygen is known. The normal dissociation curve, however, is constructed with the assumption that the only hemoglobins present are oxyhemoglobin and reduced hemoglobin. If the assumption were not valid because of the presence of significant concentrations of other hemoglobin species, then the oxygen saturation would be overestimated. For example, a blood sample with 20 per cent carboxyhemoglobin can have at most an 80 per cent oxyhemoglobin, even though both methods would have measured the oxygen saturation to be 100 per cent.

Oximetrix Inc. and American Edwards Laboratories have added to the triple lumen thermodilution flotation catheter a fiberoptic system that provides a continuous, real time measurement of mixed venous oxygen saturation. This capability is in addition to the catheter's sampling, pressure monitoring, and thermodilution cardiac output capabilities. The smallest size currently available is 7.5F (Table 8–1). Readings from this instrument are also based on the assumption that hemoglobin is either reduced or combined with oxygen.

Arterial oxygen content can be obtained indirectly with transcutaneous monitors[14] or ear oximeters.[15] With both methods, the area where the transducer is to be placed is prepared by brisk rubbing. Once in place, the devices warm the skin to be tested. The hyperthermia results in vasodilation and an increased blood flow to the skin. Transcutaneous monitors typically utilize an electrode system (e.g., Clark electrode) for sensing the diffused oxygen. Ear oximeters are optoelectronic devices that transmit light pulses through the ear lobe; the resulting transmissions are measured at several wavelengths, many times per second, and then processed to obtain oxygen saturation. When compared with arterial blood, ear oximetry has been found to provide a sufficiently accurate estimate of arterial oxygen saturation. Transcutaneous values in adults have been reported to underestimate the actual values[16] and are slower to respond to changes in saturation than the ear oximeter. We have had the opportunity to use the Hewlett Packard (4720A) and the Biox (Bioximetry Technology, Inc.) ear oximeters. Both performed satisfactorily during exercise except in patients with deeply pigmented skin.

BLOOD LACTATE CONCENTRATION

Venous blood lactate levels provide useful information regarding the onset of lactate production by working muscle (Chapter 2). In addition, by proper placement of a sampling catheter one can examine lactate production, release, and clearance in a particular working muscle group, such as femoral venous lactate. Such information may prove useful when evaluating the efficacy of vasodilator or inotropic drug therapy.[17, 18] For example, if a drug increases cardiac output, one could evaluate whether the flow to working muscle is also increased and whether the onset of lactate production is delayed.

Recently the Yellow Springs Instrument Company developed a system for rapid determination of L-lactate. Results are displayed in 45 seconds after injection of a 25 microliter sample. The instrument is extremely easy to operate and requires no special operator training. Because of the rapid response, it is possible to assay blood for lactate while the patient is exercising and, therefore, to have another method for documenting whether a patient has crossed the anaerobic threshold. This is of particular importance when the patient response to prolonged submaximal anaerobic exercise is being assessed (Chapter 10).

ELECTROCARDIOGRAM AND HEART RATE

All exercise tests should include electrocardiographic and heart rate monitoring. The American Heart Association has recommended standards that an ECG recorder should satisfy in order to insure ECG information of acceptable diagnostic quality.[19] The ECG machine should have a flat frequency response of between 0.14 to 50 Hz with no more than 3dB drop-off at 0.05 and 100 Hz. For an extensive list of manufacturers of ECG analyzers and heart rate meters, see the annual review in Medical Electronics.[20, 21]

Although the exercise test is usually performed with a multiple-lead system, it has been shown that approximately 80 per cent of the abnormal ST segment responses to exercise can be detected by lead V_5.[22] We have also found the V_5 lead to be adequate when exercising patients with chronic stable heart failure, regardless of etiology. Additional leads will depend of course on the nature of the exercise test, the type of patient, and the extent of impairment. For example, a patient with severe coronary artery disease would require 12 leads, with 3 leads displayed simultaneously at any given time.

With proper skin preparation (abrading the outer layer of skin and cleansing with alcohol) and modern ECG electrodes, cables, and electronics, motion artifact during exercise is negligible. Occasionally, however, we encounter motion artifact, particularly in obese patients or in patients who perspire excessively. In these instances, relocating one or more of the electrodes or having the patient wear a stretchable fishnet vest may correct the problem.

MANUFACTURERS CITED

1. American Edwards Laboratories
   Box 11150
   1923 S.E. Main Street
   Irvine, California 92714
2. Bioximetry Technology, Incorporated
   4765 Walnut Street
   Boulder, Colorado 80301
3. Camino Laboratories
   7550 Trade Street
   San Diego, California 92121
4. Gould Incorporated
   Medical Products Division
   1900 Williams Drive
   Oxnard, California 93030
5. Hewlett-Packard Company
   Medical Products Group
   100 Fifth Avenue
   Waltham, Massachusetts 02254
6. Hyatt Esophageal Balloon
   Vacumed (Distributor)
   2261 Palma Drive
   Ventura, California 93003
7. Instrument Laboratory Incorporated
   Biomedical Division
   113 Hartwell Avenue
   Lexington, Massachusetts 02173
8. Lexington/Evans Instruments
   Box 566
   221 Crescent Street
   Waltham, Massachusetts 02254
9. Millar Instruments, Incorporated
   P.O. Box 18227
   6001 Gulf Freeway
   Houston, Texas 77223
10. Oximetrix Incorporated
    1212 Terra Bella Avenue
    Mountain View, Massachusetts 02254
11. Radiometer A/S
    72 Emdruprej
    DK-2400
    Copenhagen NV, Denmark
12. Yellow Springs Instrument Company, Incorporated
    Box 279
    Yellow Springs, Ohio 45387

REFERENCES

1. Aronson MH (ed). Catheters and catheterization systems. Med Electronics Issue 89:164–169, 1984.
2. Milic-Emili J, Mead J, Turner JM, Glauser EM. Improved technique for estimating pleural pressure from esophageal balloons. J Appl Physiol 19:207–211, 1964.
3. Aronson MH (ed). Blood pressure. Med Electronics Issue 86:93–104, 1984.
4. Laskey WK, Kussmaul WG, Martin JL, Kleaveland JP, Hirshfeld JW Jr, Shroff S. Characteristics of vascular hydraulic load in heart failure. Circulation 72:61–71, 1985.
5. Guyton AC, Jones CE, Coleman TG. Circulatory Physiology: Cardiac Output and Its Regulation. WB Saunders, Philadelphia, 1973, pp 21–134.
6. Forrester JS, Ganz W, Diamond G, McHugh T, Chonette DW, Swan HJC. Thermodilution cardiac output determination with a single flow-directed catheter. Am Heart J 83:306–311, 1972.
7. Aronson MH (ed). Cardiac output. Med Electronics Issue 86:105–107, 1984.
8. Jones NL, Robertson DG, Kane JW. Difference between end-tidal and arterial PCO_2 in exercise. J Appl Physiol 47:954–960, 1979.
9. McHardy GJ. The relationship between the differences in pressure and content of carbon dioxide in arterial blood and venous blood. Clin Sci 32:299–309, 1967.
10. Magel JR, Andersen KL. Cardiac output in muscular exercise measured by the CO_2 rebreathing procedure, *in* Denolin H, Konig K, Messin R, Degre S (eds). Ergometry in Cardiology. Boeringer, Mannheim, 1968, pp 147–156.
11. Jones NL, Campbell EJM, McHardy GJ, et al. The estimation of carbon dioxide pressure of mixed venous blood during exercise. Clin Sci 32:311–327, 1967.
12. Godfrey S, Wolfe E. An evaluation of rebreathing methods for measuring mixed venous PCO_2 during exercise. Clin Sci 42:345–353, 1972.
13. Clausen JP, Lassen NA. Muscle blood flow during exercise in normal man studied by the [133]xenon clearance method. Cardiovasc Res 5:245–254, 1971.
14. McDowell JW, Thiede WH. Usefulness of the transcutaneous PO_2 monitor during exercise testing in adults. Chest 78:853–855, 1980.
15. Saunders NA, Powles ACP, Rebuck AS. Ear oximetry: Accuracy and practicability in the assessment of arterial oxygenation. Am Rev Respir Dis 113:745–749, 1976.
16. Beyerl D. Non-invasive measurement of blood oxygen levels. Am J Med Tech 48:355–359, 1982.
17. Wilson JR, Martin JL, Ferraro N, Weber KT. Effect of hydralazine on perfusion and metabolism in the leg during upright bicycle exercise in patients with heart failure. Circulation 68:425–432, 1983.
18. Siskind SJ, Sonnenblick EH, Forman R, Scheuer J, LeJemtel TH. Acute substantial benefit of inotropic therapy with amrinone on exercise hemodynamics and metabolism in severe congestive heart failure. Circulation 64:966–973, 1981.
19. Hellertstein HK. Specifications for exercise testing equipment. Circulation 59:849A–854A, 1979.
20. Aronson MH (ed). ECG analyzers. Med Electronics Issue 88:176–180, 1984.
21. Aronson MH (ed). Heart rate meters. Med Electronics Issue 88:184–189, 1984.
22. Koppes G, McKiernan T, Bassan M, Froelicher VF. Treadmill exercise testing. Part I. Curr Probl Cardiol 7:1–44, 1977.

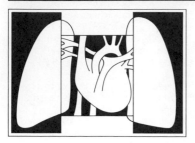

JOSEPH S. JANICKI
KARL T. WEBER

9

Equipment and Protocols to Evaluate the Exercise Response

The physiologic stress of exercise is a simple, efficient means to elicit abnormalities that may exist within the cardiopulmonary unit—abnormalities that compromise its performance. In patients with advanced expressions of a disease there is often little reason to recommend that an exercise test be performed, although there are important exceptions. In patients with less severe disease, the stress of an exercise test can be invaluable in establishing objective information about the nature and severity of the disease as well as their responses to therapy. Some patients may have coexistent heart and lung disease that compromises the cardiopulmonary unit. In these patients an exercise test can be used to evaluate the nature and severity of each disease and to identify the relative dominance of one disease over the other. As a result, therapeutic strategies can be based on the relative importance of each disease.

In Chapter 2 we identified the forms of exercise as being either isotonic or isometric in nature. Many different types of exercise tests utilize isotonic or isometric exercise, including incremental or steady state, submaximal or maximal, and symptom- or non-symptom-limited types. The test may be designed to examine a small or large muscle mass or one specific for a particular muscle group that relates to an occupation or athletic activity.

The purpose of this chapter is to identify the types of equipment and the various protocols that can be used in the clinical laboratory to perform these tests, as well as their relative merits and disadvantages. We begin by first defining work and power.

WORK AND POWER

Work is defined as the product of the force that acts to displace a body and the distance through which the body is displaced; work is force times distance. One unit of work, typically expressed in *joules*, is performed when a force of 1 newton (kg · m/sec²) displaces a body a distance of 1 meter (that is, 1 newton-meter = 1 joule). If a mass of 1 kilogram is moved vertically a distance of 1 meter against the force of gravity, the work performed is referred to as a *kilopond-meter* (kpm) (that is, 1 kilopond-meter = 9.8 joules).

Dynamic exercise, such as bicycle or treadmill exercise, is actually work performed per unit of time. It therefore represents work rate or power. If the unit of work is measured in joules, then the unit of power or work rate is the *watt* (w); 1 watt equals 1 joule per second. It is also common to express work in terms of the kilopond-meter. In this case the unit of power is the kilopond-meter per minute (kpm/min). The relation between watt and kilopond-meter/min is expressed as: 1 w = 6.12 kpm/min (Table 9–1).

Other units of power commonly used in exercise physiology are the oxygen equivalent of power (ml/min/kg) and mets. A *met* is the resting oxygen uptake ($\dot{V}O_2$) of an average 70 kg man, or 3.5 ml/min/kg. Accordingly, 2 mets is equivalent to the work rate or power that would produce a $\dot{V}O_2$ of 7.0 ml/min/kg in an average man.

To measure a force exerted by a machine, physicists and engineers use the *dynamometer*. When this force measurement is com-

Table 9–1. *Units of Work Rate or Power*

Watts (w)	Kilopond-meter/min (kpm/min)	Watts (w)	Kilopond-meter/min (kpm/min)
5	30.6	150	918
10	61.2	200	1224
15	91.8	250	1530
20	122.4	300	1836
25	153.0	350	2142
50	306.0	400	2448
75	459.0	450	2754
100	612.0	500	3060

bined with a velocity measurement, the resultant test apparatus becomes a device for measuring power. The *ergometer* is an example of a device for measuring power or work rate. By applying a controllable load in the form of resistance to a turning shaft, power can be computed from the resistance and the number of shaft revolutions per unit of time. Thus, the ergometer is an instrument used to impose a known work rate on a group of exercising muscles.

EQUIPMENT FOR ISOTONIC EXERCISE

The general requirements for the design of an exercise method and protocol that are suitable for the evaluation of the cardiopulmonary system are the involvement of large muscle groups and an ability to incrementally increase the workload in a reproducible fashion to a level where the oxygen uptake becomes maximal. The exercise test should not involve types of work to which the individual is not accustomed, and it should be tolerable and safe. For example, a bicycle test is not appropriate for an elderly patient who has not bicycled in over 30 years. A patient with severe claudication or a painful arthritic hip would be a candidate for exercise that involved only the upper body and arms, such as arm ergometry (to be discussed). Other considerations in choosing an exercise method are practical in nature and include available space and equipment cost, durability, portability and ease of operation.

In the exercise laboratory, the three most popular methods of producing standard, reproducible isotonic work loads are (1) a series of steps of variable height and number; (2) the bicycle ergometer with variable resistance; and (3) the treadmill with variable speeds and grades.

Steps

With steps the workload can be varied by changing the number and height of the steps as well as the rate of climbing and descending. Steps are inexpensive to purchase and there are no maintenance costs. In addition, climbing steps represents a form of work that is familiar to everyone. To perform this exercise, however, the patient cannot be encumbered with the various tubes and cables necessary for monitoring respiratory gas exchange and hemodynamics. In fact, with the exception of an electrocardiogram and heart rate reading, it is virtually impossible to make any measurements during the exercise test. Another disadvantage is the difficulty in quantifying work rate.

The types of steps that have been utilized for clinical testing include a fixed height single or double step arrangement,[1] the climbing step, and the variable height step (Fig. 9–1). All steps should be stable and covered with a nonslip surface. A handrail is recommended for elderly patients. Typical dimensions of a step are height, 23 to 25 cm; width, 50 to 60 cm; and depth, 25 cm. The single step is used in conjunction with the Harvard step test and the Pitteloud and Forster one-step test.[7] The Master's two step test utilizes the double step configuration shown in Figure 9–1.[3] The climbing step has been developed and used in over 50,000 patients by Kaltenbach.[2] Finally, the variable height step or adjustable platform apparatus has been developed and used extensively by Nagle et al.[4] It consists of a platform that can be elevated either manually or with a motor, from a minimum height of 2 cm to a maximum of 50 cm. Changes in height are made without disrupting the exercise cadence. The general aspects of the protocols associated with step exercise are discussed later in this chapter.

Recently Tri-Tech Incorporated introduced a step-climbing device that permits the individual to perform a continuous climbing exercise without having to step backward or turn around (Fig. 9–2). This device, called the StairMaster 6000 ergometer, consists of a series of revolving steps that are powered by the weight of the individual. Climbing rates can be varied from 45 to 115 steps per minute, and body weight is the resistance. Speed and thereby work rate are continuously monitored. Since there is no forward motion, respiratory gas exchange and hemodynamics can be monitored without difficulty.

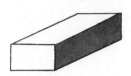

ONE – STEP

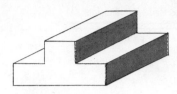

TWO – STEP

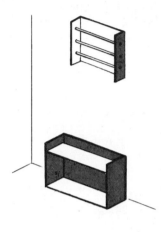

CLIMBING STEP

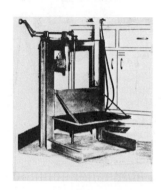

FIGURE 9–1. Four types of steps used for exercise testing. (The adjustable height step is reprinted with permission from Nagle FJ, Balke B, Naughton JP. Gradational step tests for assessing work capacity. J Appl Physiol 20:745–748, 1965.)

ADJUSTABLE
HEIGHT STEP

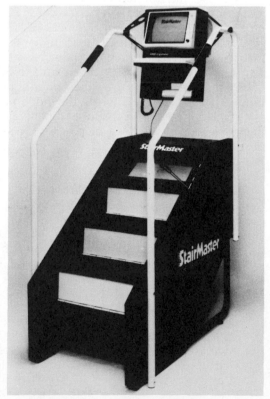

FIGURE 9–2. StairMaster 6000 ergometer, consisting of a series of revolving steps that are powered by the weight of the individual.

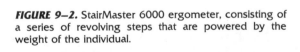

Bicycle Ergometers

A wide assortment of bicycle ergometers are commercially available for the clinical laboratory. A listing of available models and their manufacturers can be found elsewhere.[5]

The bicycle ergometer is a stationary device that consists of a mainframe, an adjustable seat, adjustable handlebars, pedal-crank assembly, and a flywheel (Fig. 9–3). Work load is a function of an adjustable resistance that is applied to the flywheel. This resistance is created either mechanically, using braking pads or braking straps, or electromechanically, whereby work is performed against an electrically produced resistance. The mechanically braked bicycle ergometer is less expensive than the electromechanically braked system and does not depend on the availability of electrical power. Work load, however, is influenced by pedalling rate, and care must be taken to have the patient maintain the rate recommended by each manufacturer. The electromechanical bicycle ergometer, on the other hand, is less sensitive to variations in pedalling frequency. For example, work load is not significantly affected with variations in rate between 40 and 70 revolutions per minute. In addition, smaller, more accurate increments in resistance are possible in the electromechanical system. Regardless of type, bicycle ergometers require frequent calibration, especially when used for clinical purposes. Most manufacturers recommend annual recalibration at a minimum. When recalibrating, the bicycle ergometer should be tested over a full range of work loads. For the calibration procedure of any particular model, the reader should refer to the operating manual or consult the manufacturer.

Oxygen uptake is determined by both work load and pedalling frequency. For this reason, a fixed pedalling rate, such as 50 revolutions per minute, is recommended. Most bicycle ergometers include a gauge to monitor revolutions per minute, which the exercising patient can use as an aid in maintaining a constant pedalling rate.

When compared with either steps or the treadmill, the bicycle ergometer has several advantages. Work rate can be easily varied and accurately quantified. Consequently, for aerobic work loads, VO_2 can be approximated with a reasonable degree of confidence in those patients in whom it is not possible to measure gas exchange. This is not the case for step or treadmill exercise, where work performed depends in part on patient weight. Bicycle ergometers are also less expensive, less bulky, and less noisy than treadmills. Many bicycle ergometers can be used in either the upright or supine position; it is also possible to modify the bicycle ergometer for use as an arm ergometer.[6] For the patient who has difficulty in walking or for the obese patient, the bicycle ergometer can

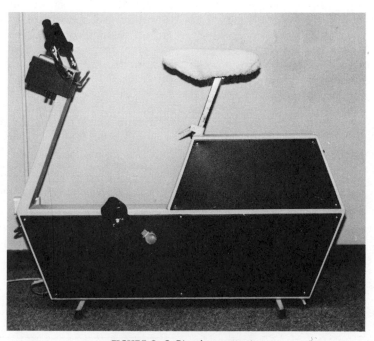

FIGURE 9–3. Bicycle ergometer.

be used to evaluate the exercise response without the fear of the patient stumbling or falling. Finally, with upright bicycle ergometry, the upper part of the body remains stationary. Accordingly, blood pressure is measured easily and motion artifact on the electrocardiogram or pressure recording is minimized.

On the other hand, many patients find it difficult to pedal smoothly and comfortably. The average American does very little cycling beyond the adolescent years. Thus, the majority of patients seen in our exercise facility have not bicycled in over 30 years and understandably their peformance on the bicycle ergometer is awkward, erratic, and often less than optimal. Bicycling is a specialized skill that often does not meet with patient acceptance. In some instances our patients have stopped exercising because of discomfort from the seat. A more common reason has been leg muscle or knee joint pain. Thus, it is not surprising to find that, in the United States 67 to 78 per cent of all exercise tests are performed on the treadmill.[7]

We are of the opinion that, for the patient population seen in our laboratory, the treadmill is a far superior form of isotonic exercise. Nevertheless, we have found that a bicycle ergometer should be available for the obese patient or the occasional patient who, for one reason or another, cannot walk on the treadmill. In an effort to obtain a useful bicycle ergometer exercise protocol, we have made the following modifications to our bicycle ergometer. First, we replaced the standard seat with one that is oversized and padded (Fitness Products); second, we installed "toe loop pedals" (Fitness Products), which prevent slippage of the foot from the pedal; and third, we modified the circuitry of our electromechanical bicycle ergometer to permit finer increments in work load (i.e., 6.25 watt as opposed to standard 25 watt increments). This is particularly helpful in patients who have more advanced chronic cardiac or circulatory failure or pulmonary disease and whose exercise tolerance is limited to low level work.

Treadmills

The work load of treadmill exercise can be varied by increasing treadmill speed or grade, or both. Of the three methods of isotonic exercise discussed in this chapter, the treadmill is the most expensive, the bulkiest (a floor space of 0.8 by 2.0 meters is

typically required), the heaviest (a treadmill weighs between 150 and 200 kg), and the least mobile. However, these are minor disadvantages in view of the fact that walking represents a form of exercise familiar to all. Moreover, walking involves more muscle groups than the bicycle and, because it incorporates body weight, it represents a larger $\dot{V}O_2$ of the various forms of exercise. In addition, because the treadmill protocol regulates the pace and grade for a particular work level, the patient's motivation need not be as strong as it would be for the step or ergometer tests. During treadmill exercise the patient should not use the handrails except for balance. The body's weight should not be distributed or supported by the arms. Tight gripping of the handrails may add an isometric component to the exercise response.

A survey of the marketplace reveals a wide choice of manufacturers who offer an equally wide range of treadmill features and costs.[5] For a clinical exercise laboratory we would recommend a treadmill of sturdy construction with handrails, side platform, and a heavy duty motor (2 or more horsepower). In addition, the treadmill should be programmable. That is, an electronic controller that makes possible the automatic variation in work load (speed/elevation) at preset time intervals should be included. Power requirements for a treadmill are usually 200 to 240 volts and 15 amperes. An easily accessible, power-off switch should be provided by the manufacturer in case of an emergency when an immediate stop is required. For most exercise protocols or routine cardiac rehabilitation programs, a treadmill with a speed range of 0 to 10 mph (or 16.0 km/hr; Table 9–2) and a grade range of 0 to 22 per cent is sufficient. The per cent grade of a treadmill is the measure of the degree of inclination.

Table 9–2. *Equivalent Units of Speed*

Miles/hour (mph)	Kilometers/hour (kmph)
1	1.6
2	3.2
3	4.8
4	6.4
5	8.0
6	9.6
7	11.2
8	12.8
9	14.4
10	16.0

That is, for a given horizontal distance from some reference point, the treadmill is inclined by an amount equal to the per cent grade times the horizontal distance (Fig. 9–4). For example, if the treadmill is 2 meters long, then for a 22 per cent grade the front of the treadmill is 0.44 meters higher than it was at a 0 per cent grade. The angle that corresponds to a 22 per cent grade is simply the inverse tangent (0.44 meters/2 meters) or 12.4°. For special purposes such as sports training, treadmills are available that have a greater range of speeds and grades (a maximum speed of 19 mph and grade of 40 per cent).[5]

Treadmill work rate cannot be directly defined in watts or kilopond-meter per minute. In addition, body weight and gait influence the work rate as the grade of the treadmill is increased. An indirect method for converting a given treadmill speed and grade into watts or kpm/min is to first obtain $\dot{V}O_2$ for the speed and grade and then find the bicycle ergometry work rate in watts or kpm/min that requires the same $\dot{V}O_2$. Table 9–3 lists the estimated, equivalent bicycle ergometry work rates, in watts, for several combinations of treadmill speed and grade.

EQUIPMENT FOR ISOMETRIC EXERCISE

An isometric effort can be defined as a sustained muscle contraction at constant muscle length; there is little or no shortening of the contracting muscle group. Isometric

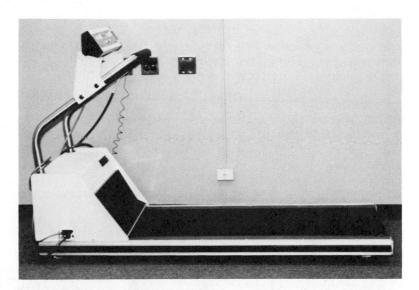

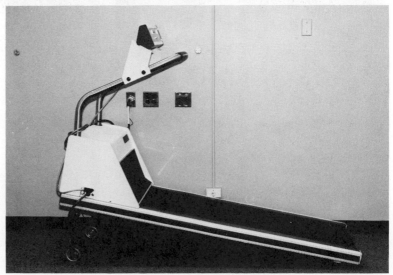

FIGURE 9–4. Treadmill at 0 per cent (top) and 22 per cent (bottom) grade. Per cent grade is the height (h) to which the treadmill is raised divided by the treadmill length (l) times 100 per cent. The corresponding angle is the inverse tangent of (h/l).

Table 9–3. Treadmill Work Rate

Speed (mph)	Grade (%)	Work Rate (watts)	Mets*
1.0	0	10	1.5
2.0	3.5	25	3.0
2.0	7.0	50	4.0
2.0	10.5	75	5.0
2.0	15.0	100	6.0
3.0	0	25	2.4
3.0	7.5	100	6.0
3.0	15.0	150	8.5
3.0	22.5	225	12.0
3.4	12.0	150	8.5
3.4	14.0	175	10.0
3.4	16.0	200	11.0
3.4	21.0	250	13.5
4.0	10.0	150	8.5
4.0	18.0	225	12.0
5.0	10.0	240	13.0
5.0	18.0	300	16.0

*Mets: The multiple of one metabolic equivalent, where $\dot{V}O_2$ = 3.5 ml/min/kg.

exercise is a common everyday activity that occurs whenever an individual lifts or pushes a heavy object. Therefore, it is often beneficial to include as part of the testing procedure an evaluation of the effects of isometric exercise. Isometric testing can be performed in a number of ways and on a variety of muscles. For example, one could use the hand dynamometer (Fitness Products). The hand dynamometer is a device that indicates the handgrip isometric effort in pounds or kilograms when squeezed (Fig. 9–5). This effort can then be maintained for a set period of time. By lifting and holding (forearm parallel to the floor) a weighted basket, a sustained isometric effort of known magnitude can be achieved.[8] Similarly, with the subject sitting, weights can be attached to the leg and the subject instructed to extend and hold the weighted leg parallel to the floor. In addition, isometric exercise testing can involve combinations of this, such as a simultaneous forearm and leg lift.[9]

The length of time an isometric contraction can be maintained depends on the magnitude of the effort with respect to the maximal voluntary contraction (MVC) of the muscle group being exercised. For work loads in the range 10 to 25 per cent MVC (that is, light static exercise), the isometric effort can be maintained for at least 10 minutes. As work load becomes greater than 25 per cent of MVC (that is, heavy static exercise), the time to exhaustion is reduced and a steady state in the hemodynamic and gas exchange parameters may not be attained.[10]

Regardless of the type of isometric testing utilized and the muscle group involved, it

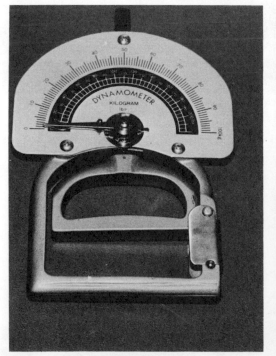 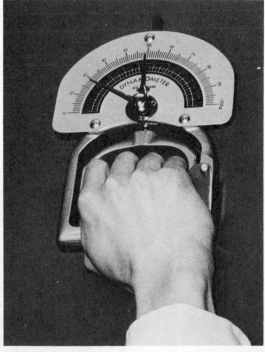

FIGURE 9–5. Hand dynamometer. Right, a patient is performing isometrics exercise at 40 per cent of his maximum voluntary contraction force of 50 kg.

should be simply and comfortably executed, quantifiable, and reproducible. In addition, it should be sustainable for the time required to make measurements.

EXERCISE TEST PROTOCOLS

As we discussed earlier in this chapter, there are several methods one can use to perform isotonic and isometric exercise and many different types of exercise tests. Regardless of the method and form of exercise, exercise testing should stress as many systems of the body as possible and should permit examination of their functional integration. Accordingly, the test should work large muscle groups at several work rates to discern the ability of the cardiopulmonary unit to maintain oxygen transport. An exercise test should also be sufficiently rigorous to allow quantitative documentation of the degree to which a given disorder has reduced the reserve capacity of the circulatory and respiratory systems.

Often these objectives may not be accomplished with a single exercise test. For this reason, Jones and Campbell have found it necessary to have four different tests.[11] The first is used as a routine screening procedure. The second through fourth tests employ increasingly complex techniques. They are used in more complicated clinical situations. Test 4 includes the measurement of pulmonary arterial pressure and the sampling of mixed venous blood.

We too have developed a series of exercise tests that employ increasingly complex techniques (Chapter 10). Our basic test is a multistage, incremental work rate treadmill exercise in which $\dot{V}O_2$, $\dot{V}CO_2$, and airflow are measured on a breath-by-breath basis to determine anaerobic threshold and aerobic capacity. These results, along with heart rate and blood pressure, are included in the patient's evaluation (Fig. 9–6). Our most complex test is similar, but it also includes a flotation catheter positioned in the pulmonary artery to continuously measure pulmonary artery and wedge pressures, right atrial pressure, and cardiac output by thermodilution and the Fick principle. In addition, the radial artery is cannulated for continuous measurement of arterial pressure and sampling of arterial blood for oxygen content, blood gases, pH, and lactate levels. Our general approach to exercise is discussed in more detail in the next chapter.

Isotonic Exercise Protocols

A survey of the literature reveals that numerous isotonic exercise protocols have been used to evaluate the status of the cardiopulmonary unit. The number of these tests is greatly reduced if one considers only those protocols that have been used in the evaluation of patients with heart, lung, or vascular disease. The most commonly used treadmill protocols in clinical cardiology are given in Tables 9–4 to 9–8.

Several criteria should be considered in choosing an exercise protocol. The test should begin with a low work load, which the patient can manage easily with little effort. We have chosen 1 mile per hour and 0 per cent grade for this purpose (Table 9–4). Aside from serving as a warm-up period, the light work load aids in relaxing the patient and permits her or him to establish an efficient rhythm. For example, we find that initially most patients tend to walk too rapidly and with a shortened stride. In addition, because of pre-exercise anxiety they may hyperventilate. Typically, the correct gait is acquired within the first 30 seconds, and by the end of the first stage most patients are breathing in a steady fashion. During the warm-up stage, the patient is instructed to use the handrail only for balance. Patients should also be told to avoid gripping the handrail tightly (thereby performing isometric exercise with the arms) and to avoid leaning on the rails (thereby reducing the weight on the lower limbs); both actions will increase $\dot{V}O_2$.

Each level of exercise should be long enough to attain a steady state. With our treadmill protocol (Table 9–4), the increments in work load are sufficiently small so that a steady state is usually attained during the first minute of each stage, whereas a 25 watt increment on the bicycle ergometer may require 1.5 minutes for a steady state to be achieved. Accordingly, we have the patient exercise for 3 minutes following each 25 watt increment on the bicycle ergometer. Recently, it has been reported that tests using equal increments of short duration (20, 30, or 50 watts per minute) provided information on ventilation, cardiovascular function, and gas exchange that was similar to information obtained from the longer, conventional 2 to 3 minute interval test.[12, 13] However, these results were obtained in normal, conditioned subjects; it remains to be seen whether such a "ramp" test would be similarly applicable

CARDIO-PULMONARY EXERCISE EVALUATION

CARDIOLOGY SECTION
MICHAEL REESE HOSPITAL

Exercise Test   : Determination of Aerobic Capacity and Anaerobic Threshold

Name: _____ Carpel #: _____ Hosp. #: _____

Date: _____ Sex: _____ Age: _____ Ht: _____ Wt: _____ BSA: _____

History and reason for test:

H R Max: _____ (bpm)   BP Max: _____ (mm Hg)

$\dot{V}O_2$ Max: _____ (ml/min/kg)

$\dot{V}O_2$ at Anaerobic Threshold: _____ (ml/min/kg)

Stage at Anaerobic Threshold: _____   (_____ mph; _____ % elevation)

Total Exercise Duration: _____ (sec)

Functional Class: _____

Reason for stopping:

Comments:

_____
Karl T. Weber, M.D.
Director, Cardiology Section

Reference: Weber KT, et al; Oxygen utilization and ventilation during exercise in patients with chronic cardiac failure.
Circulation 65: 1213, 1982.

Distribution: White - Patient Chart, Yellow - Referring Physician, Pink - Carpel File, Goldenrod - Carpel File

FIGURE 9–6. Example of an exercise evaluation form, which is sent to the referring doctor and also placed in the patient's file.

Table 9–4. Our Cardiopulmonary Exercise (CPX) Protocol for Treadmill Exercise

Stage (2 min)	Speed (mph)	Grade (%)	Mets*
Standing	0	0	1.4
1	1.0	0	2.6
2	1.5	0	3.1
3	2.0	3.5	3.8
4	2.0	7.0	4.7
5	2.0	10.5	5.4
6	3.0	7.5	6.2
7	3.0	10.0	6.9
8	3.0	12.5	7.9
9	3.0	15.0	8.7
10	3.4	14.0	9.2
11	3.4	16.0	—
12	3.4	18.0	—
13	3.4	20.0	—
14	3.4	22.0	—

*Measured $\dot{V}O_2$.

to patients with cardiopulmonary disease. These patients may require a longer time to adjust physiologically to an elevation in work load.

The total time of the test protocol should not exceed 20 minutes. Beyond this duration, factors such as discomfort with the mouthpiece or nose clamp, thirst or dryness of the throat, and boredom may cause the subject to stop prematurely. In our experience less than 1 per cent of the patients and less than 40 per cent of the normal subjects tested did not attain their anaerobic threshold and maximum oxygen uptake within 20 minutes of our treadmill protocol. Thus, although there are many advantages to having a common protocol, a second, more rigorous protocol (such as the Bruce protocol; see Table 9–5) may be necessary if the goals of the test are not attained within 20 minutes of exercise.

Table 9–5. Bruce Protocol for Treadmill Exercise

Stage (3 min)	Speed (mph)	Grade (%)	Mets†
1	1.7	10	4.8
2	2.5	12	6.8
3	3.4	14	9.6
4*	4.2	16	13.2
5*	5.0	18	—
6*	5.5	20	—
7*	6.0	22	—

*Jogging or running.
†Calculated from Bruce RA, Kusumi F, Hosmer D. Maximal oxygen intake and nomographic assessment of functional aerobic impairment in cardiovascular disease. Am Heart J 85:546–562, 1973, Table III.

Occasionally, we encounter patients who are unable to exercise beyond the first or second stage of our protocol because of the severity of their disease. Since treadmill speed cannot be adjusted below 1 mile per hour, the first stage of this protocol represents the minimum attainable level of work. In this case, it may be desirable to consider other forms of isotonic work, such as walking in place at a very slow rate. This could be done prior to stage 1 in order to acquire gas exchange data at several levels of work that are less than that associated with 1 mile per hour and 0 per cent grade or with low level (ie, 6.25 watts) bicycle ergometry.

Incremental Work Rate Treadmill Exercise

Most of the treadmill protocols described in the literature are similar in that they all utilize incremental work rates. The most commonly used treadmill protocols for cardiac patients are the Bruce,[14] Balke,[15] Naughton,[16] Ellestad,[17] and ours.[18] Results of a national survey of 1400 facilities showed that 65.5 per cent used the Bruce protocol, mostly for traditional stress testing and the evaluation of coronary artery disease.[7] As can be seen, the initial work rate of the Bruce (Table 9–5) and Ellestad (Table 9–7) protocols is quite high (5 mets or a $\dot{V}O_2$ of 17.5 ml/min/kg). Such a level of work is not achievable in heart failure class C and D patients who are defined as having a $\dot{V}O_2$ max of less than 16 ml/min/kg (see Table 10–2). For these patients, our protocol (Table 9–4), the Naughton protocol (Table 9–6), and the Balke protocol (Table 9–8), all of which

Table 9–6. Naughton Protocol for Treadmill Exercise

Stage (3 min)	Speed (mph)	Grade (%)	Mets*
1	1.0	0	2.8
2	1.5	0	2.8
3	2.0	0	3.1
4	2.0	3.5	3.4
5	2.0	7.0	4.3
6	3.0	5.0	5.1
7	3.0	7.5	6.0
8	3.0	10.0	7.1
9	3.0	12.5	8.3
10	3.0	15.0	9.7

*Calculated from Patterson JA, Naughton J, Pietras RJ, Gunnar RM. Treadmill exercise in assessment of the functional capacity of patients with cardiac disease. Am J Cardiol 30:757–762, 1972, Figure 1.

Table 9–7. *Ellestad Protocol for Treadmill Exercise*

Stage (time)	Speed (mph)	Grade (%)	Mets*
1 (3 min)	1.7	10	5.0
2 (2 min)	3.0	10	7.0
3 (2 min)	4.0	10	8.5
4 (3 min)	5.0	10	13.0

*Estimated from Table 9–3.

have a lower initial and incremental (less than 1 met per stage) work rate, are more appropriate. In fact, more than 99 per cent of our patients attain their anaerobic threshold and $\dot{V}O_2$ max within the confines of our exercise protocol. The main criticism of these three tests is their duration; healthier and fitter individuals would require 20 or more minutes of exercise, compared with 12 to 15 minutes with the Bruce protocol, to accomplish the same end-points. Thus, the decision about which exercise protocol to use depends on the fitness of the person to be tested.

If the exercise laboratory is devoted primarily to evaluating individuals who have low functional capacities (for example, elderly persons, patients with a recent myocardial infarction or surgery, and symptomatic patients with cardiopulmonary disease), then either the Naughton, Balke, or our protocol should be used. If, on the other hand, the exercise laboratory is designed primarily to screen nonsymptomatic individuals (such as persons at high cardiac risk and sedentary persons who are going to engage in highly intense activities), either the Bruce

Table 9–8. *Balke Protocol for Treadmill Exercise*

Stage (2 min)	Speed (mph)	Grade (%)	Mets*
1	3.0	0	2.4
2	3.0	2.5	4.0
3	3.0	5.0	5.0
4	3.0	7.5	6.0
5	3.0	10.0	7.0
6	3.0	12.5	8.0
7	3.0	15.0	8.5
8	3.0	17.5	10.0
9	3.0	20.0	11.0
10	3.0	22.5	12.0

*Estimated from Table 9–3 and Hellerstein HK, Franklin BA. Evaluating the cardiac patient for exercise therapy, *in* Franklin BA, Rubenfire M (eds). Symposium on Cardiac Rehabilitation. Clin Sports Med 3:371–393, 1984, Figure 1.

or Ellestad protocol is appropriate. Because the Bruce protocol has been more widely used and an abundance of published data exist that can be used for comparisons, it has an advantage over the Ellestad protocol.

Constant Work Rate Treadmill Exercise

Another treadmill exercise scheme is to maintain a constant work rate for a prolonged period of time. The level of work can be either aerobic or anaerobic. However, aerobic constant work rate exercise testing of patients with cardiac or circulatory failure has no objective end-point (Chapters 10 and 11). On the other hand, anaerobic constant work rate exercise testing is valuable as it may mimic the work rate at which effort intolerance during daily activities is encountered. Accordingly, if therapy is effective, it should ameliorate any limiting symptoms (ie, dyspnea and fatigue) experienced at this work rate level. Thus, the anaerobic constant work rate exercise test allows one to assess the efficacy of therapy using submaximal levels of work. Our experience with various exercise protocols is presented in Chapters 10 and 11.

Ergometer Exercise

Bicycle ergometer exercise protocols suitable for a wide spectrum of patients usually begin at the lowest work load setting. This is typically 15 or 25 watts (90 or 150 kpm/min). Each stage of the protocol lasts for 2 to 3 minutes provided the increment in work load is 15 to 25 watts. Larger increments in work load require a longer interval inasmuch as the time to achieve steady state is increased. Table 9–3 lists the relation between work rate in watts and mets. To find the corresponding $\dot{V}O_2$, multiply mets by 3.5 ml/min/kg.

Jones and Campbell reported three bicycle ergometer protocols that they refer to as the Scandinavian, Triangular, and Stage 1 protocols.[11] The Scandinavian protocol starts with and utilizes work rate increments of 50 w (300 kpm/min) for men and 33 w (200 kpm/min) for women, with each increment being maintained for 4 to 6 min. A 50 w increment is associated with a $\dot{V}O_2$ of 14 ml/min/kg, which exceeds the $\dot{V}O_2$ max of most Class C and all D patients. Thus, this protocol is primarily designed for nonsymptomatic individuals. The Triangular protocol consists of a continuously increasing work rate. The rate of increase is established by the person administering the test, who is attempting to elevate heart rate by 5 beats/min. The Stage 1 protocol was developed in the laboratory of Jones and uses either 8 w (50 kpm/min) or 17 w (100 kpm/min) increments, which are maintained for 1 min. The smaller increment is reserved for the extremely limited patient.

Whipp et al[12] and Davis et al[13] have recently investigated the differences between an incremental (2 to 3 min intervals) steady state exercise test and continually increasing work rates of 20, 30, and 50 w/min. Using normal, conditioned subjects, they found no major differences in the gas exchange and transport responses associated with their "ramp" test and the conventional incremental test. The advantage of the ramp, the Triangular, and the Stage 1 protocols is the reduction in total exercise time. That is, less time is required to achieve anaerobic threshold and maximum oxygen uptake.

As mentioned earlier, bicycle ergometers can be converted for use as an *arm ergometer*.[6] The same protocols recommended for bicycle ergometry can be used for arm ergometry. However, because a smaller muscle mass is used during arm ergometry, the maximum achievable $\dot{V}O_2$ is less than bicycle ergometry by about 25 per cent.[6] The arm ergometer is positioned so that the person exercising can sit with the forearm fully extended and parallel to the floor at maximal reach. The following arm ergometry protocol has been suggested by Hellerstein and Franklin:[19] The subject begins with 3 minutes of warm-up by arm pedaling at zero load. Following a 1 to 2 minute rest period, load is increased by 25 w (150 kpm/min), and the subject exercises for another 3 minute period. The cycle (ie, rest, increase load, and exercise) is then repeated until the subject can no longer maintain the correct pedal speed (maximal peak effort). Because of the continuous arm motion, measurements of cuff blood pressure and the electrocardiogram are recorded immediately at the beginning of each rest period.

The fact that arm ergometry involves a smaller muscle mass can be considered a major disadvantage of this form of exercise. Maximal achievable heart rate and $\dot{V}O_2$ are both lower than those obtained with leg exercise. Consequently, one could not use the results of an arm ergometry test to predict an individual's exercise capacity.

Step Test Exercise

A protocol for the graded step test described by Nagle, Balke, and Naughton has been recommended by the American Heart Association.[4] This protocol is designed for a step apparatus that has an adjustable step height (2 to 50 centimeters; Fig. 9–1). The step height is initially 2.0 cm, and a four count, stepping rhythm is regulated by a metronome to 30 steps/min. The patient steps up with a one-two count and back down on a three-four count. Periodically, the patient is advised to begin the four-count procedure using the opposite leg so as to prevent early fatigue of one leg. At the end of the second minute the step height is increased by 2.0 cm. Thereafter it is increased an additional 2.0 cm at the end of each minute. The test continues until the subject is no longer able to maintain the 30 steps/min rhythm.

As discussed earlier, this test is not conducive to extensive monitoring. However, it is recommended that the heart rate be continuously measured and, at each step height, that the patient stop momentarily to obtain a cuff blood pressure measurement.

Isometric Exercise Test Protocol

The usual procedure in isometric exercise testing is to first determine the maximal voluntary contraction (MVC). For example, maximum handgrip strength can be assessed on a hand dynamometer and maximal forearm lifting strength can be determined by measuring the heaviest load that could be lifted through 60°.[8] After MVC is determined, the subject is asked to repeat the isometric maneuver at a certain percentage of MVC. Usually the percentage is 25 for light and 30 to 40 for heavy isometric effort, which is sustained for at least 3 minutes for a heavy effort and as long as 6 minutes for a light effort. Gas exchange measurements are made continuously, and hemodynamic data are obtained as often as possible. Throughout the test, the subject should be encouraged to breathe freely and to avoid holding the breath and straining.

As mentioned earlier, isometric tests can involve small muscle groups such as the forearm, large muscle groups such as the legs, or combinations of both groups.[9] The hemodynamic response to isometric exercise depends on the amount of active muscle mass.[20] For example, the slope of the heart rate–absolute $\dot{V}O_2$ relationship is inversely proportional to active muscle mass, as is the work-related increase in systemic blood pressure.[20] The type of muscle that is active will dictate the length of time a particular work load can be sustained. As an example, the critical value of per cent MVC below which long-lasting (more than 10 min) static work can be maintained is 10 per cent MVC for the elbow extensors and 25 per cent for the elbow flexors. Asmussen suggested this difference to be the result of (1) the structure and placement of the muscle, and (2) the ratio of fast- to slow-twitch muscle fibers.[10] In the example just cited, the elbow extensors contain many fast fibers whereas the elbow flexors contain only a few. Therefore, if a patient is being tested to determine whether he or she could safely perform an isometric task, then the isometric test should be designed to mimic as closely as possible the actual task. That is, the test should involve the same muscle groups and a similar work load.

MANUFACTURERS CITED

Fitness Products
P.O. Box 254
Hillsday, Minnesota 49242

Tri-Tech, Incorporated
6011 N. Yorktown
Tulsa, Oklahoma 74130

REFERENCES

1. Sharrock N, Garrett HL, Mann GV. Practical exercise test for physical fitness and cardiac performance. Am J Cardiol 30:727–732, 1972.
2. Kaltenbach M. Exercise Testing of Cardiac Patients. Williams & Wilkins, Baltimore, 1976, p 17.
3. Master AM, Rosenfeld I. The two-step exercise test brought up to date. NY J Med 61:1850–1857, 1961.
4. Nagle FJ, Balke B, Naughton JP. Gradational step tests for assessing work capacity. J Appl Physiol 20:745–748, 1965.
5. Aronson MH (ed). Stress test/ergometers. Med Electronics Issue 84:187–195, 1983.
6. Sawka MN, Foley ME, Pimental NA, Toner MM, Pandolf KB. Determination of maximal aerobic power during upper-body exercise. J Appl Physiol 54:113–117, 1983.
7. Stuart RJ, Ellestad MH. National survey of exercise stress testing facilities. Chest 77:94–97, 1980.
8. DeBusk R, Pitts W, Haskell W, Houston N. Comparison of cardiovascular responses to static-dynamic effort and dynamic effort alone in patients with chronic ischemic heart disease. Circulation 59:977–984, 1979.
9. Mitchell JH, Payne FC III, Saltin B, Schibye B. The role of muscle mass in the cardiovascular response to static contractions. J Physiol (Lond) 309:45–54, 1980.
10. Asmussen E. Similarities and dissimilarities between static and dynamic exercise. Circ Res 48:I3–I10, 1981.
11. Jones NL, Campbell EJM. Clinical Exercise Testing. 2nd ed. WB Saunders, Philadelphia, 1982, pp 79–80.
12. Whipp BJ, Davis JA, Torres F, Wasserman K. A test to determine parameters of aerobic function during exercise. J Appl Physiol 50:217–221, 1981.
13. Davis JA, Whipp BJ, Lamarra N, Huntsman DJ, Frank MH, Wasserman K. Effect of ramp slope on determination of aerobic parameters from the ramp exercise test. Med Sci Sports Exerc 14:339–343, 1982.
14. Bruce RA, Kusumi F, Hosmer D. Maximal oxygen intake and nomographic assessment of functional aerobic impairment in cardiovascular disease. Am Heart J 85:546–562, 1973.
15. Balke B, Ware R. An experimental study of physical fitness of Air Force personnel. US Armed Forces Med J 10:675–688, 1959.
16. Patterson JA, Naughton J, Pietras RJ, Gunnar RM. Treadmill exercise in assessment of the functional capacity of patients with cardiac disease. Am J Cardiol 30:757–762, 1972.
17. Ellestad MH, Allen W, Wan MCK, Kemp GL. Maximal treadmill stress testing for cardiovascular evaluation. Circulation 39:517–522, 1969.
18. Weber KT, Kinasewitz GT, West JS, Janicki JS, Reichek N, Fishman AP. Long-term vasodilatory therapy with trimazosin in chronic cardiac failure. N Engl J Med 303:242–250, 1980.
19. Hellerstein HK, Franklin BA. Evaluating the cardiac patient for exercise therapy, in Franklin BA, Rubenfire M (eds). Symposium on Cardiac Rehabilitation. Clin Sports Med 3:371–393, 1984.
20. Blomqvist CG, Lewis SF, Taylor WF, Graham RM. Similarity of the hemodynamic responses to static and dynamic exercise of small muscle groups. Circ Res 48:I87–I92, 1981.

KARL T. WEBER
JOSEPH S. JANICKI
PATRICIA A. McELROY

10

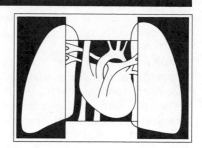

Cardiopulmonary Exercise (CPX) Testing

Exercise is a physiologic stress that can be used clinically to evaluate heart and lung function. Latent or overt abnormalities in the cardiocirculatory and respiratory systems will be manifest during the increased metabolic requirements of muscular work. The advent of rapidly responding oxygen and carbon dioxide analyzers, together with airflow-sensing devices, not only makes the noninvasive evaluation of the body's gas transport and exchange system a reality, but they also do so on a breath-by-breath basis. The continuous monitoring of oxygen uptake ($\dot{V}O_2$), carbon dioxide production ($\dot{V}CO_2$), minute ventilation ($\dot{V}E$), respiratory rate, and tidal volume at rest and during exercise can be performed simply. The former cumbersome and burdensome methods of gas collection and analysis are no longer necessary.

A variety of exercise tests can be utilized, together with the noninvasive technique of respiratory gas exchange and air flow analysis—and in selected cases invasive hemodynamic monitoring—to assess a particular clinical disorder of the cardiopulmonary unit. The choice of a cardiopulmonary exercise test and the parameters that should be measured depend on the nature and expression of the clinical disorder and the particular problem that needs to be addressed. In this chapter we will examine the various types of isotonic exercise that we have found useful in the clinical evaluation of cardiopulmonary disease. Also, the various parameters, obtained noninvasively or invasively, that can be used to evaluate various clinical problems will be discussed. Our experience with these tests in specific clinical disorders is described in greater detail in Chapters 11 through 18.

NONINVASIVE TYPES OF CPX

Exercise tests can be used to examine the response to isotonic or isometric forms of muscular work in patients with heart or lung disease or both. For most clinical evaluations we prefer isotonic forms of exercise because, first, isotonic work is an acceptable, negotiable, and reproducible form of exercise for patients with cardiovascular or respiratory disease. In contrast, with isometric exercise, patients have to be taught not to simultaneously perform the Valsalva maneuver. Second, many of the responses in respiratory gas exchange seen during the performance of isometric exercise are not temporally coincident with isometric work and only occur following the release of the muscle contraction. Third, isometric exercise is associated with a substantial increase in arterial systolic and diastolic blood pressures that may be detrimental to the patient with hypertensive cardiovascular disease, mitral regurgitation, or heart failure. Finally, less is known about the value of the isometric exercise test in the evaluation of cardiopulmonary disorders.

Incremental isotonic cardiopulmonary exercise testing (CPX), whether it be performed on the treadmill or bicycle, can be used to evaluate disorders of the cardiopulmonary unit.[1-5] In many cases, noninvasive CPX is not a diagnostic test since it will not identify the underlying mechanism responsible for the abnormal exercise response. Noninvasive CPX will identify an impaired aerobic capacity and anaerobic threshold that will indicate the functional capacity of the patient and the severity of the underlying disorder of the heart, as well as predict the cardiac reserve.

151

It will also identify abnormalities in the ventilatory response to exercise in patients with lung disease. These issues are considered more fully later in this chapter and for specific disorders of the cardiopulmonary unit in Chapters 11 to 18.

For more diagnostic information regarding a particular cardiocirculatory or respiratory disorder, complementary procedures and tests are required. For example, echocardiographic imaging of the heart may identify a thickened pericardium or stenosed mitral valve that is responsible for the impaired aerobic capacity of a particular patient. Regrettably, however, current imaging techniques cannot be utilized during exercise to identify the appearance of mitral regurgitation or myocardial wall motion abnormality. For more specific diagnostic purposes, hemodynamic monitoring, the measurement of pleural pressure, or sampling arterial blood gases during exercise will identify abnormalities that impair effort tolerance. We have considered these latter procedures to represent invasive forms of CPX. They too are reviewed later in this chapter. First, let us consider the noninvasive forms of CPX.

Incremental Treadmill Exercise

Walking is the most common form of daily exercise that each of our patients undertakes; it therefore is not a specialized skill. Moreover, if a patient can walk into the physician's office or walk the corridors of the hospital, he or she can walk on the treadmill at 1.0 or 1.5 mph, 0 per cent grade. Because most treadmills are programmable, each patient and his or her exercise capacity can be accommodated.

We have chosen a treadmill protocol of gradually progressive exercise. The protocol consists of 2 minute stages and has been presented in Table 9–4 in the preceding chapter. The levels of work represented by this protocol are expressed in terms of everyday physical activity in Table 10–1. Treadmill exercise will work a sufficiently large muscle mass to adequately stress the cardiopulmonary unit. With the monitoring of $\dot{V}O_2$, $\dot{V}CO_2$, $\dot{V}E$, and end-tidal oxygen and carbon dioxide on a breath-by-breath basis, we are able to determine the anaerobic threshold and the $\dot{V}O_2$ max (vide infra) of a patient during a single treadmill exercise test. The first two stages of exercise represent very low work loads. They can be viewed as a "warm-up" for normal subjects and patients with

Table 10–1. Our Treadmill Exercise Protocol and the Levels of Everyday Physical Activities That Are Represented in Each Stage of Work

Stage	Speed	Grade	Physical Activities
1	1.0	0	Driving a car Sitting and writing or eating
2	1.5	0	Dressing; knitting Walking to bathroom Light auto repair
3	2.0	3.5	Shave self in bathroom Wash entire body Food shopping
4	2.0	7.0	Sexual activity Raking leaves Plastering
5	2.0	10.5	Stacking firewood Mowing lawn (powered) Walking downstairs
6	3.0	7.5	Scrubbing floors Gardening Walking upstairs
7	3.0	10.0	Lifting and carrying 65–80 lbs Carpentry Climbing hills (no load)
8	3.0	12.5	Digging Snow shoveling Climbing stairs (20 lb load)
9	3.0	15.0	Beyond this level work
10	3.4	14.0	loads are compatible
11	3.4	16.0	with very vigorous
12	3.4	18.0	exercise (e.g., skiing,
13	3.4	20.0	basketball)
14	3.4	22.0	

little or no disease. On the other hand, what amounts to walking down the hall (1 or 1.5 mph, 0 per cent grade) is near maximal exercise for patients with advanced cardiac failure or pulmonary hypertension. To keep the test uniform for all patients and to draw comparisons between the normal and abnormal response, we use a common protocol for each evaluation.

Maximal oxygen uptake, or $\dot{V}O_2$ max, is defined as $\dot{V}O_2$ remaining invariant or less than 1 ml/min/kg for 30 seconds or more despite an increment in work load. We prefer to have an invariant $\dot{V}O_2$ for at least two stages of exercise whenever possible. Figure 10–1 depicts the breath-by-breath analysis of gas exchange and airflow that can be used to determine the $\dot{V}O_2$ max of a patient. The $\dot{V}O_2$ max associated with treadmill exercise provides the greatest aerobic capacity of any standard exercise test because it works the largest group of muscles.

As noted in earlier chapters, $\dot{V}O_2$ max is a function of the maximal cardiac output that the heart can generate and the maximal

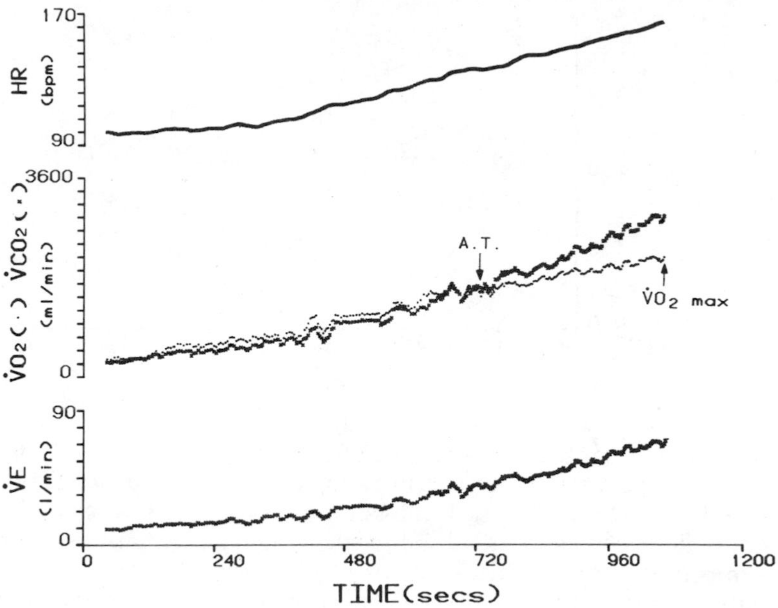

FIGURE 10–1. The breath-by-breath response in respiratory gas exchange during incremental treadmill exercise in a 43 year old man with hypertension. Note the anaerobic threshold (*A.T.*) at a $\dot{V}O_2$ of 15 ml/min/kg and an invariant $\dot{V}O_2$ for two consecutive stages of exercise and a $\dot{V}O_2$ max of 22 ml/min/kg.

amount of oxygen that the tissues can extract. We have assigned the aerobic capacity observed during an incremental treadmill exercise test into one of four classes each of which represents a given degree of functional impairment[1] (Table 10–2). We have termed the classes A, B, C, and D to avoid confusion with the New York Heart Association classification that is frequently used to derive similar information. However, unlike the objective information obtained by CPX, the Heart Association's classification is based on historical information obtained through patient interview. Our classification is the following: little or no impairment in aerobic capacity is thought to be present when $\dot{V}O_2$ max exceeds 20 ml/min/kg. We term this group functional *class A*; for age- and sex-corrected $\dot{V}O_2$ max of the normal adult population commonly seen in practice,[6] $\dot{V}O_2$ max will be above this level (Fig. 10–2). Mild to moderate impairment, termed *class B*, is present when $\dot{V}O_2$ max ranges between 16 and 20 ml/min/kg. A

moderate to severe impairment, *class C*, exists when $\dot{V}O_2$ max falls between 10 and 16 ml/min/kg. *Class D* represents a severe impairment, with $\dot{V}O_2$ max ranging between 6 and 10 ml/min/kg.

In patients with clear evidence of cardiovascular disease—for example, cardiomegaly in a patient with a dilated cardiomyopathy, we can further subdivide the class A response according to $\dot{V}O_2$ max (ml/min/kg) as 20 to 25 (class A_1), 25 to 30 (class A_2), 30 to 35 (class A_3), and 35 to 40 (class A_4).

A very severe impairment in aerobic capacity is present in *class E* patients who are markedly symptomatic and anaerobic at rest, with a $\dot{V}O_2$ max of less than 6 ml/min/kg.[7] We recommend not exercising these patients.

We do not recommend substituting the duration of symptom-free treadmill exercise for the $\dot{V}O_2$ max determination, since treadmill time is far less precise in characterizing aerobic capacity (Fig. 10–3).[1, 8] Moreover, treadmill time suffers from not having an

Table 10–2. *Functional Impairment in Aerobic Capacity and Anaerobic Threshold as Measured During Incremental Treadmill CPX*

Class	Severity	$\dot{V}O_2$ Max *(ml/min/kg)*	Anaerobic Threshold *(ml/min/kg)*
A	mild to none	> 20	> 14
B	mild to moderate	16 to 20	11 to 14
C	moderate to severe	10 to 16	8 to 11
D	severe	6 to 10	5 to 8
E	very severe	< 6	< 4

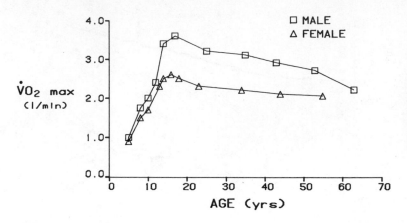

FIGURE 10–2. The age and sex predicted $\dot{V}O_2$ max to treadmill exercise for healthy subjects. (Adapted from Astrand I, Astrand P-O, Hallback I, Kilbom A. Reduction in maximum oxygen uptake with age. J Appl Physiol 35:649–654, 1973.)

objective, quantitative end-point to predict aerobic capacity. Differences in gait and body weight create different levels of work for equivalent stages of treadmill work. Finally, symptom-limited exercise time is clouded by patient and physician bias. The maximum heart rate attained with exercise is also a less precise measure of $\dot{V}O_2$ max, especially in patients with atrial fibrillation.

The $\dot{V}O_2$ max determination will identify aerobic capacity and permit a subdivision of lesser work loads into low, moderate, heavy, very heavy, and exhaustive levels of physical activity for a given individual (Fig. 10–4). The reproducibility of the treadmill $\dot{V}O_2$ max determination in patients having a wide variety of cardiovascular diseases is given in the left panel of Figure 10–5. Each value was obtained days to weeks apart. We also have had the opportunity to follow the exercise response of a number of patients (Fig. 10–6) who had agreed to participate in a controlled

clinical trial in which they received placebo in a double-blind schedule over a period of 12 weeks.[9] These findings are reviewed in Chapter 21 and again indicate the reproducibility of the aerobic capacity determination.

Patients generally adapt very rapidly to the treadmill protocol, particularly with the low level of work involved in stages 1 and 2. In the major learning portion of the test, patients become familiar with the fact that they are not expected to run, to walk too quickly, or to lean on the handrails of the treadmill. This learning curve is necessitated in part by their preconceived notion of what a treadmill exercise test represents or by the fact that they have previously been exercised with the Bruce protocol (Chapter 9) that increases energy requirements quite rapidly.

The *anaerobic threshold* determination is generally defined according to five criteria: the disproportionate rise (relative to $\dot{V}O_2$) in $\dot{V}CO_2$, $\dot{V}E$, R (or $\dot{V}CO_2/\dot{V}O_2$), and the venti-

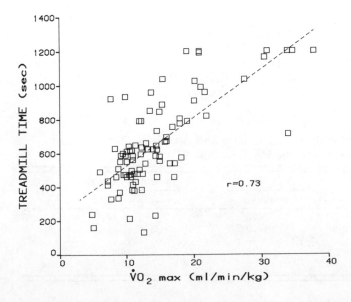

FIGURE 10–3. The relationship between aerobic capacity and treadmill time has only a weak correlation. See text for discussion.

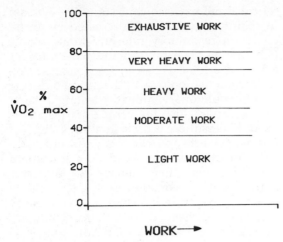

FIGURE 10–4. The intensity of muscular work can be described as a percentage of the maximal O_2 uptake ($\dot{V}O_2$ max).

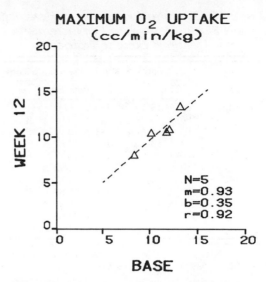

FIGURE 10–6. The reproducibility of the $\dot{V}O_2$ max determination for treadmill exercise in five patients with heart failure after 12 weeks of placebo therapy in a drug trial. (Adapted from Weber KT, Andrews V, Janicki JS, Likoff MJ, Reichek N. Pirbuterol, an oral beta-adrenergic receptor agonist, in the treatment of chronic cardiac failure. Circulation 66:1262–1267, 1982.)

latory equivalent for O_2 (or $\dot{V}E/\dot{V}O_2$), and the disproportionate rise in end-tidal O_2 relative to end-tidal CO_2. These criteria can best be applied to breath-by-breath respiratory gas exchange data. Figure 10–1 depicts the anaerobic threshold determination using breath-by-breath gas exchange during our incremental treadmill exercise protocol. We make no attempt to define the absolute time or absolute work load at which anaerobiosis occurs. Rather, we identify the stage of exercise and its corresponding level of work as being the anaerobic threshold. When it is

measured days or weeks apart, we have found the anaerobic threshold determination to be reproducible in our patients (see Fig. 10–5).[1] A further discussion of anaerobic threshold is provided later in this chapter.

The electrocardiogram, heart rate, and cuff blood pressure should be monitored with

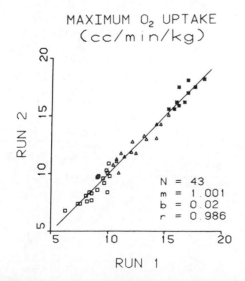

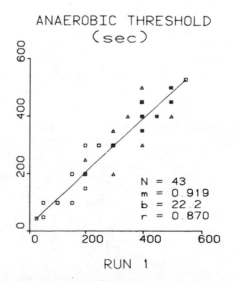

FIGURE 10–5. For patients with heart failure, the reproducibility of the treadmill $\dot{V}O_2$ max and anaerobic threshold determinations that were obtained days or weeks apart is shown. (From Weber KT, Kinasewitz GT, Janicki JS, Fishman AP. Oxygen utilization and ventilation during exercise in patients with chronic cardiac failure. Circulation 65:1213–1223, 1982.)

Table 10–3. *Normal Response in Heart Rate and Blood Pressure to Our Incremental Treadmill Exercise Protocol*

Stage	Heart Rate (bpm)	Systolic/Diastolic Pressure (mm Hg)
Standing*	86 ± 13	130 ± 8/92 ± 11
1	96 ± 15	140 ± 13/96 ± 8
2	98 ± 14	141 ± 12/93 ± 8
3	104 ± 13	145 ± 13/91 ± 7
4	110 ± 13	150 ± 13/87 ± 8
5	118 ± 14	155 ± 13/92 ± 11
6	126 ± 13	159 ± 21/87 ± 8
7	135 ± 15	168 ± 19/88 ± 9
8	144 ± 15	166 ± 19/91 ± 11
9	155 ± 14	169 ± 25/88 ± 10
10	162 ± 15	179 ± 21/86 ± 14

*The anticipatory phase of exercise is accompanied by a slight increase in blood pressure.

the patient resting (sitting and standing) throughout exercise and during a 10 minute period of recovery. The normal heart rate and blood pressure response to the first ten stages of our treadmill exercise protocol are given in Table 10–3.

Over the past 10 years we have safely and reliably monitored aerobic capacity and anaerobic threshold in many hundreds of patients with various forms of cardiovascular disease, including those with heart failure. In many of these patients the test has been performed serially over several years to monitor the natural course of their disease or their response to medical therapy (Chapter 21).

We specifically exclude exercising patients with significant aortic stenosis, hypertrophic cardiomyopathy, exertional or rest angina, significant arrhythmia, exercise-induced arrhythmia, or a history of exertional syncope.

The normal *ventilatory response* to incremental treadmill exercise consists of an increase in minute ventilation ($\dot{V}E$) created by an increase in respiratory rate and tidal volume (Chapter 5). The ratio of the maximum $\dot{V}E$ achieved with exercise to the maximal voluntary ventilation (MVV) determined during routine pulmonary function testing reflects the extent to which the ventilatory reserve is used. Unless there is coexistent lung disease, normal subjects and patients with cardiovascular disease rarely exceed 50 per cent of their MVV with their exercise $\dot{V}E$. The same is true of the maximal exercise tidal volume to vital capacity ratio. Thus, the ventilatory reserves, represented by maximal voluntary ventilation and vital capacity, are only partially utilized during light, moderate, and maximal exercise. This response appears to be consistent with the ventilatory effort that can be voluntarily sustained at rest prior to the appearance of fatigue or the sensation of breathlessness.[10, 11] Table 10–4 indicates the normal response in $\dot{V}E$, tidal volume, and respiratory rate to exercise and the proportion of the ventilatory reserves which these occupy.

The ear oximeter is an indirect, noninvasive method of monitoring *arterial oxygen saturation* that can be used as part of the treadmill test (Chapter 8). This is a particularly useful screening procedure in patients in whom oxygen desaturation might be anticipated (e.g., congenital heart disease with right to left shunt, restrictive or obstructive lung disease, or pulmonary vascular disease). We have not found normal subjects or patients with chronic cardiac failure to have a significant fall in oxygen saturation during exercise.[1] The technique, however, may give erroneous information in the hyperpigmented skin of some black patients or when the ear is pierced. In patients in whom oxy-

Table 10–4. *Normal Response in Ventilation to Our Incremental Treadmill Exercise Protocol*

Stage	Minute Ventilation (liters/min)	$\dot{V}E$/MVV (%)	VT (ml)	VT/FVC (%)	Respiratory Rate (bpm)
1	18 ± 6.1	12 ± 3.7	1153 ± 417	25 ± 7.6	17 ± 4.0
2	20 ± 5.3	14 ± 3.4	1162 ± 450	26 ± 8.2	19 ± 3.5
3	24 ± 7.2	17 ± 3.7	1270 ± 368	29 ± 6.5	20 ± 3.9
4	29 ± 8.5	20 ± 4.9	1388 ± 394	31 ± 6.2	22 ± 3.6
5	33 ± 9.3	23 ± 5.8	1468 ± 405	33 ± 6.9	24 ± 2.8
6	40 ± 12.2	27 ± 6.9	1628 ± 456	36 ± 6.9	25 ± 3.9
7	46 ± 13.7	31 ± 7.8	1776 ± 502	40 ± 7.6	27 ± 5.8
8	52 ± 17.3	35 ± 9.1	1921 ± 502	42 ± 9.8	28 ± 6.6
9	61 ± 18.9	41 ± 8.9	2153 ± 681	47 ± 9.4	29 ± 7.2
10	72 ± 25	46 ± 12.6	2216 ± 700	48 ± 9.7	33 ± 10.2

$\dot{V}E$/MVV, the ratio of minute ventilation to maximal voluntary ventilation; VT, tidal volume; and VT/FVC, the ratio of tidal volume to forced vital capacity.

gen desaturation is suspected or evident from ear oximetry, arterial blood oxygen saturation should be measured directly from an indwelling catheter.

Because of our extensive experience with treadmill exercise testing and our conviction that it is the most negotiable and reproducible exercise for our patients, we use this form of CPX in the great majority of cases referred to our Cardiopulmonary Exercise Laboratory. We have found the test to be particularly useful in the evaluation of chronic cardiac failure, valvular heart disease, pulmonary vascular disease, systemic hypertension, chronotropic dysfunction, and the response to various therapies, and in the assessment of the natural course of cardiopulmonary disease. This experience will be reviewed in subsequent chapters.

Thus, incremental treadmill exercise can be used to give the following information: (a) determination of anaerobic threshold with a submaximal test; (b) determination of anaerobic threshold and VO_2 max with a maximal test; (c) evaluation of the ventilatory response to submaximal or maximal exercise; (d) evaluation of arterial oxygen saturation during submaximal or maximal exercise. One can obviously combine each of these assessments into a single treadmill exercise test.

Incremental Bicycle Exercise

In keeping with the viewpoint that exercise testing is valuable in the evaluation of a wide spectrum of patients with cardiopulmonary disease, it is useful to have various exercise modalities available in the clinical laboratory. The bicycle ergometer is a useful device to evaluate exercise performance in patients who for one reason or another have difficulty performing treadmill exercise. These situations might include the obese patient, patients in whom a specific level of muscular work or power output is required and can easily be selected from the ergometer, circumstances in which the bicycle will be used in exercise training, or patients with far-advanced lung disease in whom only very low levels of work can be negotiated. We have chosen a program of bicycle work that represents gradually progressive increments in muscular work. Three minute levels of work are performed to permit the unfamiliar patient with sufficient time to attain pedal speed and thereby achieve a given level of work. We have modified the electronics of our ergometer to permit work load incre-

ments of 6.25 watts. Table 9–1 depicts the conversion of watts to kilopond-meters of cycle ergometer work.

Because the subject is in the sitting position, body weight is supported by the seat of the ergometer. As a result, a smaller muscle mass is used for exercise. These factors account for the lower VO_2 max (Fig. 10–7) seen at exhaustion with the bicycle ergometer in comparison with that observed with the treadmill.[12] Reproducibility of the VO_2 max determination to cycle ergometry can also be expected.

The appearance of anaerobic threshold is documented in a manner similar to that described earlier for the treadmill, as is also true for VO_2 max (Fig. 10–8). However, with bicycle ergometry a change of less than 0.75 ml/min/kg in VO_2 is used to indicate an invariant VO_2 or plateau in oxygen uptake. Special studies, such as the measurement of femoral venous blood flow and lower extremity oxygen extraction and lactate production, may also be better served and obtained more safely by the bicycle ergometer. These special procedures are discussed more fully subsequently.

The ventilatory response to cycle exercise is essentially similar to that observed for the treadmill (Fig. 10–7).

Constant Work Rate Treadmill Exercise

Constant work rate exercise can be used to assess endurance (exercise training) or in selected cases to examine ventilatory control. We have used constant work rate treadmill exercise to assess submaximal exercise capacity in patients with cardiac or circulatory failure. We found that aerobic endurance exercise (Fig. 10–9) had no symptomatic or objective end-points. The responses associated with aerobic constant work rate treadmill exercise are discussed further in Chapter 11. Anaerobic endurance exercise (Fig. 10–10), on the other hand, does have such end-points. In the anaerobic region of muscular work, representing more than 70 per cent VO_2 max, there is a progressive rise in mixed venous lactate concentration that is not seen with aerobic work. As a result of this lactate production, there is a corresponding progressive rise in VE, mediated primarily by the rise in respiratory rate. Patients discontinue walking because of the appearance of breathlessness and, in some cases, fatigue. It is quite interesting that the hemodynamic

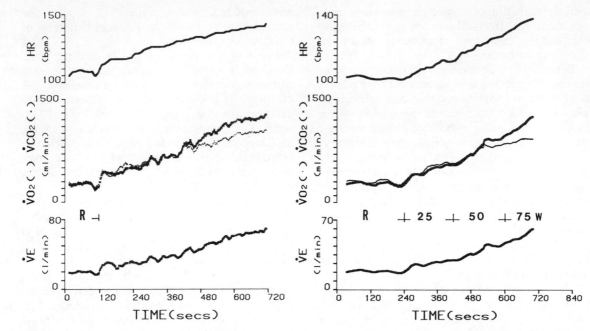

FIGURE 10–7. A comparison of the response in respiratory gas exchange and airflow of a 47 year old man with dilated cardiomyopathy who performed treadmill (left) and bicycle (right) exercise. $\dot{V}O_2$ max for the bicycle was 10 per cent less than that observed with treadmill exercise. R, standing or sitting rest; w, watts.

response to anaerobic endurance need not be different from that observed with steady state aerobic work, as will be described in Chapter 11.

We are currently evaluating the utility of the anaerobic endurance test to determine the efficacy of therapeutic interventions aimed at improving submaximal effort toler-ance. We believe this test may come closest to mimicking the effort intolerance of daily living, and if a therapeutic agent is to be effective, it should eliminate or at least atten-uate the appearance of dyspnea and fatigue during constant work rate exercise.

Many training programs are based on reg-ular exercise at 70 per cent or more of the

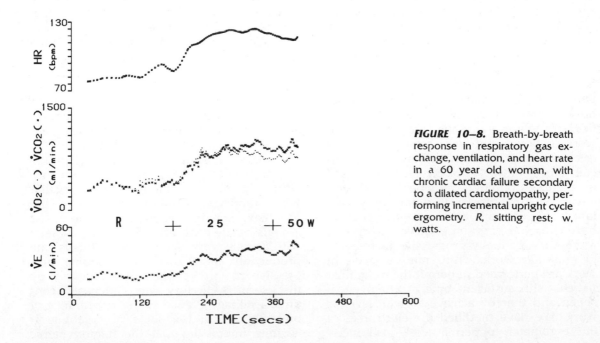

FIGURE 10–8. Breath-by-breath response in respiratory gas ex-change, ventilation, and heart rate in a 60 year old woman, with chronic cardiac failure secondary to a dilated cardiomyopathy, per-forming incremental upright cycle ergometry. R, sitting rest; w, watts.

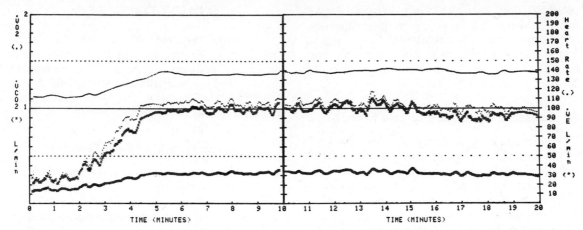

FIGURE 10–9. Submaximal aerobic constant work rate endurance treadmill exercise for a 62 year old women with chronic cardiac failure. The final 2 minutes of the exercise protocol are not shown. The first 2 minutes are at standing rest.

age- and sex-predicted maximal O_2 uptake. This will represent anaerobic work for most untrained normal subjects and patients with cardiopulmonary disease. The merit or safety of this approach in patients with heart failure is unproved and it therefore cannot be recommended at this time. We prefer an individualized exercise prescription for such patients, in the aerobic range that represents moderate to moderately heavy work loads. Depending on the nature of the clinical problem or the intended purpose for choosing this particular test, a simple gas exchange system, such as the Waters Instrument in

which $\dot{V}O_2$ alone is measured, may be sufficient for determining the $\dot{V}O_2$ for a constant rate of work. A more involved gas exchange monitoring system that includes carbon dioxide and airflow sensors is required to document the anaerobic threshold before undertaking constant-rate anaerobic work loads for a program of training or rehabilitation.

In determining the anaerobic threshold and aerobic capacity, one can also derive the heart rate–$\dot{V}O_2$ relation from direct recordings of each parameter. This relation can be subsequently used in providing heart rate–targeted levels of physical activity in the

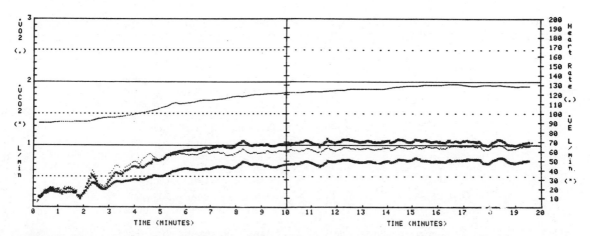

FIGURE 10–10. Submaximal anaerobic constant work rate endurance treadmill exercise for a 64 year old man with chronic cardiac failure secondary to ischemic heart disease. The appearance of a steady state in $\dot{V}O_2$ is more delayed than for aerobic endurance, and there is a progressive rise in ventilation throughout most of exercise. See text for discussion. The patient completed only 17.5 minutes of the protocol because of limiting symptoms. The first 2 minutes are at standing rest.

rehabilitation setting at the hospital or at home. Moreover, this direct determination of the heart rate–$\dot{V}O_2$ relation in each patient is a superior approach to using age, sex, and fitness predictions found in the literature and derived from population studies.

Constant Work Rate Bicycle Exercise

In a manner similar to that described for the treadmill, constant work rate exercise below or above the anaerobic threshold may be chosen for bicycle exercise testing. Wasserman et al have used this format of exercise to demonstrate the role fo the carotid bodies in dictating the ventilatory response to exercise.[13] The continual increase in $\dot{V}E$ seen with anaerobic work is related to the enhanced $\dot{V}CO_2$ that accompanies lactate buffering by bicarbonate; it is mediated by a continual rise in respiratory rate while tidal volume remains invariant or falls. In patients in whom the carotid bodies had been resected previously for the treatment of their asthma, the time constant for the ventilatory response to achieve a steady state during anaerobic work was more delayed than that observed in normal subjects (Chapter 5). These findings also emphasize the need to recognize whether the exercise work load is above or below the anaerobic threshold when examining the ventilatory response to exercise. They also underscore the important role played by the carotid bodies in mediating this response.

INVASIVE TYPES OF CPX

The same exercise tests described for noninvasive CPX can be complemented with special procedures that are by nature invasive (Table 10–5). How this is accomplished and the type of information that these procedures provide is described subsequently.

Incremental Treadmill Exercise

In patients with cardiopulmonary disease, it may be necessary to use invasive hemodynamic monitoring to define better the nature and severity of the underlying cardiopulmonary disorder. The information that can be gathered from such an approach is described later. The application of this technique to the evaluation of various clinical problems, such as heart failure and pulmonary vascular disease, is presented in the respective chapters devoted to these problems.

The advent of the flexible, triple lumen flotation catheter has simplified the process of hemodynamic monitoring in that the catheter can be inserted at the patient's bedside in the exercise laboratory without fluoroscopic imaging and can be safely used for hemodynamic monitoring during exercise,[1,14] whether it be on the treadmill or the cycle ergometer. An important fact is that an overnight hospital stay is not required. The approach we prefer to use is described in detail in Chapter 6. In brief, the triple-lumen flo-

Table 10–5. *Invasive Procedures and the Parameters Measured During Treadmill CPX*

Procedure	Parameters Measured and Derived
Catheterization of right heart	Pressures of pulmonary artery, occlusive wedge, and right atrium Thermodilution cardiac output Mixed venous blood samples for O_2 (Fick cardiac output) and lactate Pulmonary vascular resistance
Catheterization of radial or brachial artery	Systemic arterial pressure Arterial blood sampling for O_2, CO_2, and pH Systemic vascular resistance
Catheterization of esophagus	Pleural and gastric pressures Pressure-volume-flow relations of lung Transdiaphragmatic pressure Transpulmonary pressure
Catheterization of femoral vein	Femoral venous blood flow, femoral venous blood sampling for O_2 and lactate Femoral vascular resistance

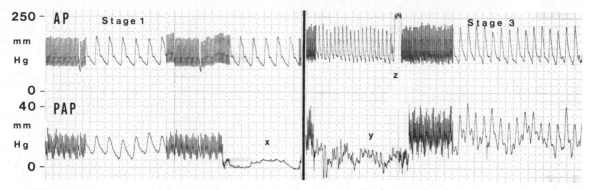

FIGURE 10–11. The hemodynamic response in pulmonary arterial, occlusive wedge (marked *x* and *y*), and arterial pressures can be monitored throughout exercise. Shown here are such data for stage 1 and 3 of treadmill work in a 64 year old woman with systemic hypertension. A flush of the arterial line is indicated by *z*.

tation catheter with thermistor is inserted via an antecubital vein and advanced into the terminal portion of the pulmonary circulation to obtain pulsatile pulmonary artery and occlusive wedge pressures (see Figure 6–7). In the process of reaching the smaller arteries of the pulmonary circulation, minimal catheter whip will be present during exercise (Fig. 10–11) unless exercise cardiac output is quite high. Right atrial pressure monitoring is obtained through the proximal port of the catheter. We also sample mixed venous blood for its oxygen saturation and the subsequent determination of cardiac output by the Fick principle. The lactate concentration of mixed venous blood can be determined at each

stage of exercise or whenever desired. Cardiac output by the thermodilution principle is obtained during each stage to indicate the direction of the flow response. However, we rely on the Fick cardiac output determination for making our final determination of the hemodynamic response to exercise (Chapter 8).

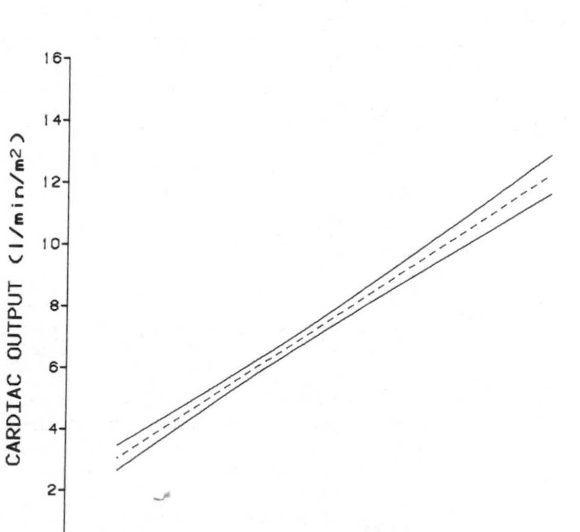

Advances in fiberoptic technology now make it possible also to monitor mixed venous oxygen saturation on a continuous basis with the flotation catheter[15] (see Chapter 8). This technique simplifies the need to obtain multiple blood samples during exercise for the Fick cardiac output determination. Finally, a catheter inserted into the radial or brachial artery of the same arm permits us to monitor arterial pressure directly and to sample arterial blood for its oxygen saturation and carbon dioxide tension. Figure 10–11 illustrates the type of hemodynamic monitoring that can be done during upright treadmill exercise.

The procedure for obtaining hemodynamic data during our incremental treadmill exercise protocol is given in Table 10–6. Each 2 minute stage of exercise is broken down according to the data acquisition process. Three trained people are involved in the test: a physician who monitors and obtains intravascular pressures, the electrocardiogram, and end-tidal oxygen, and two technicians who obtain cardiac output and blood samples, maintain catheter patency, and operate the treadmill and gas analyzer equipment.

The hemodynamic response to incremental treadmill exercise in normal subjects or those with minimal cardiovascular disease is characterized by a progressive rise in cardiac output. For every 100 ml/min/m² increase in $\dot{V}O_2$, there is a 600 ml/min/m² rise in cardiac output (Fig. 10–12). The elevation in systemic

FIGURE 10–12. The interrelationship between $\dot{V}O_2$ by working skeletal muscle and cardiac output in normal subjects. For every 100 ml/min/m² increment in O_2 uptake, the heart normally provides approximately 600 ml/min/m² of cardiac output.

Table 10–6. Protocol for Hemodynamic Monitoring During Each Two Minute Stage of Treadmill CPX

Seconds	Procedure*
0 to 45	Pulsatile pulmonary artery pressure Pulsatile radial artery pressure
45 to 60	Mean pulmonary artery and radial artery pressures
60 to 70	Resume pulsatile pressure recording Occlusive wedge pressure over 3 respiratory cycles
70 to 105	Thermodilution cardiac output Pulsatile and mean right atrial pressure Mixed venous blood sampling Arterial blood sampling
105 to 120	Thermodilution cardiac output

*The electrocardiogram and heart rate are monitored throughout each stage. Cuff arterial pressure can be obtained at 70 to 85 seconds if radial artery pressure is not being monitored.

flow is accomplished with a minimal elevation in left and right ventricular filling pressures (Fig. 10–13). The elevation in cardiac output occurs because of an increment in stroke volume, which is most apparent at low to moderate work loads, and because of an elevation in heart rate, which accompanies the entire exercise response (see Fig. 5–17). Systemic oxygen extraction rises progressively with incremental exercise. This occurs mainly because of the increased extraction of oxygen by working muscle. Figure 10–14 depicts the progressive widening of the arteriovenous oxygen difference, with exercise reaching levels of oxygen extraction in excess of 70 per cent.

Systolic and diastolic arterial pressures are increased during upright exercise (see Table 10–3); however, because of the vasodilatation that occurs in working skeletal muscle, arterial diastolic pressure remains essentially invariant. As shown in Figure 10–15, overall systemic vascular resistance falls by 50 per cent to approximately 600 dynes • sec • cm^{-5} during incremental isotonic treadmill exercise. The autoregulation of the large muscle mass involved with walking accommodates a greater proportion of systemic blood flow. Other circulatory beds, such as the splanchnic and cutaneous circulations which are less metabolically active, vasoconstrict, permitting enhanced oxygen delivery to working muscle. Table 2–7 details the reapportionment of systemic blood flow among the various organs during isotonic exercise of varying degree and indicates the rise in skeletal muscle blood flow that occurs with light, moderate, and heavy work loads.

Because of the low impedance characteristics of the pulmonary circulation (one tenth of the systemic vascular resistance), pulmonary artery systolic, mean, and diastolic pressures rise only minimally and primarily only at higher work loads (see Fig. 2–13); in Figure 10–16 the fall in pulmonary vascular resistance with exercise is demonstrated. Note that pulmonary vascular resistance, like systemic vascular resistance, falls by 50 per cent during incremental isotonic exercise. However, here the pulmonary resistance is 60 dynes • sec • cm^{-5} or less—again one tenth that in the systemic circulation at maximal exercise.

The normal relationship between the gradient in pressure across the lung and cardiac output is shown in Figure 10–17. This relationship will become quite important to the evaluation of pulmonary vascular disease that may or may not accompany other dis-

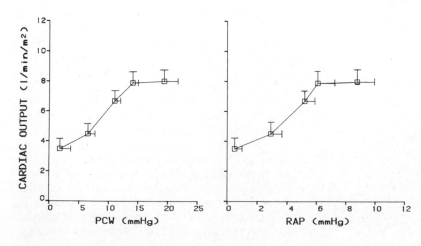

FIGURE 10–13. Exercise ventricular function curves for the left heart (left), where cardiac output and wedge pressure are compared, and the right heart (right), where right atrial pressure is used to reflect right ventricular filling pressure. Data obtained in normal subjects.

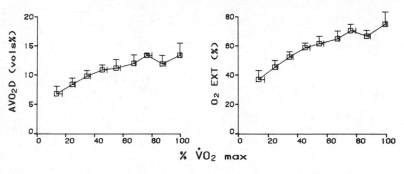

FIGURE 10–14. The normal response in arteriovenous O_2 difference (AVO_2D) on the left and systemic O_2 extraction (O_2 Ext) on the right during incremental treadmill exercise. The AVO_2D at standing rest is higher than that observed in the supine position.

orders of the cardiopulmonary unit; these are described in subsequent chapters.

Finally, the response in mixed venous lactate concentration has been monitored via the distal port of the flotation catheter. The normal resting mixed venous lactate concentration for our laboratory averages 7 to 8 mg per cent. Only when lactate exceeds 12 mg per cent, representing 2 standard deviations above resting values, do we consider lactate production to be present. As can be seen in Figure 10–18, lactate production occurs when oxygen extraction exceeds 60 per cent and when the individual is working at greater than 60 per cent of aerobic capacity.

Incremental Bicycle Exercise

Each of the invasive techniques and hemodynamic parameters noted for treadmill ex-

ercise can be measured during upright incremental cycle ergometry. In addition, it is possible to measure femoral venous blood flow by thermodilution, femoral venous oxygen extraction, and lactate production. These parameters can be obtained by percutaneously inserting a 5F catheter with thermistor into the femoral vein and advancing the catheter 15 cm antegrade into the iliac vein.[16] This technique of monitoring the response of the working leg is more safely applied to the cycle ergometer with the patient in the sitting or supine position than during upright walking on the treadmill.

The response in femoral venous blood flow to incremental cycle exercise is shown in Figure 10–19. A progressive rise in blood flow to working muscle occurs, reaching over 80 per cent of the cardiac output. Oxygen extraction also increases as exercise proceeds

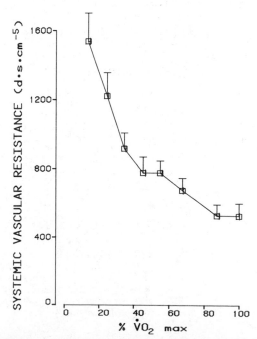

FIGURE 10–15. Systemic vascular resistance, calculated as the difference in mean arterial and right atrial pressures divided by the cardiac output (times 80 to convert to dynes • sec • cm⁻⁵), falls progressively during upright incremental treadmill exercise for normal subjects.

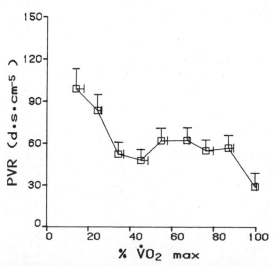

FIGURE 10–16. The normal decline in pulmonary vascular resistance (*PVR*) during upright incremental treadmill exercise is shown. PVR are calculated, as the ratio of the gradient in pressure (i.e., mean pulmonary artery minus wedge pressures) to the cardiac output, and converted to dynes • sec • cm⁻⁵.

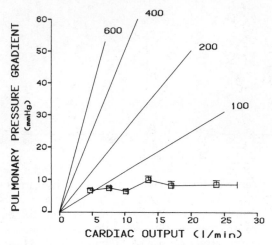

FIGURE 10–17. The interrelationship between the pressure gradient across the lung and cardiac output for normal subjects. This relationship is plotted against a background of isopleths of constant pulmonary vascular resistance (i.e., 100, 200, 400, and 600 dynes • sec • cm^{-5}).

active tissues, such as the kidney and splanchnic circulations, accounts for this difference.

The same is true for the response in lactate, in which lactate production in the leg is noted before that in the pulmonary artery (Fig. 10–20). Moreover, the rise in lactate concentration in the leg is greater than that found in the pulmonary artery, again because of the dilutional effect from other circulatory beds. Notwithstanding these differences, however, the response in the mixed venous blood lactate concentration reflects most closely the temporal response of the carotid bodies in predicting the onset of anaerobiosis during exercise.

SELECTING THE TYPE OF CPX FOR PATIENT EVALUATION

In the chapters that follow we review the utility of various forms of CPX that we have used to evaluate cardiocirculatory and pulmonary disorders. In this section we provide only a broad outline of how to select CPX for general categories of patients commonly seen in the clinical exercise laboratory. Selecting CPX is based on an evaluation of the underlying cardiopulmonary disorder for differential diagnosis, to assess disability and work capacity, and to prescribe and monitor a program of exercise training and rehabilitation. We begin by reviewing how CPX can aid in the evaluation of various disease states.

Heart Disease

Patients with documented evidence of heart disease, whether myocardial or valvular in origin, or chronotropic dysfunction (see Chapter 15) should have a noninvasive incre-

from light to moderate to heavy work loads, reaching 80 per cent with an arteriovenous oxygen difference of 15 vols per cent and a venous oxygen content of as little as 4 vols per cent. Lactate production occurs when 50 to 60 per cent of $\dot{V}O_2$ max on the ergometer has been obtained. The temporal sequence between the response in oxygen extraction and lactate production of the exercising limb relative to that of the mixed venous blood of the pulmonary artery is depicted in Figure 10–20. Clearly there is a time lag in the widening of the arteriovenous oxygen difference of the leg and that measured in the pulmonary artery. Moreover, the level of oxygen extraction in mixed venous blood never reaches that found in the working limb. The dilution of the venous blood in the central compartment by less metabolically

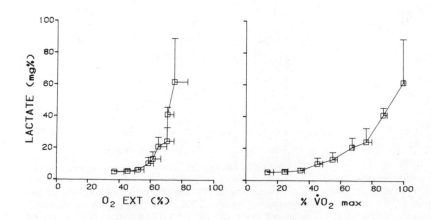

FIGURE 10–18. The response in mixed venous lactate concentration is given as a function of systemic O_2 extraction (O_2 Ext) (left) and normalized $\dot{V}O_2$ max (right) for normal subjects.

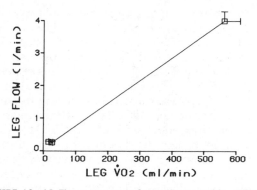
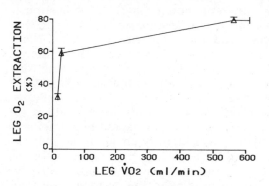

FIGURE 10–19. The response in femoral venous blood flow and arteriofemoral venous leg O_2 extraction to incremental upright bicycle ergometry for patients with coronary artery disease but no evidence of heart failure. The first value was obtained in the supine position; the second value, while sitting and resting on the bicycle; and the third value, at maximum bicycle exercise. (Adapted from Wilson JR, Martin JL, Schwartz D, Ferraro N. Exercise intolerance in patients with chronic heart failure: Role of impaired nutritive flow to skeletal muscle. Circulation 69:1079–1087, 1984.)

mental treadmill exercise test with gas exchange to determine aerobic capacity and anaerobic threshold. Implicit in this recommendation is the fact that these patients must be encouraged during the exercise test to achieve their anaerobic threshold and $\dot{V}O_2$ max. This information will indicate the severity of their disease, their cardiac reserve,

and their functional capacity. The progression of their disease can also now be monitored over time and their response to therapy assessed in an objective fashion.

Resting pulmonary function studies may need to be obtained before CPX to exclude ventilatory dysfunction, particularly in patients with a history of lung disease. If the patient has evidence of lung disease, it is wise to add ear oximetry to the exercise test to exclude exercise-induced oxygen desaturation. Our approach to the dyspneic patient with coexistent heart and lung disease is presented in Chapter 17.

The specific cardiac and circulatory diseases discussed here are considered in Chapters 11 to 17. In this section, we summarize our recommendation for CPX in each of these disorders. Based on the findings of the noninvasive CPX test and the nature of the underlying disorder, we recommend the following: (a) In patients with *dilated cardiomyopathy*, there is no need for additional testing since one can predict the cardiac reserve, the severity of cardiac failure, and functional capacity. These patients can be followed by noninvasive CPX to assess the course of their disease or their response to therapy.

(b) In patients with *ischemic heart disease* who are functional class B, C, or D, one may wish to recommend an invasive CPX with hemodynamic monitoring, either to understand why the cardiac reserve is reduced (e.g., onset of mitral regurgitation versus a noncompliant ventricle), and thereby better guide therapy, or to assess why there may be a disparity in the clinical evaluation and CPX.

(c) In *mitral* or *aortic valvular incompetence*, frequently a disparity exists between the car-

FIGURE 10–20. The temporal relationship between lactate concentration and arteriovenous O_2 difference in the femoral vein and the pulmonary artery of patients without heart failure during upright incremental ergometry. (Data courtesy of John R. Wilson, MD.)

diac catheterization findings (at rest in supine position) of the estimated severity of the disease and the response to exercise. Here an invasive CPX with hemodynamic monitoring can prove invaluable in assessing cardiac reserve and left ventricular dysfunction (both diastolic and systolic) and surgical candidacy. Moreover, the pressure gradient to cardiac output relation across the pulmonary circulation will identify an abnormal pulmonary vascular resistance that may or may not influence the decision for remedial surgery and aid in predicting the postoperative rate of recovery (that is, a slower recovery rate, the higher the vascular resistance).

(d) In patients with suspected or occult *pericardial disease*, the heightened venous return of exercise can aid in eliciting the constrictive element of the pericardium. By monitoring the response in right atrial and wedge pressures during exercise, the presence of pericardial disease and its severity in compromising the cardiac output response to exercise can be identified.

(e) In patients with *chronotropic dysfunction* at rest and during noninvasive CPX, there is no need for invasive studies. The functional capacity can be monitored in response to various therapeutic interventions (e.g., pacemaker, hydralazine, beta blockade) that are dictated by the nature of the underlying disease and the abnormality in cardiac rhythm and rate.

Vascular Disease

In patients with *systemic hypertension*, the noninvasive incremental treadmill test is recommended, with careful noninvasive monitoring of arterial blood pressure. If the patient's $\dot{V}O_2$ max is compatible with class B, C, or D, a repeat test with pulmonary artery catheter is recommended to assess the severity of left ventricular diastolic dysfunction. It appears unwise to use beta adrenergic blockage in class B, C, or D patients because their systolic function and cardiac output response to exercise are suboptimal. If a patient has a normal aerobic capacity (class A) but the arterial systolic and/or diastolic pressure response to exercise is markedly abnormal, the test should be repeated with an arterial catheter for the direct recording of arterial pressure. In class A patients, it is unlikely that the cardiac output response is impaired to any significant extent. This collected information serves as an important baseline for monitoring the response in ambulatory blood pressure to antihypertensive therapy, as well as for the correlation of the noninvasive cuff technique in subsequent follow-up tests.

Normotensive patients with *atherosclerotic cardiovascular disease* of the lower extremity may experience claudication during treadmill exercise and therefore fail to attain their anaerobic threshold and $\dot{V}O_2$ max. Here there is little reason to recommend an invasive study; however, the noninvasive test permits an objective assessment of the severity of the occlusive disease. The efficacy of various medical or surgical therapies for the vascular disease can be serially evaluated with the noninvasive CPX and the level of $\dot{V}O_2$ identified at the onset of limiting leg pain.

Patients with *pulmonary vascular disease* and pulmonary hypertension should have the invasive incremental test after the noninvasive test in which ear oximetry is included. By determining the aerobic capacity of these patients and whether or not they have arterial oxygen desaturation, the invasive test can be completed more efficiently and intelligently. An arterial line should be inserted for the invasive test to document whether there is a fall in arterial oxygen tension, and for subsequent repeat testing with supplemental oxygen if this proves to be the case. We recommend the invasive test in these patients, even if they are class A, for the following reasons: (a) to assess severity; in less severe expressions of this process it is often difficult to predict the severity of pulmonary hypertension on clinical grounds. (b) Serial noninvasive measurements of pulmonary artery pressure cannot be obtained, as is true for the systemic circulation, and this information can be invaluable to the patient's further evaluation. (c) Early detection and treatment of pulmonary hypertension with vasodilators may be effective in retarding the development of right heart failure.

We discuss our approach to assessing the pharmacoreactivity of the hypertensive pulmonary circulation in greater detail in Chapter 13. It suffices to say here that drugs can be most effectively and safely administered and their effect assessed by hemodynamic monitoring. The baseline pressure-flow relation of the diseased pulmonary circulation (at least three points are required: rest and two levels of exercise) can be compared with that following drug intervention if one of the vasodilators appears to be effective in reducing resting mean pulmonary artery pressure and pulmonary vascular resistance.

Lung Disease

Patients with *restrictive* or *obstructive lung disease* will rarely be able to cross the anaerobic threshold and attain $\dot{V}O_2$ max before becoming dyspneic (see Chapters 16 and 17). Pulmonary function studies should be obtained prior to noninvasive CPX in order to identify the ventilatory reserves (i.e., the vital capacity and maximum voluntary ventilation) so that exercise tidal volume and ventilation can be examined in relationship to these reserves. Generally speaking, these patients use over 50 per cent of these reserves during exercise when they become dyspneic (see Chapters 16 and 17). Ear oximetry should always be included with the noninvasive test to examine for arterial oxygen desaturation. If there is no evidence of cor pulmonale in these patients, there is little need to proceed to the invasive exercise test, except that an arterial line to directly quantify arterial oxygen desaturation and its severity should be performed. The line should be left in place and the exercise test repeated on supplemental oxygen.

Exertional Dyspnea

The differential diagnosis of exertional dyspnea in patients with heart or lung disease or both can be aided by CPX. The following clues help in identifying whether the exertional dyspnea is secondary to ventilatory dysfunction: (a) the appearance of arterial hypoxemia; (b) maximum $\dot{V}E$ on exercise is more than 50 per cent of MVV; and (c) the patient is unable to reach aerobic capacity when symptomatic dyspnea prohibits further exercise. This is also true in patients with coexistent heart and lung disease when the ventilatory impairment is dominant. When heart or circulatory disease is dominant, patients will be able to cross the anaerobic threshold and attain aerobic capacity. These patients do not develop arterial hypoxemia and do not use more than 50 per cent of their ventilatory reserves.

A broader discussion of the evaluation of exertional dyspnea can be found in Chapter 17.

Disability, Work Capacity, and Rehabilitation

Noninvasive CPX will permit a determination of the aerobic and anaerobic levels of work that can be invaluable in assessing disability and work capacity and prescribing individualized exercise. This information can also be followed over time to assess the results of exercise training.

REFERENCES

1. Weber KT, Kinasewitz GT, Janicki JS, Fishman AP. Oxygen utilization and ventilation during exercise in patients with chronic cardiac failure. Circulation 65:1213-1223, 1982.
2. Weber KT, Janicki JS, Fishman AP. Respiratory gas exchange during exercise in the noninvasive evaluation of the severity of chronic cardiac failure, *in* Braunwald E, Mock MB, Watson JT (eds). Congestive Heart Failure. Grune & Stratton, New York, 1982, pp 221–235.
3. Wilson JR, Martin JL, Ferraro N, Weber KT. Effect of hydralazine on perfusion and metabolism in the leg during upright bicycle exercise in patients with heart failure. Circulation 68:425–432, 1983.
4. Janicki JS, Weber KT, Likoff MJ, Fishman AP. Exercise testing to evaluate patients with pulmonary vascular disease. Am Rev Respir Dis 192:S93–S95, 1984.
5. Jones NL, Campbell EJM. Clinical Exercise Testing. WB Saunders, Philadelphia, 1982.
6. Astrand I, Astrand P-O, Hallback I, Kilbom A. Reduction in maximum oxygen uptake with age. J Appl Physiol 35:649–654, 1973.
7. Weber KT, Janicki JS. Lactate production during maximal and submaximal exercise in patients with chronic cardiac failure. J Am Coll Cardiol, 6:717–724, 1985.
8. Weber KT, Andrews V, Kinasewitz GT, Janicki JS, Fishman AP. Vasodilator and inotropic agents in the treatment of chronic cardiac failure: Clinical experience and response in exercise performance. Am Heart J 102:569–577, 1981.
9. Weber KT, Andrews V, Janicki JS, Likoff MJ, Reichek N. Pirbuterol, an oral beta-adrenergic receptor agonist, in the treatment of chronic cardiac failure. Circulation 66:1262–1267, 1982.
10. Shephard RJ. The maximum sustained voluntary ventilation in exercise. Clin Sci 32:167–176, 1967.
11. Freedman S. Sustained maximum voluntary ventilation. Respir Physiol 8:230–244, 1970.
12. Bergh U, Kanstrup I-L, Ekblom B. Maximal oxygen uptake during exercise with various combinations of arm and leg work. J Appl Physiol 41:191–196, 1976.
13. Wasserman K, Whipp BJ, Casaburi R, Golden M, Beaver WL. Ventilatory control during exercise in man. Bull Eur Physiopathol Resp 15:27–47, 1979.
14. Weber KT, Janicki JS. Cardiopulmonary exercise testing for evaluation of chronic cardiac failure. Am J Cardiol 55:22A–31A, 1985.
15. Divertie MB, McMichan JC. Continuous monitoring of mixed venous oxygen saturation. Chest 85:423–428, 1984.
16. Wilson JR, Martin JL, Schwartz D, Ferraro N. Exercise intolerance in patients with chronic heart failure: Role of impaired nutritive flow to skeletal muscle. Circulation 69:1079–1087, 1984.

KARL T. WEBER
JOSEPH S. JANICKI

11

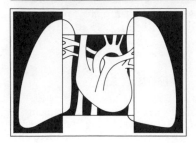

Chronic Cardiac Failure

The treatment of patients with acute cardiac failure has improved significantly over the last decade. Aided immeasurably by the development of the flotation catheter (see Chapter 6), the survival of these patients has improved. As a result, the incidence of chronic cardiac failure has increased steadily. Therefore, it has become imperative that practicing cardiologists have quantifiable and objective indices with which to grade the severity of chronic cardiac failure, including subclinical expressions of latent disease, to follow the natural course of the disease, and to monitor the patient's response to therapy.

Our approach to these issues has been to use cardiopulmonary exercise (CPX) testing. The criteria that CPX should theoretically satisfy in the evaluation of chronic cardiac failure are outlined in Table 11–1. The origins of CPX are based on the premise that the physiologic stress of exercise together with the noninvasive monitoring of respiratory gas exchange, and invasive studies of hemodynamic responses in selected patients, provides the requisite information with which to detect gross or subtle defects in cardiac performance (i.e., the cardiac reserve) as well as the means to grade the severity of chronic

cardiac failure. Because the incremental exercise test and the determination of maximal oxygen uptake and anaerobic threshold are objective quantities, they eliminate patient and physician bias in assessing the functional capacity of any given patient. CPX also provides a means with which to assess the response to various therapeutic interventions a topic that will be considered more fully in Chapter 21. Because CPX has been a fairly recent addition to the practice of cardiology, its sensitivity, specificity, and predictive value in identifying latent or early systolic ventricular dysfunction remain to be determined. Our preliminary results, however, are very encouraging.

The purpose of this chapter is first to review the underlying pathophysiology of chronic cardiac (myocardial) failure and then to review our experience with CPX in the evaluation of these patients.

PATHOPHYSIOLOGY OF CHRONIC CARDIAC FAILURE

In physiologic terms, heart failure may be defined as that condition in which the heart is unable to provide the metabolizing tissues with oxygen and substrate that are commensurate with their aerobic requirement. Many different diseases of the cardiovascular system may be responsible for the defect in oxygen supply relative to oxygen demand. As previously noted, the late Louis N. Katz[1] emphasized the need to distinguish those diseases that compromised oxygen delivery but did not affect the myocardium from those diseases that did affect the myocardium. For

Table 11–1. Objectives for Exercising the Patient with Chronic Cardiac Failure

Sensitive and specific detection of impaired
   cardiac performance (the cardiac reserve)
Gradation of the severity of chronic cardiac
   failure
Assessment of functional capacity of the patient
Monitoring of therapeutic response

example, constrictive pericardial disease, valvular heart disease, and cardiac arrhythmias will impair the ability of the heart to raise its cardiac output during physical activities. These diseases represent causes of *circulatory failure* (Table 11–2). In Chapters 12 through 15, we discuss several of these causes of circulatory failure. Ischemic and myopathic heart disease affect the myocardium directly and are considered causes of *cardiac* or *myocardial failure*. In this chapter, our attention will be directed solely to chronic cardiac failure and the circumstance in which a systolic dysfunction of the heart occurs because of a depression in myocardial contractility.

Myocardial Contractility

The physiologic characteristics of cardiac muscle and the concepts of muscle force, length, and shortening have been reviewed in Chapter 4. Here we will again use these concepts to describe abnormalities in muscle contraction that are independent of muscle length and shortening load and that are secondary to an abnormal contractile state.

Contractility is defined as that property of cardiac muscle which determines its ability to shorten independent of its shortening load and muscle length. According to this definition, contractility will describe, in mechanical terms, the biochemical characteristics of muscle (e.g., its beta$_1$ adrenergic receptor responsiveness, myosin isoform composition, or sarcolemmal/sarcoplasmic reticulum handling of calcium) and its responsiveness to neurohumoral influences (e.g., plasma norepinephrine or thyroid hormone) or exogenous substances. Drugs that alter myocardial contractility are described in terms of their inotropic properties. Drugs with *positive inotropic* properties enhance contractility, and

those with *negative inotropic* properties depress contractility.

Harrison and Reeves[2] have proposed that the concept of myocardial contractility be subdivided into two categories, which they termed *intrinsic* and *manifest contractility*. Their approach has been aimed at distinguishing the biochemical characteristics of cardiac muscle from the influences of circulating neurohumoral stimuli. Ischemic or myopathic heart disease will compromise the intrinsic contractile state, whereas endogenous catecholamines or pharmacologic agents, on the other hand, will influence manifest contractility.

In the section that follows, we provide a discussion of myocardial contractility as it relates to ischemic and myopathic heart disease. It should be clearly stated that this discussion is designed to emphasize the various concepts of contractility and is mainly based on conjecture. Our limited knowledge does not permit a more factual discourse.

In cases when the myocardium has been infarcted, that portion of the myocardium that is scarred will have little or no intrinsic contractility. The remainder of the myocardium may be reasonably normal and eventually may hypertrophy, and as a result, its contractility may actually be enhanced in response to the increased work load it must perform. The manifest contractility of the infarcted left ventricle will therefore be the summation of these two contrasting states.

With the cardiomyopathies, the cause of the defect in the contractile apparatus is usually uncertain; hence, the term *idiopathic cardiomyopathy*. Despite this uncertainty, and the fact that the intrinsic contractility of the myopathic heart is impaired, its manifest contractility may be normal or impaired depending on various compensatory mechanisms and responses and the natural history of the disease.

With either the failing ischemic or myopathic heart, a heightened activation of the adrenergic nervous system (e.g., increased plasma norepinephrine) may be present. By virtue of its positive inotropic effects, norepinephrine may enhance manifest contractility to sustain cardiac performance early in the course of the disease. Later, as the disease progresses to severe cardiac failure, plasma norepinephrine may in fact be critical to maintaining a manifest contractile state that is commensurate with adequate systemic blood flow. The heightened adrenergic state, which initially served as a compensatory re-

Table 11–2. *Examples of Circulatory and Cardiac Failure*

Circulatory Failure (Extrinsic to the Myocardium)
Constrictive pericarditis
Valvular heart disease
Pulmonary vascular disease
Hypovolemia
Anemia
Chest wall deformity
Arrhythmia
Cardiac Failure (Intrinsic to the Myocardium)
Myocardial infarction
Myocardial ischemia
Cardiomyopathy

sponse, may lead to a "down-regulation" (decreased sensitivity) of the heart's beta$_1$ adrenergic receptors.[3] In addition, the rise in plasma norepinephrine that occurs during physical activity may be excessive[4, 5] and create adverse biologic effects that have sustained consequences even after exercise has been completed. The balance between enhanced contractility and beta adrenergic receptor responsiveness may be a very delicate one—a balance between a compensated and a decompensated state.

The Clinical Assessment of Contractility

Intrinsic and manifest contractility have been examined using a variety of techniques. The extent to which intrinsic contractility is enhanced by the sympathetic nervous system and the role of the parasympathetic nervous system in modulating cardiac performance have been examined by administering the beta adrenergic receptor blocker propranolol and the parasympatholytic agent atropine. Jose and Taylor[6] have reported that the combined administration of these drugs can be used to elicit the heart's *intrinsic heart rate* and to assess the severity of cardiac failure. As ventricular pump function becomes more depressed, the intrinsic heart rate decreases (Fig. 11–1). The merits of this approach in characterizing the severity of chronic cardiac failure remains to be examined in larger clinical trials.

The relationship between wall force and the length and velocity of circumferential midwall fiber shortening represents another approach to the description of the contractile state of a given heart.[7–10] Wall *force*, which includes chamber pressure, size, and shape in its calculation, is a far better term to express shortening load in any given heart than is chamber systolic pressure. In the dilated myopathic heart, for example, left ventricular systolic pressure may be only 96 mm Hg, which in no way reflects the increased shortening load on the myopathic heart and which is present because of the increased chamber dimension (Fig. 11–2).

When comparing failing hearts among patients, wall *stress* is the proper term to represent shortening load. Unlike force, stress takes into account muscle mass and therefore is a more valid parameter to describe different degrees of left ventricular hypertrophy among patients.

Several stress-velocity-length relations may be used to describe myocardial contractile state in patients with chronic cardiac failure. The two relations that appear to be the most attractive for clinical use, because of their independence of muscle length or systolic load, are the end systolic stress-volume (or stress-length) relation and the rate-corrected velocity of shortening–end-systolic stress relation. Figures 11–3 and 11–4 describe each of these relations in diagrammatic fashion.

In patients with chronic cardiac failure, there is a depression in contractile state that can be assessed with either of these relations. Using echocardiographic techniques and pharmacologic agents (methoxamine or nitroprusside or both) to manipulate arterial pressure, Borow and co-workers[11, 12] have systematically evaluated the utility of these relationships in the evaluation of chronic

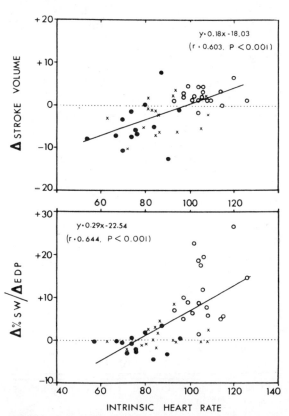

FIGURE 11–1. The relationship between the intrinsic heart rate obtained after propranolol and atropine, and the response in two indices of left ventricular function: the change in stroke volume (above) and the changes in stroke work (*SW*) relative to the change in end-diastolic pressure (*EDP*) seen below. Open circles are normal and NYHA class I patients; crosses, class II; and closed circles, classes III and IV. (From Jose AD, Taylor RR. Autonomic blockade by propranolol and atropine to study intrinsic myocardial function in man. J Clin Invest *48*:2019–2031, 1969.)

LEFT VENTRICLE

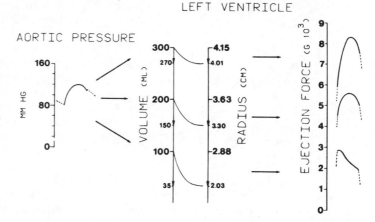

FIGURE 11–2. The response in systolic ejection wall force, or afterload, as the left ventricle enlarges to twice and three times its normal diastolic volume and its ejection fraction falls from 65 to 40 per cent and then to 10 per cent. It can be seen that the failing heart is working against itself. See text. (From Weber KT, Janicki JS. The heart as a muscle-pump system and the concept of heart failure. Am Heart J 98:371–384, 1979.)

cardiac failure. They have also used dobutamine to assess the heart's inotropic reserve. Dobutamine may or may not prove a valid pharmacologic probe to assess contractile state, in that it is dependent on the responsiveness (or down-regulation) or myocardial $beta_1$ adrenergic receptors in the chronically failing heart. Several drugs with varying mechanisms of action (e.g., dobutamine, amrinone, and MDL 17,043, a phosphodiesterase inhibitor) may provide a more complete description of inotropic reserve. In addition, these pharmacologic probes may provide us with an opportunity to better understand the biochemical alterations of the intrinsic contractile state.

Exercise activates the adrenergic nervous system; therefore, this is a natural physiologic stress that provides a broad assessment of cardiac reserve, including an indirect measure of contractility.

Hemodynamic Features of Chronic Cardiac Failure

Because of the depression in contractility, the extent and velocity of myocardial short-

ening are reduced. Accordingly, pump displacement (i.e., *stroke volume*) is reduced, the ventricle becomes dilated, and the myocardium becomes hypertrophied. The stroke volume that the ventricle can generate from any given filling volume (as reflected by filling pressure) is compromised. In other words, the ventricular function curve is depressed from normal. The extent to which contractility and the ventricular function curve are depressed will also determine to what extent the ventricle's *diastolic reserve* (i.e., an increase in stroke volume derived from an increase in diastolic volume) is reduced.

The compromise in contractility also attenuates the *systolic reserve* of the heart (i.e., the increase in stroke volume achieved by a greater extent of fiber shortening or a greater use of the end-systolic volume). As illustrated in Figure 11–5, a positive inotropic challenge will increase stroke volume by using the systolic reserve. The clinical corollary to this feature of the failing heart is that larger doses of the positive inotropic agents have to be used to effect an improvement in pump function.

FIGURE 11–3. The end-systolic stress-volume relations for the normal and failing heart. In its compensated phase, the stroke volume and end-systolic stress of the failing heart are similar to those of the normal heart. With decompensation, stress is elevated and stroke volume declines. The solid and broken lines marked normal, compensated, and decompensated represent the isovolumetric stress-volume relations and thereby the contractile state of the myocardium.

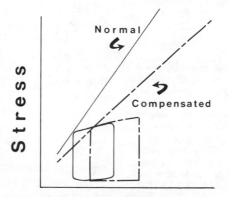

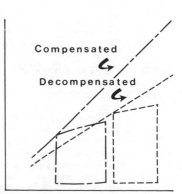

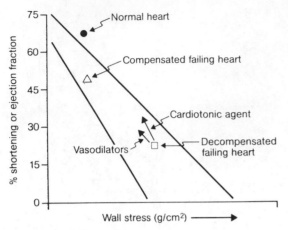

Figure 11–4. The inverse extent of circumferential fiber-shortening (ejection fraction) to systolic wall stress relation. The normal operating range for the normal heart is identified. The decompensated failing heart and its response to vasodilators and cardiotonic agents are depicted. (From Weber KT, Janicki JS, Likoff MJ, Shroff S, Andrews V. Chronic cardiac failure: Pathophysiologic and therapeutic considerations. Triangle 22:1–9, 1983.)

Exercise, with its heightened venous return and activation of the adrenergic nervous system, provides both an assessment of the diastolic and the systolic reserves of the heart and an indirect measure of contractility.

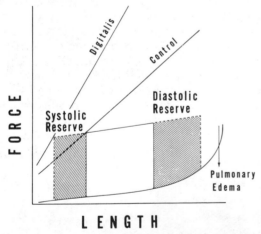

FIGURE 11–5. The diastolic and systolic reserves of the left ventricle. The increase in stroke volume that is obtained by an enhanced filling volume is termed the diastolic reserve; it is limited by the accompanying elevation in pulmonary capillary pressure and the onset of pulmonary edema. The increase in stroke volume that is obtained by having the ventricle contract to a smaller end-systolic volume is termed the systolic reserve. In the failing heart, both reserves are attenuated. (From Weber KT, Janicki JS. The heart as a muscle-pump system and the concept of heart failure. Am Heart J 98:371–384, 1979.)

Cardiac failure secondary to ischemic or myopathic disease is characterized by an *enlarged left ventricular chamber and increased left ventricular mass*. In the case of the dilated myopathic heart, hypertrophy may not be as apparent or appropriate, because the thickness of its wall is thin relative to the size of its chamber. In fact, the lower the wall thickness to chamber radius ratio (h/r), the poorer the prognosis.[13] In the myopathic heart, the *right ventricle* is also dilated and fails early in the course of the disease because of the diffuse myopathic process. In fact, clinical manifestations of right heart failure (e.g., edema, ascites, and neck vein distention) may be more dominant than those of left heart failure. This is in distinct contrast to ischemic heart disease, in which years of pulmonary venous hypertension, secondary to left ventricular failure, are required to elicit right heart failure.

The *resting filling pressure* of the enlarged left ventricle may be increased, as is usually true in more advanced cases, or it may be normal. The intrinsic stiffness of the myocardium, left ventricular chamber size, and the degree of right ventricular enlargement will determine the diastolic pressure for a given filling volume of the left ventricle. In most cases, the dilated left ventricle accommodates its enhanced filling volume under less pressure than would be present for a comparable volume in a normal-sized ventricle.

Figure 11–6 presents an augmented or amplified tracing of left ventricular pressure, which highlights the diastolic portion of the pressure tracing. Superimposed on the ventricular pressure tracing is the pulmonary capillary wedge pressure tracing with its *a* and *v* waves. A time delay in the wedge pressure tracing normally exists, because of the delay in pressure transmission from the left heart to the pulmonary circulation. The broken horizontal lines demonstrate the extent of this delay.

Typical wedge pressure tracings obtained in patients with chronic cardiac failure are shown in Figures 11–7 and 11–8. Both patients had a dilated cardiomyopathy. In the first case (Fig. 11–7), end-expiratory wedge pressure is moderately elevated to 18 mm Hg. In the second case (Fig. 11–8), end-expiratory wedge pressure is markedly elevated to 34 mm Hg, and there is mitral regurgitation with prominent *v* waves seen in the wedge pressure and pulmonary artery pressure tracings. In some patients with ad-

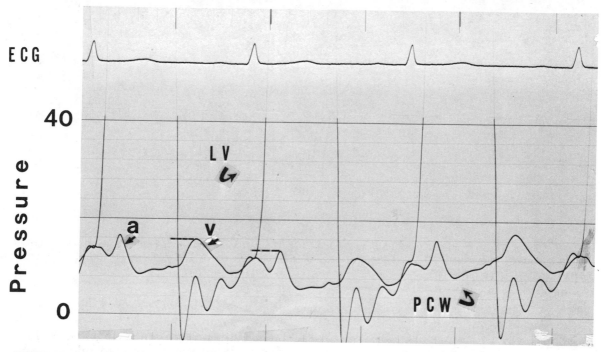

FIGURE 11—6. An amplified tracing of left ventricular (*LV*) pressure on which is superimposed the pulmonary capillary wedge (*PCW*) pressure tracing with its *a* and *v* waves.

vanced chronic cardiac failure, right ventricular pulsus alternans may be seen in the pulmonary artery systolic pressure tracing (see Figs. 6–16 and 6–22).

Cardiac output is commonly reduced at rest. Often in the compensatory phase of the disease, when cardiac dilatation preserves pump function (see Fig. 11–3), resting cardiac output is relatively normal. A normal stroke volume from an enlarged heart, however, means that its ejection fraction must be reduced. Table 11–3 reviews the typical hemo-

dynamic features of chronic cardiac failure obtained at rest. Patients have been categorized according to the severity of their failure (i.e., exercise classes A to E). In many patients, it is not possible to predict their cardiac reserve from parameters of resting cardiac output or left ventricular filling pressure.[14-18] The ejection fraction is also unreliable in predicting aerobic capacity, the severity of failure, and thereby the cardiac reserve. This disparity between resting parameters of ventricular function, as well as that of heart

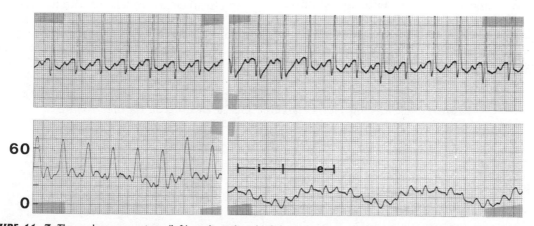

FIGURE 11—7. The pulmonary artery (left) and wedge (right) pressure recordings in a patient with chronic cardiac failure secondary to a dilated cardiomyopathy. The inspiratory (*i*) and expiratory (*e*) portions of the respiratory cycle are identified.

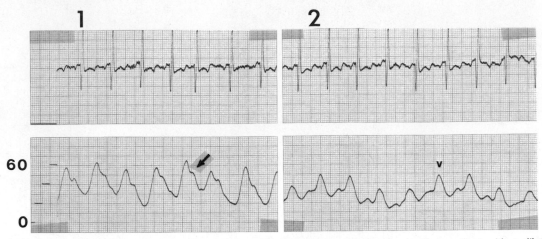

FIGURE 11–8. The pulmonary artery (left) and wedge (right) pressure tracings for another patient with a dilated cardiomyopathy, elevated wedge pressure, and mitral regurgitation (v wave). The v wave is reflected back to the pulmonary artery tracing (arrow).

size, and the cardiac reserve is illustrated in Figure 11–9.

Assessing Cardiac Reserve

Over the years, a variety of techniques have been employed to examine cardiac reserve and thereby the severity of heart failure. Each employs a challenge or stress (e.g., increased volume, systolic pressure elevation, or administration of a positive inotropic drug). A *volume challenge* is used to generate the ventricular function curve; it represents a natural extension of the experiments of Otto Frank and Ernest Starling and describes the length-dependent property of cardiac muscle. A ventricular function curve derived in a patient with acute myocardial infarction after dextran infusion[19] is given in Figure 11–10.

In more recent years, as it became apparent that afterload is an important determinant of cardiac muscle performance, studies were conducted in which the pressure term of afterload was enhanced to invoke an elevated *arterial systolic pressure* as a challenge to the failing pump. Although Ross and Braunwald[20] used an infusion of angiotensin II for this purpose, more recently Borow and associates[11, 12] have chosen methoxamine. In either case, the failing heart is sensitive to pressure loading, as indicated in Figure 11–11 and as we reviewed in Chapter 4. As a result, its output declines with increased systemic vascular resistance. Borow and coworkers[10] have also used the synthetic catecholamine dobutamine to assess the *inotropic reserve* of the heart (Fig. 11–12). Incremental exercise to determine $\dot{V}O_{2\,max}$ is another approach to assess cardiac reserve, as we will discuss further on.

Peripheral Circulation and the Neurohumoral System

In chronic cardiac failure, the intrinsic and manifest contractile states of the heart are impaired. As a result, pump performance both at rest and during exercise is reduced. When systemic blood flow and tissue perfu-

Table 11–3. Resting Hemodynamic Profile of Chronic Cardiac Failure

	Exercise Classes			
	A	B	C	D
Cardiac output (liters/min/m²)	2.7 ± 0.1	2.4 ± 0.3	2.1 ± 0.1	1.8 ± 0.1
Heart rate (bpm)	78 ± 8	89 ± 10	85 ± 2	84 ± 4
Stroke volume (ml/m²)	35 ± 5	29 ± 4	25 ± 2	20 ± 2
EF (%)	32 ± 2	25 ± 3	27 ± 2	24 ± 3
Left ventricular filling pressure (mm Hg)	6 ± 3	16 ± 4	17 ± 2	24 ± 1

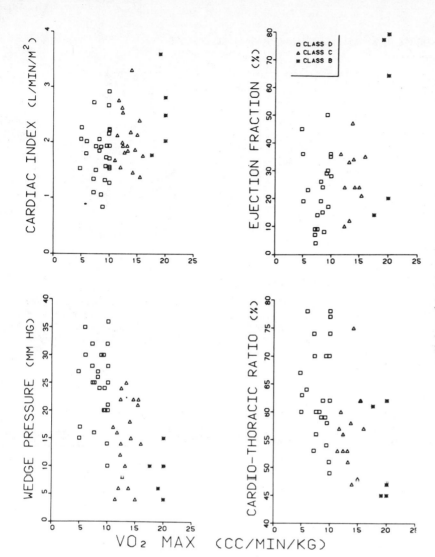

FIGURE 11–9. The relationship between indices of ventricular function measured at rest, such as cardiac output, filling pressure, ejection fraction, and overall heart size on chest x-ray, to the aerobic capacity of patients with chronic cardiac failure. (From Weber KT, Wilson JR, Janicki JS, Likoff MJ. Exercise testing in the evaluation of the patient with chronic cardiac failure. Am Rev Respir Dis *129*:S60–S62, 1984.)

FIGURE 11–10. Left ventricular function curves (i.e., cardiac output, stroke index, and stroke work index) for a patient with acute myocardial infarction who received 600 ml of dextran. Pulmonary artery diastolic pressure is given to reflect left ventricular filling pressure. (From Russell RO, Rackley CE, Pombo JH, Hunt D, Potamin C, Dodge HT. Effects of increasing left ventricular filling pressure in patients with acute myocardial infarction. J Clin Invest *49*:1539–1550, 1970.)

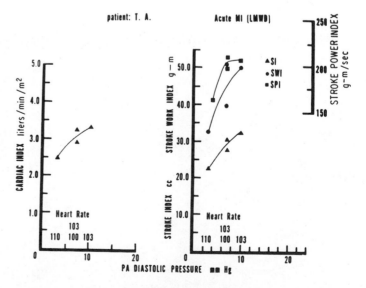

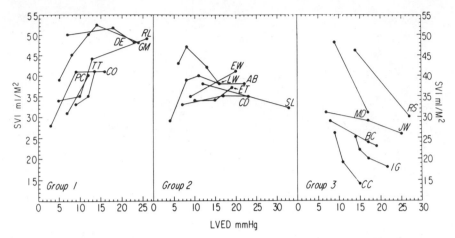

FIGURE 11–11. Left ventricular function curves (i.e., the stroke volume index, *SVI*, to end-diastolic pressure, *LVED*) for patients with minimal impairment in ventricular function (Group 1), and those with moderate (Group 2) and severe heart failure (Group 3). An infusion of angiotensin was used to construct these curves at the time of diagnostic cardiac catheterization. None were considered to have aortic or mitral regurgitation. (From Ross J, Braunwald E. The study of left ventricular function by increasing resistance to ventricular ejection with angiotensin. Circulation *29*:739–749, 1964.)

sion are compromised, a whole host of compensatory responses, primarily neurohumoral in nature, are elicited. Included here is an activation of the adrenergic nervous system, the release of arginine vasopressin, and stimulation of the renin-angiotensin-aldosterone system.[21] These various neurohu-

moral responses also interact with one another. For example, angiotensin II facilitates norepinephrine release, as well as being an intrinsically potent vasoconstrictor in its own right. Angiotensin II is also a stimulus to the release of vasopressin, whereas vasopressin, in turn, potentiates the vasoconstrictor prop-

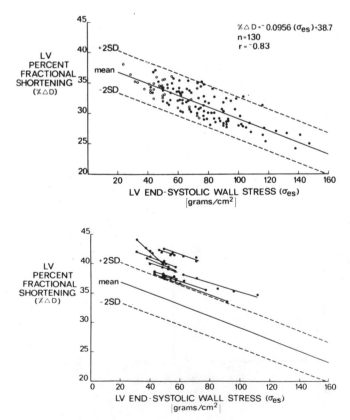

FIGURE 11–12. The percent fractional shortening to end-systolic stress relation for the left ventricle in normal subjects. Top, the control relationship obtained over a range of unmanipulated arterial pressures (solid circles) and enhanced pressure (open circles) created with methoxamine. Bottom, the enhanced shortening and contractility seen with dobutamine. (From Borow KM, Green LH, Grossman W, Braunwald E. Left ventricular end-systolic stress-shortening and stress-length relations in humans. Am J Cardiol *50*:1301–1308, 1982.)

erties of norepinephrine and angiotensin. Even though the precise signals that activate the sympathetic nervous system, the renin-angiotensin-aldosterone system, and arginine vasopressin are unknown, the net result of their activation is salt and water retention with intravascular and extravascular volume expansion and arteriolar vasoconstriction. Early in the course of heart failure, these responses are compensatory in nature; they serve a useful purpose. Later, they become detrimental and play a major role in determining the decompensated status of the patient.

The response in plasma norepinephrine to exercise in patients with chronic cardiac failure has been reported from several laboratories. Chidsey and associates[4] found norepinephrine to be greater at similar work loads in patients with cardiac failure than in healthy patients. Francis and co-workers[5] noted similar findings when $\dot{V}O_2$ was measured directly. In neither case, however, was the response in plasma norepinephrine normalized according to aerobic capacity. It is entirely possible that, as in normal patients,[22] norepinephrine is only released when >70 per cent of $\dot{V}O_2$ max has been achieved, and perhaps this activation is related to the onset of anaerobiosis in working muscle. It has been our observation[23] that resting plasma norepinephrine is only increased (654 ±58 pg/ml) in class D patients in comparison to class C (319 ±66 pg/ml) or B (283 ±47 pg/ml) patients (normal, 65 to 320 pg/ml).

Collectively, these neurohumoral responses, plus poorly defined alterations within vascular smooth muscle, serve to compromise the autoregulatory behavior of a given regional circulation, such as that of the kidney or of muscle. The consequences of this alteration in autoregulation, together with the reduction in systemic perfusion, serve to create significant alterations in oxygen delivery and oxygen availability at the tissue level.

The ability of the vasculature of working skeletal muscle to vasodilate is an important peripheral component of the exercise response that is independent of the heart. Zelis and co-workers[24] have previously shown that skeletal muscle blood flow does not rise appropriately with exercise in these patients. This flow deficit may be accounted for not only by a reduced exercise cardiac output, but also by the impairment in regional blood flow within muscle. These changes in vasoreactivity may be the result of salt retention

by the kidney with edema formation and an external compression of vessels, structural changes within the vasculature itself secondary to salt retention, as well as the elevation in circulating catecholamines that typifies the congestive state of chronic cardiac failure.

This aberration in regional blood flow has been underscored by Wilson and colleagues,[25, 26] who have demonstrated that the compromise in blood flow to working muscle is a function of the severity of heart failure. Moreover, they have shown that the reduction in limb blood flow is not simply the result of impaired cardiac output. Of equal importance, their findings have demonstrated that the pharmacologic enhancement of cardiac output and even femoral artery blood flow does not guarantee an improvement in nutritive flow to working muscle. Consequently, the aerobic capacity of the patient will be inextricably related to local phenomena within the peripheral circulation as well as to the output of the heart. Inadequate working muscle perfusion may result in a sense of muscle fatigue that these patients commonly experience with physical activity.

Thus, chronic cardiac failure is frequently accompanied by a state of congestion and hypoperfusion that eventuates in a syndrome consisting of a constellation of signs and symptoms termed *congestive heart failure*. It should be noted, however, that chronic cardiac failure does not have to be accompanied by a state of congestion; therefore, the terms are not synonymous. In addition, it should be re-emphasized that the severity of chronic cardiac failure may be mild, moderate, or severe. The physician should not wait until the patient has congestive heart failure before evaluating its severity or initiating therapy.

The Kidney

Renal blood flow normally averages 1000 to 1200 ml/min (or 600 to 700 ml/min/m²), of which 120 ml/min of plasma is filtered by the glomerular capillaries. During the course of a day glomerular filtration amounts to 180 liters, of which 178 liters are reabsorbed by the renal tubules and returned to the circulation via the peritubular capillaries. The remaining 2 liters of filtrate are excreted as urine.

In chronic cardiac failure renal blood flow is reduced.[27, 28] The accompanying reduction in renal plasma flow is in proportion to the decline in cardiac output.[27] In less severe cardiac failure, glomerular filtration is preserved because efferent peritubular arterioles vasoconstrict. This vasoconstriction may be mediated by norepinephrine and/or angiotensin II. As a consequence of this vasoconstriction, the hydrostatic pressure within the peritubular capillaries (the pressure-driving fluid from the capillaries or the pressure opposing the absorption of solute into these capillaries) is reduced. Simultaneously, and because glomerular filtration rate is preserved (a filtrate free of protein) relative to renal plasma flow, the colloidal osmotic (protein-dependent) pressure within the peritubular capillaries is increased. Collectively, these disparate responses in hydrostatic and osmotic pressures serve to enhance sodium and water reabsorption by the peritubular capillaries. Hence, the salt avid state of chronic cardiac failure has been set into motion. This salt avid state is the result of the same compensatory responses initiated by the kidney in hypovolemia or with prolonged standing.

Enhanced salt and water retention results in positive sodium balance (sodium intake greater than excretion) and expansion of plasma volume. If the heart is able to raise its cardiac output in response to the greater plasma volume, renal plasma flow will increase and the kidney will be "deactivated." Sodium and water balance will be essentially restored. A new steady state will be reached at the expense of a slight expansion of plasma and interstitial fluid volumes. If this "non-congested," compensated patient should increase dietary sodium intake relative to sodium excretion, then sodium balance would be disrupted and a state of expanded compartment volumes and congestion would ensue. The patient may then experience exertional dyspnea, orthopnea, and nocturnal dyspnea and may develop edema. This is the clinical syndrome of congestive heart failure.

Sodium balance (intake equals output) exists in most class A and B patients, with the exceptions noted above that lead to episodes of decompensation. Class C and D patients with chronic cardiac failure experience these episodes of congestion with greater frequency and require larger doses of diuretics, and in some cases multiple diuretics, to maintain sodium balance. The importance of modifying dietary sodium intake in each of these classes, particularly in classes C and D, cannot be overemphasized.

Physical activity, which reduces renal blood flow and further induces renal vasoconstriction, may also play an important role in compromising sodium balance. Renal blood flow normally is decreased with exercise. This may be accentuated in cardiac failure. Moreover, the time course to the reduction in renal plasma flow following exercise in these patients is largely unknown. If the time constant to the recovery of renal plasma flow following exercise is in fact found to require hours, or even days, then the salt-acquisitive state will be further enhanced. Frequently, our patients note that they are feeling well one day and thereby undertake more physical activity, only to develop symptoms of congestion the next day. A better understanding of the kidney and its hemodynamic and functional responses to exercise in patients with chronic cardiac failure represents a fruitful area for clinical research. Findings may suggest improved therapeutic strategies, such as pulsed diuretic therapy on more active days or routine use of drugs with selective renal vasodilatory properties to counteract these vasoconstrictive responses of the renal circulation.

In more severe cardiac failure, renal blood is reduced to an even greater extent. Renal vasoconstriction is more intense and involves both efferent and afferent arterioles. Consequently, blood flow within the kidney is redistributed away from the more numerous nephrons located within the outer or cortical layer of the kidney, toward the lesser number of juxtamedullary nephrons.[29] Thus, both filtration and pressure within the glomerular capillaries are reduced. Filtration fraction (glomerular filtration to renal plasma flow) is increased beyond that seen in milder forms of failure.[30] Here too, physical activity may adversely affect renal hemodynamics and sodium balance. In more advanced failure, potent loop diuretics and diuretics acting in the proximal and collecting tubules are required to maintain sodium balance.

EVALUATING THE SEVERITY OF CHRONIC CARDIAC FAILURE

In Chapter 2, we indicated that maximal oxygen uptake, also termed the aerobic capacity, attained by a patient with chronic cardiac failure during incremental treadmill exercise is a function of the maximal cardiac output and the maximal extraction of oxygen by the tissues. The impairment in aerobic capacity has been assigned to one of five functional classes, which were reviewed in

Chapter 10. This designation of functional exercise impairment (classes A, B, C, D, and E) will be used throughout this and subsequent chapters. We prefer this classification over that proposed by the New York Heart Association (NYHA) because it is less subjective and more quantifiable. Moreover, we have been unable to derive a significant correlation between the objective and subjective assessments.[31] We also recommend determining aerobic capacity over other indices of exercise performance, such as the duration of treadmill exercise or the maximum heart rate achieved during exercise relative to the patient's predicted maximal heart rate. Symptom-limited exercise and exercise duration are far less precise and suffer from not having objective, quantitative end points.

Aerobic Capacity

Patients with chronic cardiac failure secondary to ischemic or myopathic heart disease present with a spectrum of exercise performance and aerobic capacities. Implicit in the $\dot{V}O_2$ max determination is the fact that they are able to exercise to exhaustion. It is only in the patient who is severely symptomatic at rest and who shows evidence of pulmonary congestion on physical examination (class E) that we do not recommend exercise testing.

In order to determine if the exercise response in cardiac output and oxygen extraction correlates with the noninvasive determination of $\dot{V}O_2$ max, we studied a group of patients having chronic cardiac failure of varying severity. We monitored their responses in mixed venous oxygen saturation, cardiac output, intravascular pressures, and respiratory gas exchange during incremental treadmill exercise. Seventy-six patients with chronic cardiac failure of varying severity secondary to ischemic or myopathic heart disease were examined. There were 6 class A, 11 class B, 25 class C, and 34 class D patients in this cohort.[32]

The response in *mixed venous oxygen saturation* (SvO_2) from standing rest to maximum exercise and recovery is shown in Figure 11–13 for a class C patient; the average response for each exercise class (A, B, C, and D) is given in Figure 11–14. The data are presented according to the percentage of $\dot{V}O_2$ max that existed at rest and during exercise. That is, each aerobic capacity was set equal to 100 per cent; values less than $\dot{V}O_2$ max are equal to some fraction of the aerobic capacity. From its standing resting value, SvO_2 follows a common course, becoming progressively lower as oxygen extraction increases with higher work loads. At $\dot{V}O_2$ max, SvO_2 was 30 per cent or less. No differences were noted in SvO_2 among classes at maximum exercise.

Arteriovenous oxygen difference rose to 12 ml/dl or greater at maximum exercise, which

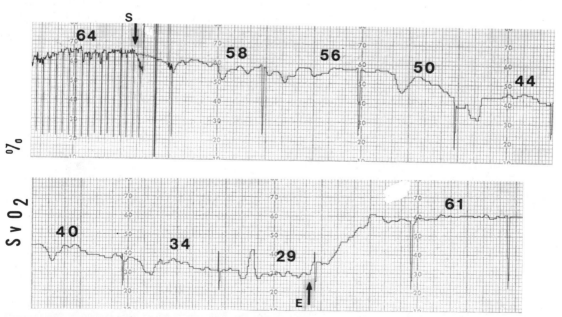

FIGURE 11–13. The response in fiberoptic venous O_2 saturation at standing rest and from the start (*S*) to maximal exercise (*E*) and during recovery for a 42 year old man with chronic cardiac failure. The transient increases or decreases in O_2 saturation reflect the periodic wedge pressure determinations, the withdrawal of mixed venous blood, and the subsequent flushing of the catheter.

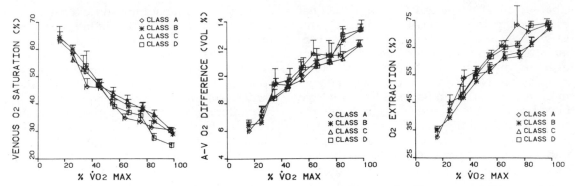

FIGURE 11–14. The response in mixed venous O_2 saturation, arteriovenous O_2 difference, and O_2 extraction to normalized aerobic capacity obtained during incremental treadmill exercise for the four functional classes of patients with chronic cardiac failure. See text for discussion. (From Weber KT, Janicki JS. Cardiopulmonary exercise testing for evaluation of chronic cardiac failure. Am J Cardiol 55:22A–31A, 1985.)

corresponds to a systemic oxygen extraction in excess of 70 per cent in each class (Fig. 11–14). These data indicate that systemic oxygen extraction increases progressively throughout exercise. The measurement of oxygen saturation and oxygen content in the femoral venous circulation of the exercising limb indicates that oxygen extraction will actually exceed 80 per cent in class C patients,[26] in whom femoral venous oxygen content can fall to as low as 1.5 to 2 ml/dl.[33] The lesser value for oxygen extraction calculated from SvO_2 of mixed venous blood is due to the dilutional effect by venous blood draining less metabolically active tissues (e.g., the splanchnic and cutaneous circulations). Thus, the extraction of oxygen approaches maximal physiologic levels in the limb, whereas the absolute level of limb blood flow is less than normal in these patients.[25, 26] Moreover, the ability of the skeletal muscle circulation to autoregulate in these patients may be impaired.[24]

Given that oxygen extraction by muscle is not impaired, the reduction in aerobic capacity of the patient with chronic cardiac failure will be primarily due to the heart's inability to sustain systemic blood flow according to the aerobic requirements of muscle. In Figure 11–15, the response in *cardiac output* to progressive treadmill exercise is given for each functional class. The resting cardiac output levels between classes A and B were not significantly different. Among classes B, C, and D, however, the resting output was significantly different. At peak exercise, differences in cardiac output were observed among the classes. Thus, it is the heart's pump reserve that is responsible for the different aerobic capacities of these patients.

Therefore, the $\dot{V}O_2$ max determination measured from respiratory gas exchange at the mouth serves as a noninvasive measure of pump reserve that can be used to predict the heart's maximal cardiac output. This relationship is shown in Figure 11–16. In this figure, we have further subdivided the class A response according to $\dot{V}O_2$ max (see Chapter 10) and predicted maximal cardiac output. Moreover, $\dot{V}O_2$ max can distinguish between defects in pump reserve that are not present at rest (e.g., between classes A and B).

The close coupling that exists between the heart and the metabolizing tissues is reflected in the interrelationship shown in Figure 11–17 between cardiac output and $\dot{V}O_2$. For each ml/min/m² increase in $\dot{V}O_2$, cardiac output rose 600 ml/min/m². This was true for normal

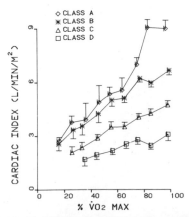

FIGURE 11–15. The response in exercise cardiac output for the four functional classes shown in the preceding figure. See text for discussion. (From Weber KT, Janicki JS. Cardiopulmonary exercise testing for evaluation of chronic cardiac failure. Am J Cardiol 55:22A–31A, 1985.)

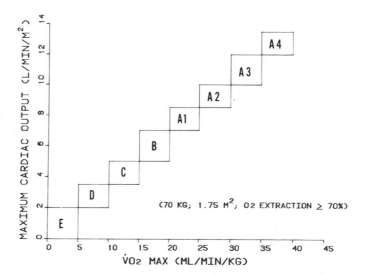

FIGURE 11–16. The predicted maximal cardiac output, or cardiac reserve, derived from the maximal O_2 uptake determination. The functional classes are identified by A to E. The Class A response has been broken down into various subgroups according to $\dot{V}O_2$ max. See text.

subjects and all exercise classes, irrespective of the severity of heart failure. Epstein and co-workers[34] have reported similar findings. Thus, the heart responds normally to the oxygen requirements of the tissues up to its maximal cardiac output. Thereafter, continued muscular work will not be accompanied by an increment in oxygen delivery.

The cardiac output response to exercise is a function of the heart's ability to raise its stroke volume and heart rate. In class A and B patients, *stroke volume* rises 50 per cent during lighter work loads that represent less than 60 per cent of $\dot{V}O_2$ max (Fig. 11–18); thereafter, at larger work loads stroke volume remains invariant. This response in stroke volume resembles that seen in normal subjects during upright exercise; however, the class B response is less in absolute value (a 45 per cent increase). In class C patients the improvement in stroke volume (25 per cent) during the transition from rest to submaximal exercise is even more reduced than in class B patients, whereas in class D patients exercise stroke volume is no different from its resting value. It appears likely that the im-

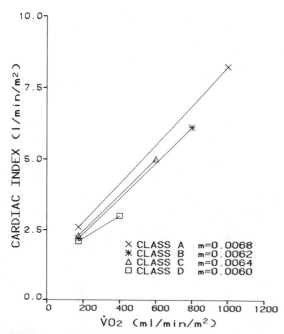

FIGURE 11–17. The relationship between cardiac output and O_2 uptake for the four functional classes. *m* equals the slope of each relation as (liter/min/m²) over (ml/min/m²). See text for discussion.

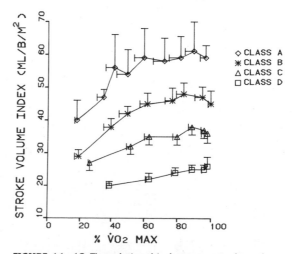

FIGURE 11–18. The relationship between stroke volume index and normalized aerobic capacity. See text for discussion. (From Weber KT, Janicki JS. Cardiopulmonary exercise testing for evaluation of chronic cardiac failure. Am J Cardiol 55:22A–31A, 1985.)

pairment in exercise stroke volume is a result of several factors, including elevated systolic wall stress and reduced systolic and diastolic reserves, that are the result of a depressed myocardial contractility (both intrinsic and manifest). In addition, however, as venous return increases during exercise in these chronically dilated hearts, the elastic limits of the pericardium may introduce a circulatory constraint on further ventricular filling.

The *heart rate* response to upright incremental exercise is shown in Figure 11–19. For each exercise class, a common slope is observed, with the maximal heart rate attained being a function of the maximal work load performed by exercising limb muscles.[35] As a result, maximal heart rate is significantly different for each class. In class D patients, the elevation in heart rate is the sole mechanism by which cardiac output is increased. These observations, which clearly indicate that the increment in heart rate is a function of work load for the limb, are contrary to traditional teaching that suggests that a more dramatic rise in heart rate should occur in class D patients. This view, however, is based largely on findings obtained during supine exercise in patients with mitral stenosis and atrial fibrillation. With normal sinus rhythm and upright exercise, this is simply not the case. The close coupling that exists between the heart and the metabolizing tissues is further reflected in the relationship that exists between $\dot{V}O_2$ and heart rate. As $\dot{V}O_2$ rises, so does the heart rate; the average slope of this relation is 3.6 beats per minute for every 1 ml/min/kg increment in

$\dot{V}O_2$, or approximately 13 bpm for each met of work, and holds true for the majority of patients in each functional class with chronic cardiac failure who are performing upright treadmill exercise. Different muscle groups, however, will elicit different heart rate responses.[36] For example, arm work is associated with a higher heart rate for any comparable $\dot{V}O_2$ attained by leg work.

In accordance with the Fick theorem, there exists a relationship among cardiac output, arteriovenous oxygen difference, and $\dot{V}O_2$. This relationship is given in Figure 11–20, where $\dot{V}O_2$ is represented as constant levels of oxygen utilization for a 70 kg individual of average body surface area (1.75 m²). This assumption of body size permits us to convert the traditional expression of cardiac output in liter/min/m² to units of $\dot{V}O_2$ in ml/min/kg. From this relationship, it is apparent that whatever the cardiac output and arteriovenous oxygen difference may be at rest, when exercise oxygen extraction exceeds 70 per cent (corresponding to an arteriovenous oxygen difference shown in the cross-hatched region in Figure 11–20), the aerobic capacity of the patient will be solely a function of cardiac output. Thus, for class D patients with $\dot{V}O_2$ max <10 ml/min/kg, maximal cardiac output will be 2 to 4 liters/min/m², whereas in classes C, B, and A it will be 4 to 6, 6 to 8, and >8 liters/min/m², respectively. These data correspond to those presented in Figure 11–16 and underscore once again that the noninvasive determination of $\dot{V}O_2$ max predicts the cardiac reserve.

Finally, we have identified a group of patients with very advanced chronic cardiac failure that are quite symptomatic at rest and should not be exercised. However, we did evaluate four such patients[32] and found them to be anaerobic at rest with mixed venous lactate concentration of 13 to 18 mg%. Their resting oxygen extraction was 52 per cent, whereas resting cardiac output was 1.5 liters/min/m². On exercise, their oxygen extraction reached 75 per cent at 1 mph, 0 grade, and their lactate concentration rose progressively; exercise cardiac output, on the other hand, never exceeded 2.1 liters/min/m². Thus, this group of patients who have very severe cardiac failure and are anaerobic at rest have been termed classed E. They should *not* be exercised.

Anaerobic Threshold

Anaerobic muscle produces lactate. In our laboratory, the normal resting mixed ve-

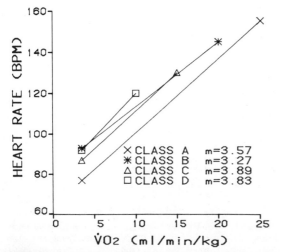

FIGURE 11–19. The heart rate to O_2 uptake relations for the four functional classes and their respective slopes (bpm/ml/min/kg). See text for discussion.

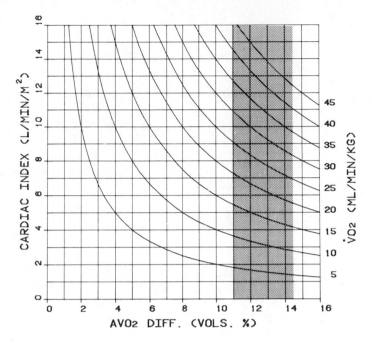

FIGURE 11–20. The interrelationship among cardiac output, arteriovenous O_2 difference (AVO$_2$ Diff), and isopleths of O_2 uptake. The shaded area indicates maximal levels of O_2 extraction and arteriovenous O_2 difference that would be observed for commonly seen levels of hemoglobin (i.e., 11 to 14 grams/dl) in clinical practice. See discussion. (From Weber KT, Janicki JS. Cardiopulmonary exercise testing for evaluation of chronic cardiac failure. Am J Cardiol *55*:22A–31A, 1985.)

nous lactate concentration averages 7 to 8 mg%.[31, 32] We have assumed that when mixed venous lactate concentration exceeds 12 mg%, which represents 2 standard deviations above the average resting value, significant lactate production and release from anaerobic muscle is present.

Figure 11–21 depicts the relationship between mixed venous lactate concentration and systemic oxygen extraction. It can be seen that when systemic oxygen extraction exceeds 60 per cent lactate production is present. The relation between mixed venous lactate and normalized aerobic capacity is shown in Figure 11–22. The appearance of anaerobiosis during exercise occurs when 60 per cent or more of the aerobic capacity has been attained. Given the differences in aerobic capacity among exercise classes, however,

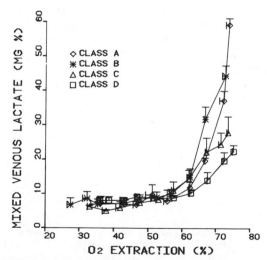

FIGURE 11–21. The response in mixed venous lactate concentration and systemic O_2 extraction during incremental treadmill exercise in patients with chronic cardiac failure. Lactate in milligrams per cent can be converted to micromoles/dl by dividing milligrams per cent by the molecular weight of lactate (90 micromoles/ml). (From Weber KT, Janicki JS. Cardiopulmonary exercise testing for evaluation of chronic cardiac failure. Am J Cardiol *55*:22A–31A, 1985.)

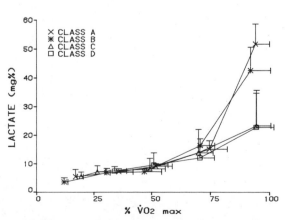

FIGURE 11–22. The response in mixed venous lactate concentration and normalized O_2 uptake (% $\dot{V}O_2$max) during incremental treadmill exercise in chronic cardiac failure. See text.

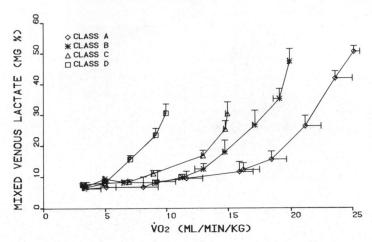

FIGURE 11–23. The response in mixed venous lactate concentration as a function of O_2 uptake observed during incremental treadmill exercise in patients with chronic cardiac failure. See text. (From Weber KT, Janicki JS. Cardiopulmonary exercise testing for evaluation of chronic cardiac failure. Am J Cardiol 55:22A–31A, 1985.)

different work loads are required for each functional class to reach its anaerobic threshold (Fig. 11–23). In class D patients whose cardiac output response is limited, lactate production occurs at very light work loads requiring only 5 to 8 ml/min/kg of $\dot{V}O_2$ (e.g., walking the corridor, dressing, or driving a car). In class C, a work load of 8 to 11 ml/min/kg is required before working muscle becomes anaerobic. In classes B and A, higher loads are tolerated before lactate production occurs (i.e., 11 to 14 ml/min/kg and >14 ml/min/kg, respectively).

Thus, the onset of anaerobiosis and the corresponding work load, or *anaerobic threshold*, reflect the severity of chronic cardiac failure. The differences observed in the absolute rise in mixed venous lactate among the classes may be related to differences in systemic and limb blood flow and the corresponding wash-out of lactate from working muscle. For example, we rarely find lactate concentration exceeding 40 mg% at end exercise, which is much less than that observed

during exhaustive exercise in normal subjects.

As with $\dot{V}O_2$ max, we can noninvasively determine the anaerobic threshold in patients with cardiac failure from their response in respiratory gas exchange to incremental treadmill exercise. We use a number of criteria for this purpose, as noted earlier in Chapter 10. During the exercise test itself, we monitor the temporal response $\dot{V}O_2$ and $\dot{V}CO_2$ (Fig. 11–24), as well as the response in end-tidal oxygen (Fig. 11–25). Consequently, we are able to determine immediately whether or not the patient has achieved an anaerobic level of work during the test. Subsequent to the test, we analyze the response according to the gas exchange criteria depicted in the remainder of Figure 11–25. Matsumura and colleagues[37] have confirmed our findings on the noninvasive determination of anaerobic threshold during treadmill exercise in patients with chronic heart failure. Their observations are quite similar to ours and support the view that the severity of

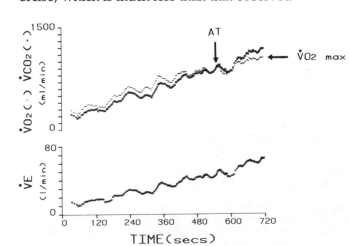

FIGURE 11–24. Breath-by-breath response in respiratory gas exchange, ventilation, and heart rate for a 72 year old man with chronic cardiac failure. The patient's anaerobic threshold (*AT*) and maximal O_2 uptake ($\dot{V}O_2$ *max*) are identified.

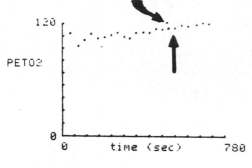

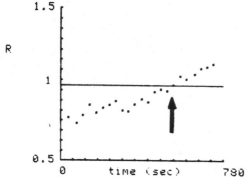

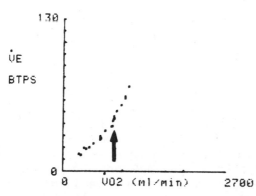

FIGURE 11–25. The exercise response in respiratory gas exchange (R) and minute ventilation ($\dot{V}_E$), which are interpreted subsequent to the exercise test to further define the anaerobic threshold. End-tidal O_2 ($P_{ET}O_2$) is used during the test to determine when the anaerobic threshold has been crossed. Data are from the patient shown in Figure 11–24. (From Weber KT, Janicki JS. Cardiopulmonary exercise testing for evaluation of chronic cardiac failure. Am J Cardiol 55:22A–31A, 1985.)

heart failure may be graded according to this measurement.

In summary, the incremental treadmill test, together with the noninvasive monitoring of respiratory gas exchange, provide objective criteria ($\dot{V}O_2$ max and the anaerobic threshold) to grade the severity of chronic cardiac failure. The test can be performed safely, is easily negotiable by most patients, and is reproducible. If the underlying nature

of the heart disease is known, no additional testing is required and the patients' exercise responses can be followed serially to determine the natural course of their disease or their response to various therapeutic interventions. We have chosen this approach to examine the long-term efficacy of various pharmacologic agents in controlled clinical trials (see Chapter 21).

Exercise Hemodynamics

In the foregoing discussion of $\dot{V}O_2$ max, we have also reviewed the response in pump performance to incremental exercise, and therefore it will not be recounted now. The remainder of the hemodynamic response will be considered here. Figure 11–26 depicts the relation between cardiac index and *left ventricular filling pressure* to exercise in these patients.

Generally speaking, class A and B patients have resting wedge pressures that are significantly lower than those in classes C and D. In fact, resting wedge pressure is normal in class A patients, while in class B patients it is only marginally elevated. However, during exercise, left ventricular filling pressure rises to a different degree in each class. In class A patients, the rise in wedge pressure during isotonic exercise rarely exceeds 18 mm Hg, resembling a normal response. In class B patients, more dramatic elevations to 25 mm Hg or more are noted frequently during exercise. When resting wedge pressure is ab-

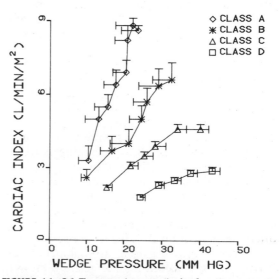

FIGURE 11–26. The exercise ventricular function curve is shown for the four functional classes with chronic cardiac failure. See text for discussion. (From Weber KT, Janicki JS. Cardiopulmonary exercise testing for evaluation of chronic cardiac failure. Am J Cardiol 55:22A–31A, 1985.)

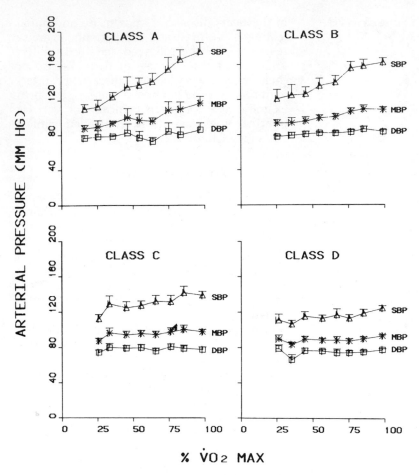

FIGURE 11–27. The response in systolic (*SBP*), mean (*MBP*), and diastolic (*DBP*) arterial pressure for treadmill exercise in the four functional classes with chronic cardiac failure. See text for discussion. (From Weber KT, Janicki JS. Cardiopulmonary exercise testing for evaluation of chronic cardiac failure. Am J Cardiol 55:22A–31A, 1985.)

normally increased in patients at rest (classes C and D), upright exercise often induces more profound elevations in wedge pressure, to levels that exceed 30 mm Hg. Despite these marked levels of pulmonary venous pressure, these patients do not develop pulmonary edema and can exercise to exhaustion without having limiting dyspnea. The pattern of ventilation in class C and D patients, however, will be quite different from that of their class A and B counterparts. When wedge pressure is markedly elevated, a pattern of rapid shallow breathing is used, as described more fully further on.

The response in arterial blood pressure from standing rest to maximal exercise is a function of the increment in cardiac output and the reduction in systemic vascular resistance. In Figure 11–27, the responses in systolic, mean, and diastolic arterial pressures during upright treadmill exercise are shown for each functional class. In class A patients, there is a normal rise in *systolic and mean arterial pressures* above their resting values

(i.e., 115 and 91 mm Hg, respectively, to 176 and 115 mm Hg, respectively) as exercise reaches maximal levels. *Diastolic arterial pressure* remains essentially invariant throughout isotonic exercise, reflecting the progressive vasodilation of working skeletal muscle. The blood pressure response in class B patients is not significantly different from that of class A patients. In class C and D patients, however, the rise in systolic pressure is significantly attenuated. This is particularly evident in class D patients and is a function of the limited elevation in systemic blood flow in the face of skeletal muscle vasodilation. None of the class C or D patients experienced lightheadedness or syncope during the exercise test or while recovering in the sitting position.

The fall in *systemic vascular resistance* that occurs from standing rest to maximum exercise is shown in Figure 11–28. At rest, patients with minimal impairment (exercise class A) had a nearly normal vascular resistance, whereas class C and D patients had

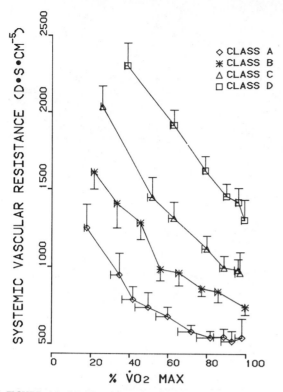

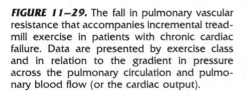

FIGURE 11–28. The fall in systemic vascular resistance that accompanies incremental treadmill exercise in patients with chronic cardiac failure. (From Weber KT, Janicki JS. Cardiopulmonary exercise testing for evaluation of chronic cardiac failure. Am J Cardiol 55:22A–31A, 1985.)

an abnormally elevated vascular resistance. During exercise, vascular resistance fell approximately 50 per cent in each class. The minimum values of vascular resistance observed at maximal exercise, however, were significantly different among all but patients in classes A and B. Even though the fall in resistance was similar in each class, the nonlinear relationship between resistance and cross-sectional area of the circulation would suggest that in patients with advanced chronic cardiac failure the degree of vasodilation of the skeletal muscle may be impaired, as Zelis and co-workers[24] suggested.

Pulmonary vascular resistance is rarely elevated above 400 dynes • sec • cm^{-5} in patients with chronic cardiac failure. This is in contradistinction to patients with much longer-standing pulmonary venous hypertension secondary to chronic mitral valve disease. During exercise, pulmonary vascular resistance falls in patients with ischemic or myopathic heart disease. This is depicted in Figure 11–29, where the relationship between the pulmonary pressure gradient (mean pulmonary artery minus wedge pressures) and pulmonary blood flow is plotted against isopleths of pulmonary vascular resistance for the four functional classes having chronic cardiac failure.

FIGURE 11–29. The fall in pulmonary vascular resistance that accompanies incremental treadmill exercise in patients with chronic cardiac failure. Data are presented by exercise class and in relation to the gradient in pressure across the pulmonary circulation and pulmonary blood flow (or the cardiac output).

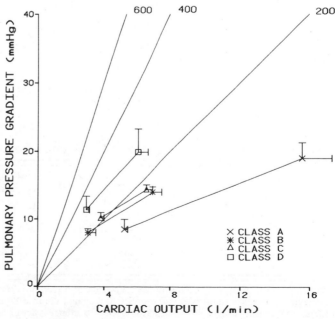

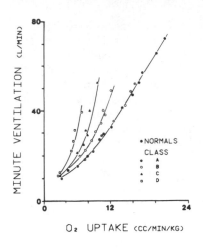 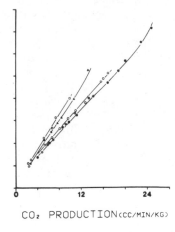

FIGURE 11–30. The exercise response in minute ventilation more closely corresponds to that of CO_2 production than O_2 uptake. (From Weber KT, Kinasewitz GT, Janicki JS, Fishman AP. Oxygen utilization and ventilation during exercise in patients with chronic cardiac failure. Circulation 65:1213–1223, 1982.)

Ventilatory Response

Minute ventilation ($\dot{V}_E$) rises appropriately during *incremental* exercise in patients with chronic cardiac failure. The response in $\dot{V}_E$ (Fig. 11–30) most closely corresponds to $\dot{V}CO_2$ throughout exercise (aerobic and anaerobic work) and is sufficient to sustain alveolar ventilation and prevent hypoxemia from occurring. This has been not only our experience, but also that of others.[38, 39] Moreover, the maximum $\dot{V}_E$ attained uses less than 50 per cent of the patient's maximal voluntary ventilation measured during routine pulmonary function testing (Table 11–4). Thus, these patients do not exhaust their ventilatory reserve in responding to exercise, even when their pulmonary compliance may be adversely elevated as a result of chronic pulmonary congestion and elevations in pulmonary venous pressure during exercise.

In order to minimize the work of breathing during exercise, class C and D patients use a pattern of rapid, shallow breathing (Fig. 11–31) to increase $\dot{V}_E$. Thus, the rise in tidal volume during exercise above its resting value is modest and compatible with a substantial portion of each breath being wasted in anatomic dead-space ventilation. The response of class A and B patients more closely approximates that of healthy individuals, in whom respiratory rate rises progressively during incremental exercise and the rise in tidal volume occurs early during the transition from rest to low-level exercise.

During *constant work rate* exercise, the ventilatory response in patients with chronic cardiac failure depends on whether or not exercise involves aerobic or anaerobic work loads.[40] During *aerobic* (<70 per cent of $\dot{V}O_2$ max) constant work rate (or endurance) treadmill exercise, patients are able to complete a full 20-minute protocol with no limiting symptoms of fatigue or breathlessness; their exercise can be electively terminated. When we measured their hemodynamic response during aerobic endurance exercise, we found the average standing cardiac output of these patients (2.12 ± 0.31 liters/min/m²) to rise to 3.90 ± 1.6 liters/min/m²

Table 11–4. Ventilatory Response to Incremental Treadmill Exercise in Chronic Cardiac Failure

	Class A	Class B	Class C	Class D
Max $\dot{V}_E$ (liters/min)	62 ± 18	44 ± 19	38 ± 17	29 ± 10
Max V_{EQ}	38 ± 7	40 ± 8	45 ± 17	38 ± 15
Max $\dot{V}_E$/MVV	0.43 ± 0.02	0.52 ± 0.45	0.34 ± 0.31	0.37 ± 0.24
Max VT (ml)	1807 ± 977	1329 ± 662	1075 ± 366	869 ± 333
Max VT/VC	0.50 ± 0.13	0.42 ± 0.15	0.38 ± 0.09	0.47 ± 0.20
Max $\dot{V}CO_2$ (liters/min)	1863 ± 485	1390 ± 569	1001 ± 362	676 ± 211
Max R	1.15 ± 0.16	1.24 ± 0.26	1.16 ± 0.35	1.22 ± 0.34

$\dot{V}_E$, maximum minute ventilation; Max V_{EQ}, maximum ventilatory equivalent for O_2; Max $\dot{V}_E$/MVV, the ratio of maximum minute ventilation at end-exercise to maximal voluntary ventilation; Max VT, maximum tidal volume; Max VT/VC, maximum tidal volume at end-exercise to vital capacity; Max $\dot{V}CO_2$, maximum CO_2 production; Max R, maximum ventilatory gas exchange ratio.

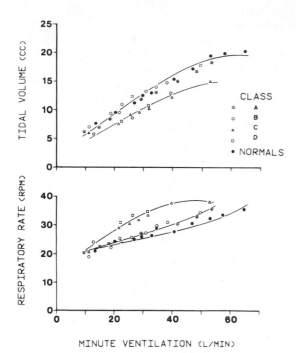

FIGURE 11–31. The pattern of ventilation during exercise differs among the four classes. See text. Shown are the response in tidal volume and respiratory rate to incremental treadmill exercise. (From Weber KT, Kinasewitz GT, Janicki JS, Fishman AP. Oxygen utilization and ventilation during exercise in patients with chronic cardiac failure. Circulation 65:1213–1223, 1982.)

(Fig. 11–32). The standing rest–to–end exercise rise in wedge pressure (from 21 ± 5 to 36 ± 8 mm Hg), heart rate (from 95 ± 17 to 117 ± 19 bpm), and right atrial pressure (5 ± 4 to 10 ± 3 mm Hg) are also given in this figure. Mixed venous lactate, which was 6.48 ± 3.06 mg% at rest, was unchanged during exercise, as depicted in Figure 11–33. From its resting level of 17 ± 3 liters/min, $\dot{V}_E$ rose to a steady state of 31 ± 6 liters/min with aerobic exercise (see Fig. 11–33). The components of the ventilatory response to aerobic endurance consisted of a steady state rise in respiratory rate from 22 ± 3 bpm at rest to 28 ± 5 bpm with exercise and in tidal volume, which rose from 762 ± 181 ml at rest to 1150 ± 170 ml with exercise; these are shown in Figure 11–34.

For patients who performed steady-state *anaerobic* constant work rate exercise (92 ± 4 percent of their $\dot{V}O_2$ max), the hemodynamic response was quite similar to their counterparts performing aerobic exercise (see Fig. 11–32). Cardiac output rose from 2.10 ± 0.17 liters/min/m² at rest to 3.85 ± 0.21 liters/min/m² with exercise; wedge pressure and right atrial pressure rose from 14 ± 11

and 7 ± 7 mm Hg at rest to 25 ± 6 and 12 ± 8 mm Hg, respectively, with exercise. Heart rate was similarly increased from 87 ± 7 to 115 ± 12 bpm with anaerobic exercise.

A progressive rise in mixed venous lactate was seen with anaerobic endurance exercise. Figure 11–33 depicts the rise in lactate that reached 26.39 ± 6.51 mg% with anaerobic exercise, from its resting level of 5.70 ± 1.38 mg%. Moreover, these patients experienced either dyspnea or fatigue as their dominant symptom, which was perceived to be of sufficient severity to make them prematurely terminate (after 10.6 ± 3.8 min) the 20-minute endurance test. As a result of the progressive rise in lactate, there was a different ventilatory response to exercise characterized by a progressive rise in $\dot{V}_E$ (Fig. 11–33) from 13 ± 3 liters/min at rest to 44 ± 11 liters/min at end exercise. The rise in $\dot{V}_E$ was achieved by a steady rise in tidal volume from 682 ± 64 to 1470 ± 360 ml and a

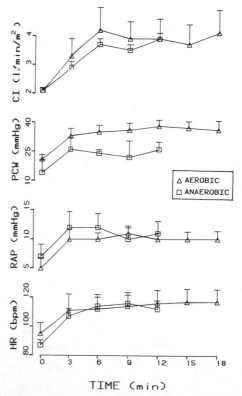

FIGURE 11–32. The average hemodynamic and heart rate response to submaximal, aerobic (five patients) and anaerobic (four patients) endurance exercise. Shown are standing rest data and data obtained at 3 minute intervals of constant level exercise for cardiac index (*CI*), wedge (*PCW*) and right atrial (*RAP*) pressures, and heart rate (*HR*). (From Weber KT, Janicki JS. Lactate production during maximal and submaximal exercise in patients with chronic heart failure. J Am Coll Cardiol 6:717–724, 1985.)

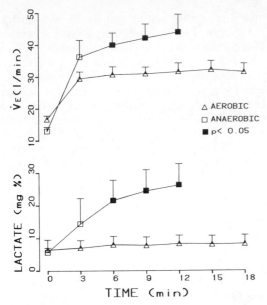

FIGURE 11–33. The response in mixed venous lactate concentration and minute ventilation ($\dot{V}_E$) during submaximal aerobic and anaerobic endurance exercise. (From Weber KT, Janicki JS. Lactate production during maximal and submaximal exercise in patients with chronic heart failure. J Am Coll Cardiol 6:717–724, 1985.)

progressive rise in respiratory rate from 19 ± 3 bpm at rest to 31 ± 4 bpm at end exercise (Fig. 11–34).

As a result of these findings, we are examining the utility of an anaerobic constant

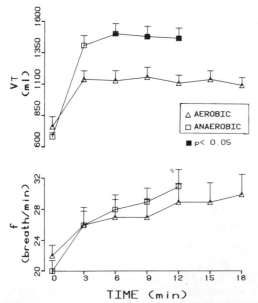

FIGURE 11–34. The response in tidal volume (VT) and respiratory rate (f) to submaximal aerobic and anaerobic endurance exercise are shown. (From Weber KT, Janicki JS. Lactate production during maximal and submaximal exercise in patients with chronic heart failure. J Am Coll Cardiol 6:717–724, 1985.)

work rate exercise test to evaluate the exertional dyspnea and submaximal effort in tolerance of the patient with chronic failure. At this point, however, we are unable to make any recommendations as to the clinical indications for this test and whether or not it will prove more effective or more sensitive than the incremental exercise test in assessing the response to therapy.

CLINICAL APPLICATIONS OF CPX

For the patient with chronic cardiac failure secondary to ischemic or myopathic heart disease, quality of life can be viewed from several vantage points. None, however, are more important than the ability of these patients to participate in symptom-free physical activities. The physician must be able to gauge objectively the effort tolerance of these patients and, in so doing, to assess the severity of disease, its progression over time, and its response to therapeutic intervention.

Several indirect methods have been used for this purpose. Each is based on obtaining historic information relating to exertional dyspnea and fatigue, through patient interview. The traditional classification of the NYHA[41] is based on a physician-dependent appraisal of physical activity. Another method[42] uses a structured questionnaire of effort tolerance that includes different levels of work to create an activity scale. Each method has been useful but suffers from its lack of objectivity. In the foregoing discussion, we have indicated that various objective parameters of left ventricular function (e.g., ejection fraction) are also poor predictors of effort tolerance or cardiac reserve.

We have found that cardiopulmonary exercise (CPX) testing and the noninvasive determination of aerobic capacity and anaerobic threshold during incremental treadmill exercise are more objective approaches to the problem. This methodology also permits us to assess noninvasively the ventilatory response to exercise, as well as to determine noninvasively arterial oxygen saturation by ear oximetry. Collectively, this information derived from CPX can be used not only to evaluate the nature of exertional dyspnea and fatigue, but also to determine the severity of the disease, to follow its progression over time, and to evaluate the patient's response to therapy. In Chapters 17 and 21, we review our respective experience with CPX in distinguishing the cause of exertional dyspnea and

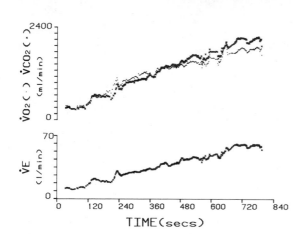

FIGURE 11–35. Respiratory gas exchange during incremental treadmill exercise for a 61 year old woman with idiopathic cardiomyopathy, who was functional class A with an anaerobic threshold and maximal O_2 uptake of 17 and 23 ml/min/kg, respectively.

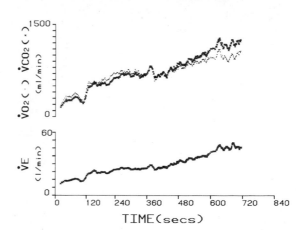

FIGURE 11–37. Another patient with dilated cardiomyopathy (a 45 year old man) but one who was functional class C to treadmill exercise. Anaerobic threshold and maximal O_2 uptake were 9 and 13 ml/min/kg, respectively.

in assessing medical therapy for chronic cardiac failure. Herein we will provide illustrative cases that highlight the clinical utility of noninvasive and invasive CPX in the evaluation of individual patients with chronic cardiac failure, including their functional status over time and their response to medical therapy.

Noninvasive CPX

The measurements of respiratory gas exchange and airflow during an incremental exercise test permit the physician to distinguish aerobic and anaerobic work loads and to determine the anaerobic threshold and maximal oxygen uptake. Figures 11–35 through 11–38 represent such data obtained

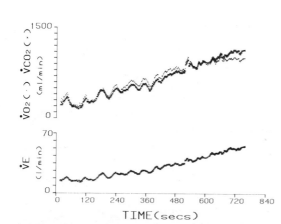

FIGURE 11–36. A class B treadmill response with anaerobic threshold and maximal O_2 uptake of 14 and 19 ml/min/kg, respectively, in a 58 year old man with dilated cardiomyopathy.

on a breath-by-breath basis in four different patients with chronic cardiac failure; each represents the four functional classes A, B, C, and D. The reproducibility of these determinations for two of these patients is shown in Figures 11–39 and 11–40.

Having documented the functional status of a patient in an objective manner, patient stability, improvement, or deterioration can be monitored over time in a manner that is free of patient or physician bias.

Figures 11–41 through 11–44 depict the results for a 45 year old man with ischemic heart disease and dyspnea on exertion that were obtained over the course of 9 months. The patient had several previous myocardial infarctions and poor left ventricular function, as indicated by an ejection fraction of *20 per cent*. His aerobic capacity, which was functional class B (Fig. 11–41), however, predicted that he had a reasonable cardiac reserve and maximal exercise cardiac output of 6 to 8 liters/min/m². The patient's diuretic therapy was altered to provide a greater saluresis. Within a month, he had improved to a class A status (Fig. 11–42). Three months later, the patient had an uneventful myocardial infarction. Three months after his discharge, even though the patient was ambulatory at home at the time, his aerobic capacity had fallen to 11 ml/min/kg (class C; Fig. 11–43), and he subsequently developed congestive cardiac failure. He now was less responsive to his previous medical regimen and was therefore placed on a new cardiotonic agent, enoximone. An improvement in the patient's aerobic capacity to class B

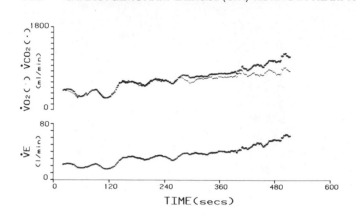

FIGURE 11–38. A treadmill class D response in a 42 year old man with cardiomyopathy. Anaerobic threshold and maximal O_2 uptake were only 6 and 9 ml/min/kg, respectively. The patient also had a straight back and demonstrated an excessive ventilatory response to exercise. Class D patients are anaerobic during stage 1 or 2 of our treadmill exercise protocol.

status (Fig. 11–44) was achieved, with an enhanced effort tolerance and resolution of the signs and symptoms of his heart failure. CPX made it possible to document a change in the progression of his disease and to assess his response to medical therapy.

Figure 11–45 depicts the CPX findings for a 47 year old man with a dilated cardiomyopathy of uncertain etiology. The patient had been referred to our laboratory for evaluation of his functional capacity. His primary physician felt that because of his previous cardiac failure symptoms (now controlled on digoxin and a diuretic), cardiomegaly, and poor ejection fraction (22 per cent), he would be unable to participate in many physical activities. CPX demonstrated his anaerobic threshold to be 13 ml/min/kg, and his aerobic capacity was 17 ml/min/kg. As a result, an intelligent regimen of physical activity, and one that exceeded the expectations of the patient or his physician, can be recommended.

A 32 year old man was referred for evaluation because of atypical chest pain and dyspnea on exertion, both of which were of uncertain origin despite standard diagnostic studies. CPX was recommended and the results are shown in Figure 11–46. The patient had a normal aerobic capacity (29 ml/min/kg), anaerobic threshold (15 ml/min/kg), heart rate (maximum 184 bpm), and ventilatory response (maximum $\dot{V}_E$ 97 liters/min) to incremental treadmill exercise. Moreover, simultaneous analysis of his electrocardiogram (three-lead system) during exercise revealed no evidence of myocardial ischemia. Based on these findings, the primary physician was able to exclude disease of the cardiopulmonary unit and to consider other causes of this man's symptoms.

A 41 year old woman with a dilated cardiomyopathy and depressed ejection fraction (31 per cent) was referred to the laboratory for evaluation of her functional status. Despite several attempts at incremental treadmill exercise, the patient was quite uncom-

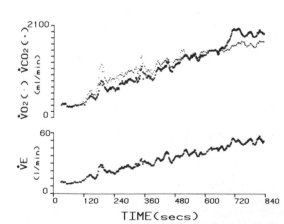

FIGURE 11–39. The reproducibility of the treadmill exercise response is shown for the patient whose record is reproduced in Figure 11–35. This one was obtained 2 weeks after her previous test.

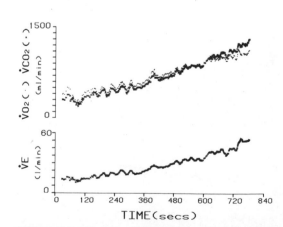

FIGURE 11–40. Reproducibility of treadmill exercise aerobic capacity for the patient whose response is shown in Figure 11–36 and obtained 2.5 months after the previous test.

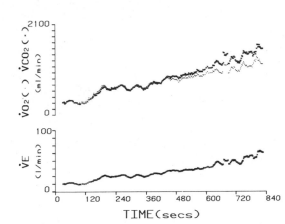

FIGURE 11–41. Initial evaluation of a 45 year old man with ischemic heart disease. See text. The next three figures relate to this patient.

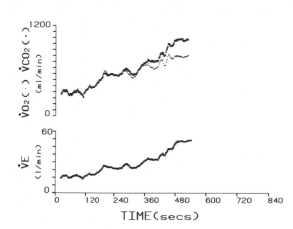

FIGURE 11–43. Aerobic capacity had declined 3 months after the patient's myocardial infarction.

fortable and anxious about the treadmill. As a result, she was exercised several days later using an incremental upright cycle ergometer, the results of which are shown in Figure 11–47. Her anaerobic threshold and maximal oxygen uptake on the bicycle were 9 and 12 ml/min/kg, respectively. These findings indicate that she is functional class C with a substantial reduction in her cardiac reserve (predicted maximal cardiac output of 4 to 6 liters/min/m²). Later the same day, she was re-exercised on the bicycle with similar outcome (Fig. 11–48).

Invasive CPX

The insertion of a pulmonary artery catheter to monitor right heart and pulmonary capillary wedge pressures may be indicated in the patient with ischemic heart disease. This circumstance may arise when there is a disparity in the clinical evaluation and examination of the patient and an unexpectedly reduced aerobic capacity on CPX. This disparity may be due to the appearance of mitral regurgitation during physical activity, which can be documented by the presence of v waves in the wedge pressure recording. A segmental wall motion abnormality that becomes dyskinetic during exercise can be inferred from a wedge pressure that rises excessively with exercise, although this would be best assessed by direct imaging. Regrettably, however, there are few techniques that have the resolution, precision, and sensitivity to document this abnormality during exercise.

Right heart pressure monitoring is rarely indicated to evaluate pulmonary vascular resistance in the patient with either ischemic or myopathic heart disease. Moreover, one can predict with relative certainty that the patient with a dilated cardiomyopathy, whose functional status is class C or D, will have a marked elevation in wedge pressure during exercise.

Other invasive techniques, such as an arterial line or an esophageal catheter, will rarely be indicated in patients with chronic cardiac failure, because they do not develop

FIGURE 11–42. The second treadmill exercise response for the patient in Figure 11–41. An improvement in aerobic capacity was noted.

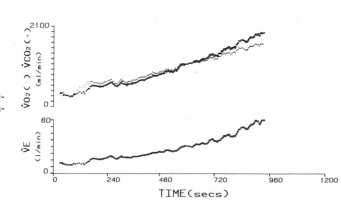

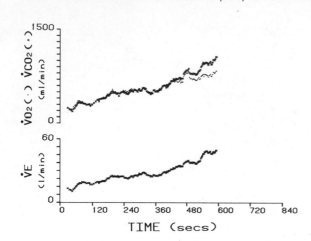

FIGURE 11—44. A return to initial functional status after revision of the patient's medical therapy.

FIGURE 11—45. The exercise response for a 47 year old man with cardiomyopathy who was referred to the laboratory for evaluation. See text. His anaerobic threshold and maximal O_2 uptake were 13 and 17 ml/min/kg, respectively.

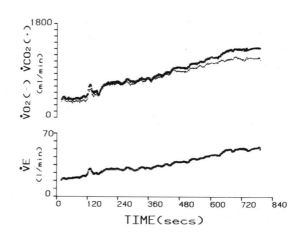

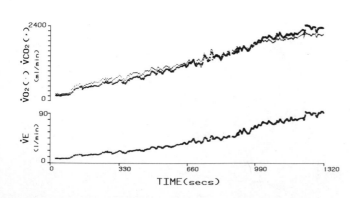

FIGURE 11—46. Response of a 32 year old man with dyspnea on exertion and atypical chest pain, who was referred to the laboratory for evaluation. See text.

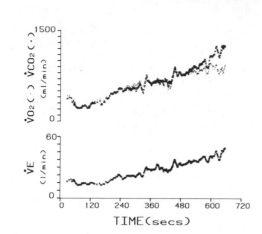

FIGURE 11–47. Response of a 41 year old female with cardiomyopathy who preferred upright cycle ergometry to treadmill exercise.

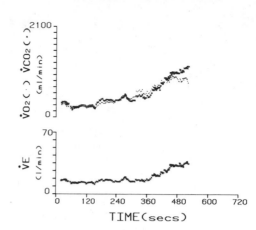

FIGURE 11–48. A repeat bicycle exercise test was obtained the same day for the patient whose response is shown in Figure 11–47.

hypoxemia or have a ventilatory impairment to exercise unless there is coexistent lung disease.

REFERENCES

1. Katz, LN, Feinberg H, Shaffer AB. Hemodynamic aspects of congestive heart failure. Circulation 21:95 111, 1960.
2. Harrison TR, Reeves TJ. Principles and Problems of Ischemic Heart Disease. Year Book Medical Publications, Inc. Chicago, 1968, p 24.
3. Bristow MR, Ginsburg R, Minobe W, Cubicciotti R, Sageman WS, Lurie K, Billingham ME, Harrison PC, Stinson EB. Decreased catecholamine sensitivity and beta adrenergic receptor density in failing human hearts. N Engl J Med 307:205–211, 1982.
4. Chidsey CA, Braunwald E, Morrow AG. Catecholamine excretion and stores of norepinephrine in congestive heart failure. Am J Med 39:442–451, 1965.
5. Francis GS, Goldsmith SR, Ziesche SM, Cohn JN. Response of plasma norepinephrine and epinephrine to dynamic exercise in patients with congestive heart failure. Am J Cardiol 49:1152–1156, 1982.
6. Jose AD, Taylor RR. Autonomic blockade by propranolol and atropine to study intrinsic myocardial function in man. J Clin Invest 48:2019–2031, 1969.
7. Ross J, Covell JW, Sonnenblick EH, Braunwald E. Contractile state of the heart characterized by force-velocity relations in variably afterloaded and isovolumic beats. Circ Res 18:149–152, 1966.
8. Weber KT, Janicki JS, Hunter WC, Shroff SG, Pearlman ES, Fishman AP. The contractile behavior of the heart and its functional coupling to the circulation. Prog Cardiovasc Dis 24:375–400, 1982.
9. Weber KT, Janicki JS. The heart as a muscle-pump system and the concept of heart failure. Am Heart J 98:371–384, 1979.
10. Borow KM, Green LH, Grossman W, Braunwald E. Left ventricular end-systolic stress-shortening and stress-length relations in humans. Am J Cardiol 50:1301–1308, 1982.
11. Borow KM, Neumann A, Wynne J. Sensitivity of end-systolic pressure-dimension and pressure-volume relations to the inotropic state in humans. Circulation 65:988–997, 1982.
12. Colan SD, Borow KM, Neumann A. Left ventricular end systolic wall stress-velocity of fiber shortening relation: a load-independent index of myocardial contractility. J Am Coll Cardiol, 4:715–724, 1984.
13. Benjamin IJ, Schuster EH, Bulkley BH. Cardiac hypertrophy in idiopathic dilated cardiomyopathy: a clinicopathologic study. Circulation 64:442–447, 1981.
14. Gelberg HJ, Rubin SA, Ports TA, Brundage H, Parmley WW, Chatterjee K. Detection of left ventricular functional reserve by supine exercise hemodynamics in patients with severe, chronic heart failure. Am J Cardiol 44:1062–1067, 1979.
15. Benje W, Litchfield RL, Marcus ML. Exercise capacity in patients with severe left ventricular dysfunction. Circulation 61:955–959, 1980.
16. Franciosa JA, Park M, Levine B. Lack of correlation between exercise capacity and indices of left ventricular performance in heart failure. Am J Cardiol 47:33–39, 1981.
17. Engler R, Ray R, Higgins C, McNally C, Buxton WH, Bhargava V, Shabetai R. Clinical assessment and follow-up of functional capacity in patients with chronic congestive cardiomyopathy. Am J Cardiol 49:1832–1837, 1982.
18. Higginbotham MD, Morris KG, Conn EH, Coleman RE, Cobb FR. Determinants of variable exercise performance among patients with severe left ventricular dysfunction. Am J Cardiol 51:52–64, 1983.
19. Russell RO, Rackley CE, Pombo JH, Hunt D, Potamin C, Dodge HT. Effects of increasing left ventricular filling pressure in patients with acute myocardial infarction. J Clin Invest 49:1539–1550, 1970.
20. Ross J, Braunwald E. The study of left ventricular function by increasing resistance to ventricular ejection with angiotensin. Circulation 29:739–749, 1964.
21. Francis GS. Neurohumoral mechanisms involved in congestive heart failure. Am J Cardiol 55:15A–21A, 1985.
22. Kotchen TA, Hartley LH, Rice TW, Mogey EH, Jones LG, Mason JW. Renin, norepinephrine, and epi-

nephrine responses to graded exercise. J Appl Physiol 31:178–184, 1971.

23. Weber KT, Janicki JS, Likoff MJ, Shroff S, Andrews V. Chronic cardiac failure: pathophysiologic and therapeutic considerations. Triangle 22:1–9, 1983.

24. Zelis R, Longhurst J, Capone RJ, Mason DT. A comparison of regional blood flow and oxygen utilization during dynamic forearm exercise in normal subjects and patients with congestive heart failure. Circulation 50:137–143, 1974.

25. Wilson JR, Martin JL, Ferraro N, Weber KT. Effect of hydralazine on perfusion and metabolism in the leg during upright bicycle exercise in patients with heart failure. Circulation 68:425–431, 1983.

26. Wilson JR, Martin JL, Schwartz D, Ferraro N. Exercise intolerance in patients with chronic heart failure: role of impaired nutritive flow to skeletal muscle. Circulation 69:1079–1087, 1984.

27. Merrill AJ. Edema and decreased renal blood flow in patients with chronic congestive heart failure: evidence of "forward failure" as the primary cause of edema. J Clin Invest 25:389–400, 1946.

28. Leithe ME, Macgorien RD, Hermiller JB, Unverferth DV, Leier CV. Relationship between central hemodynamics and regional blood flow in normal subjects and in patients with congestive heart failure. Circulation 69:57–64, 1984.

29. Kilcoyne MM, Schmidt DH, Cannon PJ. Intrarenal blood flow in congestive heart failure. Circulation 47:786–797, 1973.

30. Cannon PJ. The kidney in heart failure. N Engl J Med 296:26–33, 1977.

31. Weber KT, Kinasewitz GT, Janicki JS, Fishman AP. Oxygen utilization and ventilation during exercise in patients with chronic cardiac failure. Circulation 65:1213–1232, 1982.

32. Weber KT, Janicki JS. Cardiopulmonary exercise testing for evaluation of chronic cardiac failure. Am J Cardiol 55:22A–31A, 1985.

33. Kugler J, Maskin C, Frishman WH, Sonnenblick EH, LeJemtel TH. Regional and systemic metabolic effects of angiotensin-converting enzyme inhibition during exercise in patients with severe heart failure. Circulation 66:1256–1261, 1982.

34. Epstein SE, Beiser GD, Stampfer M, Robinson BF, Braunwald E. Characterization of the circulatory response to maximal upright exercise in normal subjects and patients with heart disease. Circulation 35:1049–1062, 1967.

35. Weber KT, Wilson JR, Janicki JS, Likoff MJ. Exercise testing in the evaluation of the patient with chronic cardiac failure. Am Rev Respir Dis 129:S60–S62, 1984.

36. Vokac Z, Bell H, Bautz-Holter E, Rodahl K. Oxygen uptake/heart rate relationship in leg and arm exercise, sitting and standing. J Appl Physiol 39:54–59, 1975.

37. Matsumura N, Nishijima H, Kojima S, Hashimoto F, Minami M, Yasuda H. Determination of anaerobic threshold for assessment of functional state in patients with chronic heart failure. Circulation 68:360–367, 1983.

38. Rubin SA, Brown HV, Swan HJC. Arterial oxygenation and arterial oxygen transport in chronic myocardial failure at rest, during exercise and after hydralazine treatment. Circulation 66:143–148, 1982.

39. Wilson JR, Ferraro N. Exercise intolerance in patients with chronic left heart failure: relation to oxygen transport and ventilatory abnormalities. Am J Cardiol 51:1358–1363, 1983.

40. Weber KT, Janicki JS. Lactate production during maximal and submaximal exercise in patients with chronic heart failure. J Am Coll Cardiol 6:717–724, 1985.

41. Freidberg CK. Diseases of the Heart. WB Saunders, Philadelphia, 1966, p 241–242.

42. Goldman L, Hashimoto B, Cook EF, Loscalzo A. Comparative reproducibility and validity of systems for assessing cardiovascular functional class: advantages of a new specific activity scale. Circulation 64:1227–1234, 1981.

KARL T. WEBER
JOSEPH S. JANICKI

12

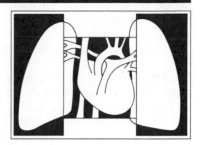

Valvular Heart Disease

Valvular heart disease can lead to *chronic circulatory failure*. The clinical course of the patient with mitral or aortic valve disease will be determined by the nature and severity of the disease, the ability of the left and right heart to compensate for the hemodynamic abnormality created by the diseased valve, and the extent to which the vascular resistance of the pulmonary circulation is elevated. Mitral and aortic valve disease alters the functional integrity of the cardiopulmonary unit by impairing its ability to raise systemic blood flow in accordance with the oxygen requirements of the tissues. Secondary pathophysiologic alterations that occur within the unit as a result of valvular disease also will influence the clinical outcome of valve replacement. The more marked the preoperative impairment in cardiac reserve, the poorer the long-term prognosis. Similarly, the greater the elevation in pulmonary vascular resistance, the more delayed its return to normal levels and the slower the postoperative improvement in symptoms. The decision for the best timing for surgical intervention, therefore, requires a sensitive and objective measure of cardiopulmonary status, one that can be reliably and noninvasively repeated, and that detects even the most subtle decline in performance. Serial echocardiographic measurements of left ventricular size and systolic shortening have been suggested as one way of deciding on the timing of valve replacement.

Our approach to the patient with valvular heart disease has been to use cardiopulmonary exercise (CPX) to determine the patient's maximal oxygen uptake, anaerobic threshold, and ventilatory response to incremental treadmill exercise. In Chapter 11, in which we reviewed our experience with pa-

tients with chronic cardiac failure secondary to ischemic heart disease or dilated cardiomyopathy, we indicated that noninvasive CPX allowed us to predict maximal cardiac output (that is, cardiac reserve) and at the same time objectively assess functional status. The purpose of this chapter is to review our experience with noninvasive CPX in patients with mitral or aortic regurgitation or both. We describe the interrelationship between aerobic capacity and other hemodynamic characteristics of the left and right heart and the pulmonary circulation in these patients when invasive measurements are made during CPX. We also review how similar techniques have been used by others in the evaluation of patients with mitral stenosis.

Because of the heightened risk of syncope, myocardial ischemia, and arrhythmias that might occur during exercise in patients with aortic stenosis, we specifically exclude exercising these patients and therefore will not consider the condition in this chapter.

ASSESSMENT OF MITRAL AND AORTIC VALVULAR INCOMPETENCE

Incompetence of the mitral and aortic valves creates a volume overload on the left ventricle. When valvular incompetence develops gradually, the volume overload on the ventricle is accommodated initially by chamber enlargement and myocardial hypertrophy without a serious compromise in the pumping function of the left ventricle. Chamber dilatation and myocardial hypertrophy serve as compensatory responses. In addition, and because the left ventricle now ejects blood into the left atrium or a decompressed central aorta, instantaneous shortening load (or afterload) is reduced in both mitral and aortic regurgitation.[1] Thus the ventricle accommodates to the volume overload while sustaining systemic blood flow. This is true both at rest and during physical activity. Eventually, however, for unknown reasons, the left ventricle begins to fail. The onset of ventricular dysfunction is generally unpredictable. Generally speaking, initially this will be apparent only during vigorous levels of physical activity. Later, as the disease becomes more severe, the patient is symptomatic at lower levels of activity; finally, the patient is disabled at rest.

Also, it must be recognized that the hemodynamic overload of mitral or aortic regurgitation is not confined to the left ventricle. As left ventricular filling and left atrial pressures rise, so too must pulmonary venous, capillary, and arterial pressures rise. As a result, an additional pressure load is placed on the right heart and pulmonary circulation. The right ventricle must enlarge and hypertrophy to accommodate this extra load. Moreover, because small pulmonary arteries and arterioles develop smooth muscle hypertrophy and some degree of intimal proliferation in response to the increased pulmonary artery pressure, the vascular resistance of the pulmonary circulation will be increased.[2] The functional status of a patient, as well as the possibility of operation, therefore, must be considered in light of the function of the overloaded left and right ventricles and the resistance of the pulmonary circulation. A broader perspective of the clinical entities of mitral and aortic valvular incompetence can be found in Braunwald.[3]

For the most part, the current approach to the evaluation of mitral or aortic regurgitation is based on hemodynamic measurements obtained in the resting supine position, together with an angiographic assessment of the severity of valvular incompetence and left ventricular ejection fraction. However, a number of investigators have indicated that this approach is not sufficiently sensitive to predict the cardiac reserve or to detect a subtle defect in ventricular function.[4-8] Therefore exercise to stress the cardiopulmonary unit in these patients has been used with increasing frequency.

We have had the opportunity to evaluate with noninvasive and invasive CPX a number of patients with mitral (11 patients) or aortic (6 patients) valvular incompetence or both (5 patients). Their mean age was 53 ± 15 years (15 to 78 years); 9 were women. Fifteen patients were in sinus rhythm, whereas the remainder had atrial fibrillation. From historical information given, all were considered to have either class II, III, or IV heart failure by New York Heart Association criteria. Each patient had a cardiothoracic ratio of more than 50 per cent on standard chest roentgenograph and left ventricular hypertrophy by electrocardiographic criteria. All patients were stable and treated with oral digoxin and one or more diuretics. The objective of our evaluation was to assess cardiac reserve, right and left ventricular function, and pulmonary vascular resistance. We graded their functional status according to their aerobic capacity, as described in Chapter 10.

Cardiac Reserve by Determining Maximal Oxygen Uptake

Table 12–1 presents the resting hemodynamic profile of patients with valvular heart disease studied in our laboratory. At standing rest, the cardiac output was not distinguishable among classes A, B, C, or D with either regurgitant lesion (Fig. 12–1). The exercise response in cardiac output is shown in

Table 12–1. Resting Hemodynamic Profile of Patients with Mitral or Aortic Valvular Regurgitation

	Cardiac Output (liters/min/m²)	Mean PAP (mm Hg)	PCW (mm Hg)	PVR (dynes·sec·cm⁻⁵)	RAP (mm Hg)
Mitral regurgitation (N = 11)	2.4 ± 0.7	16 ± 15	20 ± 12	147 ± 45	6 ± 3
Aortic regurgitation (N = 6)	2.4 ± 0.5	18 ± 7	14 ± 6	71 ± 17	2 ± 3
Combined (N = 5)	2.0 ± 0.4	32 ± 19	20 ± 7	355 ± 260	2 ± 3

PAP, pulmonary artery pressure; PCW, wedge pressure; PVR, pulmonary vascular resistance; RAP, mean right atrial pressure.

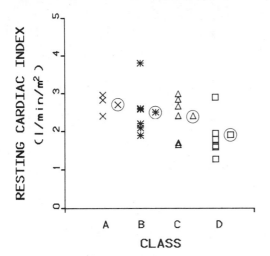

FIGURE 12–1. The resting cardiac index for patients with valvular incompetence is shown for each exercise class, irrespective of the nature of the valvular incompetence. The average values for each class are shown as the circled symbol. The classes could not be distinguished from one another by the resting cardiac output measurement.

Figure 12–2 for the four exercise classes. In *A*, the regression line for cardiac output is given as a function of the level of work performed where work is expressed as a per cent of aerobic capacity. During exercise, there was a progressive rise in cardiac output in each functional class irrespective of the nature of the underlying valvular heart disease. In class D patients, however, the rise in exercise cardiac output did not exceed 4 liters/min/m² at maximal exercise. In classes A, B, and C, peak cardiac output was more than 8, 6 to 8, and 4 to 6 liters/min/m²,

respectively. As in patients with chronic cardiac failure (see Chapter 11), $\dot{V}O_2$ max was an indicator of maximal cardiac output and thereby one measure of cardiac reserve.

The relationship between the cardiac output response and absolute $\dot{V}O_2$ is given in *B* of Figure 12–2. The slope of this relation was not statistically different among classes and was approximately 600 ml/min/m² for every dl/min/m² rise in $\dot{V}O_2$. This is the normal "gain" setting of the cardiac output response and once again emphasizes that the close coupling between the heart and tissues is preserved in these patients. Because of the valvular disease, however, the heart's reserve is reduced and, consequently, so is the patient's aerobic capacity. Chronic mitral and aortic regurgitation, therefore represent examples of chronic *circulatory* failure.

Maximal cardiac output response to exercise is impaired for two reasons: (1) the inability of the heart to appropriately raise its forward stroke volume in the presence of mitral or aortic regurgitation (Fig. 12–3, left panel); and (2) a component of chronic cardiac failure as left ventricular dysfunction appears. In either case, the extent of the impairment in forward stroke volume determines the decline in aerobic capacity.

The heart rate response to exercise in these patients, even those with atrial fibrillation, falls within the range seen for patients with chronic cardiac failure of varying severity (3 bpm per 1 ml/min/kg increment in $\dot{V}O_2$), as discussed in Chapter 11. Like the patients with chronic cardiac failure, peak heart rate

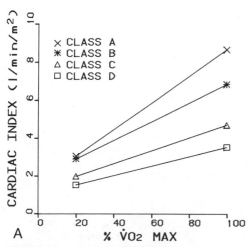
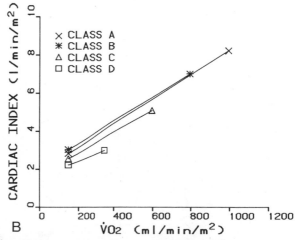

FIGURE 12–2. The relationship between cardiac index and $\dot{V}O_2$ attained during incremental treadmill exercise in patients with mitral or aortic valvular incompetence, or both, who are categorized according to their aerobic capacity. *A*, $\dot{V}O_2$ uptake is normalized according to maximum O_2 uptake. *B*, $\dot{V}O_2$ is given in absolute units, expressed in terms of body surface area (m²). Maximal exercise cardiac output was significantly different between classes. The slope of the cardiac output-$\dot{V}O_2$ relation, however, was not different among the classes.

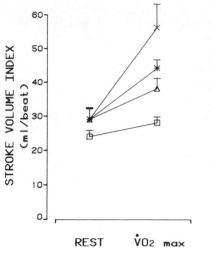
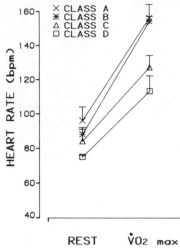

FIGURE 12–3. The response in stroke volume and heart rate from standing rest to maximal treadmill exercise is given for patients with valvular incompetence presented according to their aerobic capacity. See text.

in these patients with chronic circulatory failure is related to the $\dot{V}O_2$ max attained (Fig. 12–3, right panel).

A progressive rise in arteriovenous oxygen difference accompanies incremental exercise in these patients. The response in oxygen extraction, or the ratio of arteriovenous oxygen difference to arterial oxygen content, to exercise is shown in Figure 12–4 for each class having mitral, aortic, or combined valvular incompetence. As 80 per cent or more of the patient's aerobic capacity is reached, systemic oxygen extraction exceeds 70 per cent. There is no impairment on the part of exercising muscle to extract oxygen. Thus, the observed decreases in aerobic capacity are primarily related to the decline in maximal forward cardiac output that the heart can generate, or the cardiac reserve.

In patients with valvular incompetence we have found no relationship between $\dot{V}O_2$ max—and by inference cardiac reserve—and the usual indices of left ventricular function, such as resting cardiac output (Fig. 12–5) or resting left ventricular filling (wedge) pressure (Fig. 12–6). These findings underscore the uncertainty surrounding the estimated severity of mitral or aortic regurgitation, which is based solely on resting supine hemodynamic data obtained in the cardiac catheterization laboratory. It is therefore important to recognize that the cardiac reserve can be noninvasively assessed during maximal exercise by the determination of $\dot{V}O_2$ max.

Although the noninvasive determination of aerobic capacity is a sensitive descriptor of cardiac reserve, it does not specifically iden-

FIGURE 12–4. The response in O_2 extraction to incremental treadmill exercise for patients with valvular incompetence presented according to aerobic capacity.

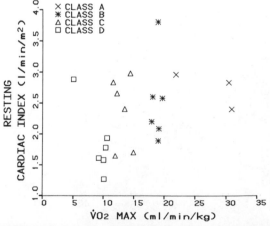

FIGURE 12–5. The poor correlation that exists between resting cardiac index and aerobic capacity is demonstrated. As in chronic cardiac failure, the cardiac reserve in circulatory failure cannot be predicted from resting cardiac output.

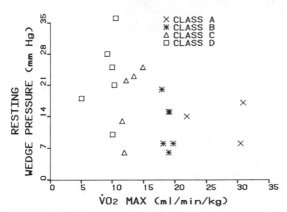

FIGURE 12–6. A poor correlation exists between resting wedge or left ventricular filling pressure and $\dot{V}O_2$ max, emphasizing again that resting indices of ventricular function do not predict the pumping reserve of the heart.

for example, are anaerobic walking the corridor with a $\dot{V}O_2$ of approximately 6 ml/min/kg. These findings on the lactate response correlate well with the noninvasive respiratory gas exchange response and our previous findings in chronic cardiac failure. Thus, the anaerobic threshold predicts the severity of the deficit in systemic blood flow because it represents a relatively fixed percentage (>60 per cent) of the aerobic capacity.

tify the cause of the abnormality in cardiac reserve. It is not possible from the $\dot{V}O_2$ max determination to distinguish between the inability of the cardiac output to rise appropriately because of valvular incompetence or left ventricular dysfunction. $\dot{V}O_2$ max also does not distinguish among limitations to cardiac output that are posed by the left ventricle, right ventricle, or pulmonary circulation. Therefore, right heart catheterization for hemodynamic monitoring during incremental isotonic exercise should be performed to elucidate further the functional status of each ventricle and the vascular resistance of the pulmonary circulation.

Cardiac Reserve by Determining Anaerobic Threshold

Maximal oxygen uptake will predict the heart's cardiac reserve, as we have just indicated. The anaerobic threshold alone can be determined for similar purposes. Figure 12–7 pictures the response in mixed venous lactate concentration to progressive treadmill exercise for patients with valvular incompetence. At 60 to 70 per cent of patients' aerobic capacity, lactate production occurs; this corresponds to a level of systemic oxygen extraction of 60 or more per cent. Figure 12–8 depicts the rise in mixed venous lactate concentration as a function of absolute treadmill work for each exercise class. As in patients with chronic cardiac failure (see Chapter 11), the anaerobic threshold occurs at progressively lower levels of work as the severity of valvular disease increases. Class D patients with mitral or aortic valvular incompetence,

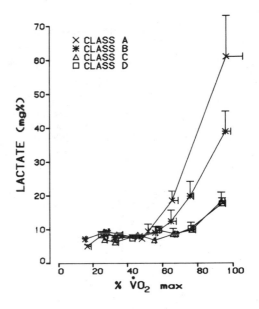

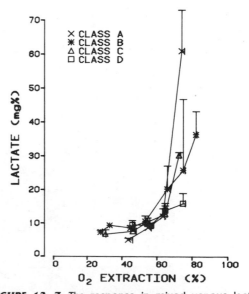

FIGURE 12–7. The response in mixed venous lactate concentration is given as a function of normalized aerobic capacity or $\dot{V}O_2$ max (upper panel) and systemic O_2 extraction (lower panel) for patients with mitral or aortic valvular incompetence, or both. See text.

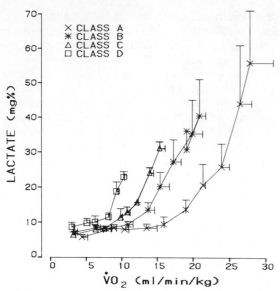

FIGURE 12–8. As in chronic cardiac failure, the onset of lactate production (> 12 mg per cent) in valvular incompetence and chronic circulatory failure occurs at different workloads, depending on the severity of the impairment in aerobic capacity.

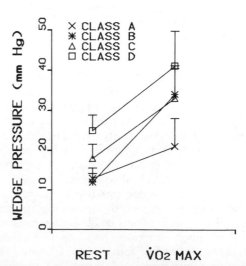

FIGURE 12–10. The response in wedge pressure from rest to maximum exercise is shown for patients with mitral (*VMR*) or aortic (*VAR*) regurgitation or both (*VARMR*).

Ventricular Function

In patients with mitral or aortic valvular incompetence, a certain portion of left ventricular ejection is diverted to the left atrium in systole or the left ventricle in diastole; both the left atrium and *left ventricle* enlarge with time, and each becomes more distensible. Therefore it is not possible to suggest that a reduction in systemic blood flow in these patients is due solely to an impairment in left ventricular function. On the other hand, because systemic vascular resistance falls progressively during isotonic exercise (Fig. 12–9) as working skeletal muscle vasodilates, either left ventricular emptying should be

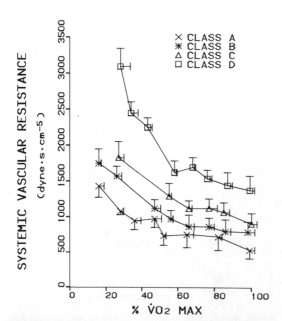

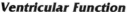

FIGURE 12–9. The response in systemic vascular resistance according to normalized aerobic capacity for patients with mitral or aortic valvular incompetence. See text.

FIGURE 12–11. The response in wedge pressure to exercise is presented for patients with mitral or aortic valve incompetence who were categorized according to aerobic capacity.

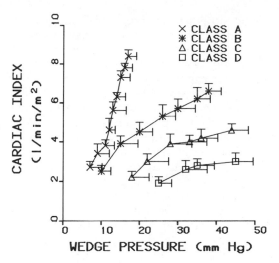

FIGURE 12–12. The relation between cardiac index and wedge (left ventricular filling) pressure during upright, isotonic exercise for patients with mitral or aortic regurgitation or both.

facilitated in mitral regurgitation or the regurgitant volume into the left ventricle caused by aortic incompetence should be reduced.

A marked rise in left ventricular filling pressure with exercise may indicate intrinsic left ventricular dysfunction.

The left ventricular filling pressure response to exercise in these patients can be estimated by monitoring occlusive wedge pressure with invasive CPX. In aortic insufficiency particularly, however, one must remember that the true left ventricular end-diastolic pressure may be higher than the wedge pressure as a result of premature closure of the mitral valve. The rise in wedge pressure that occurs with exercise is greatest in combined aortic and mitral regurgitation (Fig. 12–10). Nevertheless, as shown in Figure 12–11, the response in occlusive wedge or left atrial pressure is quite different for each exercise class, regardless of the nature of the valvular lesion. The greatest rise in exercise wedge pressure is seen in class D patients with mitral or aortic valvular incompetence or both, suggesting that left ventricular dysfunction is present. From the rise in left ventricular filling pressure it also appears likely that class C and B patients have an element of ventricular dysfunction.

Ventricular pump function has traditionally been described in terms of the relationship between ventricular displacement (e.g., cardiac output or forward stroke volume) or work (e.g., stroke work) and the filling volume (or pressure) of the corresponding ventricle. To obtain this information, invasive hemodynamic monitoring during upright exercise is required. In Figure 12–12, the left ventricular function curve comparing cardiac output with left ventricular filling pressure at rest and throughout exercise is shown for class A to D patients with mitral or aortic regurgitation or both. Once again, it is apparent that, despite large elevations in left ventricular filling pressure, class C and D patients with either lesion have a greater impairment in left ventricular pump function. Thus, based on indices of pump function, class C and D patients have left ventricular dysfunction.

However, indices of left ventricular pump function in mitral or aortic regurgitation will also be influenced by the regurgitant lesion. The ejection fraction, for example, may remain in the normal range because of the incompetent valves even when there is left ventricular dysfunction. Indices of myocardial contractility based on concepts of cardiac muscle (see Chapters 4 and 11) have been derived to circumvent this problem. Carabello and coworkers have demonstrated the utility of the end-systolic stress to end-systolic volume ratio in the evaluation of chronic mitral regurgitation and the prediction of surgical outcome.[8] A reduced ratio was strong evidence of left ventricular dysfunction.

Because of the pulmonary venous hypertension that accompanies chronic mitral or aortic incompetence, the *right ventricle* has to generate a larger systolic pressure to maintain pulmonary blood flow; as a result, it will hypertrophy and enlarge. Eventually the right ventricle will fail, and tricuspid valvular incompetence may appear at rest or during exercise. The marked levels of right ventricular pressure work that occur in chronic valvular incompetence are often overlooked in these patients; the relevance of right ventricle function to the immediate postoperative course must be recognized. In Figure 12–13, the response in right ventricular systolic and filling pressures is shown according to the nature of the valve lesion. The right heart in patients with mitral or aortic regurgitation is placed under a larger hemodynamic overload than that seen in chronic cardiac failure.

Right ventricular filling pressure, or right atrial pressure, also may rise considerably during exercise. In Figure 12–14 the response in right atrial pressure to upright exercise is shown for two patients. Tricuspid regurgitation can be detected during exercise by the

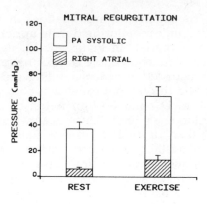

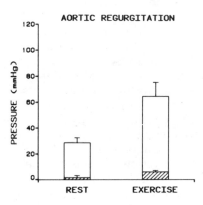

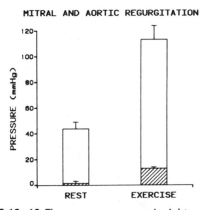

FIGURE 12–13. The average response in right ventricular and diastolic and systolic pressures to incremental, upright treadmill exercise in patients with mitral or aortic regurgitation or both. Right ventricular systolic pressure is inferred from the response in pulmonary artery (PA) systolic pressure.

marked and abrupt elevation in right atrial pressure.

Pulmonary Vascular Resistance

The level of preoperative pulmonary vascular resistance is important in determining the surgical outcome of valve replacement. When vascular resistance is elevated, symptomatic improvement after valve replacement

will be slower to evolve, which in all likelihood reflects the gradual regression of medial hypertrophy in the pulmonary circulation.

The *pressure-flow relation* of the pulmonary circulation can be characterized by invasive hemodynamic monitoring during exercise. Pulsatile and mean pulmonary artery and occlusive wedge pressures should be determined at each stage of treadmill exercise. These data, together with the corresponding monitoring of cardiac output, will characterize the pressure-flow relation of the pulmonary circulation, as well as permit the calculation of pulmonary vascular resistance. This topic is considered in detail in Chapter 13, in which we review the topic of pulmonary hypertension.

Figure 12–15 depicts the pressure-flow relation for the pulmonary circulation in patients with mitral or aortic regurgitation or both. The pressure-flow relation for each functional class is plotted against isopleths of constant pulmonary vascular resistance. With chronic mitral or aortic regurgitation, pulmonary vascular resistance does not exceed 600 dynes • sec • cm $^{-5}$. Class A, B, and C patients generally have a resistance of less than 200 dynes • sec • cm $^{-5}$. During isotonic exercise pulmonary vascular resistance falls for each of these classes. Because of the more marked pulmonary venous hypertension that exists in class D patients, the absolute level of their vascular resistance is severalfold higher than that normally found at rest (less than 120 dynes • sec • cm^{-5}) and during

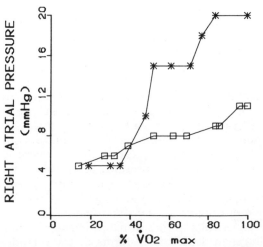

FIGURE 12–14. Responses in right atrial pressure to progressive upright exercise for two patients with chronic mitral regurgitation. Note that one of these patients develops tricuspid regurgitation during exercise, with marked elevation in right atrial pressure.

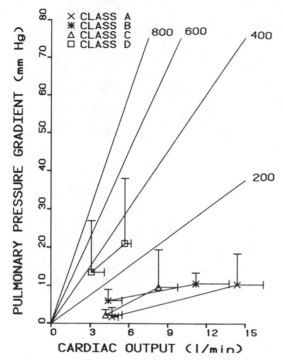

FIGURE 12–15. The gradient in pressure across the pulmonary circulation to cardiac output relation for patients who have mitral or aortic valvular incompetence. Values for the standing resting position and maximum exercise are presented for each exercise class against a background of isopleths of constant pulmonary vascular resistance.

day. By the tenth postoperative day, the average mean pulmonary artery pressure was 35 mm Hg, representing a 51 per cent decrease.[10] In another series[9] in which similar patients received a mitral valve replacement, pulmonary artery systolic pressure was found to average 36 mm Hg and the pressure gradient averaged 15 mm Hg 2 months following operation; the average preoperative pulmonary vascular resistance in these patients was shown to fall from 774 to 245 dynes · sec · cm^{-5}.

The only means with which to identify this subset of patients with mitral regurgitation and excessive pulmonary vascular resistance is invasive hemodynamic monitoring. Even though one would expect their exercise cardiac output response and aerobic capacity to be significantly reduced and compatible with functional class D, it appears unlikely that the explanation for the reduced aerobic capacity (left ventricular dysfunction versus elevated pulmonary vascular resistance) could be inferred from noninvasive CPX. Invasive CPX is therefore of diagnostic value in this setting.

THE ASSESSMENT OF MITRAL STENOSIS

The reduced mitral valve orifice that accompanies rheumatic mitral valvular stenosis leads to left atrial distention and chamber enlargement, pulmonary venous hypertension, and right heart pressure overload. Pulmonary vascular resistance in most patients ranges between 200 and 600 dynes · sec · cm^{-5}. In all likelihood this elevation in resistance reflects the longstanding nature of the mitral valve obstruction and the fact that some degree of smooth muscle hypertrophy has occurred in the pulmonary circulation. Wood[12] estimated that approximately 12 per cent of patients with mitral stenosis, predominantly women, will have an even greater elevation in pulmonary vascular resistance, with values exceeding 700 dynes · sec · cm^{-5}.

Taken collectively or individually, each of the hemodynamic abnormalities associated with mitral stenosis is responsible for a reduction in left ventricular filling. As a result, resting cardiac output may be reduced or, if preserved, may fail to rise appropriately with exercise.

Transmitral flow primarily depends on the cross-sectional area of the mitral valve and to a lesser extent on the gradient in pressure

exercise (60 dynes · sec · cm^{-5}), or that found in class D patients with ischemic or myopathic heart disease in whom pulmonary vascular resistance averages 200 to 400 dynes · sec · cm^{-5}. Even in class D patients with valvular incompetence, pulmonary vascular resistance falls during exercise because the rise in cardiac output is greater than the elevation in the pressure gradient across the pulmonary circulation.

A number of laboratories have reported that a small subset (less than 10 per cent) of patients with mitral regurgitation have a disproportionately elevated pulmonary vascular resistance (more than 700 dynes · sec · cm^{-5}) relative to their pulmonary venous hypertension.[9–12] The resting systolic pulmonary artery pressure in these patients—a reflection of the right ventricular systolic pressure—averages 70 to 80 mm Hg whereas the pressure gradient across the lung ranges in most cases from 15 to 30 mm Hg. Surgical replacement of the mitral valve in these patients is associated with a decline in these pressures. Mean pulmonary artery pressure, which averaged 71 mm Hg preoperatively, fell to 47 mm Hg by the first postoperative

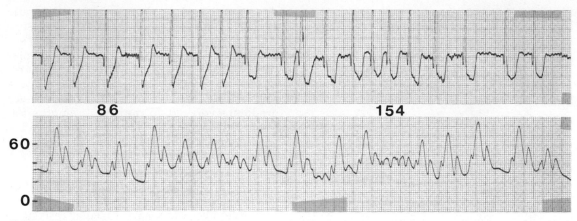

FIGURE 12–16. A 62 year old woman with rheumatic mitral valve disease and chronic atrial fibrillation that was difficult to control on oral digoxin therapy alone. A chest lead electrocardiogram and pulmonary artery pressure tracing are shown. When the ventricular response averaged 86 bpm, the pulsatile nature of pulmonary artery pressure is apparent and consistent with right ventricular ejection. In addition, the respiratory variation in pressure can be appreciated. For more rapid rates (e.g., 154 bpm), effective right ventricular ejection was minimal, as evidenced by the absence of pulmonary artery systolic pressure.

between the atrium and ventricle (the square root of this gradient) and the length of diastole.[13] When heart rate rises, as it does with exercise, diastole is shortened and left ventricular filling is compromised further. The appearance of atrial fibrillation, which is common in patients with longstanding mitral stenosis, adds yet another confounding variable that reduces left ventricular filling on the basis of the lost atrial contraction and the irregularly irregular, frequently rapid rhythm that abbreviates diastole (Fig. 12–16 and 12–17).

Hence, mitral valvular stenosis and its companion abnormalities of the pulmonary circulation and cardiac rhythm create a state of chronic *circulatory* failure. Surgical intervention can provide marked improvement in these disturbances and clinical status. But, as was true for mitral valvular incompetence, candidates for operation in mitral stenosis must have a preoperative assessment not only of the severity of the stenosis but also the cardiac reserve, right and left ventricular function, and pulmonary vascular resistance. In this segment of the chapter we will focus on these issues and the role of noninvasive and invasive CPX in making these assessments. A detailed discussion of the disease entity can be found elsewhere.[3]

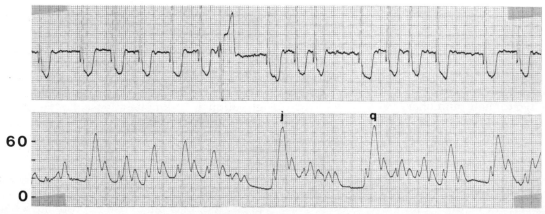

FIGURE 12–17. Data from the patient discussed in Figure 12–16. Following a premature ventricular contraction, there was no substantial ejection of blood. The subsequent postpotentiated beat (*j*) was associated with an elevation in pulmonary artery systolic pressure. Thereafter, pump function was impaired by the rapid ventricular response. The q beat that followed a long RR interval was associated with a greater ejection volume and corresponding pulmonary artery pressure.

Cardiac Reserve by Determining Maximal Oxygen Uptake and Anaerobic Threshold

Between 1920 and 1965, mitral stenosis was probably the most frequently studied circulatory disorder of the cardiopulmonary unit. The introduction of mitral commissurotomy in 1952 only heightened the interest in this condition, as had the development of cardiac catheterization in 1947. Most clinical studies utilized exercise to estimate the severity of the disease.

Before the advent of cardiac catheterization evaluation of cardiac reserve was approached by indirect methods. Spurred by the studies and techniques of Hill and coworkers on oxygen utilization during muscular exercise and the accompanying appearance of lactic acid,[14] a number of investigators undertook clinical studies in patients with mitral stenosis. Exercise was used to raise oxygen requirements while respiratory gas exchange was monitored. Meakins and Long found that when the patients walked (3.5 miles per hour) or ran in place (184 steps/min), their oxygen uptake was less than that of normal subjects.[15] Moreover, their rise in blood lactic acid was greater for any given work load. Harrison and Pilcher extended these observations to patients with more advanced disease and peripheral edema.[16] In their study, patients were exercised by ascending and descending stairs. An excessive degree of ventilation and carbon dioxide production was noted to accompany muscular work and recovery in these patients. Cotes verified that the release of lactic acid observed during a standardized step test accounted for this ventilatory response.[17] Hence, even before cardiac catheterization, respiratory gas exchange techniques and exercise testing had identified the circulatory failure characteristic of the patient with mitral stenosis.

Invasive hemodynamic monitoring during exercise provided the means of determining the mechanism responsible for the circulatory failure and the earlier appearance of anaerobiosis during exercise. In 1951, Gorlin et al reported on the circulatory dynamics seen in mitral stenosis during symptom-limited supine bicycle exercise.[18] For most patients in this study, cardiac output failed to rise appropriately because of the inability of the heart to raise its stroke volume (Fig. 12–18); systemic oxygen extraction, on the other hand, increased markedly with exercise. In addition, pulmonary capillary wedge and mean pulmonary artery pressures rose excessively (Fig. 12–19) during supine exercise.

Donald, Bishop and Wade[19] measured the interrelationship among cardiac output, arteriovenous oxygen difference, and oxygen consumption during symptom-limited supine exercise in 14 patients with mitral stenosis.[19] The results of their study have been adapted for the format in Figure 12–20. Based on their findings, which described a spectrum of cardiac output responses, these investigators categorized the severity of mitral stenosis as grades 1, 2, and 3 according to the impairment in cardiac reserve and aerobic capacity.

Donald and coworkers[20] further identified that the rise in arterial lactate concentration during exercise was a function of the graded severity of the impairment in cardiac reserve (Fig. 12–21). Lactate production was noted to occur when mixed venous oxygen saturation fell below 40 per cent (Fig. 12–22).

Using an incremental treadmill exercise protocol and respiratory gas exchange technique, Chapman et al determined the $\dot{V}O_2$ max of 15 men with mitral stenosis.[21] The aerobic capacity of these patients averaged 22 ml/min/kg and would lead one to predict that for the average-sized individual in this study, the peak cardiac index would be approximately 8 to 9 liters/min/m². This prediction in fact correlates closely with the measured values of systemic blood flow in this study. As was true of the supine exercise studies, the defect in the cardiac output response to upright exercise was due to the impairment in the stroke volume response to exercise. Blackmon and coworkers studied a similar group of patients in whom aerobic capacity averaged 23 ml/min/kg.[22] The subnormal cardiac output response to exercise is shown in Figure 12–23 for these patients; the heightened level of oxygen extracted and the greater arteriovenous oxygen difference at lesser work loads are shown in Figure 12–24. Lactate production occurred when 60 to 70 per cent of $\dot{V}O_2$ was achieved (Fig. 12–25), which could be detected noninvasively from the response in respiratory gas exchange (Fig. 12–26).

Ventricular Function

The assessment of *left ventricular* function in mitral stenosis has followed traditional lines of inquiry (a) regarding systolic pump function, as well as (b) according to concepts of cardiac muscle. This latter approach has

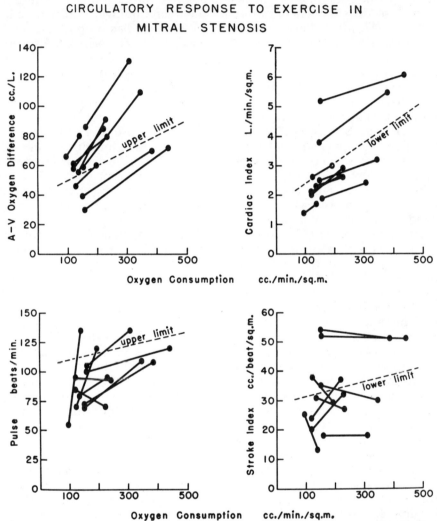

FIGURE 12–18. The response in arteriovenous (A-V) O_2 difference, cardiac index, heart rate or pulse, and stroke index to elevations in O_2 consumption resulting from progressive supine bicycle exercise. The dotted line represents the limits of variation seen in Dr. Gorlin's laboratory. (From Gorlin R, Sawyer CG, Haynes FW, Goodale WT, Dexter L. Effects of exercise on circulatory dynamics in mitral stenosis. Am Heart J 41:192–203, 1951.)

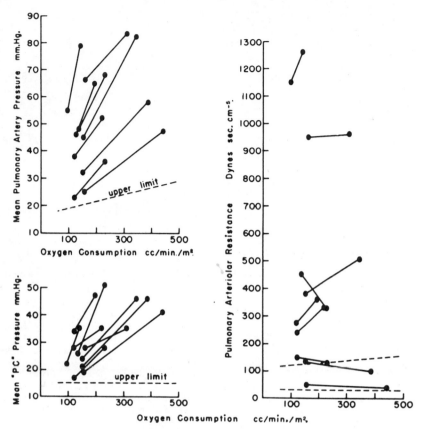

FIGURE 12–19. The response in mean pulmonary artery and wedge pressures and pulmonary arteriolar resistance to increments in O_2 consumption resulting from supine bicycle exercise. The dotted lines are defined in Figure 12–18. (From Gorlin R, Sawyer CG, Haynes FW, Goodale WT, Dexter L. Effects of exercise on circulatory dynamics in mitral stenosis. Am Heart J *41*:192–203, 1951.)

FIGURE 12–20. Three grades of severity (groups I to III) of mitral stenosis, reported by Donald and coworkers. Their data were adapted for presentation here. The severity of the disease was based on maximum exercise cardiac output and thereby $\dot{V}O_2$ attained during supine cycle ergometry. (Adapted from Donald KW, Bishop JM, Wade OL. A venous oxygen content difference, oxygen uptake and cardiac output and rate of achievement of a steady state during exercise in rheumatic heart disease. J. Clin Invest *33*:1146–1167, 1954.)

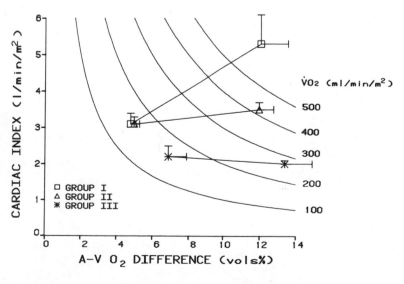

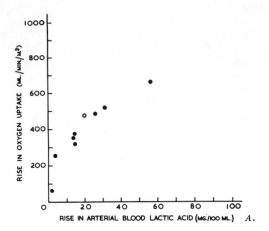

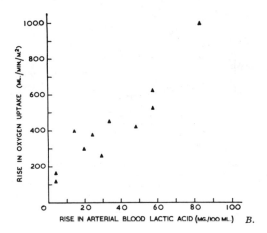

FIGURE 12–21. The relationship between the rise in arterial lactate concentration and the increment in O_2 uptake during supine exercise is shown for the three grades of mitral stenosis described in Figure 12–20 (top, group I; middle, group II; bottom, group III). (From Donald KW, Gloster J, Harris EA, Reeves J, Harris P. The production of lactic acid during exercise in normal subjects and in patients with rheumatic heart disease. Am Heart J 62:494–510, 1961.)

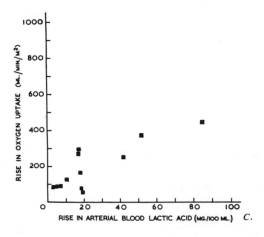

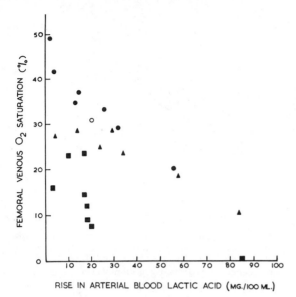

FIGURE 12–22. Arterial lactate concentration began to rise once femoral venous O_2 saturation fell below 40 per cent during supine exercise in patients with mitral stenosis. Symbols as shown in Figure 12–21 for the three groups. (From Donald KW, Gloster J, Harris EA, Reeves J, Harris P. The production of lactic acid during exercise in normal subjects and in patients with rheumatic heart disease. Am Heart J 62:494–510, 1961.)

been chosen, based on the well-recognized alterations in left ventricular chamber–loading conditions (both diastolic and systolic) that exist in mitral stenosis. Thus, to assess myocardial contractility, these abnormalities in loading must be excluded.

Ross and colleagues utilized supine exercise and left ventricular catheterization to examine the issue of systolic pump function in mitral stenosis (group 2 in Fig. 12–27).[23] They found that cardiac index increased normally (group 1) or nearly so (left panels), whereas end-diastolic pressure fell in their patients with mitral stenosis. The same was true of the change in stroke volume relative to the change in end-diastolic pressure (right panels). Moreover, these findings were consistent with the response of these patients to angiotensin (see Chapter 11).

In a recent study conducted by Gash and coworkers in which indices of cardiac muscle were obtained at the time of cardiac catheterization, there was no evidence of impaired fiber-shortening velocity in many patients.[24] In those in whom shortening velocity was reduced (and ejection fraction was reduced), end-systolic stress (as a measure of afterload) was increased. This was found to be secondary to lower myocardial wall thickness.

In general, it is believed that there is little abnormality in the intrinsic contractile state of the myocardium with mitral stenosis.

Right ventricular pressure work was derived by Gorlin and coworkers for patients with mitral stenosis performing supine exercise.[18] The left hand panel of Figure 12–28 depicts these findings and the increased levels of pressure work that the right ventricle has to generate. This is in distinct contrast to left ventriclar pressure work (right panel), which was generally below normal.

Pulmonary Vascular Resistance

In the right panel of Figure 12–19, which depicts the experience of Gorlin et al,[18] it is apparent that for most patients with mitral stenosis pulmonary vascular resistance is less than 600 dynes · sec · cm^{-5} at rest and during exercise. Our observations for patients with mitral regurgitation are similar. In Gorlin's series, a small subset of patients with mitral

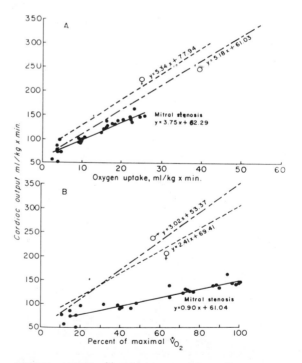

FIGURE 12–23. The response in cardiac output (ml/min/kg) to $\dot{V}O_2$ uptake (A) and normalized aerobic capacity (B) seen during upright incremental treadmill exercise in patients with mitral stenosis. The broken lines and regression line equations are for young men and women studied by Astrand and coworkers (J Appl Physiol 19:268, 1964). (From Blackmon JR, Rowell LB, Kennedy JW, Twiss RD, Conn RD. Physiological significance of maximal oxygen intake in "pure" mitral stenosis. Circulation 36:497–510, 1967.)

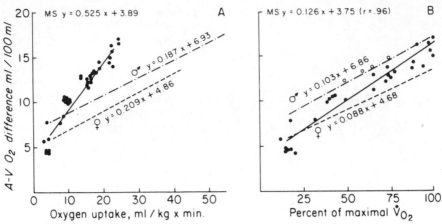

FIGURE 12–24. The response in arteriovenous O_2 difference during incremental treadmill exercise in patients with mitral stenosis. A greater degree of O_2 extraction occurs at lighter work loads (A), but the extent of O_2 extraction relative to normalized $\dot{V}O_2$ (B) is no different from normals (Astrand et al, J Appl Physiol *19*:268, 1964). (From Blackmon JR, Rowell LB, Kennedy JW, Twiss RD, Conn RD. Physiological significance of maximal oxygen intake in "pure" mitral stenosis. Circulation *36*:497–510, 1967.)

stenosis displayed an abnormal elevation in pulmonary vascular resistance (more than 900 dynes • sec • cm^{-5}) and, as a result, right ventricular pressure work was elevated. This hyperreactivity of the pulmonary circulation mirrors that found in a subset of patients with mitral valvular incompetence.[9] The experience with mitral valve replacement in these patients has been detailed earlier in the chapter. The message from this surgical experience is similar to that in mitral stenosis. Mitral valve replacement will lead to a reduction in pulmonary vascular resistance[25] but not to the same level seen in the more usual case, in which preoperative pulmonary vascular resistance is less than 600 dynes • sec • cm^{-5}. Moreover, this decline may require weeks (as opposed to hours) to reach levels of several hundred dynes • sec • cm^{-5}.

VENTILATION IN PATIENTS WITH VALVULAR HEART DISEASE

Peabody et al in 1917 reported that in symptomatic patients with valvular heart disease, tidal volume was reduced and respiratory rate increased (in comparison with asymptomatic patients).[26] In addition, $\dot{V}_E$ in dyspneic patients was increased while their vital capacity was reduced. These findings have been reproduced by many investigators.

Christie and Meakins demonstrated that the lungs were stiffer in patients with symptomatic heart failure.[27] They arrived at these findings by measuring intraesophageal pressure—to reflect intrapleural pressure—and tidal volume. They found that a larger intrapleural pressure had to be generated to produce a given tidal volume, implying that a greater respiratory muscle effort was required. Marshall and coworkers extended

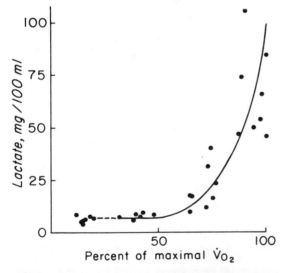

FIGURE 12–25. Arterial lactate concentration rose in patients with mitral stenosis walking on the treadmill when greater than 60 per cent of $\dot{V}O_2$ max was attained. (From Blackmon JR, Rowell LB, Kennedy JW, Twiss RD, Conn RD. Physiological significance of maximal oxygen intake in "pure" mitral stenosis. Circulation *36*:497–510, 1967.)

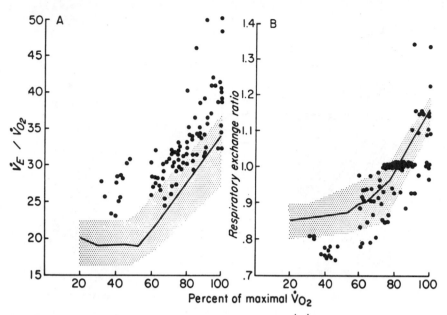

FIGURE 12–26. A, The response in the ventilation, relative to O_2 uptake ($\dot{V}_E/\dot{V}O_2$), and B, the respiratory gas exchange ratio ($\dot{V}CO_2/\dot{V}O_2$ or R), are shown for patients with mitral stenosis performing treadmill exercise. Patient data are presented as solid circles; normal response is shown as the shaded area and solid line. (From Blackman JR, Rowell LB, Kennedy JW, Twiss RD, Conn RD. Physiological significance of maximal oxygen intake in "pure" mitral stenosis. Circulation 36:497–510, 1967.)

these observations to periods of symptom-limited exercise on a bicycle ergometer.[28] In patients with mitral stenosis, a marked increase in lung stiffness was noted, unlike the fall seen in normal subjects. Moreover, even if the elasticity of the lung were normal at rest in these patients, it was quite abnormal on exercise. Hence, the work of breathing for any given level of $\dot{V}_E$ in these patients was two-to threefold greater than that required by normal subjects. As a result, a pattern of rapid, shallow breathing is adopted to minimize work and increase efficiency. Marshall et al called attention to the fact that this same increase in respiratory muscle work, or force generation in displacing air, increases the levels of negative intrapleural pressure that must be generated.[29] In patients with mitral stenosis, -45 cm H_2O appeared to be the maximum intrapleural pressure that could be generated by breathing through graded reductions in the inspiratory orifice during treadmill exercise before the patient became dyspneic. The same values were observed in normal subjects, except that in them larger volumes of air could be mobilized each minute.

In studies in which pulmonary compliance and pulmonary capillary wedge pressures were recorded during supine exercise in patients with mitral stenosis awaiting valvulot-omy, Saxton et al found a close correlation between the fall in compliance and the level of wedge pressure in most patients.[30] Moreover, following operation, lung compliance and wedge pressure had returned toward normal. In their review of the subject, Turino and Fishman summarized these findings and indicated that the work of breathing is increased in the patient with mitral stenosis.[31] This may be true at rest in the more severely compromised patient and in all patients with mitral stenosis during exercise when pulmonary compliance is reduced. As a result, a pattern of rapid, shallow breathing is adopted to minimize the work of breathing.

Wood and coworkers have shown recently that the specific abnormality in ventilatory mechanics in these patients is focused on the static pressure-volume relation of the lung.[32] At small lung volumes, lung recoil is diminished, presumably because of vascular congestion. At larger volumes, because of the chronic interstitial edema and fibrosis that these patients develop, increased recoil and a high transpulmonary pressure were noted.

The alterations in $\dot{V}_E$ that accompany the appearance of anaerobiosis during exercise in these patients was reviewed earlier in this chapter. As in chronic cardiac failure, a pattern of rapid, shallow breathing is

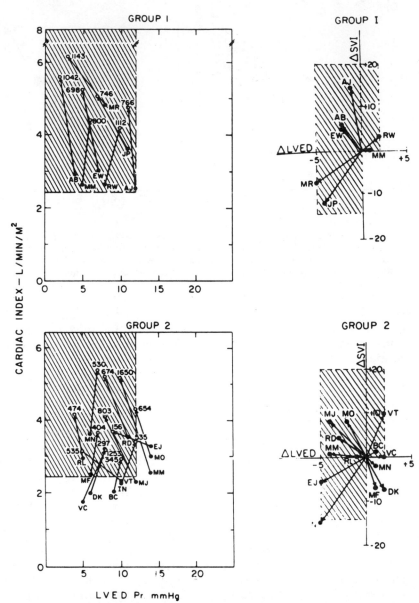

FIGURE 12–27. The response in left ventricular pump function to supine bicycle exercise in normal subjects (group 1) and in patients with mitral stenosis (group 2). The left panels depict the relations between cardiac index and left ventricular end-diastolic pressure (*LVEDPr*) from rest (solid circle) to peak exercise (open circle). Right, the change in stroke volume (△ *SVI*) to the change in end-diastolic pressure (△ LVED) during exercise for these two groups. (From Ross J, Gault JH, Mason DT, Linhart JW, Braunwald E. Left ventricular performance during muscular exercise in patients with and without cardiac dysfunction. Circulation *34*:597–608, 1966.)

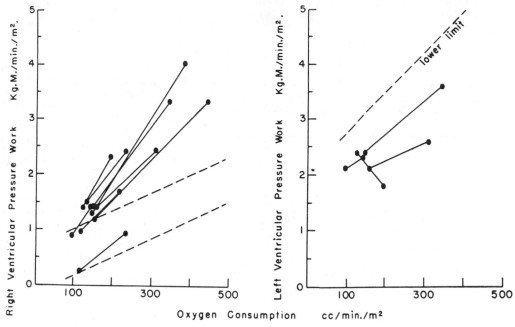

FIGURE 12–28. Right and left ventricular pressure work and their relationship to O_2 consumption during supine bicycle exercise. The dotted lines are defined in Figure 12–18. (From Gorlin R, Sawyer CG, Haynes FW, Goodale WT, Dexter L. Effects of exercise on circulatory dynamics in mitral stenosis. Am Heart J *41*:192–203, 1951.)

characteristic during physical activity when pulmonary venous pressure is elevated. Consequently, the proportion of the tidal volume that occupies the dead space at rest (approximately 30 per cent) does not fall with exercise as is normally the case.

CLINICAL APPLICATIONS

It is recognized that the clinical New York Heart Association classification of the severity of circulatory failure is subjective and therefore of limited value. These discrepancies have been identified by Krause and Rudolph in patients with regurgitant or stenotic lesions of the mitral or aortic valves.[33] Their findings are shown in Figure 12–29, which indicates that there is no interrelationship between the mean pulmonary artery pressure to cardiac output relation and the corresponding clinical classification. These data also show that the cardiac output response to 50 watts of upright bicycle exercise cannot be predicted on clinical grounds.

Figure 12–30 depicts CPX data for a patient with valvular heart disease who was referred to our laboratory for evaluation. The patient was thought to have significant mitral valvular incompetence, based on historical information relating to effort tolerance and the

presence of significant angiographic valvular regurgitation. The results of the CPX test, however, indicated that he had a substantial cardiac reserve and rated a very high functional class B. Valve replacement was not recommended.

This patient's history is described further in Figures 12–31, 12–32, and 12–33, in which serial CPX test results are shown. These data provided valuable insights into the patient's evaluation and management over the course of a year. For example, he was re-exercised 2 and 3 months after his baseline study to assess the stability of his functional status. The reproducibility of the aerobic capacity and anaerobic threshold obtained in these tests (Fig. 12–31), in comparison to his first CPX testing, was quite good. The patient became more self-assured about his exercise capacity and took comfort in the fact he would not require valve replacement. As a result, he liberalized his dietary salt intake; within 1 month of his last CPX test, a decline in functional status was apparent (Fig. 12–32). At this point, there was no clinical evidence of congestion and the importance of dietary sodium restriction was re-emphasized. Within 3 weeks he required hospitalization for overt congestive heart failure, with orthopnea, bibasilar rales, and peripheral edema. His congestive symptoms were re-

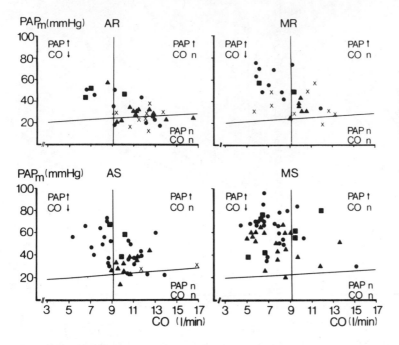

FIGURE 12–29. The response in mean pulmonary artery pressure (PAP_m) and cardiac output (*CO*) to 50 watts of upright cycle ergometry. Patients with aortic (*AR*) or mitral (*MR*) regurgitation and aortic (*AS*) and mitral (*MS*) stenosis are shown and categorized according to clinical severity by NYHA criteria (class I, X; class II, ▲; class III, ●; and class IV, ■). (From Krause F, Rudolph W. Symptoms, exercise capacity and exercise hemodynamics: Interrelationships and their role in quantification of the valvular lesion. Herz 9:187–199, 1984.)

solved by the administration of diuretics and reduction of sodium intake. One month later (upper panel, Fig. 12–33) he had returned to his baseline functional status where he remained over the next 6 months. His repeat CPX test 6 months after discharge is shown in the lower panel of Figure 12–33.

Figure 12–34 depicts the CPX results of a patient with aortic regurgitation and mitral valve replacement. The patient's two exercise studies were separated by 1 year; her functional capacity was quite stable (class C). With the advent of a paraprosthetic valvular leak 6 months later, her functional capacity declined significantly, with aerobic capacity and anaerobic threshold becoming compatible with class D. Surgical correction of the prosthetic defect was performed, resulting in a return to the previous baseline in aerobic capacity. Thus, her CPX test served to identify the severity of the valvular heart disease and, together with clinical evaluation, pointed up the need for surgical repair. CPX was also useful in monitoring her response to surgical intervention.

A knowledge of the vascular resistance of the pulmonary circulation in patients with valvular heart disease is also invaluable in assessing their operative candidacy and response to surgery. Figure 12–35 discloses the hemodynamic data for a 45 year old woman seen in this hospital with signs and symptoms of congestive heart failure and a history of a heart murmur for several years. Her vital signs were within normal limits, and she was noted to be in atrial fibrillation. Neck vein distention to the angle of the jaw was observed with the patient sitting at 45 degrees. A right ventricular lift and an accentuated pulmonic component of the second heart sound were noted. A murmur of mitral regurgitation and a short diastolic rumble were heard, together with an S3 gallop. Echocardiography revealed that the mitral valve leaflets were sclerotic, but no stenosis was pres-

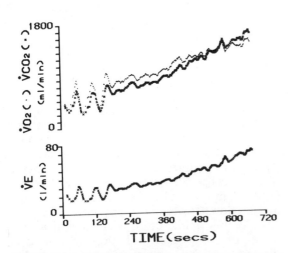

FIGURE 12–30. A 66 year old patient with mitral and aortic regurgitation. Depicted is the patient's response to treadmill exercise. His baseline anaerobic threshold and $\dot{V}O_2$ max were 13 and 18 ml/min/kg, respectively. Surgery was not recommended in view of his adequate cardiac reserve.

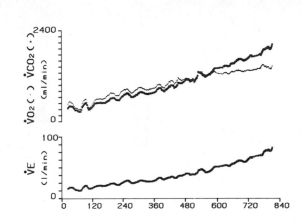

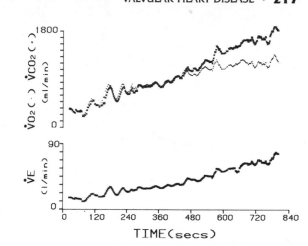

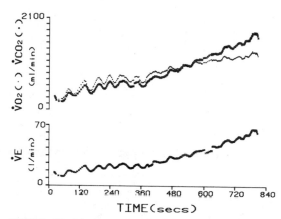

FIGURE 12–31. The reproducibility of the anaerobic threshold (13 ml/min/kg) and aerobic capacity (17 and 18 ml/min/kg) for the patient described in Figure 12–30 was demonstrated at 2 (upper panel) and 3 (lower panel) months, respectively.

FIGURE 12–32. One month after the last exercise test, shown in Figure 12–31, the patient demonstrated a deterioration in his functional status (anaerobic threshold and aerobic capacity of 12 and 15 ml/min/kg, respectively) that predated any decline in clinical status. See text for discussion.

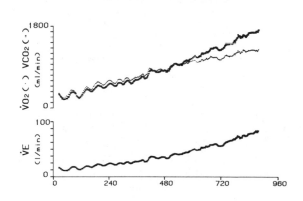

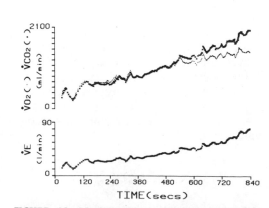

FIGURE 12–33. Following a brief hospitalization and increase in diuretics, the patient returned to his previous baseline functional status (threshold and capacity of 14 and 18 ml/min/kg, respectively) as shown in the upper panel. He remained stable over the next 6 months (lower panel).

ent; a ruptured cord of the anterior leaflet was noted, and the left ventricle was hyperdynamic. The right ventricle was markedly enlarged. The patient was unable to exercise because of an arthritic complaint.

Cardiac catheterization found marked pulmonary hypertension, with a pulmonary vascular resistance of 1040 dynes • sec • cm^{-5} and a mean pulmonary artery pressure of 72 mm Hg (Fig. 12–35); her mean wedge pressure was 35 mm Hg with v waves to 44 mm Hg. Coronary arteriography revealed normal coronary arteries. Pulmonary angiography was not performed because of her markedly elevated vascular resistance. A vasodilator trial with supplemental oxygen and then isoproterenol was given in the catheterization laboratory without a reduction in pulmonary artery pressure. However, we did not want to conclude that the patient had a "fixed" pulmonary vascular resistance, and based on the presumption that by lowering her wedge

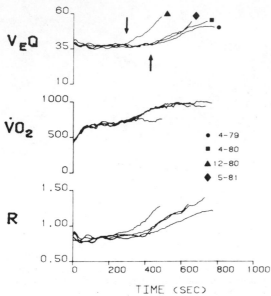

FIGURE 12–34. The response of a 62 year old woman, who had mitral valve replacement and aortic regurgitation. Her aerobic capacity was stable between April, 1979, and April, 1980. In December, 1980, she had a decline in $\dot{V}O_2$ max secondary to the appearance of a paravalvular leak. After surgical correction, her baseline functional status was restored by May, 1981. Shown are her responses in respiratory gas exchange ratio (*R*), O_2 uptake ($\dot{V}O_2$), and ventilatory equivalent to O_2 (V_EQ). (From Weber KT, Kinasewitz GT, Janicki JS, Fishman AP. Oxygen utilization and ventilation during exercise in patients with chronic cardiac failure. Circulation 65:1213–1223, 1982.)

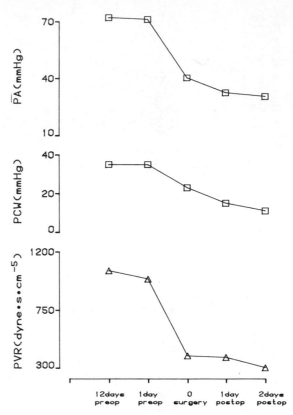

FIGURE 12–35. The mean pulmonary artery (*PA*) and wedge (*PCW*) pressures and pulmonary vascular resistance (*PVR*) in a 45 year old woman with rheumatic mitral valve disease and disproportionate pulmonary hypertension, on days 12 and 1 before surgery (preop), the day of surgery, and 2 days postoperative, following mitral valve replacement. Note the fall in PVR and PA pressure following valve replacement. PVR, however, does not fall within the normal range, which suggests that there must be a residual element of pulmonary vascular smooth muscle hypertrophy.

pressure a reduction in pulmonary vascular resistance would ensue, we advised her to have mitral valve replacement.

The results of hemodynamic monitoring prior to and following mitral valve replacement are shown in Figure 12–35. Wedge pressure fell to 23 mm Hg the day of operation and to 11 mm Hg on day 2. Even though her pulmonary vascular resistance fell by over 70 per cent within the first 2 postoperative days, it still remained elevated at 350 dynes • sec • cm^{-5}, suggesting that a residual element of smooth muscle hypertrophy was present that would require several weeks to resolve. The remainder of the patient's recovery was uneventful.

REFERENCES

1. Urschel CW, Covell JW, Sonnenblick EH, Ross J, Braunwald E. Myocardial mechanics in aortic and valvular regurgitation: The concept of instantaneous impedance as a determinant of the performance of the intact heart. J Clin Invest 47:867–873, 1968.

2. Heath D, Edwards JE. The pathology of hypertensive pulmonary vascular disease. A description of six grades of structural changes in the pulmonary arteries with special reference to congenital cardiac septal defects. Circulation 18:533–547, 1958.

3. Braunwald E. Valvular heart disease, *in* Braunwald E. (ed): Heart Disease. A Textbook of Cardiovascular Medicine. WB Saunders, Philadelphia, 1984, pp 1063–1135.

4. Bonow R, Rosing DR, Kent KM, Epstein SE. Timing of operation for chronic aortic regurgitation. Am J Cardiol 50:325–336, 1982.

5. Firth BG. The value of rest and exercise radionuclide ventriculography as compared to echocardiography and angiography in the detection of left ventricular dysfunction in patients with chronic aortic regurgitation. Herz 9:279–287, 1984.

6. Shen WF, Roubin GS, Choong CYP, Hutton BF, Harris PJ, Fletcher PJ, Kelly DT. Evaluation of relationship between myocardial contractile state and left ventricular function in patients with aortic regurgitation. Circulation 71:31–38, 1985.

7. Borer JS, Bacharach SL, Green MV, Kent KM, Henry WL, Rosing DR, Seides SF, Johnston GS, Epstein

SE. Exercise-induced left ventricular dysfunction in symptomatic and asymptomatic patients with aortic regurgitation: Assessment with radionuclide cineangiography. Am J Cardiol 42:351–357, 1978.

8. Carabello BA, Nolan SP, McGuire LB. Assessment of preoperative left ventricular function in patients with mitral regurgitation: Value of the end-systolic wall stress–end-systolic volume ratio. Circulation 64:1212–1217, 1981.

9. Braunwald E, Braunwald NS, Ross J, Morrow AG. Effects of mitral-valve replacement on the pulmonary vascular dynamics of patients with pulmonary hypertension. N Engl J Med 273:509–514, 1965.

10. Dalen JE, Matloff JM, Evan GL, Hoppin FG, Bhardwaj P, Harken DE, Dexter L. Early reduction of pulmonary vascular resistance after mitral-valve replacement. N Engl J Med 277:387–394, 1967.

11. Ward C, Hancock BW. Extreme pulmonary hypertension caused by mitral valve disease. Br Heart J 37:74–78, 1975.

12. Wood P. Pulmonary hypertension with special reference to the vasoconstrictive factor. Br Heart J 19:557–570, 1957.

13. Gorlin R, Gorlin SG. Hydraulic formula for calculation of the area of the stenotic mitral valve, other cardiac valves and central circulatory shunts. Am Heart J 41:1–29, 1951.

14. Hill AV, Long CNH, Lupton H. Muscular exercise, lactic acid, and the supply and utilization of oxygen. Proc R Soc Lond 96:438–475, 1924.

15. Meakins J, Long CNH. Oxygen consumption, oxygen debt and lactic acid in circulatory failure. J Clin Invest 4:273–293, 1927.

16. Harrison TR, Pilcher C. Studies in congestive heart failure. II. The respiratory exchange during and after exercise. J Clin Invest 8:291–315, 1930.

17. Cotes JE. The role of oxygen, carbon dioxide and lactic acid in the ventilatory response to exercise in patients with mitral stenosis. Clin Sci 14:317–328, 1955.

18. Gorlin R, Sawyer CG, Haynes FW, Goodale WT, Dexter L. Effects of exercise on circulatory dynamics in mitral stenosis. Am Heart J 41:192–203, 1951.

19. Donald KW, Bishop JM, Wade OL. A study of minute to minute changes of arterio-venous oxygen content difference, oxygen uptake and cardiac output and rate of achievement of a steady state during exercise in rheumatic heart disease. J Clin Invest 33:1146–1167, 1954.

20. Donald KW, Gloster J, Harris EA, Reeves J, Harris

P. The production of lactic acid during exercise in normal subjects and in patients with rheumatic heart disease. Am Heart J 62:494–510, 1961.

21. Chapman CB, Mitchell JH, Sproule BJ, Polter D, Williams B. The maximal oxygen intake test in patients with predominant mitral stenosis. Circulation 22:4–13, 1960.

22. Blackmon JR, Rowell LB, Kennedy JW, Twiss RD, Conn RD. Physiological significance of maximal oxygen intake in "pure" mitral stenosis. Circulation 36:497–510, 1967.

23. Ross J, Gault JH, Mason DT, Linhart JW, Braunwald E. Left ventricular performance during muscular exercise in patients with and without cardiac dysfunction. Circulation 34:597–608, 1966.

24. Gash A, Carabello BA, Cepin D, Spann JF. Left ventricular ejection performance and systolic muscle function in patients with mitral stenosis. Circulation 67:148–154, 1983.

25. Zener JC, Hancock EW, Shumway NE, Harrison DC. Regression of extreme pulmonary hypertension after mitral valve surgery. Am J Cardiol 30:820–826, 1972.

26. Peabody FW, Wentworth JA, Barber BI. Clinical studies on respiration. V. The basal metabolism and the minute-volume of the respiration of patients with cardiac disease. Arch Intern Med 20:468–478, 1917.

27. Christie RV, Meakins JC. The intrapleural pressure in congestive heart failure and its clinical significance. J Clin Invest 13:323–331, 1934.

28. Marshall R, McElroy MB, Christie RV. The work of breathing in mitral stenosis. Clin Sci 13:137–146, 1954.

29. Marshall R, Stone RW, Christie RV. The relationship of dyspnea to respiratory effort in normal subjects, mitral stenosis and emphysema. Clin Sci 14:626–631, 1955.

30. Saxton GA, Rabinowitz M, Dexter L, Haynes F. The relationship of pulmonary compliance to pulmonary vascular pressures in patients with heart disease. J Clin Invest 35:611–618, 1956.

31. Turino GM, Fishman AP. The congested lung. J Chron Dis 9:510–524, 1959.

32. Wood TE, McLeon P, Anthonisen NR, Macklem PT. Mechanics of breathing in mitral stenosis. Am Rev Respir Dis 104:52–60, 1971.

33. Krause F, Rudolph W. Symptoms, exercise capacity and exercise hemodynamics: Interrelationships and their role in quantification of the valvular lesion. Herz 9:187–199, 1984.

KARL T. WEBER
JOSEPH S. JANICKI

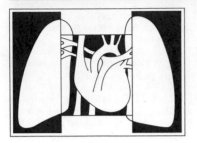

Pulmonary Hypertension

Pulmonary hypertension can be defined as an abnormal elevation in mean and pulsatile pulmonary artery pressures that exceeds the expected upper range of normal (18 and 30/12 mm Hg, respectively) at rest. Left heart failure with its attendant elevation of pulmonary venous pressure remains the most common cause of pulmonary hypertension and right heart failure. Several causes of pulmonary venous hypertension have been considered in Chapters 11 and 12, in which we reviewed ischemic, myopathic, and valvular heart disease. In this chapter we focus on pulmonary arterial hypertension, which accompanies intrinsic pulmonary vascular disease secondary to such disorders as collagen-vascular disease, recurrent thromboembolic disease, and primary pulmonary hypertension. Pulmonary arteriolar vasoconstriction that accompanies the hypoxemia of intrinsic lung disease is also considered. In each of these circumstances small and medium-sized pulmonary arteries are involved. Vascular smooth muscle may be hypertrophied whereas the intima may fibrose. Each of these structural changes leads to luminal narrowing and eventual occlusion of these vessels. As a result, pulmonary vascular resistance is elevated. This serves to create a pressure overload on the right ventricle, and when of sufficient severity, right heart failure ensues. This condition is termed *cor pulmonale*. Because of the impediment to left ventricular filling, systemic blood flow will also be compromised and aerobic capacity will decline. Pulmonary hypertension therefore represents another example of chronic *circulatory* failure.

We begin this chapter by briefly examining the pathophysiology of cor pulmonale. Next, the hemodynamic evaluation of pulmonary vascular disease is reviewed. We will indicate how the pressure-flow relation of the pulmonary circulation can be obtained during exercise to assess the severity of pulmonary hypertension. Finally, we will consider the ventilatory response to exercise that these patients demonstrate.

PATHOPHYSIOLOGY OF COR PULMONALE

Cor pulmonale is defined as right ventricular hypertrophy, dilatation, and failure due to pulmonary hypertension secondary to the involvement of pulmonary arteries. Many disease states of diverse etiology may cause cor pulmonale. The fundamental point to recognize here is that the pulmonary circulation is involved directly and the right heart failure is not secondary to left heart or mitral valve disease. In most cases, the pulmonary arteries are the primary target of the disease process and the site of the elevated pulmonary vascular resistance.

The impedance characteristics of the normal pulmonary circulation are such that the right ventricle rarely has to generate more than 30 mm Hg systolic pressure in order to provide 5 liters/minute of pulmonary blood flow. As pulmonary blood flow increases twofold with low-level exercise, the systolic pressure of the right heart rises to only 35 or 40 mm Hg. It is not until the cardiac output reaches 20 liters/min with heavy exercise that right ventricular systolic pressure may reach 50 mm Hg. Nevertheless, in contrast to the systemic circulation, the impedance of the normal pulmonary circulation is modest, even to 20 liters/min of blood flow. This is so because the pulmonary circulation being encased within the compressible air-filled lungs is very distensible and because additional segments of its circulation can be recruited to accommodate the increase in blood flow. This point can be further underscored by the fact that it is possible to occlude the right pulmonary artery and have all pulmonary blood flow pass through the left lung without significantly raising right ventricular or pulmonary artery pressure.[1] Thus, the right ventricle remains much thinner with a mass of only one-third that of the left ventricle.

Pulmonary vascular disease must be extensive, be widespread, and involve both lungs, in order for significant pulmonary hypertension to be present. As we will indicate later in the chapter, the earliest manifestations of pulmonary vascular disease and elevated pulmonary vascular resistance will be noted during incremental isotonic exercise when pulmonary blood flow is increased. Under these circumstances, an abnormal elevation in right ventricular and pulmonary artery systolic pressures will be apparent.

Right Ventricular Pressure Overload

The determinants of right ventricular pump performance are similar to those of the left ventricle.[2] Filling volume, ejection pressure, myocardial contractile state, and heart rate determine the stroke volume that the right ventricle can produce.[3] The greater the systolic pressure that the right ventricle must generate from any given filling volume, the less its stroke volume. Thus, acute increments in right ventricular systolic pressure, such as that seen with an acute pulmonary embolus, will depress right heart pump function. This represents an example of *acute cor pulmonale*. It would be unusual for the normal, thin-walled right ventricle to sustain pulmonary blood flow when its systolic pressure must exceed 60 mm Hg.

Under circumstances when right ventricular systolic pressure rises gradually (e.g., in chronic obliterative pulmonary vascular disease), the right ventricle will hypertrophy and dilate. It will then be able to generate much higher systolic pressures and sustain its stroke volume. In fact, once hypertrophied and enlarged, the right ventricle is capable of generating systemic and even suprasystemic levels of systolic pressure to maintain pulmonary blood flow. These marked elevations in right ventricular pressure work will be particularly evident during incremental isotonic exercise.

Eventually, however, the chronically pressure-overloaded right ventricle will fail. This is termed *chronic cor pulmonale*. Under these circumstances it would be preferable to increase right ventricular emptying by the vasodilation of the pulmonary circulation rather than with positive inotropic agents (e.g., digitalis), which raise myocardial contractility thereby raising right ventricular stroke volume. This may only compound the pressure overload on the right ventricle by driving it to increase pulmonary blood flow against an abnormally elevated pulmonary vascular resistance.

Pulmonary hypertension and cor pulmonale are known to be reversible in certain patients with chronic bronchitis or emphysema or both. In these patients, the presence of hypoxia (arterial oxygen saturation <90 per cent) will induce pulmonary vasoconstriction and raise mean pulmonary artery pressure (Fig. 13–1).[4] The correction of the gas exchange abnormality will produce vasodilation and a fall in pulmonary artery pressure.

THE EVALUATION OF PULMONARY VASCULAR DISEASE

In comparison to the other cardiocirculatory disorders that are considered in this section of the text, the incidence of pulmonary vascular disease appears to be relatively low. The true prevalence and incidence of pulmonary vascular disease, however, are difficult to estimate. This is in large part the result of having no effective noninvasive techniques to measure pulmonary artery pressure in large patient populations. Clinicians, therefore, rarely see or are aware of the early or milder expressions of pulmonary vascular disease.

We have had the opportunity to evaluate patients with pulmonary vascular disease but without hypoxemia at rest or during exercise, as well as patients who have had pulmonary hypertension secondary to hypoxic (arterial oxygen saturation of <90 per cent) vasoconstriction that accompanied their chronic lung or pulmonary vascular disease.

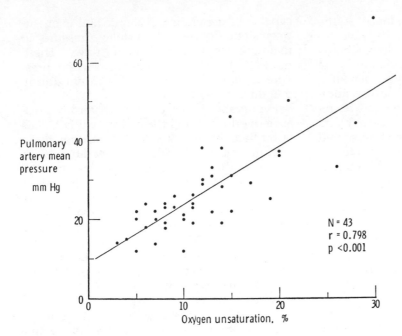

FIGURE 13–1. The relationship between mean pulmonary artery pressure and arterial oxyhemoglobin unsaturation (100 minus the per cent saturation) is shown for patients with chronic lung disease. (From Enson Y, Giuntini C, Lewis ML, Morris TQ, Ferrer MI, Harvey RM. The influence of hydrogen ion concentration and hypoxia on the pulmonary circulation. J Clin Invest 43:1146–1161, 1964.)

Clinical Characteristics of Pulmonary Hypertension

The clinical features of our patients with *nonhypoxic pulmonary vascular disease* and pulmonary hypertension were quite similar to those described in several other large series.[5-8] Twenty to 35 year old women were seen most frequently—three to four times more frequently than men. Patients most commonly presented with the symptom of exertional breathlessness; chest pain, exertional fatigue and syncope were also noted, but less frequently. These symptoms, which were first noted during physical activity, had been present for only a few years in each patient. Evidence of pulmonary hypertension and right ventricular pressure overload were characteristic at the time of clinical presentation. Except for a few patients with collagen-vascular disease or recurrent emboli, the etiology of the pulmonary hypertension was unclear. Even in those patients having a disease such as cirrhosis, or a relevant drug history (e.g., oral contraceptives or amphetamines) suspected to be associated with pulmonary vascular disease, the relationship between the two conditions remained uncertain. Thus, in our patients with nonhypoxic pulmonary vascular disease, primary pulmonary hypertension was the rule.

Clinical examination, including the chest roentgenogram and electrocardiogram, was compatible with right ventricular pressure overload. For example, the electrocardiogram showed right axis deviation and right ventricular hypertrophy. One quarter of the patients had tricuspid valvular incompetence; only one patient, however, had enlargement of the liver with ascites and peripheral edema. Standard chest radiographs revealed no abnormalities of the lungs in the patients with nonhypoxic pulmonary vascular disease. However, they did show a prominence of the main pulmonary artery and its major trunks in conjunction with obliteration of peripheral pulmonary vessels.

These patients typically do not have evidence of obstructive airway disease; inspiratory and expiratory flow rates on pulmonary function testing were normal. This is in contradistinction to patients with hypoxic pulmonary vasoconstriction, which we will discuss shortly. One abnormality shared by all patients with nonhypoxic pulmonary vascular disease and pulmonary hypertension was a reduction in the diffusing capacity for carbon monoxide (D_{LCO}).

Patients with *hypoxic pulmonary vasoconstriction* secondary to intrinsic disease of the pulmonary parenchyma or airways also were symptomatic, particularly noting breathlessness with exertion that curtailed their effort tolerance and quality of life. Clinical and laboratory evaluation were compatible with right heart enlargement or hypertrophy or both. Unlike the nonhypoxic group, there was no predilection for young women, and the age distribution was quite broad.

Table 13–1. Resting and Peak Exercise Hemodynamics for Patients with Nonhypoxic Pulmonary Vascular Disease and Pulmonary Hypertension

		Resting	Exercise
PA	(mm Hg)	29 ± 9	47 ± 20
RVSP	(mm Hg)	52 ± 30	86 ± 37
RVDP	(mm Hg)	7 ± 4	16 ± 10
PCW	(mm Hg)	10 ± 3	22 ± 14
PVR	(dynes·sec·cm^{-5})	412 ± 319	302 ± 331
CO	(l/min/m^2)	2.8 ± 1.6	5.3 ± 2.2
AP	(mm Hg)	106 ± 6	130 ± 8
Art O$_2$ sat (%)		97 ± 2	96 ± 2

PA, mean pulmonary artery pressure; RVSP and RVDP, right ventricular systolic and diastolic pressures, respectively; PCW, wedge pressure; PVR, pulmonary vascular resistance; CO, cardiac output; AP, mean arterial pressure.

Resting Hemodynamics

All patients with pulmonary hypertension underwent elective right heart catheterization with a triple-lumen flotation catheter; many were then exercised. The average resting and peak exercise hemodynamic responses for patients with *nonhypoxic pulmonary vascular disease* are given in Table 13–1. At rest, the mean pulmonary arterial pressure was elevated exceeding 18 mm Hg (the upper range of normal). The average right ventricular systolic pressure at rest was in excess of 50 mm Hg, and in one quarter of the patients it approximated or exceeded left ventricular (and systemic arterial) systolic pressure. The resting wedge pressure was normal in these patients. Figure 13–2 depicts

the resting, supine hemodynamic data from one of these patients. Calculated pulmonary vascular resistance exceeded 170 dynes · sec · cm^{-5} and in over 30 per cent of the patients resistance was extremely high, (i.e., >1000 dynes · sec · cm^{-5}), approximating normal levels of systemic vascular resistance.

Table 13–2 summarizes the resting and peak exercise hemodynamic responses for patients with *hypoxic pulmonary vasoconstriction*. As in the patients with nonhypoxic pulmonary vascular disease, pulmonary hypertension was present at rest in all patients with hypoxic pulmonary vasoconstriction. Figure 13–3 depicts the resting, supine hemodynamic data from one of these patients.

Exercise Hemodynamics

During upright treadmill exercise (see Table 13–1), pulmonary arterial systolic pressure (or right ventricular systolic pressure) rose to levels in excess of 80 mm Hg (range 43 to 138 mm Hg) in patients with *nonhypoxic pulmonary vascular disease*. The ratio of pulmonary arterial systolic pressure to systolic arterial pressure was <1.0 at rest and frequently >1.0 at peak exercise. Peak cardiac output during exercise rose approximately twofold in those patients in whom resting pulmonary vascular resistance was <1000 dynes · sec · cm^{-5}. For those in whom resistance was extremely high (>1000 dynes · sec · cm^{-5}), cardiac output failed to increase during exercise.

The response in cardiac output expressed as a function of the normalized aerobic capacity is shown in Figure 13–4 for patients

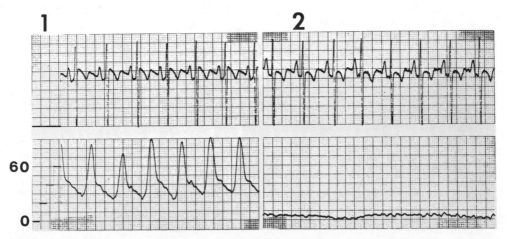

FIGURE 13–2. The resting, supine pulmonary artery pressure (tracing 1) and wedge pressure (tracing 2) and electrocardiogram of a 34 year old woman with nonhypoxic pulmonary vascular disease and pulmonary hypertension. End-expiratory pulmonary artery pressure was 90/30 mm Hg; wedge pressure was 6 mm Hg.

Table 13–2. *Resting and Peak Exercise Hemodynamics for Patients with Hypoxic Pulmonary Vasoconstriction*

		Resting	Exercise
PA	(mm Hg)	36 ± 16	61 ± 16
RVSP	(mm Hg)	55 ± 32	104 ± 37
RVDP	(mm Hg)	4 ± 2	14 ± 6
PCW	(mm Hg)	12 ± 5	24 ± 12
PVR	(dynes·sec·cm^{-5})	656 ± 424	545 ± 319
CO	(l/min/m²)	2.1 ± 0.7	4.2 ± 1.6
AP	(mm Hg)	102 ± 18	120 ± 25
Art O$_2$ sat (%)		87 ± 2	76 ± 12

PA, mean pulmonary artery pressure; RVSP and RVDP, right ventricular systolic and diastolic pressures, respectively; PCW, wedge pressure; PVR, pulmonary vascular resistance; CO, cardiac output; AP, mean arterial pressure.

with nonhypoxic pulmonary vascular disease. It can be seen that, in a manner similar to chronic cardiac failure or valvular incompetence, the peak cardiac output response to exercise determined $\dot{V}O_2$ max. Irrespective of their impairment in aerobic capacity the heart rate response to treadmill exercise in these patients fell within the expected range for normal subjects and patients with chronic cardiac or circulatory failure (Fig. 13–5, *A*). The stroke volume response to treadmill exercise was impaired in proportion to the functional capacity of these patients in a manner similar to that observed for patients with ischemic or myopathic heart disease and mitral or aortic valvular incompetence (Fig. 13–5, *B*).

The severity of the nonhypoxic pulmonary hypertension and circulatory failure can be predicted from the aerobic capacity, given that the impairment in the cardiac output response to exercise is a function of the severity of the pulmonary vascular disease. Patients having a markedly elevated resting pulmonary vascular resistance (>1000 dynes · sec · cm^{-5}) will fall into functional exercise class D (Fig. 13–6).

By definition, no patient in our group with nonhypoxic pulmonary hypertension demonstrated a fall in arterial oxygen saturation during exercise. The response in systemic oxygen extraction to progressive treadmill exercise is presented in Figure 13–7. Each patient representing a different functional class follows a single relation reaching ever increasing levels of oxygen extraction, as aerobic capacity is approached. Thus, these patients with pulmonary vascular disease and no evidence of arterial oxygen desaturation during exercise demonstrate that their predominant impairment to physical activity is primarily a function of their compromised cardiac output response. This defect is a function of the inability of the right ventricle to generate sufficient pulmonary blood flow to sustain left ventricular filling and systemic blood flow.

Because of the elevation in pulmonary vascular resistance the right heart must generate systemic or suprasystemic levels of systolic pressure. Figure 13–8 depicts the rise in right ventricular systolic and right atrial pressures that the four functional classes with nonhypoxic pulmonary hypertension develop during incremental exercise. In order to unload the right heart and prevent its progression to chronic cor pulmonale, effective vasodilation of the diseased pulmonary circulation is warranted. This strategy, however, must be considered with due regard for the systemic vascular resistance that has become elevated in response to the limited systemic blood flow (Fig. 13–9) and is critical to maintaining

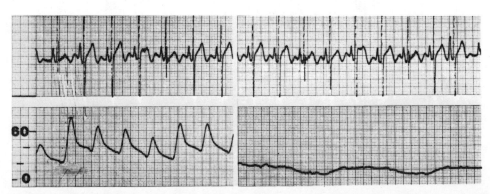

FIGURE 13–3. Supine hemodynamic data and the electrocardiogram for a 46 year old woman with chronic airway disease. Large variations in pleural pressure are apparent during the respiratory cycle and are reflected in the pulmonary artery (left) and wedge (right) pressure tracings. End-expiratory pressures were 70/32 and 12 mm Hg, respectively.

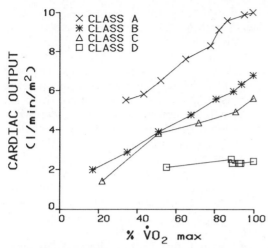

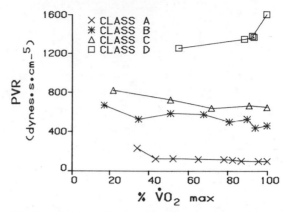

FIGURE 13–4. The response in cardiac output to upright incremental treadmill exercise in patients with pulmonary hypertension secondary to nonhypoxic pulmonary vascular disease. As in other forms of circulatory failure, the maximal O_2 uptake ($\dot{V}O_2$max) determination reflects the maximal cardiac output response to exercise.

FIGURE 13–6. Resting pulmonary vascular resistance (PVR) and its response to incremental treadmill exercise in patients with nonhypoxic pulmonary vascular disease and pulmonary hypertension. Patients are divided according to their aerobic capacity.

systemic arterial pressure. Vasodilators carry the potential for systemic vasodilation and thereby may lead to systemic hypotension and circulatory collapse.

Patients with nonhypoxic pulmonary vascular disease stopped exercising because of breathlessness or fatigue or both; none experienced retrosternal chest pain, lightheadedness, or syncope, or developed arrhythmias. In most, it was possible to determine their $\dot{V}O_2$ max, and in all the anaerobic threshold could be attained (vide infra).

In patients with *hypoxic pulmonary vasoconstriction*, upright isotonic exercise also results in an increase in mean pulmonary artery and right ventricular systolic and diastolic pressures (Table 13–2). In many of these patients pulmonary vascular resistance actually rose during exercise because of their marked hypoxemia (arterial oxygen saturation of 70 to 80 per cent).

During exercise testing with supplemental oxygen (because of the vasodilatory effects

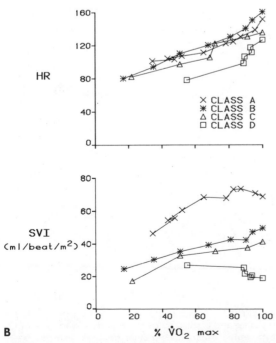

B

FIGURE 13–5. The response in heart rate (HR) and stroke volume index (SVI) to incremental treadmill exercise is shown for patients with pulmonary hypertension secondary to nonhypoxic pulmonary vascular disease.

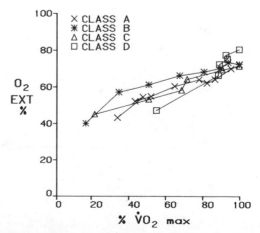

FIGURE 13–7. The response in systemic O_2 extraction to incremental treadmill exercise for patients shown in Figures 13–4, 13–5, and 13–6.

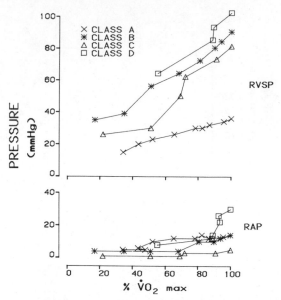

FIGURE 13–8. Systolic (*RVSP*) and diastolic (*RAP*) pressures of the right ventricle, which exist at rest and during incremental treadmill exercise in patients with pulmonary hypertension secondary to nonhypoxic pulmonary vascular disease.

with either nonhypoxic pulmonary vascular disease or hypoxic pulmonary vasoconstriction, physical activities at home should be curtailed to modest levels of muscular work. Collectively, these patients would not appear to benefit from regular exercise. Instead, the progressive pressure overloading of the right ventricle that accompanies exercise should be forestalled in the hope that the relentless downhill course of chronic cor pulmonale may be attenuated. An effort should also be made to determine whether or not an effective program of pharmacologic pulmonary vasodilation can be established without systemic hypotension or increased venous admixture.

We can use our observations in the individual patients with nonhypoxic pulmonary vascular disease of varying severity to reconstruct the progression of the hemodynamic overload that is placed on the right heart as the severity of pulmonary vascular disease becomes more advanced. Early in the course of the disease, structural changes within the intima and/or media of the small and medium-sized pulmonary arteries impede only high levels of pulmonary blood flow associated with significant levels of physical activity. As the severity of these vascular abnormalities progresses, or as they become

of oxygen), pulmonary vascular resistance does not rise but remains constant or falls. As a result, mean pulmonary artery and right ventricular systolic and diastolic pressures rise less dramatically with exercise; resting pulmonary artery pressure will also be reduced (Fig. 13–10). Thus, the acute therapeutic benefits of ambulatory oxygen are apparent. Moreover, based on the dramatic pressure overload that confronts the right ventricle during exercise in patients

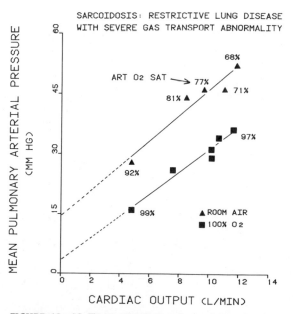

FIGURE 13–10. The response in mean pulmonary artery pressure and cardiac output for a patient who developed hypoxemia during incremental treadmill exercise while breathing room air. The attenuation in pressure for comparable levels of pulmonary blood flow is shown for a repeat exercise test in which the patient was receiving supplemental oxygen.

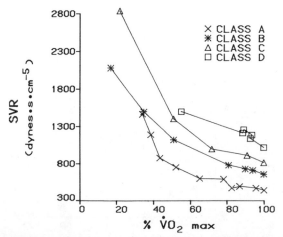

FIGURE 13–9. Systemic vascular resistance (*SVR*) and its response from rest and throughout incremental treadmill exercise in patients with nonhypoxic pulmonary vascular disease.

widespread and fixed anatomic lesions, or both, a larger vascular resistance to blood flow is apparent with only modest levels of muscular work. Thus, in the majority of patients with pulmonary vascular disease symptoms first appear with exertion. Finally, when the disease is far advanced, vascular resistance is elevated at rest for normal or even subnormal levels of pulmonary blood flow. The advanced stage of pulmonary hypertension secondary to nonhypoxic vascular disease, therefore, would generally appear to require months to years to develop. It is here, in the more advanced stages of the disease, that patients most often present with clinical evidence of right ventricular hypertrophy and enlargement.

The explanation for the exertional fatigue that these patients experience with low or moderate levels of physical work would appear related to the failure of cardiac output to rise appropriately during exercise and the resultant decline in aerobic capacity. Once again, this represents an example of chronic *circulatory* failure. As the cardiac output response to exercise becomes more compromised, these patients develop an increasing dependence on systemic vascular resistance to maintain arterial blood pressure during exercise. In the advanced cases, cardiac output fails to rise during exercise or may even fall if tricuspid regurgitation appears to further limit the cardiac output response to exercise. Such a restriction in systemic blood flow in the face of vasodilation of working skeletal muscle is the expected setting for a fixed or falling arterial blood pressure and sets the stage for the appearance of near-syncope or syncope during or immediately following physical activity. Moreover, these findings of a limited cardiac output response to exercise in more advanced stages of the disease process indicate the important role that systemic vascular resistance plays in maintaining arterial blood pressure in these patients.

The mechanism responsible for the exertional breathlessness that patients with pulmonary vascular disease experience, despite normal pulmonary venous pressure, is less clear. Later in this chapter, the ventilatory response of these patients will be reviewed and will shed more light on this issue.

Exertional chest pain or angina most likely results from several factors favoring ischemia of the hypertrophied right ventricular myocardium. These are as follows: (1) right ventricular systolic pressure exceeds mean aortic systolic pressure, thereby throttling right coronary artery flow and confining right ventricular perfusion to diastole, as is normally the case for left coronary artery blood flow and left ventricular perfusion; and (2) the elevation in right ventricular diastolic pressure during exercise may restrict right ventricular subendocardial blood flow throughout the cardiac cycle.

Pressure-Flow Relation

The hemodynamic behavior of the pulmonary circulation and its vascular resistance can be characterized by the relationship between the pressure gradient driving blood flow across the lung and the corresponding pulmonary blood flow. In the absence of external forces, such as those related to tissue pressure, the pressure gradient across the pulmonary vasculature is simply the difference between the upstream (or arterial) and the downstream (or venous) pressures. However, because the pulmonary vasculature is contained within the parenchyma of the lung, as depicted in Figure 13–11, it is subjected to an extravascular (e.g., alveolar) pressure, which results in blood vessel closure when the extravascular pressure exceeds the intravascular pressure; alveolar pressure would therefore represent the *critical closing pressure*, and not venous pressure. Under these circumstances, the true gradient in pressure exists between the pulmonary artery pressure and tissue pressure.

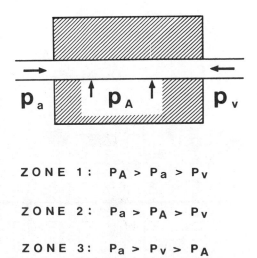

ZONE 1: $P_A > P_a > P_v$

ZONE 2: $P_a > P_A > P_v$

ZONE 3: $P_a > P_v > P_A$

FIGURE 13–11. Pulmonary arteries and their intravascular pressure (P_a) are subjected to a tissue (alveolar) pressure (P_A) that may exceed pulmonary venous pressure (P_v). The relationship among these pressures determines the various zones of the lung.

It is not certain whether tissue pressure normally exceeds the venous pressure in the human lung; therefore, the calculation of the true pressure gradient of the pulmonary circulation has been uncertain. In the isolated lung preparation,[9] in which a curvilinear relationship exists between arterial pressure and blood flow, the nonlinear portion of the relation is most evident at either low levels of blood flow or high lung volumes. In intact ventilated animals, where it is possible to control and keep constant both pulmonary venous and alveolar pressures, the pressure gradient to flow relation is linear over a wide physiologic range of blood flow.[10]

The nature of the pressure-flow relation in the pulmonary circulation of humans has been examined using various techniques that alter pulmonary blood flow, such as exercise,[11] balloon-occlusion of a segment of the pulmonary circulation,[12] or crystalloid infusion.[13] However, few observations on this relation for the abnormal pulmonary circulation are available in which cardiopulmonary disease has created either pulmonary arterial or venous hypertension.

We chose to estimate the average closing pressure and to characterize the relationship between pressure gradient and blood flow in the pulmonary circulation of patients with and without pulmonary arterial or venous hypertension of varying severity.[14] In order to obtain multiple pressure-flow points, invasive CPX testing was performed using a treadmill and our incremental work protocol.

Figure 13–12 depicts the exercise hemodynamic response for a 32 year old woman with nonhypoxic pulmonary vascular disease and pulmonary hypertension. Fifty-one patients were examined. Forty-two had chronic, stable pulmonary venous hypertension of varying severity secondary to either idiopathic cardiomyopathy, valvular heart disease, or ischemic heart disease. Nine other patients had biopsy-proven intrinsic pulmonary vascular disease and pulmonary arterial hypertension.

The average closing pressure for the pulmonary circulation was estimated in the following manner: cardiac output and mean pulmonary arterial pressure, at rest and for each level of exercise, were plotted and the best fit line determined by linear regression. The extrapolated, zero-flow pressure intercept of this relation, which has been shown to approximate the average closing pressure for the pulmonary circulation,[9] was then used as an estimate of closing pressure. Finally, this intercept pressure was compared with the resting pulmonary wedge pressure to determine if the wedge pressure was higher or lower than the closure pressure. A higher wedge pressure would imply that it should be used as the downstream pressure when calculating the pressure gradient.

Patients with pulmonary venous hypertension secondary to heart disease were subdivided according to whether or not their resting mean pulmonary arterial pressure was less than (mild), or greater than (moderate

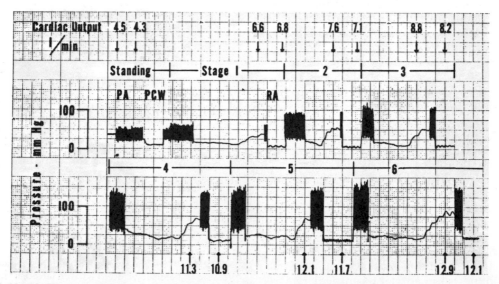

FIGURE 13–12. The hemodynamic response from standing rest to incremental treadmill exercise for a 32 year old woman with nonhypoxic pulmonary hypertension. Pulsatile pulmonary artery (*PA*), wedge (*PCW*), and right atrial (*RA*) pressures were obtained during each stage of exercise, as was cardiac output.

to severe) the upper-normal value of 19 mm Hg. Patients with nonhypoxic pulmonary vascular disease and pulmonary arterial hypertension were considered separately. Regardless of etiology, all patients were able to exercise beyond their anaerobic threshold and to attain their maximal oxygen uptake.

The upright resting hemodynamics for these patients with venous or arterial pulmonary hypertension are summarized in Table 13–3. The average group responses to exercise in terms of pulmonary arterial systolic, diastolic and mean pressures, and pulmonary capillary wedge pressure, and cardiac index are shown in Figure 13–13. All parameters increased as the level of work was raised.

The relationship between mean pulmonary arterial pressure and cardiac output during exercise was linear in the majority of patients. The average mean pressure to flow relationship for each group is given in Figure 13–14, along with the slope (±95 per cent confidence limit) and correlation coefficient for each relationship; each slope differed significantly (p <0.01) from the others. The pressure-flow relationship of the pulmonary circulation tended to be shifted upward and became steeper as the level of resting pulmonary artery pressure increased.

The zero-flow pressure intercept of the mean pressure-flow relation was used to ap-

Table 13–3. *Resting and Peak Exercise Hemodynamics for Patients with Pulmonary Venous or Arterial Hypertension*

		Rest	Exercise
		Mild Pulmonary Venous Hypertension	
PAS	(mm Hg)	21 ± 4	51 ± 12
PAD	(mm Hg)	10 ± 3	27 ± 9
PA	(mm Hg)	14 ± 4	37 ± 11
PCW	(mm Hg)	8 ± 4	21 ± 12
CO	(l/min/m²)	2.2 ± 0.6	6.8 ± 1.4
PVR*	(dynes·sec·cm⁻⁵)	215 ± 65	140 ± 40
		Moderate to Severe Pulmonary Venous Hypertension	
PAS	(mm Hg)	42 ± 9	68 ± 14
PAD	(mm Hg)	24 ± 8	40 ± 11
PA	(mm Hg)	32 ± 8	52 ± 13
PCW	(mm Hg)	21 ± 3	37 ± 11
CO	(l/min/m²)	1.9 ± 0.6	3.6 ± 1.4
PVR*	(dynes·sec·cm⁻⁵)	305 ± 150	215 ± 105
		Pulmonary Arterial Hypertension	
PAS	(mm Hg)	63 ± 25	124 ± 27
PAD	(mm Hg)	35 ± 12	58 ± 9
PA	(mm Hg)	43 ± 16	81 ± 16
PCW	(mm Hg)	8 ± 5	18 ± 7
CO	(l/min/m²)	1.9 ± 0.3	5.0 ± 1.5
PVR*	(dynes·sec·cm⁻⁵)	695 ± 270	575 ± 230

*Excluding patients who did not have a fall in PVR during exercise.

PAS, pulmonary arterial systolic pressure; PAD, pulmonary arterial diastolic pressure; PA, mean pulmonary artery pressure; PCW, wedge pressure; CO, cardiac output; PVR, pulmonary vascular resistance.

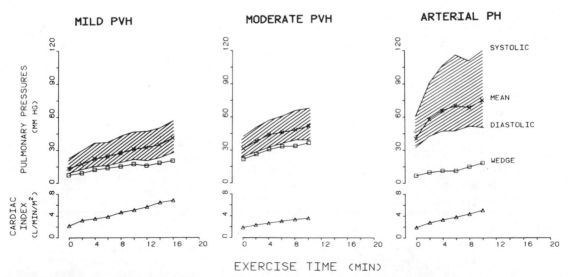

FIGURE 13–13. The response in pulmonary arterial systolic, mean, and diastolic pressures; pulmonary capillary wedge pressure; and cardiac output to incremental treadmill exercise for patients with mild and moderate pulmonary venous hypertension (*PVH*) and nonhypoxic pulmonary artery hypertension (*PH*). (From Janicki JS, Weber KT, Likoff MJ, Fishman AP. The pressure-flow response of the pulmonary circulation in heart failure and pulmonary vascular disease. Circulation 72:1270–1278, 1985.)

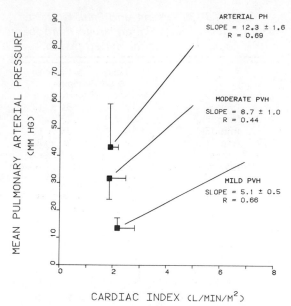

FIGURE 13–14. The relation between mean pulmonary artery pressure and cardiac output during incremental treadmill exercise for the three patient groups described in Figure 13–13. Solid squares and bars represent resting data and standard deviations. (From Janicki JS, Weber KT, Likoff MJ, Fishman AP. The pressure-flow response of the pulmonary vascular disease. Circulation 72:1270–1278, 1985.)

proximate the average closing pressure for the pulmonary circulation. In order to investigate whether average closing pressure exceeded the resting pulmonary capillary wedge pressure in these patients, the resting wedge pressure was compared with the extrapolated y-intercept pressure for each patient. The results are shown in Figure 13–15. Eighty-five per cent of the points lie on, or to the left of, the line of identity, indicating that resting wedge pressure was equal to or exceeded the average closure pressure. Accordingly, wedge pressure can be used as the downstream pressure in calculating the

pressure drop and vascular resistance of the pulmonary circulation.

Pressure Gradient–Flow Relation

In Figure 13–16, the average relationship between the gradient in pulmonary artery pressure and cardiac output is shown both at rest and at peak of exercise for patients with *nonhypoxic pulmonary hypertension*. Pulmonary vascular resistance decreased significantly during exercise in the majority of patients.

For all patients, the average decrease in vascular resistance was approximately 20 per cent. Patients who had a resting pulmonary vascular resistance >850 dynes $\cdot$ sec $\cdot$ cm^{-5} did not have a fall in resistance during exercise; all were functional class D. If these patients in whom pulmonary vascular resistance failed to decline during exercise are excluded from the analysis, then the average resting and peak exercise resistances are those shown in Table 13–3.

If one assumes pulmonary vascular resistance to be proportional to 1/(effective pulmonary vascular cross-sectional area)^2, then the exercise-induced reductions in resistance were associated with increases in effective area of 11, 9, and 5 per cent for both groups with venous pulmonary hypertension and for the group with arterial pulmonary hypertension, respectively. Although these responses do not indicate whether the increase in pulmonary vascular area was the result of a passive or an active process or both, the magnitude of increase and the fact that both pulmonary arterial and venous pressures increased during exercise suggest that the increase in pulmonary vascular area is predominantly a passive process secondary to recruitment and distension. The findings of Hopkins and co-workers[15] in the conscious

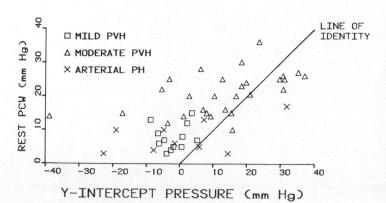

FIGURE 13–15. The mean pulmonary artery pressure at zero cardiac output (e.g., the y-intercept in Fig. 13–14), representing the critical closing pressure, and resting wedge pressure (PCW). Note that in the great majority of cases, wedge pressure was higher than the closing pressure, and therefore PCW represents the appropriate downstream pressure in the calculation of the pressure gradient in the derivation of pulmonary vascular resistance. (From Janicki JS, Weber KT, Likoff MJ, Fishman AP. The pressure-flow response of the pulmonary circulation in heart failure and pulmonary vascular disease. Circulation 72:1270–1278, 1985.)

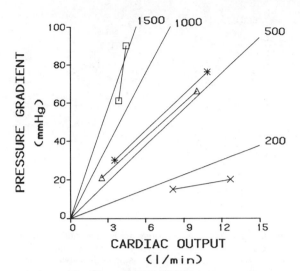

FIGURE 13–16. The relationship between the gradient in pressure (pulmonary artery minus wedge pressure) across the pulmonary circulation and cardiac output to incremental exercise in patients with nonhypoxic pulmonary vascular disease.

dog support this view. These investigators reported that pulmonary vascular resistance decreased after acute increments in left atrial pressure. An analysis of the impedance spectra revealed that capillary recruitment had occurred as a result of acute pulmonary venous hypertension. This conclusion is further supported by our findings in a patient with primary pulmonary hypertension (Fig. 13–17). Before administering isoproterenol intravenously, exercise evoked a 29 per cent decrease in pulmonary vascular resistance from a resting value of 620 dynes • sec • cm^{-5};

the administration of isoproterenol (1 µg/min for 3 min) at rest evoked a 58 per cent decrease in vascular resistance; with exercise, a further decrease in resistance of 23 per cent was noted. It would have been surprising for this additional decrease in resistance to occur following active pharmacologic vasodilation, if it were solely the result of an active process; thus, the fact that resistance declined with exercise before and after isoproterenol administration by approximately the same amount is consistent with the concept that this is a passive process.

VENTILATORY RESPONSE TO EXERCISE

Regardless of the nature or severity of the pulmonary vascular disease, most of our patients with nonhypoxic pulmonary hypertension were able to attain their $\dot{V}O_2$ max, and all were able to attain their anaerobic threshold. There was no evidence of a ventilatory impairment to exercise. In patients with hypoxic pulmonary vasoconstriction, on the other hand, most were unable to attain their anaerobic threshold because of a primary ventilatory limitation to exercise. These responses are described more fully further on.

The responses of minute ventilation and carbon dioxide production to increments in oxygen use are shown in Figure 13–18 for patients with *nonhypoxic pulmonary vascular disease* and pulmonary hypertension.[16] By definition, these patients did not develop arterial oxygen desaturation during exercise. The

FIGURE 13–17. The relationship between the pulmonary pressure gradient and cardiac output at rest and during supine bicycle exercise (25 watts) before (Control) and following the administration of isoproterenol (Isuprel) in a patient with nonhypoxic pulmonary vascular disease. Control exercise evoked a 29 per cent decrease in pulmonary vascular resistance from a resting value of 620 dynes • sec • cm^{-5}. Isoproterenol at rest produced a 58 per cent decrease in PVR, and with exercise a further decrease of 23 per cent.

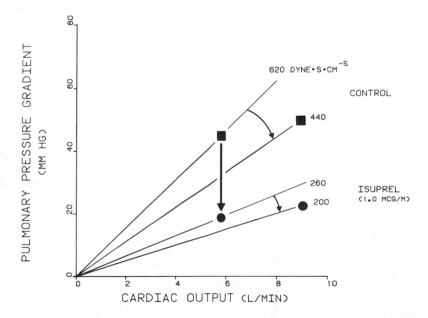

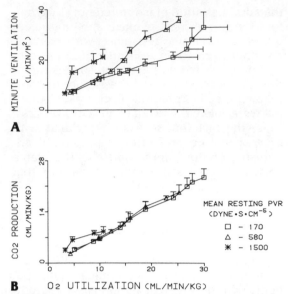

A

B O₂ UTILIZATION (ML/MIN/KG)

FIGURE 13–18. The response in CO₂ production ($\dot{V}CO_2$), and minute ventilation ($\dot{V}E$) during incremental treadmill exercise for patients with moderately severe and severe elevations in pulmonary vascular resistance secondary to nonhypoxic pulmonary vascular disease. Normal subjects are also shown. (From Janicki JS, Weber KT, Likoff MJ, Fishman AP. Exercise testing to evaluate patients with pulmonary vascular disease. Am Rev Respir Dis *129*:S93–S95, 1984.)

more severe the elevation in pulmonary vascular resistance in the nonhypoxic group, the greater $\dot{V}_E$ for any level of $\dot{V}O_2$ and muscular work (*A*). The associated increase in $\dot{V}CO_2$ primarily accounts for the abnormal elevation in minute ventilation (*B*).

The ventilatory response in the *hypoxic*

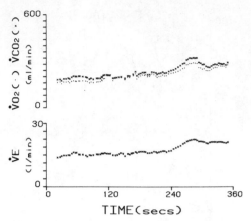

FIGURE 13–20. The response to incremental treadmill exercise for a 37 year old woman with sarcoidosis. The patient had pulmonary hypertension and hypoxemia during exercise, which commenced after 4 minutes of standing rest.

group is considered in Chapter 16. Herein, individual examples of their response are shown in Figures 13–19 and 13–20, where the stimulus to ventilation in these patients was hypoxia. In the first case, hypoxia was the result of thromboembolic disease in major segments of the pulmonary circulation, and in the second case it was secondary to severe interstitial lung disease and sarcoidosis. Hence, abnormalities in the perfusion or the ventilation of the lung can create hypoxia, and the ventilatory response reflects the body's compensatory response, which is designed to maintain alveolar ventilation at a rate that would sustain oxygenation.

CLINICAL APPLICATIONS

The overall incidence of nonhypoxic pulmonary hypertension is difficult to estimate. Because we do not have an "inflatable cuff" to place around the pulmonary artery and noninvasively to detect pulmonary artery pressure, we must rely on the physical examination to detect right ventricular enlargement and pulmonary hypertension. Regrettably, the sensitivity and specificity of the physical examination are not adequate to detect a subtle increase in pulmonary artery pressure that might occur early in the course of the disease. Various laboratory tests have been proposed, such as detection of midsystolic closure of the pulmonic valve on the echocardiogram. But once again, this parameter and other methods have lacked the necessary characteristics to prove useful as a screening device.

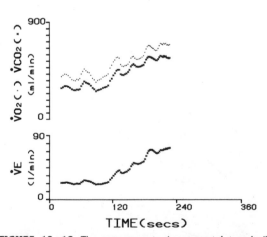

FIGURE 13–19. The response to incremental treadmill exercise for a 36 year old man with recurrent pulmonary emboli, pulmonary hypertension, arterial O₂ desaturation with exercise, and exertional dyspnea. Note the marked elevation in minute ventilation with low level physical activity (1 mph, 0 per cent grade).

A decline in the diffusing capacity for carbon monoxide (D_{LCO}), without other abnormalities in pulmonary function, could be a useful screening tool to signal the physician of a gas-transfer abnormality that accompanies pulmonary vascular disease. However, the reliability of using the sensitivity and specificity of the D_{LCO} determination as a means to detect pulmonary hypertension in large patient populations is unproven.

Cardiopulmonary exercise testing, by increasing pulmonary blood flow and the oxygen requirements of working skeletal muscle, may provide a noninvasive method to detect structural and/or vasomotor abnormalities in the pulmonary circulation. A reduction in aerobic capacity and anaerobic threshold and/or the appearance of arterial oxygen desaturation during exercise may be indicative of pulmonary vascular disease and pulmonary hypertension. A major problem arises in identifying which patient to exercise. Perhaps the screening of susceptible populations, such as young women on oral contraceptives who are dyspneic on exertion or with Raynaud's phenomenon would be a reasonable starting point. Further study will

be necessary to determine whether or not these suggestions have any merit.

In patients with pulmonary hypertension previously established via ventilation/perfusion scintigraphy, pulmonary angiography, echocardiography, or all three techniques, noninvasive CPX can be valuable in establishing the severity of the circulatory failure, which could then serially be monitored to assess the progression of the disease.

Invasive CPX to characterize the pressure-flow relation of the pulmonary circulation can be useful in assessing pulmonary vascular resistance at rest and during exercise. From this information, one can infer whether or not vascular resistance is "fixed" secondary to a widespread structural deformity within the circulation or "nonfixed" as a result of abnormal vasomotor reactivity or less-extensive disease. For example, a small subset (6 to 15 per cent) of patients with mitral valve disease will have a hyper-reactive pulmonary circulation with advanced pulmonary hypertension (see Chapter 12). Even though vascular resistance may exceed 1000 dynes $\cdot$ sec $\cdot$ cm^{-5}, this does not prohibit their having mitral valve replacement. On

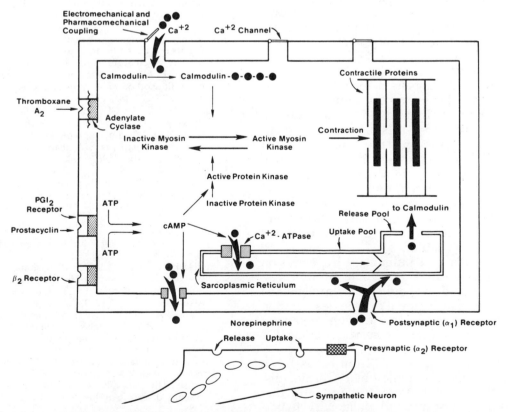

FIGURE 13–21. The schematic representation of vascular smooth muscle and the various pharmacodynamic and biochemical events involved in smooth muscle contraction and relaxation.

Table 13—4. *Pharmacologic Agents That May Be Useful in Promoting Vasodilatation of the Diseased Pulmonary Circulation*

Agent	Mechanism of Action
Isoproterenol	beta$_2$ agonist
Phentolamine	alpha antagonist
Verapamil	Ca^{+2} channel blocker
Nifedipine	Ca^{+2} channel blocker
Nitroprusside	prostaglandin-mediated (?)
Hydralazine	prostaglandin-mediated (?)

the other hand, patients with intrinsic, non-hypoxic pulmonary vascular disease whose pulmonary vascular resistance exceeds 1000 dynes • sec • cm^{-5} will not have a reduction in resistance with exercise. This finding would suggest far-advanced, widespread structural disease of the pulmonary circulation.

An invasive CPX should be timed with respect to any attempts at pharmacologic manipulation of the vasomotor reactivity of the diseased pulmonary circulation. Each test should be performed in sequence to maximize assessment while minimizing patient inconvenience and medical costs. Moreover, if a vasodilator agent proves useful in reducing pulmonary artery pressure, it should unload the right heart at rest and during exercise. A follow-up invasive CPX may therefore be warranted.

Figure 13—21 depicts a model of vascular smooth muscle and various intracellular biochemical events that would mediate vasodilatation. Table 13—4 lists a number of pharmacologic agents and their mechanism of action that may serve to promote vasodilation of the diseased pulmonary circulation. A more extensive description of the issues and problems associated with the assessment of the pharmacoreactivity of the abnormal pulmonary circulation is beyond the intended scope of this chapter.

Hypoxemia and pulmonary hypertension that apper during exercise and are not present at rest, and the addition of supplemental oxygen to retard arterial oxygen desaturation with its accompanying elevation in pulmonary artery pressure, can best be documented by invasive CPX.

Finally, an invasive CPX can be useful in excluding occult expressions of cardiac disease that are not present at rest and that account for unexplained pulmonary hyper-

tension. For example, we have seen a number of patients with systemic hypertension who develop mitral regurgitation during exertion when systemic arterial pressure rises excessively (see cases 3 and 5 in Chapter 18).

REFERENCES

1. Harris P, Heath D. The Pulmonary Circulation. New York, Churchill-Livingstone, 1977.
2. Weber KT, Janicki JS, Reeves RC, Hefner LL. Factors influencing left ventricular shortening in the isolated canine heart. Am J Physiol 230:419–426, 1976.
3. Weber KT, Janicki JS, Shroff S, Fishman AP. Contractile mechanics and interaction of the right and left ventricles. Am J Cardiol 47:685–695, 1981.
4. Enson Y, Giuntini C, Lewis ML, Morris TQ, Ferrer MI, Harvey RM. The influence of hydrogen ion concentration and hypoxia on the pulmonary circulation. J Clin Invest 43:1146–1161, 1964.
5. Dresdale DT, Schultz M, Michtom RJ. Primary pulmonary hypertension. Am J Med 11:686–705, 1951.
6. Shepherd JT, Edwards JE, Burchell HB, Swan HJC, Wood EH. Clinical, physiological, and pathological considerations in patients with idiopathic pulmonary hypertension. Br Heart J 19:70–81, 1957.
7. Sleeper JC, Orgain ES, McIntosh HD. Primary pulmonary hypertension. Review of clinical features and pathologic physiology with a report of pulmonary hemodynamics derived from repeated catheterization. Circulation 26:1358–1369, 1962.
8. Walcott G, Burchell HB, Brown AL. Primary pulmonary hypertension. Mayo Clin Proc 49:70–79, 1970.
9. Graham R, Skoog C, Oppenheimer L, Rabson J, Goldberg HS. Critical closure in the canine pulmonary vasculature. Circ Res 50:566–572, 1982.
10. Hyman AL. Effects of large increases in pulmonary blood flow on pulmonary venous pressure. J Appl Physiol 27:179–185, 1969.
11. Epstein SE, Beiser GD, Stampfer M, Robinson BF, Braunwald E. Characterization of the circulatory response to maximal upright exercise in normal subjects and patients with heart disease. Circulation 35:1049–1062, 1967.
12. Harris P, Segel N, Bishop JM. The relation between pressure and flow in the pulmonary circulation in normal subjects and in patients with chronic bronchitis and mitral stenosis. Cardiovasc Res 2:73–83, 1968.
13. Fowler NO. The normal pulmonary arterial pressure-flow relationships during exercise (editorial). Am J Med 47:1–6, 1969.
14. Janicki JS, Weber KT, Likoff MJ, Fishman AP. The pressure-flow response of the pulmonary circulation in heart failure and pulmonary vascular disease. Circulation 72:1270–1278, 1985.
15. Hopkins RA, Hammon JW Jr, McHale PA, Smith P, Anderson RW. An analysis of the pulsatile hemodynamic responses of the pulmonary circulation to acute and chronic pulmonary venous hypertension in the awake dog. Circ Res 47:902–910, 1980.
16. Janicki JS, Weber KT, Likoff MJ, Fishman AP. Exercise testing to evaluate patients with pulmonary vascular disease. Am Rev Respir Dis 129:S93–S95, 1984.

KARL T. WEBER
PATRICIA A. McELROY

14

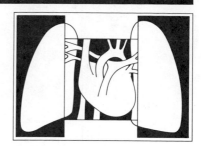

Systemic Hypertension

Systemic hypertension represents a hemo-dynamic abnormality of the cardiocirculatory system, and by definition it is an abnormal elevation in arterial blood pressure above the expected range of normal. In practical terms, this means that for adult men and women at rest, systolic arterial pressure will be greater than 140 mm Hg and diastolic pressure higher than 90 mm Hg. In cases when arterial blood pressure is only occasionally greater than 140/90, but less than 160/100, the hyper-tensive state is said to be *labile*, or of *borderline* severity. *Established* hypertension is present when arterial pressure is consistently ele-vated above these values. Early in the course of established hypertension, end-organ in-volvement (e.g., left ventricular hypertro-phy) or damage (e.g., vascular changes within the retinal circulation) are absent, and therefore this phase is considered to repre-sent *mild* hypertension. Later in the course of the disease, multisystem involvement ap-pears to parallel the severity of the disease. The World Health Organization has graded the severity of systemic hypertension accord-ing to three stages: *stage 1* exists when there are no complications of the disease; *stage 2* is present when left ventricular hypertrophy alone is present; and *stage 3* represents a more extensive form of the disease with left ventricular hypertrophy and organ damage.

The pressure in the arterial circulation is a function of systemic blood flow and the impedance characteristics of the arterial cir-culation. Thus, at rest, the hemodynamic abnormalities of systemic hypertension in-clude elevations in cardiac output, vascular resistance, or both. During the physiologic stress of isotonic exercise oxygen delivery and thus cardiac output must increase. An excessive rise in cardiac output relative to the oxygen requirements of the tissues, or a defect in the vasomotor reactivity of the re-sistance vessels (the arterioles), will be ac-companied by an abnormally elevated arterial pressure.

Exercise testing to maximum aerobic ca-pacity has been performed safely in hundreds of patients with systemic hyperten-sion, particularly in Scandinavian countries. The results of one landmark study[1] in which upright cycle ergometry was used to assess the response in arterial blood pressure rela-tive to $\dot{V}O_2$ in normal subjects and patients with hypertension are given in Figures 14–1 and 14–2. Regrettably, however, confidence limits for the normal response were not pro-vided and therefore cannot be included in these or subsequent figures taken from this study. Except in stage 1 men, there was little overlap in blood pressure at any level of $\dot{V}O_2$ when hypertensive patients were compared with healthy individuals. In healthy men systolic blood pressure at maximum exercise remains below 230 mm Hg, and in healthy women it remains below 200 mm Hg. In another large trial[2] where patient age was taken into consideration, similar results were found. The responses in arterial pressure in this study are shown in Figures 14–3 and 14–4. Note that control subjects for the 50 to 66 year old group were not included in this elegant study.

An invasive isotonic exercise test currently represents one means of assessing the rela-tive contribution of the heart (i.e., its cardiac output response) and circulation (i.e., its impedance) to the genesis, maintenance, and severity of hypertension. Although nonin-vasive exercise testing may prove useful in assessing the effectiveness of antihyperten-sive therapy, the application of noninvasive

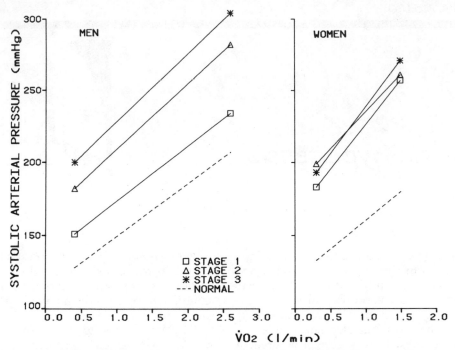

FIGURE 14–1. The response in systolic arterial pressure to upright bicycle exercise and incremental work or O_2 uptake ($\dot{V}O_2$) for patients with stage 1, 2, or 3 hypertension and normal subjects. (Adapted from Sannerstedt R. Hemodynamic response to exercise in patients with arterial hypertension. Acta Med Scand *180* (Suppl 458):7–101, 1966.)

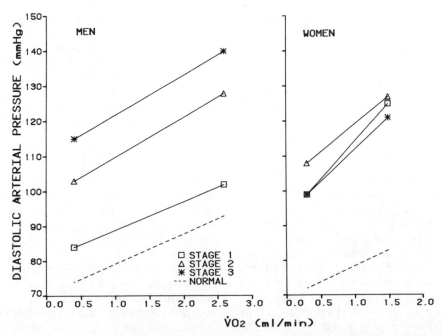

FIGURE 14–2. The response in diastolic arterial pressure to incremental exercise in the same group of patients shown in Figure 14–1. (Adapted from Sannerstedt R. Hemodynamic response to exercise in patients with arterial hypertension. Acta Med Scand 180 (Suppl 458):7–101, 1966.)

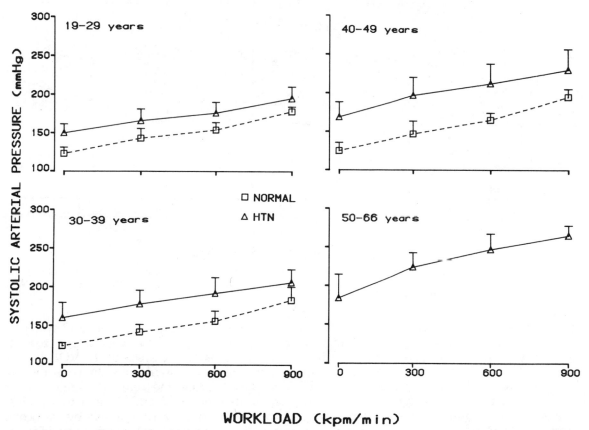

FIGURE 14–3. The response in systolic arterial pressure (SBP) to incremental cycle ergometry in patients with systemic hypertension. The patients are divided according to age, with age-matched controls. (Adapted from Lund-Johansen P. Hemodynamics in early essential hypertension. Acta Med Scand *183* (Suppl 482):1–105, 1967.)

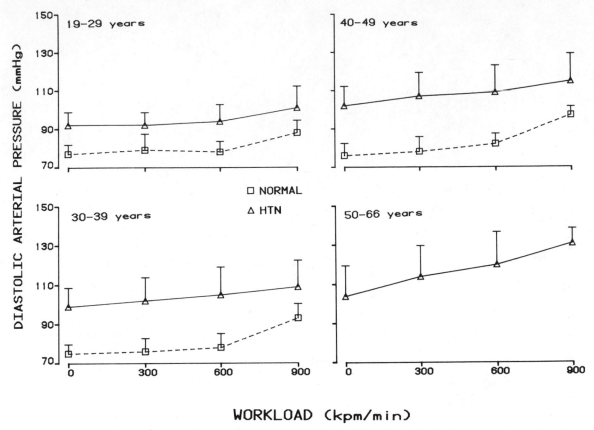

FIGURE 14–4. The response in diastolic arterial pressure to incremental bicycle exercise in the same group of patients shown in Figure 14–3. (Adapted from Lund-Johansen P. Hemodynamics in early essential hypertension. Acta Med Scand *183* (Suppl 482):1–105, 1967.)

techniques to monitor cardiac output (e.g., carbon dioxide rebreathing) may permit one to characterize the role of the heart in future studies. In this connection, Devereux and co-workers[3] have shown that the presence of left ventricular hypertrophy is most closely correlated with ambulatory blood pressure, particularly blood pressure during regularly occurring stresses, such as going to work. The purpose of this chapter will be to review how cardiopulmonary exercise (CPX) testing may be used in the evaluation and management of systemic hypertension. Before discussing these issues, however, it is worth reviewing the evolution of the control systems for cardiac output and vascular resistance, and thereby blood pressure control, a perspective that emphasizes that each system evolved based on oxygen delivery.

PHYSIOLOGIC CONTROL OF CARDIAC OUTPUT

Separate physiologic controls, often having common input moduli, are responsible for the regulation of cardiac output and systemic vascular resistance. Cardiac output, for example, is matched precisely to $\dot{V}O_2$. In the same manner, vascular resistance is related to $\dot{V}O_2$ because the redistribution of large quantities of blood and oxygen to working muscle must be accompanied by vasoconstriction of other vascular beds (e.g., kidney) in order to prevent an abnormal fall in arterial pressure. Several clinical studies have shown cardiac output to be elevated in patients with borderline hypertension, even though vascular resistance is "normal".[2,3] Later, as the disease becomes established, cardiac output returns to normal, whereas structural changes within arterioles raise their resistance to flow. Eventually, the heart fails, its output declines, and vascular resistance rises even further.

Given that cardiac output is so closely coupled to tissue $\dot{V}O_2$, why should it be increased early in hypertension unless $\dot{V}O_2$ is also proportionally elevated? Many theories have been proposed to account for this presumably hyperdynamic heart; few have been examined critically relative to $\dot{V}O_2$, the primary determinant in the cardiac output control system. In addition, compensatory adjustments in neural control, regional autoregulation, and renal function under these circumstances should return blood pressure to the physiologic range in such cases. If not, why? Similar questions may be asked of the vascular resistance control system. It would appear useful to examine these issues in hypertensive subjects, but first the normal response must be reviewed.

The Normal Response

Phylogenetically, the origin of the physiologic control systems for the regulation of cardiac output and systemic vascular resistance can be traced to the need for oxygen, which arose as animal life evolved from water, where oxygen was derived by diffusion and convection, to a terrestrial existence. This evolutionary process not only altered the source of oxygen and the process of ventilation, it also raised the overall need for oxygen as land living animals became warm-blooded.[4] The oxygen uptake ($\dot{V}O_2$) of resting warm-blooded mammals, for example, is higher than that of fish (3.5 to 8 versus 0.5 to 1 ml/min/kg). The mobility and survival of these mammals were dependent on their capacity to perform muscular work and to use oxidative metabolism as a source of energy. A system of oxygen transport was therefore needed to meet the aerobic requirements of the tissues on a moment-to-moment basis. The heart and lungs assumed this role. Given that the resting $\dot{V}O_2$ of warm-blooded mammals is ten times that of fish, mammals had to have a greater systemic blood flow (70 to 150 versus 10 to 40 ml/min/kg). The heart and its cardiac output are therefore closely coupled to the tissues and their $\dot{V}O_2$. The control logic of the oxygen transport system, however, has not been well characterized. Input signals to the heart may originate from the central nervous system; reflexes initiated from within active skeletal muscle, the sympathetic nervous system, and/or various cardiovascular reflexes.

In normal subjects, it is well known that cardiac output will rise in proportion to the prevailing $\dot{V}O_2$. As shown in Figure 14–5, for every 100 ml/min/m² rise in $\dot{V}O_2$ above its resting value, systemic blood flow is increased approximately 600 ml/min/m² above the resting cardiac output.[5] This value, which represents the slope of the cardiac output − $\dot{V}O_2$ relation, has also been reported by others for normal individuals.[6] Each increment in blood flow is achieved by an elevation in heart rate, which occurs at all levels of $\dot{V}O_2$, and an increase in stroke volume, which is most apparent at lighter work loads. Eventually, however, $\dot{V}O_2$ rises to a level that exceeds the pumping capacity of the heart; cardiac output fails to rise any further. Thus, there exists a *maximal oxygen uptake*, or $\dot{V}O_2$ max, the absolute level of which is based on

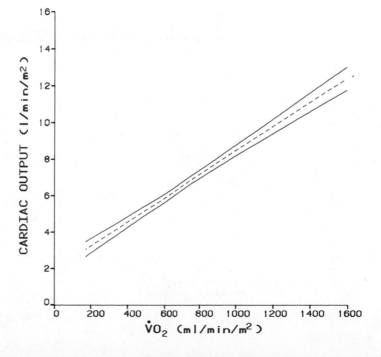

Figure 14–5. The normal response in cardiac output to incremental treadmill exercise. The slope of this relation indicates the rise in cardiac output to increasing muscular work (see text).

the maximal cardiac output and the maximal level of oxygen extraction (the arteriovenous oxygen difference). $\dot{V}O_2$ max is also dependent on the age, sex, and level of physical training of the individual.[7]

In considering this relationship between cardiac output and $\dot{V}O_2$, the resting cardiac output and the cardiac output response to isotonic exercise can be viewed as the *"intercept"* and *slope* of this relation, respectively; together, they represent the *"gain"* of the cardiac output control system. A number of possible combinations for resting and exercise cardiac output can be predicted (Fig. 14–6), many of which may create abnormalities in systemic blood flow leading to an abnormal elevation in arterial pressure.

The specific manner in which the oxygen requirements of the tissues regulate cardiac output is not well known. Other responses that may or may not be independent of the tissues are also operative in raising cardiac output during exercise. For example, an increase in venous return elicits an increase in both stroke volume by the Frank-Starling mechanism and heart rate mediated by the Bainbridge reflex. On the other hand, vagal tone falls, while the sympathetic nervous system is activated. Plasma norepinephrine rises during bicycle exercise when work loads representing >70 per cent of $\dot{V}O_2$ max are attained. This response in norepinephrine underscores the fact that the choice of work load relative to $\dot{V}O_2$ is fundamental to assessing the responsiveness of the sympathetic nervous system during exercise in patients with systemic hypertension.

Borderline Hypertension

In patients with essential hypertension, cardiac output system gain, or flow relative to $\dot{V}O_2$, has been examined during upright progressive bicycle exercise. In 18 patients

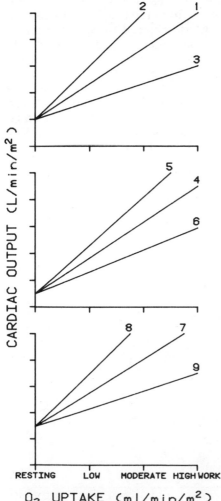

	CO	
	RESTING	**EXERCISE**
1	N	N
2	N	↑
3	N	↓

	CO	
	RESTING	**EXERCISE**
4	↓	N
5	↓	↑
6	↓	↓

	CO	
	RESTING	**EXERCISE**
7	↑	N
8	↑	↑
9	↑	↓

CARDIAC OUTPUT (L/min/m²)

RESTING   LOW   MODERATE HIGH WORK

O₂ UPTAKE (ml/min/m²)

FIGURE 14–6. Theoretic combinations of resting cardiac output ("intercept") and exercise cardiac output (slope), many of which may exist in systemic hypertension.

with stage 1 hypertension (mean age, 37 years), Sannerstedt[1] reported a significant elevation in resting $\dot{V}O_2$ compared with age- and sex-matched normotensive control subjects (296 versus 270 ml/min, respectively). Resting cardiac output (7.19 versus 6.03 liters/min) (Fig. 14–7) and heart rate (82 versus 67 bpm) were also elevated in these patients, although there was no difference in their stroke volume, vascular resistance, or arteriovenous oxygen difference compared with those of control subjects. It is difficult to reconcile how the modest elevation in resting $\dot{V}O_2$ of 26 ml/min was responsible for these patients having a greater cardiac output (1.16 liters/min) and heart rate (15 bpm) at rest. When exercised to their symptomatic (not aerobic) maximum, these patients demonstrated a wide range of $\dot{V}O_2$ at peak exercise (760 to 2260 ml/min); and their exercise response in blood pressure, heart rate, vascular resistance, and arteriovenous oxygen difference were similar to those of control subjects. On the other hand, their increment in cardiac output (Fig. 14–7) and stroke volume were reported to be significantly less than those of the control subjects.

Lund-Johansen[2] studied 93 patients with essential hypertension, of whom 19 were less than 30 years of age and had stage 1 hypertension. In this group, the average intra-arterial blood pressure was 146/86, whereas the average cuff blood pressure was 145/90. Lund-Johansen found that the $\dot{V}O_2$ at rest tended to be higher in these patients than in control normotensive subjects (164 versus 147 ml/min/m²), although the difference was not

statistically significant. The resting cardiac output (Fig. 14–8, *upper left*) also tended to be elevated in these patients compared with control subjects (3.70 versus 3.29 liters/min/m²), and again the difference did not reach significance. The increase in exercise cardiac output in these patients under 30 years of age was due to a significantly increased heart rate; stroke volume was unchanged. Although resting cardiac output was elevated, exercise cardiac output was slightly reduced at all work loads compared with that of control subjects (Fig. 14–8), the mechanism being a compromised elevation in exercise stroke volume. In hypertensive patients over 30 years, the cardiac output response to exercise (Fig. 14–8) was reported to be lower than in normotensive control subjects.

Thus, according to these two studies, in young patients (under 40 years) with hypertension, many of whom have borderline hypertension, resting cardiac output is elevated, predominantly owing to an increased heart rate with normal stroke volume. As $\dot{V}O_2$ increases during isotonic exercise, cardiac output rises less than normal owing to a reduced stroke volume response.

Established Hypertension

In established hypertension, the cardiac output response to exercise is reported to be both normal and depressed.[1,2] Differences in age, sex, and aerobic capacity, however, make interpretation difficult. Moreover, the response in left ventricular filling or wedge

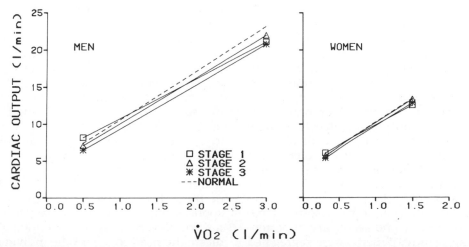

FIGURE 14–7. The response in cardiac output to incremental ergometric work is shown for patients with systemic hypertension. See legend for Figure 14–1. (Adapted from Sannerstedt R. Hemodynamic response to exercise in patients with arterial hypertension. Acta Med Scand 180 (Suppl 458):7–101, 1966.)

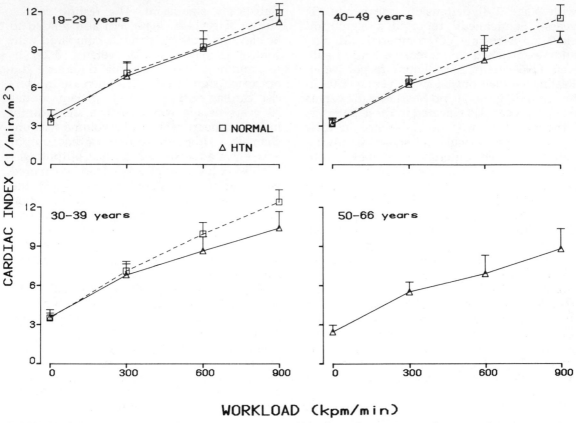

FIGURE 14–8. The response in cardiac output to incremental bicycle work in patients with systemic hypertension. See legend for Figure 14–3. (Adapted from Lund-Johansen P. Hemodynamics in early essential hypertension. Acta Med Scand *183* (Suppl 482):1–105, 1967.)

pressure has not been measured. In Sannerstedt's experience,[1] in which the mean age of men and women with stage 2 and stage 3 disease was 47 and 50 years, respectively, the resting cardiac output was the same (stage 2) or slightly less (stage 3) than in control subjects (see Fig. 14–7). In neither case, however, was the resting cardiac output significantly different from that of control subjects. During bicycle exercise, cardiac output in hypertensive men and women rose in a manner that was equivalent to that found in the control population. In Lund-Johansen's experience,[2] on the other hand (Fig. 14–8), the cardiac output response to exercise was reported to be lower than controls, particularly in the older subjects (50 to 66 years) and at the higher work loads in those patients between 30 and 49 years of age.

Amery and co-workers[8] examined the response to upright bicycle exercise in 61 patients with primary and secondary hypertension; in their study, patients were segregated according to age. A decline in $\dot{V}O_2$ max and exercise cardiac output was observed with advancing age; however, a greater arterial pressure (systolic, diastolic, and mean) response to exercise and a lesser reduction in vascular resistance were noted in all hypertensive subjects, irrespective of their age. The resting cardiac output was normal for all patients including those between 19 and 34 years of age.

In a preliminary study of 12 patients with established hypertension, we have also found the resting cardiac output to be normal in 75 per cent and elevated in 25 per cent of the patients, who ranged in age from 33 to 61 years (mean 48 years). Although in most of these patients (five of nine) the response in cardiac output to exercise was normal, an interesting subgroup of four patients had a heightened cardiac output response to exercise (Fig. 14–9). The therapeutic implications of these heterogeneous cardiac output responses during exercise remain to be determined. Nevertheless, these findings may indicate the need to determine individually the pathophysiologic response to exercise in order to provide the most logical therapeutic

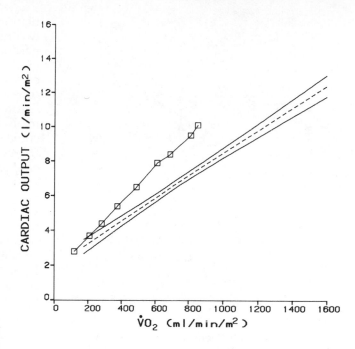

FIGURE 14–9. Examples of the response in cardiac output to incremental treadmill exercise observed in patients with systemic hypertension (open squares) compared with normals (broken line ± solid line confidence intervals).

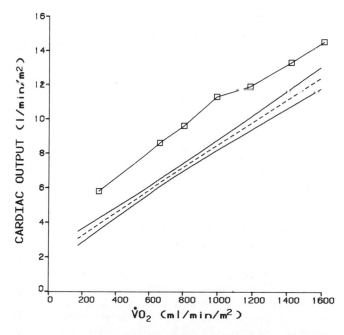

strategy. This issue is discussed in more detail subsequently.

From our observations on systemic oxygen extraction (Fig. 14–10), there is a normal progressive widening of the arteriovenous oxygen difference during incremental treadmill exercise in hypertension, and there appears to be no grossly apparent defect in tissue oxygen extraction. These findings are also in agreement with the findings of others.[1,2,8]

In summary, the resting cardiac output response may be altered in essential hypertension. A number of different theoretical combinations of the "intercept" and slope are possible (see Fig. 14–6). Existing information as to the incidence of each of these is limited, particularly the relationship between exercise cardiac output and $\dot{V}O_2$ in individual patients. For example, it is not clear whether or not patients with borderline hypertension will routinely fall into responses 7, 8, or 9. It is attractive to speculate that patients having an elevated cardiac output gain would be

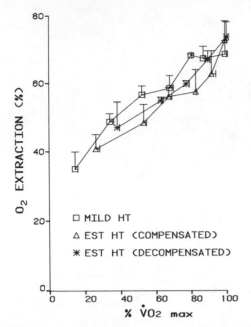

FIGURE 14–10. The response in systemic O_2 extraction (arteriovenous O_2 difference/arterial O_2 content) to incremental treadmill exercise in patients with hypertension who are either compensated (no clinical heart failure) or decompensated.

candidates for selective beta$_1$ adrenergic receptor blockade. Alternatively, such therapy may be less than ideal for subjects having responses 4 or 6, where resting or exercise cardiac output is less than normal. Here, there would be little advantage to decoupling of the heart further relative to the oxygen requirements of the tissues.

PHYSIOLOGIC CONTROL OF VASCULAR RESISTANCE

Mean resting arterial pressure averages 80 mm Hg in mammals, whereas in fish and reptiles it is only 30 mm Hg, owing to the correspondingly lower cardiac output; the vascular resistance of each species, however, is similar. Guyton[9] has suggested that one explanation for this difference in pressure relates to the position of the head of mammals, which is above the level of the heart. Other factors, however, must also be operative in the origins of blood pressure control. The need to redistribute large quantities of blood with exercise provides another explanation. During isotonic exercise, the vascular resistance of skeletal muscle falls dramatically, while other vascular segments vasoconstrict to maintain blood pressure. This mod-

ulation of vascular resistance is produced by two neurohumoral systems: the sympathetic nervous system primarily and the renin-angiotensin system to a lesser extent. As in the control of cardiac output, oxygen delivery is central to vascular resistance control. The autoregulatory vasodilation of muscle normally over-rides the vasoconstrictive effect of circulating norepinephrine and angiotensin II and permits oxygen delivery to match oxygen demand.

In a manner analogous to that developed for the cardiac output control system, resting vascular resistance and its response to isotonic exercise represent the *"gain"* of this control system (Fig. 14–11). Because of the curvilinear response in vascular resistance we have taken its reciprocal to create a linear relationship (Fig. 14–12), which is termed systemic vascular *conductance*.[1] The resting and exercise response in conductance represent the "intercept" and slope, respectively, of system gain, and once again there are multiple theoretic combinations of each of these variables (Fig. 14–13). Armed with these concepts, we can now examine the normal response in systemic vascular resistance to exercise, as well as that seen in hypertensive patients.

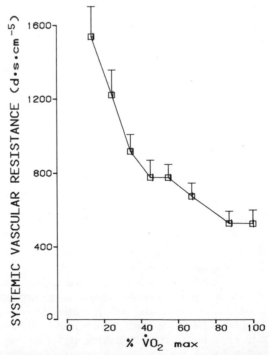

FIGURE 14–11. The response in systemic vascular resistance (mean arterial minus right atrial pressures/cardiac output) for normal subjects and class A patients with minimal cardiovascular disease performing incremental treadmill exercise.

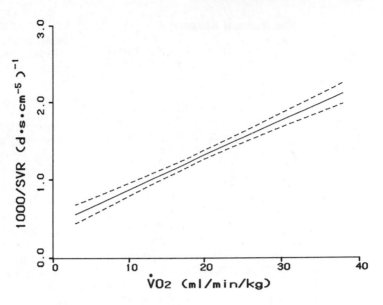

FIGURE 14–12. The reciprocal of systemic vascular resistance (*SVR*), termed systemic vascular conductance, and its response to incremental treadmill exercise in normal subjects and class A patients with minimal cardiovascular disease. Broken lines represent confidence intervals.

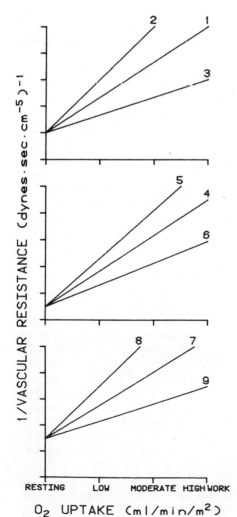

FIGURE 14–13. Theoretic combinations in vascular conduction (slope and intercept), many of which may be present at rest and during exercise in systemic hypertension. See text.

The Normal Response

In normal subjects (patients with minimal cardiovascular disease performing upright, progressive isotonic exercise on the bicycle or treadmill), arterial systolic and mean pressures increase, while diastolic pressure remains unchanged or falls slightly.[10] The response in arterial pressure for bicycle exercise has been presented in Figures 14–1 through 14–4. The response to treadmill exercise shown in Figure 14–14 is quite similar. This response in arterial pressure is, in part, a result of the progressive increment in cardiac output as higher work loads are achieved. Neurohumoral, reflexive, and autoregulatory adjustments in regional vascular resistance permit a massive redistribution of blood flow to muscle without adversely lowering arterial pressure. Skeletal muscle blood flow can reach 22 liters/min or 88 per cent of systemic blood flow (see Table 2–8) at maximal exercise. Other organs, such as the kidney and splanchnic circulation, will have a 10- to 20-fold reduction in their apportionment of the cardiac output. Blood flow to the kidney has been measured during upright cycle ergometry in healthy persons averaging 28 years of age.[11] A 10 per cent reduction in renal flow was observed at 450 kpm/min, while at 600 kpm/min flow fell to 15 per cent of its resting value. $\dot{V}O_2$ was not recorded in this study, however, and heart rate rose to only 100 and 115 bpm, respectively, for each load, suggesting that these were low levels of work for these subjects. After 40 minutes of recov-

ery, it is important to note that renal flow had nearly returned to baseline levels. A similar response in the rate of glomerular filtration was observed.

Borderline Hypertension

In patients with essential hypertension, abnormalities in the neurohumoral and reflexive control of blood pressure and vascular resistance have been a subject of considerable interest. This section will focus on the studies that have directed their attention to these issues during the course of upright isotonic exercise when $\dot{V}O_2$ was measured.

In patients with borderline hypertension, recall that Sannerstedt[1] reported that the blood pressure response to upright, symptom-limited bicycle exercise of variable loads (220 to 1200 kpm/min) was no different from that of control subjects. This was not the case for patients with established hypertension, in whom systolic and mean pressure rose abnormally with similar levels of exercise. Vascular resistance, which was normal at rest, fell normally during exercise in patients with borderline hypertension (Fig. 14–15). It therefore would follow that systemic vascular conductance in these male patients was no different from that of normal control subjects at rest; it too rose with exercise, but not to the same extent as that seen in control subjects, with the difference in response (less vasodilatation) being significant (Fig. 14–16). In the younger age group, Lund-Johansen[2] also found vascular resistance to decline with upright exercise but not to the extent found in normal subjects (Fig. 14–17). This retarded fall in resistance became greater with advancing age.

Amery and colleagues[8] found that in 19 to 32 year old patients with resting diastolic pressure >90 mm Hg, systolic pressure response to bicycle exercise was no different from that of control subjects. In older (35 to 69 year old) patients with hypertension, on the other hand, the rise in systolic pressure during exercise was greater than that of their age-matched controls, and the fall in systemic resistance was never as great as that of their controls. No information is given, however, as to the level of exercise used relative to $\dot{V}O_2$ max. Henquet and co-workers[12] found that at 50 per cent and 75 per cent of $\dot{V}O_2$ max, and at $\dot{V}O_2$ max, 18 to 30 year old men with borderline hypertension demonstrated greater systolic and diastolic pressures than those of healthy individuals. Here, however,

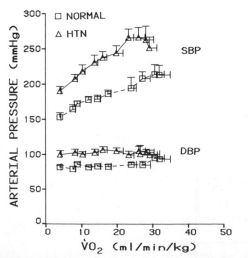

FIGURE 14–14. The response in invasive arterial systolic (*SBP*) and diastolic (*DBP*) arterial pressures to incremental treadmill exercise for normal and class A subjects and patients with systemic hypertension.

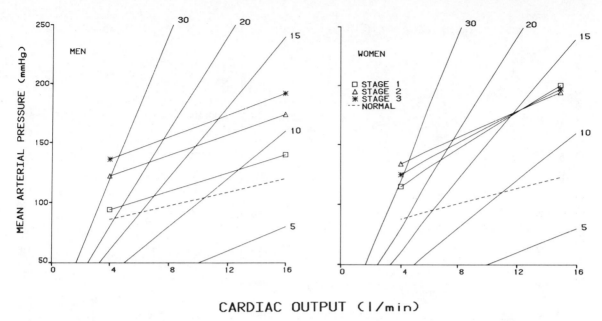

FIGURE 14–15. The response in mean arterial pressure and cardiac output during incremental bicycle exercise for patients with hypertension and normal subjects. The data are plotted against isopleths of total peripheral resistance in Wood units (e.g., 5 and 10 mm Hg/liters·min^{-1}). See legend of Figure 14–1 for symbols. (Adapted from Sannerstedt R. Hemodynamic response to exercise in patients with arterial hypertension. Acta Med Scand *180* (Suppl 458):7–101, 1966.)

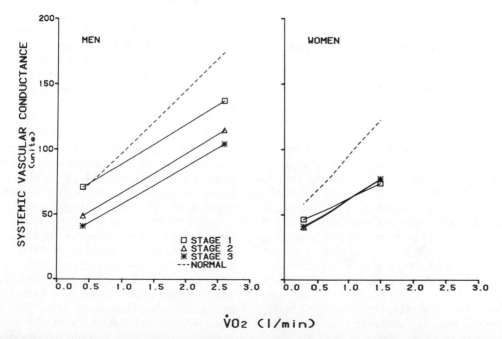

FIGURE 14–16. The response in vascular conductance to incremental cycle ergometry for normal subjects and patients with hypertension. See legend of Figure 14–1. (Adapted from Sannerstedt R. Hemodynamic response to exercise in patients with arterial hypertension. Acta Med Scand *180* (Suppl 458):7–101, 1966.)

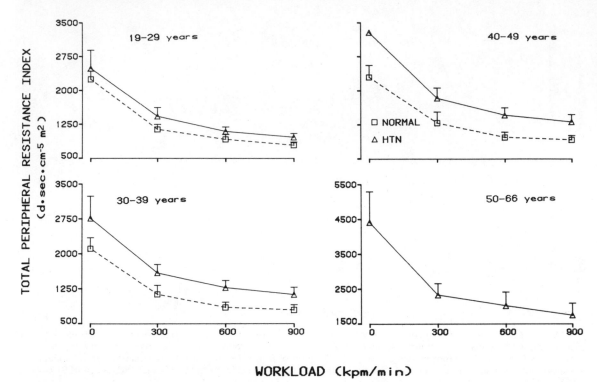

FIGURE 14—17. The response in total peripheral resistance to incremental bicycle work for normal individuals and patients with hypertension. See legend of Figure 14–3. (Adapted from Lund-Johansen P. Hemodynamics in early essential hypertension. Acta Med Scand *183* (Suppl 482):1–105, 1967.)

blood pressure was measured only indirectly by sphygmomanometry. In Henquet's study, the responses in plasma norepinephrine, epinephrine, and renin to all levels of exercise were measured, and there was found to be no difference between those of the hypertensive patients and those of the control subjects.

Established Hypertension

In patients with established hypertension, the fall in vascular resistance during exercise is compromised. Sannerstedt[1] found that in stage 2 or 3 of the disease, resting resistance was significantly elevated, particularly in women. During exercise, resistance fell (but not to the extent seen in control subjects), with the difference being significant in men and women with stage 2 or 3 hypertension (see Fig. 14–15). Not unexpectedly, the same was true of the response in vascular conductance (see Fig. 14–16). Lund-Johansen[2] observed a similar compromise in the vasodilatation in exercise that was most apparent with advancing age (Fig. 14–17).

In our own experience using incremental treadmill exercise in normal subjects or patients with minimal cardiovascular disease, we find that vascular resistance has declined by 50 per cent at $\dot{V}O_2$ max (see Fig. 14–11); conductance, therefore, must rise twofold (see Fig. 14–12). In patients with established hypertension, we find that resting resistance is significantly increased and during treadmill exercise there is a fall in resistance, which primarily takes place at lower work loads (<60 per cent $\dot{V}O_2$ max). Even though the degree of vasodilation in these patients may appear to be comparable to that in control subjects (Fig. 14–18), differences in the cross-sectional area of the systemic circulation dictate that this is not so.

Folkow[13] has repeatedly emphasized that vascular structure, including the ratio of wall thickness to lumen diameter of arterioles, will determine the absolute response in resistance and cross-sectional area of the circulation to any neurohumoral stimulus or to exercise. In established hypertension, structural alterations within arterioles retard the ability of skeletal muscle circulation to vasodilate to the same extent as normal vessels.

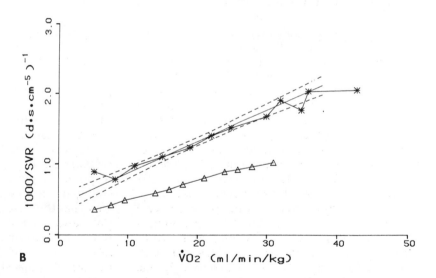

FIGURE 14–18. The response in systemic vascular resistance (*SVR*), shown in *A*, and in conductance (1000/SVR), shown in *B*, to incremental treadmill exercise for normal subjects (open squares in *A* and solid line plus confidence intervals in *B*) and two patients with hypertension.

NEUROHUMORAL ACTIVATION DURING EXERCISE

The Adrenergic Nervous System

The sympathetic and renin-angiotensin systems are each thought to contribute to the exercise-induced redistribution of blood flow that shunts blood flow away from less metabolically active tissues in favor of those of working muscle. Several studies in *normal subjects* have emphasized that although these two systems are activated during upright isotonic exercise, they mainly participate in blood pressure control associated with higher levels of muscular work. At >70 per cent $\dot{V}O_2$ max, Kotchen and associates[14] noted a 50 per cent increase in plasma norepinephrine; plasma epinephrine rose to a lesser extent and only at $\dot{V}O_2$ max. Sleight[15] has suggested that baroreceptor sensitivity will determine the absolute rise in catecholamines with exercise. Plasma renin activity behaves in a manner similar to that of norepinephrine.[14]

Various pharmacologic antagonists have been used to examine the contribution of these neurohumoral substances to the arterial pressure response to exercise. Epstein and associates[16] chose intravenous propranolol (0.15 mg/kg) to examine the beta adrenergic responses to submaximal and exhaustive treadmill exercise in seven healthy individuals. Significant reductions in exercise heart rate, cardiac output, mean arterial pressure, and peak $\dot{V}O_2$ were observed at maximal exercise; similar findings were noted during submaximal levels of work. A greater degree of oxygen extraction by the tissues was therefore needed to sustain oxidative metabolism during beta blockade.

The role of the adrenergic nervous system in mediating the abnormal response in vascular resistance to exercise has been examined by the measurement of plasma catecholamines or pharmacologic blockade. The determination of plasma norepinephrine is a very indirect measure of sympathetic nervous system activity. Local norepinephrine levels, neuronal uptake and clearance, as well as receptor number, affinity, and sensitivity may each influence the biologic effects of norepinephrine.[17]

Pharmacologic blockade of autonomic influences, together with plasma determination of the catecholamines, is a more direct approach to the problem. Reybrouck and colleagues[18] used the beta$_1$ blocker atenolol to assess the role of the heart in mediating the abnormal blood pressure response to progressive bicycle exercise in patients with *hypertension*. They observed a decrease in exercise heart rate, cardiac output, and blood pressure, but the fall in systemic vascular resistance in treated patients was similar to that of control subjects, and peak exercise $\dot{V}O_2$ was unchanged as tissue oxygen extraction was increased with muscular work. Once again, however, the level of $\dot{V}O_2$ achieved during exercise relative to $\dot{V}O_2$ max was not given; neither was the response in plasma norepinephrine.

Fagard and co-workers[19] also examined the response to labetalol, a compound with beta$_1$, beta$_2$, and alpha receptor antagonistic properties. The response in norepinephrine to exercise was unchanged after therapy; again, $\dot{V}O_2$ was not determined. Nevertheless, vascular resistance fell to a greater extent during exercise, emphasizing the role of the alpha receptor in mediating blood pressure in the upright position.

In essential hypertension, there are various theoretic combinations of resting and exercise vascular resistance to describe the underlying pathophysiology from which therapeutic strategies may be derived. Once again, however, such information is not available, particularly as it relates to $\dot{V}O_2$. In patients with responses 4 or 6 (see Fig. 14–6), an alpha$_1$ receptor antagonist may be more effective in normalizing vascular resistance, and thereby resting and ambulatory pressure, than a beta blocker, which might unmask the alpha receptor response and therefore be less than ideal under these circumstances.

The studies cited typify those wherein autonomic blockade was used together with exercise to determine the neurogenic component of blood pressure regulation. One has to conclude that either a substantial proportion of patients with hypertension do not have a neurogenic component to their elevated blood pressure or that there are too many unresolved issues, particularly those surrounding exercise methodology, the level of work chosen, and its relevance to neurohumoral system activation, to permit drawing any meaningful conclusions.

The Renin-Angiotensin System

Fagard and co-workers[20] used the angiotensin II antagonist saralasin to examine the role of this vasoactive octapeptide during progressive upright bicycle exercise in *normal subjects*. Following saralasin administration, there was only a modest reduction in the blood pressure response to exercise, which occurred only at higher levels of work corresponding to 75 per cent $\dot{V}O_2$ max. The response in plasma norepinephrine was unchanged after saralasin administration, as was also the case for heart rate, cardiac output, and plasma renin activity. Thus the renin-angiotensin system may not play an important role in blood pressure regulation in normal subjects.

The renin-angiotensin system also has been examined during exercise in *hypertensive patients*, both before and after pharmacologic blockade. Pedersen and co-workers[21] examined this system in young hypertensive patients during 75 and 100 watts of upright bicycle exercise. $\dot{V}O_2$ was not measured, but for each work load, heart rate rose to 108 and 128 bpm, respectively, suggesting that only light to moderate levels of work were achieved. Plasma renin activity increased at the lower work load, but not at 100 watts, whereas in healthy volunteer individuals it increased at both loads. This was interpreted as an abnormality in the patients. However, the wide variation in renin levels seen in both the patients and the control subjects and the modest levels and increments of work, representing in all likelihood <50 per cent $\dot{V}O_2$ max in both cases, make the interpretation of these findings difficult.

Manhem and associates[22] examined the role of angiotensin II during exercise by evaluating patients with hypertension before and after 1 week of captopril (600 mg daily) therapy. Captopril is an inhibitor of the angiotensin-converting enzyme. Upright bicycle exercise was conducted at both 40 and 70 per cent of the maximum work capacity, while arterial blood pressure was measured indirectly. Systolic and diastolic blood pressures were significantly reduced from pretreatment levels at the 40 per cent work load but less so at the higher load. The response in plasma norepinephrine to exercise was unchanged after captopril administration. The authors therefore concluded that the sympathetic nervous system is dominant in blood pressure regulation. Given that plasma renin activity does not normally increase until >70 per cent $\dot{V}O_2$ max, these results would appear either to be inconsistent or to represent an abnormality specific to hypertension; more likely neither of these is the case. Since the response in renin and angiotensin II to exercise has not been systematically examined in highly defined, hypertensive populations, this would appear to be the next logical step before drawing conclusions as to its contribution to blood pressure regulation during exercise in these patients.

The Renal Circulation

Pedersen[11] has raised several other pertinent issues that may be operative during exercise. In young *borderline hypertensive* patients, he found resting renal plasma flow to be normal but to be decreased significantly after salt loading or during upright bicycle exercise (450 and 600 kpm/min); this response was not seen as dramatically in control subjects. Thus, an abnormality in regulation of the renal circulation may require exercise in order to be elicited. Moreover, propranolol therapy accentuated this abnormality during exercise but not at rest (supine position). Of equal interest is the fact that these abnormalities were seen at low work loads in the patients but not in the control subjects. The recovery in renal flow following exercise was also significantly delayed and was prolonged even more with administration of propranolol.

These findings emphasize the need to examine (1) the hemodynamic behavior of two important regional circulations (i.e., muscle and kidney), under the physiologic stress of exercise of variable loads and during recovery; (2) their alpha and beta receptor responsiveness; and (3) their vascular structure.

Central Nervous System

The role of the central nervous system in mediating blood pressure control during exercise adds another confounding variable that should also be taken into consideration. Manhem and Hökfelt[23] have examined the results of 8 to 20 weeks of clonidine therapy on the exercise response of the autonomic nervous system in *hypertensive* patients. Clonidine is a central alpha receptor agonist that decreases sympathetic tone while increasing vagal activity. A bicycle work load, based on 80 per cent of the predicted maximum heart rate–work capacity relation, was chosen from a nomogram. After clonidine administration (daily dose, 300 to 600 μg), systolic and diastolic blood pressures and heart rate were reduced during rest and during submaximal exercise. Plasma norepinephrine, which rose severalfold during exercise before the administration of clonidine, was now significantly reduced (40 to 50 per cent). The influence of the central nervous system across the spectrum of systemic hypertension remains to be elucidated.

CLINICAL APPLICATION OF CPX

Incremental CPX testing with the monitoring of arterial blood pressure provides a means to assess the "gain" setting of the cardiac output and vascular resistance control systems, as well as the information to devise more physiologically oriented therapeutic strategies.

The determination of aerobic capacity in patients with hypertension will noninvasively predict the *maximal* cardiac output response to isotonic exercise, because at maximal work loads and with normal oxygen extraction, maximal cardiac output is directly related to maximal $\dot{V}O_2$. However, at submaximal levels of exercise, the cardiac output in patients with hypertension is not easily predicted, because there appears to be considerable heterogeneity in the cardiac output–$\dot{V}O_2$ relation among patients. Thus, the presence of an abnormally elevated blood pressure during the early stages of exercise could be due to an inappropriate rise in cardiac output relative to $\dot{V}O_2$, an inappropriate fall in vascular resistance, or both. Thus, isotonic exercise testing allows one to determine the adequacy of blood pressure control. A measurement of cardiac output (invasively or noninvasively measured with the carbon dioxide rebreathing technique), however, is needed to determine the hemodynamic mechanism responsible for the elevation in blood pressure.

Nevertheless, the noninvasive measurement of aerobic capacity and blood pressure can guide therapeutic decisions, as illustrated in the next two cases.

Figure 14–19 depicts the exercise response for a 61 year old woman with established hypertension. Her aerobic capacity on incremental cycle ergometry was 13 ml/min/kg (class C), whereas her systolic arterial pressure rose from 157 mm Hg at rest to 237 mm Hg at maximum exercise. Because this patient's predicted maximal cardiac output was 4 to 6 liters/min/m², leading us to assume that her systemic vascular resistance would be abnormally elevated, she was given an alpha receptor antagonist, prazosin, for the treatment of her hypertension. Over the next 2 months her resting blood pressure and her systolic and diastolic blood pressure response to exercise were normalized. Shortly thereafter, and because of increased dietary sodium intake, her blood pressure control became less favorable. A repeat CPX demonstrated a fall in aerobic capacity (Fig. 14–20) to 7.5 ml/min/kg (class D). As a result, a diuretic was added to her regimen with the restoration of her functional status to class C

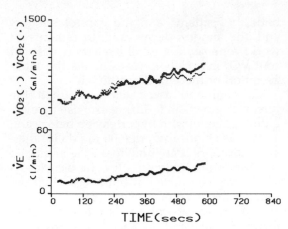

FIGURE 14–20. The same patient shown in Figure 14–19 after a decline in aerobic capacity to cycle exercise. See text.

and the normalization of her resting and exercise arterial pressures.

Class A patients, who comprise the majority of patients with systemic hypertension (Fig. 14–21), have a predicted maximal cardiac output of greater than 8 liters/min/m². Here, class A should be broken down into subgroups A_1, A_2, A_3, and A_4, as indicated in Chapter 11, to better define their maximal cardiac output. An excessive cardiac output gain may be present in both younger and older patients and if so, beta$_1$ blockade would appear to be a logical, albeit unproven therapeutic choice. A noninvasive method of assessing the cardiac output response to exercise, such as that offered by the carbon dioxide rebreathing method,[24] may be a useful approach in the class A patient with essential hypertension.

THERAPEUTIC IMPLICATIONS

A better understanding of the pathophysiologic mechanisms responsible for the appearance of hypertension, as well as the abnormalities that exist in the control logic of cardiac output and vascular resistance throughout the natural course of the disease, would provide useful information from which to develop a more physiologic approach to the management of hypertension and one that could be individualized for any given patient.

Maximum systolic blood pressure during symptom-limited treadmill testing is an important predictor of increased left ventricular mass on 2D echocardiography.[25] This may have important therapeutic implications, as

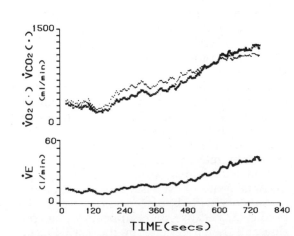

FIGURE 14–19. A class C patient with systemic hypertension performing upright cycle ergometry. See text.

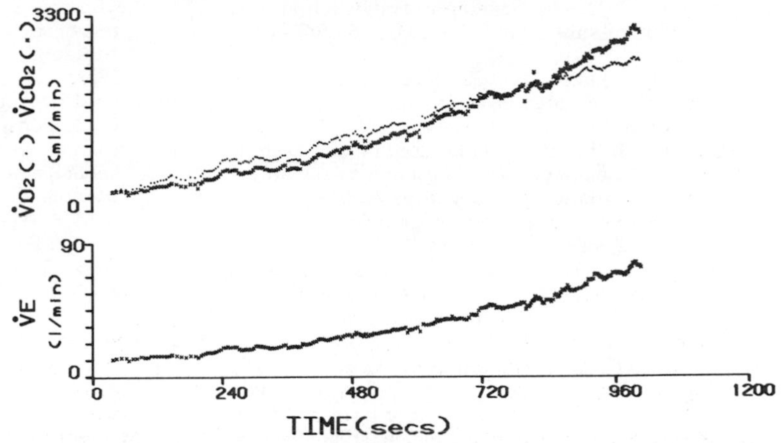

FIGURE 14–21. A patient with systemic hypertension who was functional class A. See text.

many antihypertensive agents do not favorably affect the exercise blood pressure response.

We and others have identified heterogeneity in invasively measured resting and exercise cardiac output and vascular resistance responses during exercise. As noted before, the slope of the cardiac output–$\dot{V}O_2$ relation cannot be predicted from the resting cardiac output. Thus, a noninvasive method of measuring cardiac output during exercise, such as carbon dioxide rebreathing, may provide useful information about an individual patient's cardiac output gain. When combined with the measurement of blood pressure, the individual's entire hemodynamic response at rest and throughout exercise can be determined. What remains to be determined, is whether or not therapy directed at normalizing resting and exercise hemodynamics is more effective than current antihypertensive therapy.

Our therapeutic objective, however, should not be simply to lower blood pressure either during activity or during rest. Our objective should be to *control pressure* and to do so *at rest and during physical activity*. Unfortunately, it is during exercise that our understanding of blood pressure control and its management is weakest. The importance of blood pressure control during the physiologic stress of exercise is underscored by the fact that left ventricular hypertrophy correlates best with ambulatory systolic and diastolic arterial pressures, not with resting systolic pressure.

In simple physiologic terms, hypertension may be viewed as representing an abnormality in the control systems that regulate cardiac output and vascular resistance and in the physiologic variables that are the input

moduli to these systems. In much of this discussion, we have taken a global view of the circulation. The regional responses in vascular resistance, however, are variable. In the kidney, for example, resistance actually rises during exercise, whereas in working muscle it must fall. These discordant responses preserve oxygen delivery relative to oxygen demand, while maintaining arterial blood pressure. Isotonic exercise, which is a useful means of assessing the individual gain settings of these two important regional circulations that participate in blood pressure regulation, may have major therapeutic implications.

REFERENCES

1. Sannerstedt R. Hemodynamic response to exercise in patients with arterial hypertension. Acta Med Scand *180*(Suppl 458):7–101, 1966.
2. Lund-Johansen P. Hemodynamics in early essential hypertension. Acta Med Scand *183*(Suppl 482): 1–105, 1967.
3. Devereux RB, Savage DD, Sachs I, Laragh JH. Relation of hemodynamic load to left ventricular hypertrophy and performance in hypertension. Am J Cardiol *51*:171–176, 1983.
4. Harris P. Evolution and the cardiac patient. Cardiovasc Res *17*:373–378, 1983.
5. Weber KT, Kinasewitz GT, Janicki JS, Fishman AP. Oxygen utilization and ventilation during exercise in patients with chronic cardiac failure. Circulation *65*:1213–1223, 1982.
6. Epstein SE, Beiser GD, Stampfer M, Robinson BF, Braunwald E. Characterization of the circulatory response to maximal upright exercise in normal subjects and patients with heart disease. Circulation *35*:1049–1062, 1967.
7. Astrand P-O. Quantification of exercise capability and evaluation of physical capacity in man. Prog Cardiovasc Dis *19*:51–67, 1976.
8. Amery A, Julius S, Whitlock LS, Conway J. Influence of hypertension on the hemodynamic response to exercise. Circulation *36*:231–237, 1967.

9. Guyton AC. The relationship of cardiac output and arterial pressure control. Circulation 64:1079–1088, 1981.

10. Weber KT, Janicki JS. Cardiopulmonary exercise testing for evaluation of chronic cardiac failure. Am J Cardiol 55:22A–31A, 1985.

11. Pedersen EB. Effect of sodium loading and exercise on renal hemodynamics and urinary sodium excretion in young patients with essential hypertension before and during propranolol treatment. Acta Med Scand 201:365–373, 1977.

12. Henquet JW, Kho TL, Schols M, Thijssen H, Rahn KH. The sympathetic nervous system and the renin-angiotensin system in borderline hypertension. Clin Sci 60:25–31, 1981.

13. Folkow B, Hallback M, Lundgren Y, Sivertison R, Weiss L. Importance of adaptive changes in vascular design for establishment of primary hypertension, studied in man and in spontaneously hypertensive rats. Circ Res 32(Suppl I):I2–I16, 1973.

14. Kotchen TA, Hartley LH, Rice TW, Mougey EH, Jones LG, Mason JW. Renin, norepinephrine and epinephrine responses to graded exercise. J Appl Physiol 31:178–184, 1971.

15. Sleight P, Floras JS, Hassan MD, Jones JV, Osikowska BA, Sever P, Turner KL: Baroreflex control of blood pressure and plasma noradrenaline during exercise in essential hypertension. Clin Sci 57:1695–1715, 1979.

16. Epstein SE, Robinson BF, Kahler RL, Braunwald E. Effects of beta-adrenergic blockade on the cardiac response to maximal and submaximal exercise in man. J Clin Invest 44:1745–1751, 1965.

17. Ibsen H, Julius S. Pharmacologic tools for assessment of adrenergic nerve activity in human hypertension. Fed Proc 43:67–71, 1984.

18. Reybrouck T, Amery A, Billiet L. Hemodynamic response to graded exercise after chronic beta adrenergic blockade. J Appl Physiol 42:133–138, 1977.

19. Fagard R, Amery A, Reybrouck T, Lijnen P, Billiet L. Response of the systemic and pulmonary circulation to alpha- and beta-receptor blockade (labetalol) at rest and during exercise in hypertensive patients. Circulation 60:1214–1219, 1979.

20. Fagard R, Amery A, Reybrouck T, Lijnen P, Moerman E, Bogaert M, de Schaepdryver A. Effects of angiotensin antagonism on hemodynamics, renin, and catecholamines during exercise. J Appl Physiol 43:440–444, 1977.

21. Pedersen EB, Kornerup HJ, Larsen JS. Responsiveness of the renin-aldosterone system during exercise in young patients with essential hypertension. Eur J Clin Invest 11:403–408, 1981.

22. Manhem P, Bramnert M, Hulthen UL, Hökfelt B. The effect of captopril on catecholamines, renin activity, angiotensin II and aldosterone in plasma during physical exercise in hypertensive patients. Eur J Clin Invest 11:389–395, 1981.

23. Manhem P, Hökfelt B. Prolonged clonidine treatment: Catecholamines, renin activity and aldosterone following exercise in hypertensives. Acta Med Scand 209:253–260, 1981.

24. Guyton AC, Jones CE, Coleman TG. Circulatory Physiology: Cardiac Output and its Regulation. WB Saunders, Philadelphia, 1973, pp 38–39.

25. Ren J, Hakki A, Kotler M, Iskandrian A. Exercise systolic blood pressure: a powerful determinant of increased left ventricular mass in patients with hypertension. J Am Coll Cardiol 5:1224–1231, 1985.

ANDREW C. EISENHAUER
PATRICIA A. McELROY
KARL T. WEBER

15

Chronotropic Dysfunction and Exercise

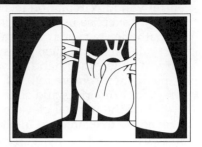

The increase in the oxygen requirements of working skeletal muscle must be accompanied by a proportionate elevation in oxygen delivery. The cardiac output response to exercise is mediated largely by an elevation in heart rate, a response that is well recognized in clinical medicine. Although it is known that pulse rate increases with exercise, the mechanism responsible for this close coupling between heart rate and $\dot{V}O_2$ remains to be elucidated.

Heart rate has been available for study for thousands of years. However, appreciation of the importance of atrial and ventricular synchrony in cardiac rhythm remained obscure until relatively recently. Shortly after electrocardiographic rhythm disturbances were identified, it was recognized that alterations in cardiac rhythm could significantly affect cardiac performance. Conversely, it has become apparent that exercise itself may affect cardiac rhythm. With the advent of antiarrhythmic drugs, artificial cardiac pacemakers, and implantable antitachycardia devices, the examination of the relative contributions of heart rate and rhythm to exercise capacity has taken on new importance.

Based on the concepts developed in previous chapters, it should be apparent that the heart and lungs must function as an integrated metabolic unit to satisfy the gas transport requirements of the tissues. Thus, it is not possible to isolate completely cardiac performance from that of the entire cardiopulmonary unit. In fact, the response of the respiratory system may provide valuable indirect but highly predictive information about the appropriate heart rate response in patients with chronotropic dysfunction. This chapter will review what is known about the normal heart rate response to exercise and its inter-relationship with the other responses of the cardiopulmonary unit during exercise. Abnormalities in cardiac rate or rhythm that compromise the heart's ability to satisfy the oxygen requirements of muscle during physical activity (i.e., *circulatory* failure) will also be considered.

THE NORMAL HEART RATE RESPONSE TO EXERCISE

As indicated in Chapter 1, the sino-atrial (SA) node has the greatest intrinsic automaticity of the heart's pacemaker tissue. It therefore is normally the dominant pacemaker and determines the frequency of the heart's contraction. Depending on a variety of factors, including the patient's posture and arterial blood pressure, the SA node is under varying degrees of sympathetic and parasympathetic control. Hence, at any moment in time, heart rate is an integrated response to multiple contrasting influences. Input moduli to the SA node include those that arise from the central nervous system, peripheral reflexes (e.g., circulatory and visceral reflexes), and circulating humoral substances. Many of these reflexes are pertinent to the control of heart rate during exercise. The *baroreceptor reflex* arises via signals transmitted from the central aorta. It serves to adjust heart rate in inverse proportion to arterial pressure. For example, when arterial pressure rises, heart rate falls, because of enhanced parasympathetic nervous system activity. Alternatively, when pressure falls, a reflexive increase in sympathetic nervous system activity causes an increased heart rate.[1] The *Bainbridge reflex*, which arises from within the central venous circulation, produces a tachycardia as the central venous circulation is distended.

During exercise in the upright posture, the sympathetic nervous system's control of heart rate predominates; parasympathetic activity, on the other hand, is withdrawn. At 70 per cent or more of $\dot{V}O_2$ max, plasma norepinephrine rises and sinus rate increases further. If the normal elevation in heart rate in response to exercise is inhibited (e.g., beta blockade or sinus node dysfunction), the overall circulatory response and delivery of oxygen to working muscle may be compromised. Cardiac output fails to rise appropriately.

The type of exercise, whether isotonic or isometric, also will influence the heart rate response. The heart rate response to each of these forms of exercise needs to be reviewed if diagnostic studies designed to elucidate abnormalities in the chronotropic response to exercise are to be considered.

Isotonic Exercise

During incremental treadmill exercise or cycle ergometry, there is a progressive rise in heart rate with each increment in work load. Heart rate appears to be a linear function of $\dot{V}O_2$. In Figure 15–1, the relationship between heart rate and $\dot{V}O_2$ is given for our incremental treadmill exercise protocol. The protocol has been reviewed in Chapter 9. For patients with cardiac or circulatory failure, a

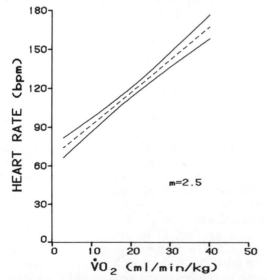

FIGURE 15–1. The linear relation between heart rate and O_2 uptake is shown (broken line) for normal subjects performing incremental treadmill exercise. Solid lines represent confidence interval; m, slope.

similar relation between heart rate and $\dot{V}O_2$ holds true. Thus, the maximum heart rate achieved during treadmill exercise is a function of the maximum work load attained.

Patients with an impaired cardiac output response to exercise (e.g., functional classes C and D) may have a slightly but not dramatically increased heart rate response to treadmill exercise. This finding is in conflict with more traditional views, which suggested that such patients would have a marked tachycardia during all levels of exercise. This finding does not imply that class C and D patients are not dependent on their heart rate response to increase cardiac output; because of their limited stroke volume response, this is indeed the case. However, patients with abnormally elevated heart rate response to exercise (e.g., inappropriate sinus tachycardia) should be identified and considered for pharmacologic therapy, which is aimed at normalizing the resting and exercise heart rate to improve functional status. These issues are discussed more fully hereafter.

In addition to the influence of maximum work load on the maximum heart rate, other factors such as age, sex, the level of physical fitness, and the type of exercise (e.g., arm work versus leg work) are known to be operative in determining the maximum heart rate achieved with exercise.

The effects of cardiac rhythm and rate on the preservation of the cardiac output response to exercise have been examined, but not in a comprehensive fashion. Many of these studies have been performed on subjects at the extreme ends of the spectrum of cardiac performance. Conditioned athletes, for example, may show marked increases in cardiac output with exercise (e.g., a ninefold increase in flow has been recorded).[2] Because cardiac output is the product of heart rate and stroke volume, the augmentation in cardiac output can be accomplished by increases in either or both. Stroke volume can be increased three times in trained athletes and perhaps one and a half times in normal young adults. Given a normal chronotropic response of about threefold at maximum exercise (i.e., a maximum rate of 180 bpm), a normal adult may increase cardiac output four- to fivefold. Thus, in trained athletes and normal subjects, heart rate can account for a 300 per cent increase in cardiac output. In contrast, the augmentation of stroke volume accounts for only a 150 per cent increase in normal subjects.[3]

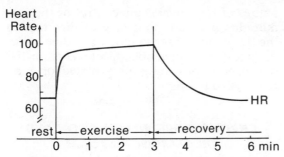

FIGURE 15–2. The response in heart rate to heavy isometric exercise. (From Asmussen E. Similarities and dissimilarities between static and dynamic exercise. Circ Res 48:I3–II0, 1981.)

Isometric Exercise

Isometric exercise is also accompanied by an elevation in heart rate. The extent of this elevation will be a function of the percentage of the maximum voluntary contraction that is achieved. Contractions of 10 to 25 per cent of the maximum are considered *light* work loads; contractions above this value are *heavy* forms of static work. With the onset of either a light or heavy isometric contraction, there is a very prompt elevation in heart rate (Fig. 15–2); as the contraction is sustained, heart rate continues to rise, but more slowly.

For a contraction representing 30 per cent or more of maximum, the initial rapid increase in heart rate is mediated by a withdrawal of vagal tone. Thereafter, the remainder of the slowly progressive tachycardia occurs as a result of enhanced sympathetic activity.[4,5] In all cases, the heart rate response to isometric exercise is greater than that seen for comparable levels of $\dot{V}O_2$ during isotonic exercise. The extent of the elevation in heart rate at the onset of an isometric contraction appears to be a function of the percentage of the maximum contraction that is exerted rather than the muscle mass that is involved in the contraction.

Predicting the Heart Rate Response

Owing to the close functional integration of the heart and lungs based on $\dot{V}O_2$, it is not surprising that isotonically mediated elevations in $\dot{V}O_2$ are accompanied by both an enhanced heart rate and an increased ventilatory response that includes minute ventilation ($\dot{V}_E$). Figure 15–3 depicts the relationship among heart rate, $\dot{V}O_2$, and $\dot{V}_E$ for aerobic levels of isotonic work. It can be seen that the correlation between $\dot{V}_E$ and heart rate is quite good. For anaerobic work loads, a disproportionate rise in $\dot{V}_E$ occurs as a result of lactate production and its buffering by bicarbonate to raise carbon dioxide production. Here, however, the correlation between $\dot{V}_E$ and heart rate is only slightly less precise.

Other physiologic parameters that are closely coupled to the heart rate response to exercise include cardiac output (Fig. 15–4) and mixed venous oxygen saturation (SvO_2) (Fig. 15–5). As $\dot{V}O_2$ rises with exercise, so must oxygen delivery. In order to sustain oxygen transport at a rate that is commensurate with prevailing $\dot{V}O_2$, cardiac output and thereby heart rate must rise accordingly.

FIGURE 15–3. Response to incremental treadmill exercise for a normal subject. The relation between heart rate, $\dot{V}_E$, and $\dot{V}O_2$ is shown for aerobic and anaerobic levels of isotonic (treadmill) exercise. The first 120 seconds are at standing rest.

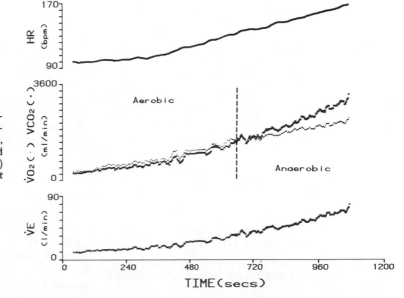

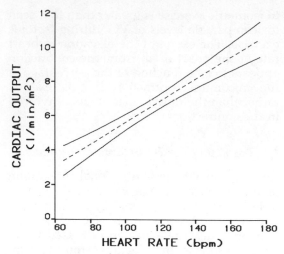

FIGURE 15—4. A direct linear relation exists between isotonic exercise cardiac output and heart rate.

Thus, since mixed venous blood and its percentage saturation of oxygen will reflect oxygen delivery and oxygen extraction (see Chapter 2), any link between the tissues and heart that is mediated by oxygen delivery will be depicted by this relation.

Other parameters, such as mixed venous pH and temperature, may predict heart rate but are likely to be less sensitive than SvO_2 and $\dot{V}_E$, because they will be significantly altered only with heavy work loads.

The relationships among minute ventilation, cardiac output, and heart rate are presented, to demonstrate the highly integrative

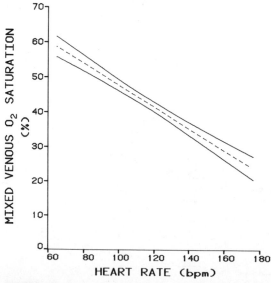

FIGURE 15—5. An inverse relation exists between the isotonic exercise response in mixed venous O_2 saturation and heart rate.

nature of the physiologic control of the cardiopulmonary unit and to give direction to the discussion of sensors that could be incorporated into implantable pacemakers for the purpose of providing physiologic or rate-responsive pacing.

CHRONOTROPIC DYSFUNCTION AND THE EXERCISE RESPONSE

The heart rate response to isotonic exercise should be appropriate for the level of muscular work and $\dot{V}O_2$. In order for this to occur, the SA node must function normally, and the delivery of its impulses to the atrioventricular (AV) node and His-Purkinje system must be appropriate and orderly. When the intrinsic automaticity of the SA node is compromised secondary to ischemic heart disease or an infiltrative myopathic process, heart rate will not rise appropriately. Alternatively, enhanced automaticity, secondary to extraneous factors such as heightened sensitivity of the beta adrenergic receptors of the SA node, will cause an abnormally accelerated sinus rate for any level of work. This circumstance may compromise myocardial relaxation and ventricular filling in patients with heart disease. As a result, their aerobic capacity may be reduced. In patients with atrial fibrillation, effective atrial contraction is lost; this condition may represent an example in which the heart rate response to exercise is too great and in which the effects of the loss of the contribution of the atria to ventricular filling can be examined.

Alternatively, the synchrony of atrial and ventricular contraction may be compromised by disease within the AV node or His bundle. In such atrioventricular block, ventricular and atrial contraction may bear no relation to one another, and as a result, cardiac output falls.

Next, we will review the influences of abnormalities in rate and rhythm on the response to exercise. Each is considered to be an example of chronotropic dysfunction.

Inappropriate Sinus Tachycardia

During the past several years, we have come to recognize a subgroup of patients with chronic stable cardiac failure, often secondary to a dilated cardiomyopathy, who have a resting sinus tachycardia.[6] During low-level treadmill exercise, they have a marked elevation in heart rate. For example, when such patients walk at 1 mph, 0 per cent grade (stage 1), their sinus rate may reach 150 bpm and may rise even further during stages 2 and 3. This is inappropriate in view of the mechanical function and energetics of the failing myocardium. The mechanism of the inappropriate sinus tachycardia at rest and during exercise has not been elucidated, but possible clinical causes, such as hyperthyroidism, anemia, infection, hypoxemia, arteriovenous fistula, pharmacologic agents, or an exacerbation of heart failure, have been excluded. The role of circulating catecholamines, the responsiveness of beta adrenergic receptors, and vagal tone remain to be clarified. Figure 15–6 depicts the heart rate response from standing rest to end exercise for two patients with inappropriate sinus tachycardia. Both had pulse rates of 150 bpm at stage 1 and of 170 bpm at the symptomatic end point (i.e., fatigue) of exercise.

We have been impressed by the response of these patients to small doses of beta adrenergic receptor antagonists, which can be used to normalize the resting and exercise heart rate response. Dramatic, prompt improvements in exercise performance can be seen. The open symbols in Figure 15–6 depict the heart rate response of these patients to low-dose beta blockade with propranolol or metoprolol. In one of the patients, the blockade was effective through several of the early stages of exercise, but heart rate exceeded the expected normal range (broken lines) toward the end of exercise.

Perhaps patients with cardiomyopathy who have been reported to have a beneficial response to beta blockade[7] have a normalization of their heart rate response to exercise; however, this has not been examined. Further study will be needed to determine the pathophysiologic mechanism(s) responsible for inappropriate sinus tachycardia in these patients. Only then can the best therapeutic approach be identified. In the meantime, it is worth evaluating patients with inappropriate sinus tachycardia at rest with incremental, low-level exercise to determine their heart rate response to physical activity. If their heart rate response is dramatically increased, as in the aforementioned patients, then low-dose oral metoprolol (6.25 mg) or propranolol (5 mg) could be given under close clinical observation and dosage titrated upward over the next several days to normalize the resting and exercise heart rate responses.

Atrial Fibrillation

In atrial fibrillation, the atria beat in a rapid, uncoordinated fashion in excess of 340 bpm and no longer serve their transport function to the ventricles. As a result, ventricular filling becomes an entirely passive event. Through a normal mitral valve, this filling is a function of the gradient in pressure

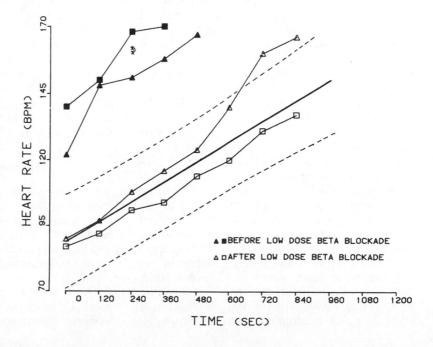

FIGURE 15–6. The heart rate response to incremental treadmill exercise in patients with chronic cardiac failure who had an inappropriate sinus tachycardia at rest and during exercise. Following low dose beta adrenergic receptor blockade, the heart rate response to exercise was normalized. (From Weber KT, Likoff MJ, McCarthy D. Low-dose beta blockade in the treatment of chronic cardiac failure. Am Heart J *104*:877–879, 1982.)

between the atrium and the ventricle. Incomplete transmission of atrial impulses through the AV node retards the ventricular rate somewhat; but without additional pharmacologic suppression of AV conduction, ventricular rate will be inappropriately high (at least 120 bpm). Drugs such as the digitalis glycosides may be used to further suppress AV conduction, which may reduce the resting ventricular rate to 70 to 80 bpm. However, it may be worth examining the heart rate response to exercise in patients with atrial fibrillation in order to judge better the adequacy of atrioventricular blockade.

Occasionally, we have been surprised by patients with long-standing mitral valve disease receiving therapeutic levels of digoxin, who have a dramatic rise in heart rate with low-level exercise. Additional daily doses of digoxin or the addition of small doses of the calcium channel blocker verapamil can be used effectively to slow AV conduction further, which leads to a more appropriate heart rate response to exercise.

Atrial fibrillation is commonly seen in patients with chronic rheumatic mitral valve disease. The characteristics of the mitral valve orifice area are important in determining the hemodynamic consequences of atrial fibrillation and its influence on exercise performance. In patients with mitral valve stenosis and rapid heart rates, reduced left ventricular diastolic filling time becomes the dominant factor in restricting transvalvular flow; the pressure gradient across the valve is of less importance (i.e., flow is proportional to the square root of this gradient). In the clinical setting, the onset of atrial fibrillation in patients with mitral stenosis will often usher in symptoms of pulmonary congestion on exertion that were previously absent.[8] A further analysis of the hemodynamic consequences of atrial fibrillation in these patients may be instructive.

In patients with severe mitral stenosis, obstruction to emptying of the left atrium increases mean left atrial pressure and ultimately results in pulmonary venous and capillary hypertension. Insufficient left ventricular filling may undermine the ability of the ventricle to generate an appropriate forward output or arterial pressure or both. Of course, the degree of impairment of "atrial emptying" or "ventricular filling" depends on transvalvular flow, which is in turn a function of cardiac output, the length of diastole, and mitral valve orifice area. As heart rate increases and diastole shortens, the transval-

vular flow rate must increase in order to maintain constant cardiac output. Obstruction to this flow increases atrial pressure, and if sufficient ventricular filling cannot occur in the diastolic time available, output will fall. In practice, poor forward output is usually associated with left atrial and pulmonary capillary hypertension.

In those patients with mitral stenosis and atrial fibrillation at opposite ends of the spectrum of clinical functional status (asymptomatic patients versus those with pulmonary edema and hypotension), the relative contributions of heart rhythm (loss of atrial transport) and rate (rapid ventricular response) are difficult to study and may not be important. Digoxin probably improves the symptoms from mitral stenosis primarily by slowing the ventricular response. One assumes that a rapid rate may result in a decreased left ventricular filling time. But is this important? Does rate slowing improve cardiac performance? If so, does it improve it to the level of sinus rhythm at an equivalent heart rate, and at what energy cost? Exercise testing may aid in addressing some of these issues.

Figure 15–7 presents the response in respiratory gas exchange during exercise for a patient with mitral stenosis. At the time of the first test, atrial fibrillation was the cardiac rhythm. Exercise duration was short (7 min), the anaerobic threshold occurred early, and maximal oxygen uptake was low. Sinus rhythm had been restored at the time of the second test (Fig. 15–8), without a change in medication. In this case, the exercise duration increased to 17 minutes, maximal oxygen uptake was augmented, and the anaerobic threshold was delayed. In each case, the patient stopped exercising because of fatigue. Note that the maximum ventricular rate achieved during exercise while atrial fibrillation was present exceeds that achieved when the patient was in sinus rhythm.

Atrioventricular Block

An increase in heart rate is important in mediating the normal rise in cardiac output that occurs during physical activities. Patients with complete atrioventricular block and limited chronotropic response to exercise would be expected to have impaired exercise capacity.

There are two general categories of complete AV block: congenital and acquired. The block in the *congenital* form is usually in the

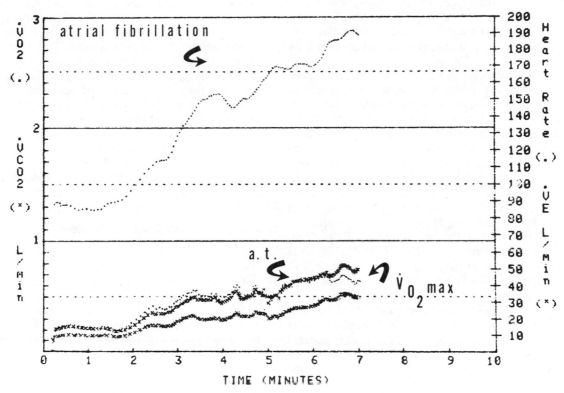

FIGURE 15–7. Response to incremental treadmill exercise in a 32 year old woman with mitral stenosis and atrial fibrillation. Note the rapid elevation in heart rate with low level exercise. a. t., anaerobic threshold.

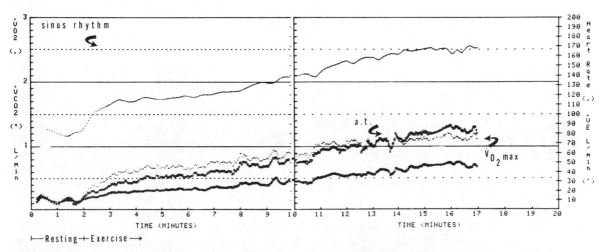

FIGURE 15–8. Response to incremental treadmill exercise for the patient whose record was shown in Figure 15–7 after normal sinus rhythm had been restored. Exercise capacity is significantly improved.

AV node, with the resting ventricular rate between 40 to 60 bpm. In *acquired* AV block, which normally occurs in adults, the defect is usually in the Purkinje system and may be accompanied by trifascicular conduction disturbances. Here the resting ventricular rate is most often <40 bpm.

The management of the neonate with profound bradycardia and symptoms (such as syncope or seizures) is not problematic; pacemaker insertion is indicated. Likewise, in the adult with marked bradycardia (<40 bpm) and symptoms of inadequate cardiac output at rest (e.g., mental sluggishness, congestive heart failure, syncope), treatment is not controversial. Exercise testing may be difficult to perform in these patients, and pacing will markedly improve their functional status.

However, in the less severely ill patient, exercise testing can provide useful insights into the pathophysiology of AV block and the patient's objective functional status.

A limited number of hemodynamic or exercise studies have been performed in children and young adults with congenital heart block.[9-11] The resting cardiac output is normal in most patients. In the presence of bradycardia, normal flow is maintained by cardiac enlargement, with a resultant increase in stroke volume. The resting heart rate, cardiac output, and stroke volume do not predict the response in these parameters during exercise. In general, all patients with congenital AV block will have some increase in ventricular rate and cardiac output during exercise. Stroke volume may increase or remain unchanged. Aerobic capacity, which is a function of maximal cardiac output,[12] is thus related to the combined increases in stroke volume and heart rate. The most limited exercise capacity will be found in patients whose ventricular rate or stroke volume fail to increase with exercise. Exercise testing, with measurement of respiratory gas exchange, is a useful method of objectively assessing functional cardiovascular impairment in terms of aerobic capacity, anaerobic threshold, and heart rate and rhythm responses. Correlation of patient symptoms with these objective measurements may guide therapeutic decisions.

Acquired AV block usually occurs in the adult in the setting of other cardiac disease. The causes of acquired AV block are diverse. Most commonly, AV block is due to coronary artery disease, drug toxicity, or degenerative processes in the conduction system.[13] How-

ever, many other inflammatory and infiltrative processes may cause complete heart block. The resting heart rate is slower than in the congenital form of AV block; often the left ventricle and occasionally the aortic and mitral valves are also diseased. The rise in cardiac output during exercise may then be even more impaired because the diseased ventricle may have limited or no capacity to increase stroke volume. With no ability to increase stroke volume, forward flow is completely dependent on heart rate. Simple ventricular pacing, without rate responsiveness, may result in continued impaired aerobic capacity. Rate-responsive pacing would be most important in these patients.

Sick Sinus Syndrome

Sick sinus syndrome is a disease of the entire pacemaker and conducting systems of the heart, which manifests itself as tachycardia, bradycardia, and combinations of these arrhythmias. It is usually a disease of the elderly, caused by inflammatory or degenerative changes involving the sinus node, AV node, and bundle of His and its branches or distal subdivisions.[14,15] Because it usually affects patients over 50 years old, the majority of these patients will have additional heart disease, most often coronary artery disease.[16]

During supraventricular tachyarrhythmias, the ventricular response may be either rapid or inappropriately slow. At other times, the patient may experience persistent sinus bradycardia or combinations of sinoatrial and atrioventricular block. Thus, the patient may become symptomatic from tachycardia, bradyarrhythmias, or both. Drug suppression of the tachyarrhythmias may exacerbate the bradycardias; therefore, many of these patients require pacemaker insertion in order to control symptoms from slow heart rates and to allow antiarrhythmic therapy to control rapid heart rates.

Exercise testing is a useful method of stressing the cardiovascular system in the patient with sick sinus syndrome and unclear symptoms during physical activity. By monitoring the rhythm during the test, one can determine whether tachycardia or inappropriately slow heart rate occurs with activity. The measurement of aerobic capacity, with the use of breath-by-breath measurement of respiratory gases, allows an assessment of the patient's overall cardiopulmonary function.

CARDIAC PACING

Current cardiac pacemakers, unlike early devices, may be adjusted to affect both heart rate and AV synchrony. The development of this technology has intensified interest in the interrelationship of rate and rhythm. Current cardiac pacing permits management of these two parameters in ways not previously possible. Although the heart and other muscles were known to respond to electrical stimuli since the time of Galvani, electrical therapy for bradyarrhythmia (e.g., primary complete heart block) was first proposed by Hyman in 1930.[17] Zoll[18] developed external transthoracic pacing in 1952. The first "permanent" implantable epicardial fixed rate ventricular pacemaker was developed in the late 1950s.

In subsequent years, however, exercise response in paced patients was of little interest. Clinicians and patients alike were only too happy to have been able to avert the episodic hypotension and seizures that resulted from untreated profound bradycardia. In 1958, Folkman and colleagues[19] published observations on an external device to link ventricular stimulation with atrial contraction, thus creating an "artificial AV node." Interest in this technique heightened when advances in electronics permitted this type of device to be of implantable size. Unfortunately, early experiences with atrial leads were not positive, and the development of a reliable, practical, implantable "AV sequential" device was delayed until the 1970s.

A standardized code for the description was developed,[20] which is given in Table 15–1. Early AV sequential devices were not coupled to atrial activity (DVI; see Table 15–1). Thus, they maintained AV synchrony at rest but could not provide rate responsiveness during exercise. As atrial lead technology and microelectronics improved, a variety of different modes of pacing was developed. In addition, external programming has reached a level of sophistication that permits noninvasive external adjustment of nearly all pacing parameters. The modern dual-chamber device can be programmed to the DDD (see Table 15–2) mode. It can respond to intrinsic atrial or ventricular activity, or both, to preserve AV synchrony and the ventricular response to the atrial rate (Fig. 15–9). However, this sophistication is costly, and therefore investigation of the concepts that support its use has been prompted.

AV Synchrony versus Rate Responsiveness

Normally, the heart maintains a synchronized sequential contraction of the atria and ventricles. Atrial contraction helps to eject blood into the ventricles, augmenting their filling in the later portion of diastole. This contraction produces a transient rise in atrial and ventricular pressures, or the familiar *a* wave seen in atrial pressure tracing, or in the diastolic portion of ventricular pressure tracing (see Fig. 11–6). The preservation of ap-

Table 15–1. *Five-Position Pacemaker Code*

Position	I	II	III	IV	V
Category	*Chamber(s) Paced*	*Chamber(s) Sensed*	*Mode of Response(s)*	*Programmable Functions*	*Special Tachyarrhythmia Functions*
Letters used	V—Ventricle	V—Ventricle	T—Triggered	P—Simple programmable (rate and/or output)	B—Bursts
	A—Atrium	A—Atrium	I—Inhibited	M—Multiprogrammable	N—Normal rate competition
	D—Double	D—Double	D—Double*	C—Multiprogrammable with telemetry	S—Scanning
		0—None	0—None R—Reverse†	0—None	E—External
Manufacturer's designation only	S—Single-chamber‡	S—Single-chamber‡			

*Atrial triggered and ventricular inhibited.
†Activated by tachycardia and (usually) bradycardia.
‡Can be used for atrial or ventricular pacing; a manufacturer's designation.

Table 15–2. Pacing Rate Control Parameters

Parameter	Available Sensor	Pace-maker
Primary Metabolic		
Catecholamines	N/A	N/A
Oxygen consumption	N/A	—
Secondary Metabolic		
Sinus rate	Atrial elecrode	DDD
QT interval	RV electrode	CE
Stroke volume	RV dipole	Ext
Oxygen saturation	RV oximeter	Ext
pH	RV pH electrode	CE
Temperature	RV thermister	Ext
Respiratory Rate	Thoracic dipole	CE
Exercise		
Body motion	Piezoelectric sensor	CE

CE = Experimental device undergoing clinical evaluation.
Ext = External experimental system.
N/A = None available.
DDD = Standard dual chamber devices.

propriately timed atrial contraction can serve to augment cardiac performance. This graphic observation has been made repeatedly since the beginning of cardiac catheterization, and its clinical importance was recognized as early as 1916 by Gessell.[21] It has been shown that atrial or appropriate atrioventricular (DVI) pacing generally improves mean arterial pressure in patients requiring pacing for peri-operative bradycardia or AV block.[22] In these patients, it is important not only that AV synchrony be maintained but also that the timing of atrial contraction be appropriate. Occasionally, physicians may institute atrial pacing for postoperative bradycardia, secure in the hope that atrial pacing with 1:1 AV conduction will be beneficial. However, if severe first-degree AV block also exists, atrial contraction may come too early (i.e., against a closed AV valve) to preserve effective atrial transport. DVI pacing with an appropriate "physiologic" AV delay can restore the benefits of AV synchrony.

Similar observations have been made relating improved cardiac output with preservation of AV synchrony in patients with myocardial infarction,[23] hypertrophic cardiomyopathy,[24] and dilated cardiomyopathy.[25]

Observations in the catheterization laboratory or the postoperative cardiac unit, however, may not be representative of what occurs in awake, active, upright individuals. Parameters of primary importance during cardiac illness normally assume secondary roles. Further, parameters that appear important when changed acutely may be unimportant chronically when normal compensatory mechanisms are operative. For example, syncope is usually the result of episodic high-degree AV block in the ambulatory patient. Yet many patients with transient high-degree AV block during the course of an inferior myocardial infarction do not develop symptoms. Typically, acute high-degree AV block may be much more significant in the awake, otherwise-well ambulatory patient than in the patient who is supine and at rest. In addition, there exist patients (infant and adult) with congenital complete heart block and normal ventricular function who are completely without symptoms. The implications and consequences of this chronic rhythm differ from those whose occurrence is episodic and acute in the presence of left ventricular dysfunction. Further, in third-degree AV block, although AV *dissociation* exists, there is frequently fortuitous *association* of atrial and ventricular contractions. This can occur in as many as 30 to 40 per cent of systoles (Fig. 15–10). The onset of atrial fibrillation, with its abolition of effective atrial contraction, removes these fortuitous events. Therefore, clinical deterioration of patients with chronic third-degree AV block may coincide with the development of atrial fibrillation.

There also may exist differences in chronicity, venous capacity, reflex vascular tone, myocardial contractility, or tissue require-

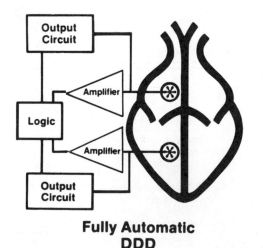

Fully Automatic DDD

✱ = **Stimulation**
○ = **Sensing**

FIGURE 15–9. A modern dual chamber pacing system can be programmed to the DDD mode. It can sense and pace both atria and ventricles. In addition, logic circuitry relates and coordinates these activities.

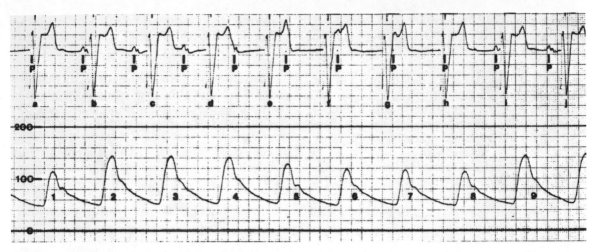

FIGURE 15–10. Fortuitous A-V association. Tracing from a patient with VVI pacemaker and 3 degree A-V block. Note P waves preceding QRS complexes b, c, d, and i, and the corresponding aortic systolic pressure of 150 mm Hg in beats 2, 3, 4, and 9. Functional "normal sinus rhythm" is present in four of nine complexes.

ments that determine the consequences of a bradyarrhythmia. Thus, rather than simply considering arterial pressure or cardiac output in supine acute observations, it is much more appropriate to examine the effects of heart rate and rhythm on cardiac performance in ambulatory individuals. In this regard, although DVI pacing has been shown to be of benefit in supine patients, no reliable studies have shown acute improvement in the exercise capacity of patients with DVI versus VVI pacing (see Table 15–1). Further, no studies of chronic benefits are available. It should be remembered that neither of these modes of pacing permits atrial "tracking" or the timely stimulation of the ventricle in response to an increase in atrial rate.

The development of VAT, VDD, and finally, DDD pacing permitted the maintenance of AV synchrony *and* rate responsiveness. Serious doubts still remain about which patients benefit from these devices versus the simpler (and less expensive) VVI systems. Further, questions exist concerning whether this benefit is the result of AV synchrony or of rate responsiveness.

A pioneering study in this regard is that of Kruse and co-workers.[26] Sixteen patients with programmable pacing systems were randomly assigned to VVI or VDD for 3-month periods in a single-blind protocol. Chest x-rays and exercise tests were done and a subjective questionnaire administered. Several days later, catheterization was performed and hemodynamic data recorded at rest and exercise. Reprogramming to the alternative mode (VVI to VDD, or VDD to VVI)

was accomplished and a repeat invasive study performed in 2 hours. The entire process was repeated 3 months later.

Patients chronically paced in the VVI mode showed significantly poorer symptom-limited work capacity than did those in chronic VDD, in which atrial transport and rate responsiveness were preserved. The comparison of chronic VDD with acute VVI revealed less of a difference. The authors concluded that, rather than adapting to simple ventricular pacing, the cardiovascular system continuously deteriorated. Interestingly, the exercise stroke volume (at a given work load) of VVI patients exceeded that of VDD patients. In contrast, the stroke volume of VDD patients at rest exceeded that of VVI patients, suggesting that with VVI pacing the heart attempted to compensate for a lack of rate responsiveness with an increase in stroke volume. Cardiac output was higher in VDD patients at rest and during all phases of exercise. Eleven of 16 patients reported subjective improvement in their general condition during their randomization to the VDD mode. Considerable increases in arteriovenous oxygen difference and lactate accumulation were noted with exercise in the VVI mode, commensurate with compromised cardiac output response. $\dot{V}O_2$ unfortunately was not measured, and thus, the level of work at the subjective cessation of exercise was not precisely determined. However, this study provides convincing evidence in this group of patients that VDD pacing improved cardiovascular performance.

Additional studies have shown improved

Doppler cardiac output at rest with DDD pacing compared with VVI pacing[27] and an improvement in exercise duration in the DDD mode, but without significant increase in maximal oxygen uptake or delay of anaerobic threshold.[28]

Although hemodynamic improvement at rest from dual-chamber pacing may be from preservation of atrial transport, hemodynamic improvement with exercise may be related to heart rate responsiveness. Fananapazir and colleagues[29] demonstrated identical improvement in work capacity when patients' ventricular pacing rates were adjusted externally and asynchronously to equal those of VAT pacing. Although muscular work was estimated from patients' body weight, speed, and treadmill incline and not measured by determining $\dot{V}O_2$, this landmark study clearly suggested that the chronotropic response is a more important determinant of work capacity than the maintenance of AV synchrony.

Several studies of patients done in our laboratory suggest that these data can be confirmed when respiratory gas exchange is measured, as illustrated in Figure 15–11.

Unfortunately, the controversy between

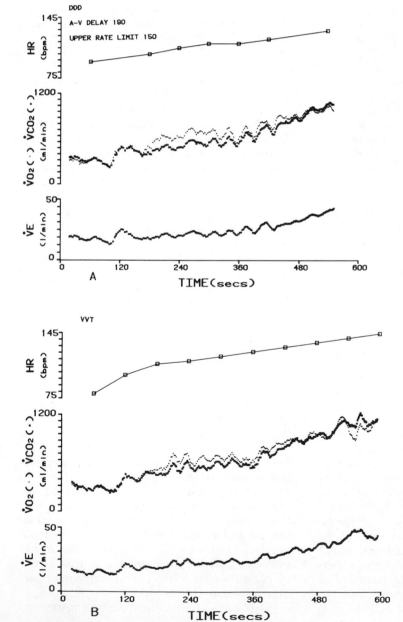

FIGURE 15–11. In A, cardiopulmonary exercise testing was performed on a patient with a dual chamber pacemaker programmed to the DDD mode with an upper rate limit of 150. In B, the heart rate was externally altered with the pacemaker in the VVT mode (triggered by skin electrodes and an external pacing device) to stimulate the rate response in A. The CPX results are similar, suggesting in this patient a greater contribution of heart rate than A-V synchrony to the preservation of cardiac performance.

the importance of AV synchrony and rate responsiveness is yet more complicated. Nearly every exercise study of exercise pacing hemodynamics employs patients with a variety of cardiac diseases. Variations in ventricular function, intrinsic inotropic reserve, sinus node responsiveness, degree of pacemaker dependence and presence of retrograde ventriculo-atrial (VA) conduction are commonly not addressed in such studies. In addition, little information is known concerning how to optimize AV delay, and thus "normal" values of 150 to 200 msec are usually employed. Individualized adjustment of this interval, however, may be appropriate given our observations depicted in Figure 15–12.

It is therefore possible that certain patients with dual-chamber devices are deriving benefits only from the rate-responsiveness of these devices and that atrial contraction cannot augment the stroke volume of an already diseased heart during exercise.

On balance, the evidence suggests that atrial transport is most important at rest and that adequate exercise performance is most closely correlated with an appropriate rate response.

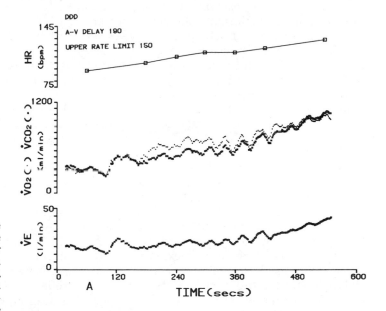

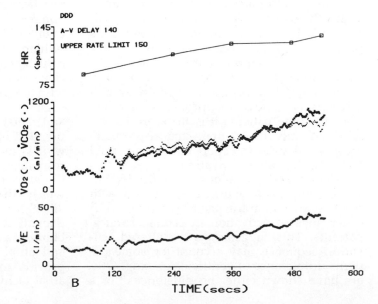

FIGURE 15–12. Cardiopulmonary exercise tests at different A-V delays (upper rate limits) in a patient with a dual chamber pacemaker programmed to the DDD mode. Note the reduced anaerobic threshold in B, where the A-V delay is inappropriately short. This testing may permit more accurate individualized selection of A-V delay (see text).

The Role of Vascular Reflexes

Despite the general conclusion reached earlier, there may be individual patients in whom the atrial "kick" provides additional benefit other than that of simply augmenting ventricular filling. Why is it, for example, that many patients with VVI devices function normally with normal exercise tolerance for many years, whereas others are burdened by fatigue, exercise intolerance, and even dizziness or syncope that coincide with the onset of ventricular pacing. Still others develop the "pacemaker syndrome" of extreme fatigue, exercise intolerance, a fixed cardiac output, and cannon *a* waves in the jugular venous pulse. Perhaps, in these groups, the loss of atrial transport is less important than the interruption of the normal pattern of vascular reflexes or ventricular activation.

Alicandri and associates[30] proposed that the pacemaker syndrome exists in patients with sustained retrograde (VA) conduction during ventricular pacing and that it is mediated via atrial stretch receptors that reduce peripheral vascular resistance inappropriately. It was further postulated that VA conduction creates an inappropriately timed atrial contraction and pressure profile that accounts for cannon *a* waves and reflex hypotension. Similarly, patients with carotid sinus hypersensitivity may still suffer syncope or lightheadedness (despite pacemaker therapy), owing to a vasodepressor reflex that is activated. It remains unexplained why these reflex mechanisms, if they are responsible, do not fatigue after repeated stimulation. Of further interest is the observation that the onset of atrial fibrillation may ameliorate the symptoms of the pacemaker syndrome.[31] Erlebacher and colleagues[32] have postulated a direct atrial vasodepressor reflex activated by inappropriately timed atrial stretch to explain this response. Atrial fibrillation might interrupt such a pathway and could thus remove inappropriate vasodilation. In some patients it is therefore important not only to maintain the appropriate mechanical atrial transport but also to avoid inappropriate atrial activation.

Raichlen and colleagues[33] recently demonstrated improved ventricular function with right ventricular apical pacing compared with other sites of activation in cardiac surgical patients. This suggests that an altered activation sequence may account for some patients' intolerance of ventricular pacing. Others have shown either no differences[34] or a significant alteration in cardiac index,[35] with varying sites of activation.

For the most part, aerobic capacity is determined by appropriate heart rate response to exercise rather than by maintenance of atrial transport. There remain individuals, however, whose hearts require AV synchrony for adequate exercise performance. There is a complex interplay of atrial and ventricular contractile reserve, diastolic mechanics, cardiac reflexes, and heart rate in the patient's response to exertion. The challenge of the next decade will be to identify and study these interactions and to develop therapy of bradyarrhythmias that more nearly simulates the normal physiologic mechanisms.

Criteria for Physiologic Pacing

In most instances, appropriate heart rate response is one of the most important factors in maintaining exercise capacity. It is unknown what parameters best reflect optimal heart rate at a given level of exercise. The answer has obvious implications in the design of rate-responsive pacemakers.

Table 15–2 presents a summary of current parameters that have been shown by various investigators to reflect the heart's rate response to exercise. The sympathetic nervous system is responsible, in part, for mediating this response in upright human beings. Monitoring of catecholamine levels or actual measurements of sympathetic drive could reflect a factor with a significant influence on sinus rate and inotropy. No real-time sensors for these parameters exist; however, development of these sensors is not inconceivable. Of interest is that a pacemaker driven in this fashion would respond not only to exercise-related changes in catecholamines but also to changes related to anxiety, elation, or drugs with adrenergic activity.

Other less direct measurements of neural and metabolic controls already exist. Measurement of atrial rate is, of course, the most widely used technique for providing rate responsiveness. In patients with heart block, the *atrial* rate has been assumed to be that which the cardiovascular system would "like" for ventricular contraction. However, patients with DDD pacemakers may have a blunted sinus rate increase[36] with exercise and atrial tracking and may therefore not provide an optimal rate profile. In addition, atrial tachyarrhythmias may be sensed, and

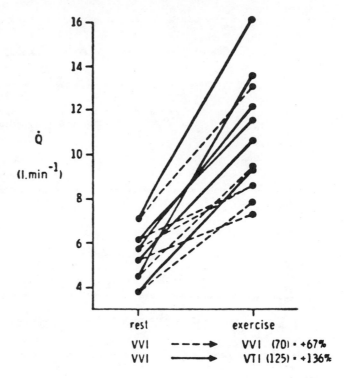

$\dot{Q}$

$(l.min^{-1})$

rest   exercise

VVI - - - → VVI (70) · +67%
VVI ———→ VTI (125) · +136%

FIGURE 15–13. Marked improvement in exercise cardiac output is noted in these patients with QT scanning rate-responsive pacing. (From Rickards AF, Norman J. Relation between QT interval and heart rate. New design of physiologically adaptive cardiac pacemaker. Br Heart J 45:56–61, 1981.)

inappropriately rapid ventricular pacing may result. Also, atrial sensing is not possible in the patient with atrial fibrillation. Nevertheless, atrial sensing remains the primary method by which rate responsiveness is achieved.

A simple impedance system has been developed[37] that can measure instantaneous intracardiac volume. It has the potential to be adapted to control cardiac pacing. This concept, although simple in theory, relies on volume changes induced by circulating catecholamines, sympathetic drive, or increased venous return.

The QT interval of the electrocardiogram or cardiac electrogram is controlled by intrinsic heart rate and circulating catecholamines. Thus, changes in QT interval reflect heart rate response, and this ultimately can be used to drive a pacemaker. The interval can be measured accurately using the same electrode for pacing and sensing. Rickards and Norman[38] have developed an implantable system undergoing clinical trials. This system has resulted in impressive improvements in exercise cardiac output thus far (Fig. 15–13). Despite the fact that the absolute QT interval varies among individuals and that the QT interval may be affected by drugs (e.g., quinidine), QT interval change appears to be a promising rate-related parameter.

Most aerobic exercise involves body mo-

tion. Activity sensors have been developed that detect muscular activity, filter the resulting signal, and employ certain frequencies to judge the level of patient activity.[39] An implantable system has shown good correspondence with the normal sinus node rate in continuous monitoring tests (Fig. 15–14), and clinical trials are underway. Possible disadvantages to such a system include poor sensitivity to isometric exercise and oversensitivity to local effects (e.g., tapping the area of implant).

Other exercise-related parameters, including mixed venous pH,[40] oxygen saturation,[41] and respiratory rate[42] have been proposed. To date, the activity related, QT interval, and respiratory rate sensing pacemaker systems are the only rate-responsive systems undergoing significant clinical trials.

In most instances, exercise is the major circumstance requiring an increased heart rate. Fever, anxiety, and hypovolemia are all less common and less important. Parameters that reflect exercise response are therefore logical to consider when planning control of pacing rate. Many physiologic parameters appear to reflect changes corresponding with exercise-related heart rate. In addition, the type of exercise itself will influence the heart rate response. The challenge of the future will be to continue to study the interaction of exercise with cardiac performance and to

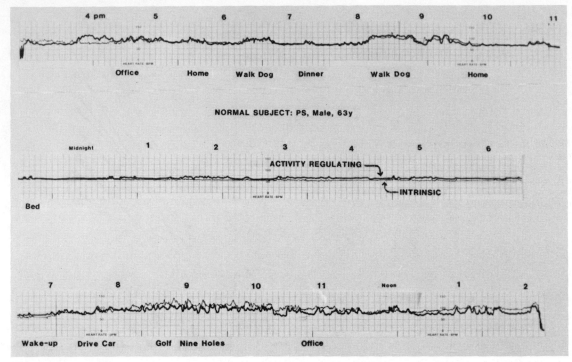

FIGURE 15–14. Rate output of an activity-related pacemaker strapped to a normal subject's chest compared with his heart rate histogram (i.e., Holter monitor). Note good correlation of rates with gross physical activity. Less correlation is obtained with other stresses.

design more physiologically appropriate pacemaker therapy.

REFERENCES

1. Bard P. Regulation of the systemic circulation, *in* VB Mountcastle, (ed). Medical Physiology. CV Mosby Co, St Louis, 1968, pp 178–208.
2. Hermansen L, Ekblom B, Saltin B. Cardiac output during submaximal and maximal treadmill and bicycle exercise. J Appl Physiol 29:82–89, 1973.
3. Rickards AF, Donaldson RM. Rate responsive pacing. Clin Prog Pac Electrophysiol 1:12–19, 1983.
4. Asmussen E. Similarities and dissimilarities between static and dynamic exercise. Circ Res 48:I3–I10, 1981.
5. Martin CE, Shaver JA, Leon DF, Thompson ME, Reddy PS, Leonard JJ. Autonomic mechanisms in hemodynamic responses to isometric exercise. J Clin Invest 54:104–115, 1974.
6. Weber KT, Likoff MJ, McCarthy D. Low-dose beta blockade in the treatment of chronic cardiac failure. Am Heart J 104:877–879, 1982.
7. Waagstein F, Hjalmarson A, Varnauskas E, Wallentin I. Effect of chronic beta-adrenergic receptor blockade in congestive cardiomyopathy. Br Heart J 37:1022–1028, 1975.
8. Wood P. An appreciation of mitral stenosis. Br Med J 1:1051–1113, 1954.
9. Taylor MRH, Godfrey S. Exercise studies in congenital heart block. Br Heart J 34:930–935, 1972.
10. Manno BV, Hakki AH, Eshaghpour E, Iskandrian AS. Left ventricular function at rest and during exercise in congenital complete heart block: a radionuclide angiographic evaluation. Am J Cardiol 52:92–94, 1983.
11. Ikkos D, Hanson JS. Response to exercise in congenital complete atrioventricular block. Circulation 22:583–590, 1969.
12. Weber KT, Janicki JS. Cardiopulmonary exercise testing for evaluation of chronic cardiac failure. Am J Cardiol 55:22A–31A, 1985.
13. Zipes DP. Specific arrhythmias: diagnosis and treatment, *in* Braunwald E (ed). Heart Disease, A Textbook of Cardiovascular Medicine. WB Saunders, Philadelphia, 1985, pp 735–736.
14. Bharati S, Nordenberg A, Bauernfiend R, Varghese JP, Carvalho AG, Rosen KM, Lev M. The anatomic substrate for the sick sinus syndrome in adolescents. Am J Cardiol 46:163–172, 1980.
15. DeMoulin JC, Kulbertus HE. Histopathological correlates of sinoatrial disease. Br Heart J 40:1384–1389, 1978.
16. Simonsen E, Nielson JS, Nielson BL. Sinus node dysfunction in 128 patients: a retrospective study with follow-up. Acta Med Scand 208:343–348, 1980.
17. Hyman AS. Resuscitation of the stopped heart by intracardiac therapy. Arch Int Med 46:553–557, 1930.
18. Zoll PM. Resuscitation of the heart in ventricular standstill by external electric stimulation. N Engl J Med 247:768–771, 1952.
19. Folkman MJ, Watkins E Jr. An artificial conduction system for the management of experimental complete heart block (abstr). Surg Forum 8:331, 1958.

20. Parsonnet V, Furman S, Smyth NPD. A revised code for pacemaker identification. PACE 4:400–403, 1981.

21. Gessell RA. Cardiodynamics in heart block as affected by auricular systole, auricular fibrillation and stimulation of the vagus nerve. Am J Physiol 40:267–313, 1916.

22. Hartzler GO, Maloney JD, Curtis JJ, Barnhorst DA. Hemodynamic benefit of atrioventricular sequential pacing after cardiac surgery. Am J Cardiol 40:232–236, 1977.

23. Chamberlain DA, Leinbach RC, Vassaux CE, Kasktor JA, DeSanctis RW, Sanders CA. Sequential atrioventricular pacing in heart block complicating acute myocardial infarction. N Engl J Med 282:577–582, 1970.

24. Shemin, RJ, Scott WC, Kaste DG, Morrow AG. Hemodynamic effects of various modes of cardiac pacing after operation for idiopathic hypertrophic subaortic stenosis. Ann Thorac Surg 27:137–140, 1979.

25. Benchimol A, Ellis JC, Dimond EG. Hemodynamic consequences of atrial and ventricular pacing in patients with normal and abnormal hearts. Am J Med 39:911–922, 1965.

26. Kruse I, Arnman K, Conradson TB, Ryden L. A comparison of the acute and long-term hemodynamic effects of ventricular inhibited and atrial synchronous ventricular inhibited pacing. Circulation 65:846–855, 1982.

27. Stewart WJ, DiCola VC, Harthrone JW, Gillam DL, Weyman AE. Doppler ultrasound measurement of cardiac output in patient with physiologic pacemakers: effects of left ventricular function and retrograde ventriculoatrial conduction. Am J Cardiol 54:308–312, 1984.

28. DiCola VC, Hand R, Boucher CA, Kanarek D, Okada R, Pohost GM, Harthrone JW. Exercise cardiopulmonary assessment with dual chamber versus ventricular pacing (abstr). 7th World Congress of Pacing. Vienna, Austria. PACE 6:311, 1983.

29. Fananapazir L, Bennett DH, Monks P. Atrial synchronized ventricular pacing: Contribution of the chronotropic response to improved exercise performance. PACE 6:601–608, 1983.

30. Alicandri C, Fouad FM, Tarazi RC, Castle L, Morant F. Three cases of hypotension and syncope with ventricular pacing. Possible role of atrial reflexes. Am J Cardiol 42:137–142, 1978.

31. Vera Z, Mason DT, Awan NA, Mueller RR, Tarrzen D, Tonken M, Visman LA. Improvement of symptoms in patients with sick sinus syndrome by spontaneous development of stable atrial fibrillation. Br Heart J 39:160–165, 1977.

32. Erlebacher JA, Danner R, Stelzer PE. Hypotension with ventricular pacing: an atrial vasodepressor reflex in human beings. JACC 4:550–555, 1984.

33. Raichlen JS, Campbell FW, Edie RN, Josephson M, Harken A. The effect of site of placement of temporary epicardial pacemakers on ventricular function in patients undergoing cardiac surgery. Circulation 70:I118–I123, 1984.

34. Benchimol A, Liggett MS. Cardiac hemodynamics during stimulation of the right atrium, right ventricle and left ventricle in normal and abnormal hearts. Circulation 33:933–944, 1966.

35. Barold S, Linhart J, Hildner F, Samet P. Hemodynamic comparison of endocardial pacing of outflow and inflow tracts of the right ventricle. Am J Cardiol 23:697–701, 1969.

36. Griffin JC, Spencer WH, Castrion R, Nelson AP, Schwenemeyer T. Exercise capacity of patients receiving DDD pacemakers (abstr). PACE 7:40, 1984.

37. Baan J, Jong TT, Kerkhoe PM, Moene RJ, Van Dijk AD, van der Velde ET, Koops VJ. Continuous stroke volume and cardiac output from intraventricular dimensions obtained with an impedance catheter. Cardiovasc Res 15:328–334, 1981.

38. Rickards AF, Norman J. Relation between QT interval and heart rate. New design of physiologically adaptive cardiac pacemaker. Br Heart J 45:56–61, 1981.

39. Anderson K, Humen D, Klein GJ, Brumwell D, Huntley S. A rate variable pacemaker which automatically adjusts for physical activity (abstr). PACE 6:A12, 1983.

40. Camilli L, Alcidi L, Papeschi G. A new pacemaker autoregulating the rate of pacing in relation to metabolic needs (abstr). in Cardiac Pacing. Proceedings of the 5th International Symposium. Excerpta Medica, Amsterdam, p 414, 1977.

41. Wirtzfeld A, Goedel-Meinen L, Block T, et al. Central venous oxygen saturation for the control of automatic rate responsive pacing. PACE 5:829–835, 1982.

42. Ionescu VL. An "on demand pacemaker" responsive to respiratory rate (abstr). PACE 3:375, 1980.

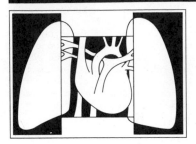

16

LARRY C. CASEY
KARL T. WEBER

Chronic Lung Disease and Chest Wall Deformities

As we indicated in Chapter 5, there is a linear relationship between minute ventilation and oxygen consumption for aerobic levels of work. For anaerobic work, $\dot{V}_E$ increases out of proportion to $\dot{V}O_2$, because of increased lactic acid production, lactate buffering by bicarbonate, and the corresponding increase in carbon dioxide production. The increase in $\dot{V}_E$, therefore, is more in proportion to $\dot{V}CO_2$.

In a normal subject at the end of maximal exercise, $\dot{V}_E$ is approximately 50 per cent of the maximal voluntary ventilation (MVV) achieved at rest, and the maximum tidal volume is about 50 percent of the vital capacity. These responses indicate the large ventilatory reserve that normally exists and that is not entirely used. Thus, exercise is not normally limited by ventilation. In patients with lung disease, these ventilatory reserves are reduced and other factors may be responsible for the limitation to exercise. Under these circumstances, exercise is ventilation limited. This chapter will examine the respiratory factors that may limit exercise performance and review the response to exercise in patients with various expressions of lung disease. Finally, we will consider how deformities of the thorax, such as kyphoscoliosis or pectus excavatum, also create a ventilation-limited response to exercise.

RESPIRATORY FACTORS LIMITING EXERCISE

The cardiovascular system normally limits maximal aerobic exercise, as we have shown in earlier chapters. In patients with lung disease, exercise performance may be limited by the ventilatory system for several reasons:[1] (1) altered lung mechanics, (2) impaired gas exchange, (3) the development of pulmonary hypertension, and/or (4) respiratory muscle fatigue.

Lung Mechanics

In normal subjects, resting $\dot{V}_E$ occupies a small fraction of the MVV; at maximum levels of work, the ratio of maximum $\dot{V}_E$ to MVV is 50 per cent, or in most cases <60 per cent, again indicating a large ventilatory reserve. Maximum exercise ventilation can be predicted from the FEV_1 (see Chapter 5) obtained by standard pulmonary function testing or by comparison with the MVV. In normal individuals, the maximal predicted exercise $\dot{V}_E$ is approximately equal to 35 percent of FEV_1. In patients with a reduced FEV_1, maximum $\dot{V}_E$ is also reduced. Since there is a linear relationship between $\dot{V}_E$ and $\dot{V}O_2$ for aerobic levels of work, if patients stop exercising as a result of having reached their maximal ventilation, then this will occur at a reduced level of $\dot{V}O_2$. In fact, frequently, patients with lung disease will not even reach an anaerobic threshold and rarely, if ever, their $\dot{V}O_2$ max.

During normal breathing at rest, the flow-volume loop of a tidal volume is well within the maximal forced expiratory flow-volume loop. In patients with airway obstruction, the flow-volume loop may approach the loop generated during a maximal effort (Fig. 16–1), even during tidal breathing at rest.[2] During exercise, there is a proportional increase in both respiratory rate and tidal volume in normal subjects (Fig. 16–2).[3] In patients with airway disease, because of abnormal elast-

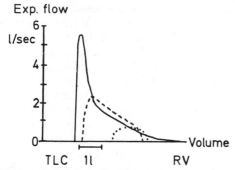

FIGURE 16–1. Maximal expiratory flow-volume curve (solid line), together with the flow-volume curve during breathing at rest (dotted line) and during exercise (dashed line), in a patient with obstructive lung disease. TLC, total lung capacity; RV, residual volume. (From Grimby G, Elgefors B, Oxhoj H. Ventilatory levels and chest mechanics during exercise in obstructive lung disease. Scand J Respir Dis 54:45–52, 1973.)

ance and resistance of the lung, an increased time is required for adequate inflation and deflation. It therefore can be expected that the increased respiratory rate seen during exercise will result in areas of the lung being inadequately ventilated. Also, it is possible that the next breath will occur prior to the completion of exhalation, thus leading to air trapping.

The prospect of air trapping is further supported by examining the response in intrapleural pressure during exercise. Normally, during maximal exercise, transpulmonary pressure does not exceed that generated during a forced vital capacity. In patients with airflow obstruction, there is a reduced maximal recoil pressure of the lung and a leftward shift of its pressure-volume curve. Since elastic recoil pressure is a major determinant of maximal expiratory flow, this

may account for the reduced expiratory flow rate. The reduced expiratory flow rate in conjunction with the increased respiratory rate contributes to air trapping. This circumstance has also been confirmed by demonstrating an increase in intrapleural pressure in patients with obstructive lung disease.[3]

Gas Exchange

During exercise, arterial hypoxemia has been demonstrated in healthy persons exercising at high altitudes, and in patients with either restrictive or obstructive lung disease exercising at sea level. An increase in alveolar-arterial oxygen gradient can result from any combination of worsening ventilation/perfusion inequality, anatomic shunt, diffusion limitation, or all three. Diffusion limitation is unlikely to play a significant role except in extreme situations, such as severe restrictive lung disease during maximal exercise or maximal exercise in normal subjects at high altitude. In patients with obstructive airway disease, there is no demonstrable diffusion limitation to oxygenation.

In patients with airway disease, the primary mechanism for exercise-induced hypoxemia is ventilation/perfusion mismatch. This occurs as the result of the abnormal time constants for airflow, which lead to areas of the lung that are underventilated with respect to their perfusion (low $\dot{V}/Q$ ratio).

The abnormally low $\dot{V}/Q$ ratios can contribute to carbon dioxide retention and hypercapnia at rest, or during exercise, or both. The development of carbon dioxide retention depends on a complex relationship between the ventilatory drive (i.e., sensitivity to in-

FIGURE 16–2. Changes in tidal volume and breathing frequency with increasing levels of ventilation during exercise. (From Pardy RL, Hussain SNA, Macklem PT. The ventilatory pump in exercise. Clin Chest Med 5:35–49, 1984.)

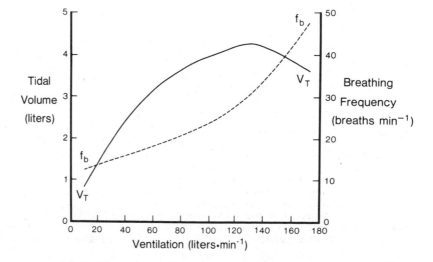

creased carbon dioxide production), and the ventilatory capacity of these patients. An increase in carbon dioxide production would require an increase in alveolar ventilation and $\dot{V}_E$ in order to maintain a constant $PaCO_2$ (Fig. 16–3). The increase in $\dot{V}_E$ required to maintain a normal $PaCO_2$ requires an increase in the work of breathing, and thus in $\dot{V}O_2$. Interestingly, some patients "choose" to adopt a higher $PaCO_2$, rather than to increase their ventilation to a rate necessary to maintain $PaCO_2$ within normal limits. The explanation for this divergent response remains to be elucidated. A reduced ventilatory response at a higher $PaCO_2$ results in a reduced level of work of breathing compared with that of patients who have similar degrees of airway obstruction and increased dead space–to–tidal volume ratio but who "choose" to maintain a normal $PaCO_2$. Generally speaking, the development of hypercapnia does not result in limitation of exercise, whereas the development of hypoxemia may contribute to exercise limitation.

Pulmonary Hypertension

Normally, during exercise, the increase in cardiac output results in an insignificant increase in pulmonary artery pressure, as noted in Chapter 2. The modest degree of pulmonary vascular impedance has been postulated to be the result of both an increase

in the diameter of the perfused blood vessels (*horizontal recruitment*) and an increase in the number of perfused capillaries (capillaries that were not perfused at a lower cardiac output, and termed *vertical recruitment*). Patients with lung disease may have a decrease in the capillary bed of the pulmonary circulation, thus limiting the number of capillaries available for vertical recruitment or decreased distensibility of existing vessels, or both, where horizontal recruitment would be limited. Patients who develop arterial oxygen desaturation during exercise have hypoxia-mediated pulmonary vasoconstriction. In either case, the net result is an increase in pulmonary vascular resistance, which, for a given pulmonary blood flow, results in a higher pulmonary artery pressure. Pulmonary vascular resistance has been described more fully in Chapter 13.

An increase in pulmonary vascular resistance can result in decreased left ventricular filling, both through a decreased volume reaching the left ventricle and a decreased end-diastolic volume of the left ventricle secondary to displacement of the interventricular septum by the high right ventricular pressure. In addition, in patients with airway disease who develop air trapping and an increase in their functional residual capacity (FRC), the increased pleural pressure will also be transmitted to the pulmonary arteries, thus contributing to an increase in the pulmonary artery pressure and pulmonary vascular resistance. Collectively, these disturbances in the ventilatory system would create a state of circulatory failure at rest or, more commonly, during exercise.

An increase in pulmonary artery pressure may contribute to the limitation of exercise performance by a stretch receptor mechanism leading to the sensation of dyspnea and/or by a decreased cardiac output leading to a decreased mixed venous oxygen tension, which exacerbates the $\dot{V}/Q$ mismatch resulting in arterial hypoxemia.[3]

Respiratory Muscle Fatigue

Another mechanism by which exercise may be limited is via fatigue and/or weakness of the respiratory muscles.[1, 3, 4] During ventilation at rest or even during moderately increased ventilation (as with exercise in patients with normal lungs) the respiratory muscles consume little oxygen. During strenuous exercise, however, the $\dot{V}O_2$ of the respiratory muscles may increase to as much as

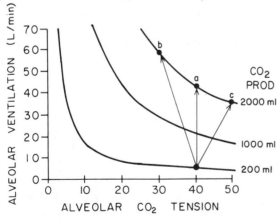

FIGURE 16–3. Relationship between alveolar ventilation and alveolar CO_2 tension for various rates of CO_2 production. Point *a* denotes the increase in alveolar ventilation that must occur when there is a tenfold increase in CO_2 production in order to maintain a constant $PaCO_2$; point *b* illustrates the increase in aveolar ventilation when the $PaCO_2$ is decreased by 10 mm Hg; and point *c* is the response when the $PaCO_2$ is allowed to increase by 10 mm Hg. (From Wasserman K. Breathing during exercise. N Engl J Med 298:783, 1978.)

1.0 liter/min. On the other hand, in patients with obstructive lung disease, the $\dot{V}O_2$ of the respiratory muscles increases rapidly with increasing $\dot{V}_E$ (see Fig. 5–11) and may represent 40 per cent of the total body $\dot{V}O_2$. In order to achieve this increased $\dot{V}_E$, oxygen delivery (blood flow) must also increase. Here, the respiratory muscles may "steal" blood flow and oxygen that is potentially available for other working muscles, and thus may contribute to exercise limitation.[3, 4]

Respiratory muscle fatigue is defined as the inability of the respiratory muscles to continue generating a given pleural pressure. Many studies have demonstrated that normally the MVV is sustainable for only 15 to 30 sec, whereas 75 per cent of the MVV can be sustained for 4 minutes and 60 per cent of the MVV can be sustained for 15 minutes (Fig. 16–4). It is obvious that patients with lung disease who have a reduced FEV_1 will exceed 50 per cent of their MVV very quickly and that they may have limited exercise capacity on the basis of respiratory muscle fatigue.

The precise mechanism of respiratory muscle fatigue is unknown but could include (1) inhibition of neural drive, (2) failure of transmission across neuromuscular junctions, (3) excessive force and duration of contraction, (4) impaired muscle blood supply, (5) impaired excitation-contraction coupling, or (6) depletion of muscle energy stores.[4] The major cause of fatigue appears to be within the cell, involving the excitation-contraction coupling mechanism and muscle energy metabolism.[4]

A final mechanism by which respiratory muscle function may become impaired during exercise in patients with airway disease is via lengthening of the muscle fibers. The force-length relationship indicates that a muscle that is stimulated at its optimal length produces its maximum contractile force. If the muscle either is stretched beyond the optimal resting length or is foreshortened prior to contraction, maximal stimulation produces submaximal force.[3, 4] At lung volumes above FRC, the diaphragm and the other inspiratory muscles are foreshortened, and thus their maximal contractile force is reduced. In contrast, at low lung volumes, expiratory muscle force is reduced. In patients with airway disease, the increased FRC will place the respiratory muscles in an unfavorable length-tension relationship and thus reduce the generated muscular force.[3, 4]

EXERCISE TESTING IN OBSTRUCTIVE LUNG DISEASE

At the present time, insufficient information is available to provide true guidelines for determining when, or which, patients with airway disease should have a cardiopulmonary exercise test. In general, the most common evaluation for CPX in patients with airway disease is to determine if they develop arterial oxygen desaturation during exercise.

Oxygen therapy decreases pulmonary artery pressure and hematocrit, improves psychologic function, and decreases mortality in patients with obstructive lung disease.[3, 5] Generally, it is recommended that patients with a resting PaO_2 of less than 55 mm Hg should receive oxygen therapy. Those patients who have an arterial PaO_2 of greater than 55 mm Hg while breathing room air may also benefit from home oxygen therapy if they develop arterial oxygen desaturation during exercise or during sleep. Recently, it has been demonstrated that a measured diffusing capacity (D_{LCO}) of less than 55 per cent of the predicted value is a good predictor of arterial oxygen desaturation during exercise.[3, 5] An alternative method for selecting those patients with airway disease who should undergo exercise testing is to evaluate the patient for signs of chronic hypoxemia. If there is cor pulmonale, pulmonary hypertension, an elevated hematocrit, or alterations in higher cortical neurologic function,

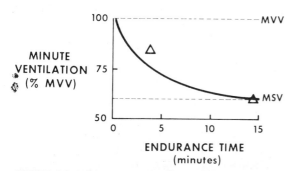

FIGURE 16–4. The relationship between minute ventilation and endurance time. The dotted lines represent 60 and 100 per cent of the maximal voluntary ventilation (*MVV*). The triangles represent data from patients with obstructive airway disease. The solid line is the best fit curve of data from normal subjects, which appears to asymptotically approach 60 per cent of the MVV; this is designated the maximum sustainable ventilation (*MSV*). (From Rochester DF, Arora NS, Braun NM, Goldberg SK. The respiratory muscles in chronic obstructive pulmonary disease (COPD). Bull Physiopathol Respir (Nancy) *15*:951–975, 1979.)

then exercise testing and sleep studies should be performed to determine if oxygen desaturation occurs.

There are a variety of different methods of performing exercise tests, including steady state or progressive incremental bicycle and treadmill exercise. These are discussed in Chapter 9. The optimal method for testing patients with airway disease is not well defined. In general, several factors must be kept in mind. First, depending on the severity of the obstructive lung disease, the test may be over within 2 to 3 minutes after starting exercise. In general, we use an incremental work load every 1 minute while on a cycle ergometer. The increments in work load are 6.25 watts and represent the lowest amount of work to which the ergometer can be adjusted. In some patients, we have found it advantageous simply to perform endurance testing with the patient pedaling under no load.

An additional technical problem that must be considered in patients with a reduced FEV_1 is the difference between breath-by-breath analysis versus analysis of mixed expired gas. While breath-by-breath analysis is preferable, the equipment is more expensive and may not be available. The problem with the analysis of mixed expired gas is the size of the mixing chamber. The average volume of a mixing chamber is 5 liters. The volume of the mixing chamber influences the time that is required for a change in exhaled oxygen/carbon dioxide at the mouth piece to be reflected by a change in exhaled oxygen/carbon dioxide at the mixing chamber. This means that 15 liters of ventilation (3 × volume of the box) is required before the oxygen/carbon dioxide analyzers will detect such a change. At low levels of ventilation, this can produce a substantial phase-lag, wherein the changes in the analyzer oxygen/carbon dioxide do not correspond with the measured changes in tidal volume, respiratory rate, and arterial oxygen saturation. To correct this problem, a phase-lag correction must be made, or the volume of the mixing chamber must be decreased. These modifications need to be evaluated and verified prior to conducting an exercise test in the clinical laboratory.

In 1971, Jones and associates[6] reported the effects of exercise in 50 men with obstructive lung disease. They found relationships among the maximal work load, the patients' ages, and the severity of their airway obstruction, as assessed by the FEV_1 (Fig. 16–5) and

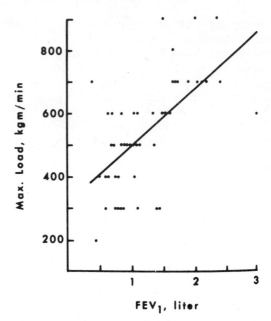

FIGURE 16–5. Relationship of maximal work in the progressive step test to FEV_1 in 50 patients with COPD. (From Jones N, Jones G, Edwards R. Exercise tolerance in chronic airway obstruction. Am Rev Respir Dis *103*:477–491, 1971.)

D_{LCO} (Fig. 16–6). A multiple linear regression analysis was performed, which demonstrated that maximal work = $563 - (5.4 \cdot age) + (142\ FEV_1) + (7.5\ D_{LCO})$. In addition, there was a relationship between the pa-

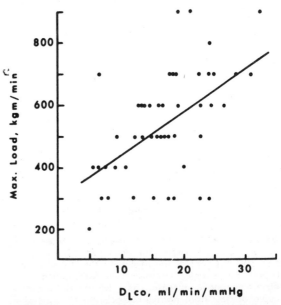

FIGURE 16–6. Relationship of maximal work in the progressive exercise test to pulmonary diffusing capacity for carbon monoxide (D_{LCO}) in 50 patients with COPD. (From Jones N, Jones G, Edwards R. Exercise tolerance in chronic airway obstruction. Am Rev Respir Dis *103*:477–491, 1971.)

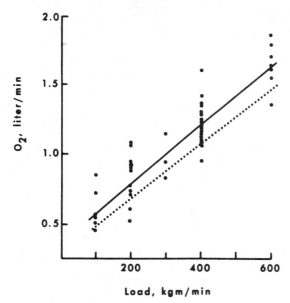

FIGURE 16–7. Oxygen consumption related to steady state work. The regression lines are for 50 patients with COPD (solid line) and normals (dotted line). (From Jones N, Jones G, Edwards R. Exercise tolerance in chronic airway obstruction. Am Rev Respir Dis *103*:477–491, 1971.)

tient's dyspnea grade index and the resulting maximum load. These findings demonstrate an inter-relationship among symptoms, work capacity, and exercise performance, which is one that has not been established for pulmonary function testing performed at rest.

Figure 16–7 shows the change in $\dot{V}O_2$ with increasing load for both normal subjects and patients with airway disease.[6] The patients with airway disease had a higher $\dot{V}O_2$ at rest, and their $\dot{V}O_2$ remained greater than that of the control subjects during increasing work loads. One aspect of this relationship not presented in this graph is that because of ventilatory limitation, patients with airway disease stop at a reduced level of $\dot{V}O_2$, whereas the normal subjects could have continued to a higher level of work.

Figure 16–8 shows the changes in $\dot{V}_E$ with increasing $\dot{V}O_2$ in patients with airway disease.[7] Patients with emphysema (closed circles) had a higher ventilation for a given level of $\dot{V}O_2$ than did patients with chronic bronchitis. Again, the reader is referred to Figure 5–11, which illustrates the relationship be

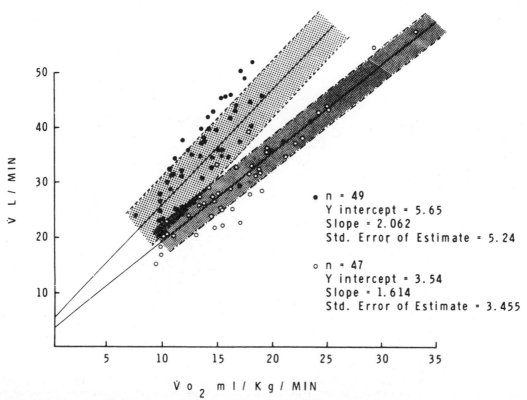

FIGURE 16–8. The relationship between ventilation and oxygen consumption in patients with emphysema (solid circles) and chronic bronchitis (open circles). (From Marcus J, McLean R, Duffell G, Ingram R. Exercise performance in relation to the pathophysiologic types of chronic obstructive pulmonary disease. Am J Med *49*:14–22, 1970.)

tween $\dot{V}_E$ and $\dot{V}O_2$ in normal subjects, in order to appreciate that in patients with airway disease there is a reduced effort tolerance or $\dot{V}O_2$ and that for any given level of $\dot{V}O_2$, $\dot{V}_E$ is greater than in normals. Furthermore, it should be appreciated that these patients will have reached their maximal predicted $\dot{V}_E$, whereas normal subjects will have reached only approximately 50 per cent of their MVV.

The changes in the volume contribution of the rib cage versus those of the abdomen are shown in Figure 16–9. This figure demonstrates that patients with airway disease have a greater increase in FRC than do healthy individuals during exercise.[2] This is consistent with the previously explained mechanism of air trapping during exercise.

The pattern of breathing in patients with obstructive lung disease can be derived from the relationship between tidal volume and $\dot{V}_E$ (Fig. 16–10). In patients with airway dis-

ease, tidal volume increases progressively to its maximum (approaching FVC), with a slower rise in respiratory rate compared with the normal response.[8] In patients with severe airway disease, a further increase in $\dot{V}_E$ is not possible by an increase in respiratory rate, and as a result exercise ceases.

Jones,[9] in 1966, described the changes in arterial blood gases during exercise in patients with emphysema or chronic bronchitis. He found that patients with severe emphysema had a significant fall in PaO_2, whereas patients with chronic bronchitis actually had an increase (Fig. 16–11). The patients with severe emphysema had a lower D_{LCO}, suggesting more alveolar capillary destruction. The improvement in oxygenation in patients with chronic bronchitis was thought to be the result of improved ventilation in areas of the lung that had had low $\dot{V}/\dot{Q}$ ratios.

The D_{LCO}, as previously discussed, is a good predictor of those patients who will

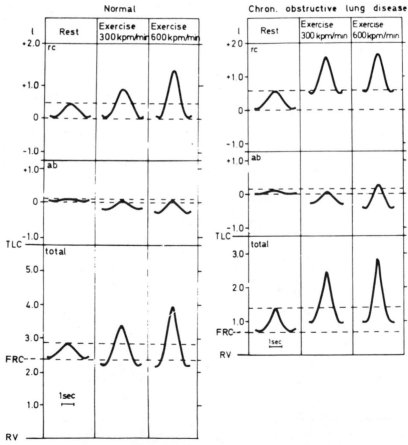

FIGURE 16–9. Changes in the volume contribution of the rib cage (*rc*) and the abdomen (*ab*) at rest and with exercise in normal subjects and patients with COPD. The dashed lines represent the end-expiratory and end-inspiratory levels during tidal breathing at rest. Note that in patients with COPD there is an increase in the functional residual capacity (*FRC*) during exercise. (From Grimby G, Elgefors B, Oxhoj H. Ventilatory levels and chest mechanics during exercise in obstructive lung disease. Scand J Respir Dis 54:45–52, 1973.)

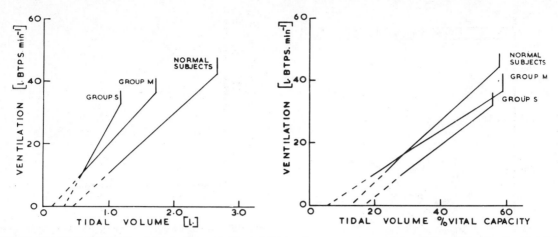

FIGURE 16–10. Relationship of tidal volume (left) and tidal volume as a percentage of the vital capacity (right) in normal subjects and in patients with mild (Group M) or severe (Group S) obstructive lung disease. (From Spiro S, Hahn H, Edwards R, Pride N. An analysis of the physiologic strain of submaximal exercise in patients with chronic obstructive bronchitis. Thorax 30:415–425, 1975.)

develop exercise-induced arterial oxygen de-saturation.[3, 5] Those patients with a D_{LCO} less than 55 per cent of predicted will most likely have desaturation with exercise. Thus, most patients with significant emphysema will de-velop arterial oxygen desaturation with ex-ercise. In patients with chronic bronchitis, the response is much more variable and seems to depend on the severity of the air-way obstruction as well as on the presence of resting hypoxemia and hypercapnia.

Patients with airway disease frequently have an elevated dead space–to–tidal volume ratio (VD/VT) at rest. With exercise, because of the increased tidal volume, the VD/VT ratio usually decreases. However, in some patients, the VD/VT ratio actually increases. When this occurs, it is an indicator of a ventilatory rather than a cardiac limitation to exercise.

Patients with airway disease tend to have a higher heart rate at rest than do age-matched normals.[8] During exercise, the heart rate for a given level of $\dot{V}O_2$ tends to be higher in patients with airway disease than in normals (Fig. 16–12). However, it should

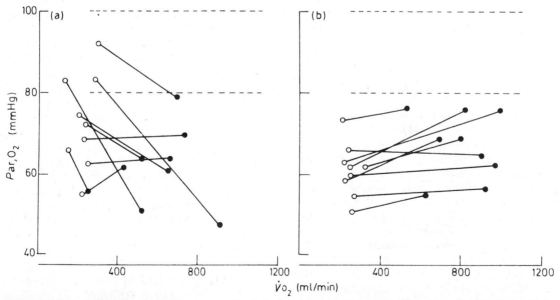

FIGURE 16–11. Arterial PaO$_2$ at rest (open circles) and during exercise (solid circles) in patients with emphysema (left) and chronic bronchitis (right). (From Jones N. Pulmonary gas exchange during exercise in patients with chronic airway obstruction. Clin Sci 31:39–50, 1966.)

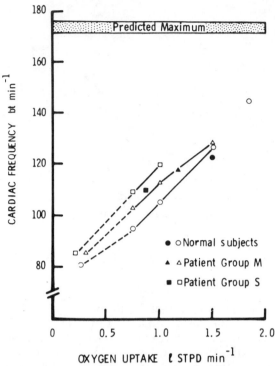

FIGURE 16–12. Cardiac frequency as a function of oxygen consumption in normal subjects and in patients with mild (Group M) or severe (Group S) COPD. Patients with COPD tend to have a higher heart rate than do normal subjects. (From Spiro S, Hahn H, Edwards R, Pride N. An analysis of the physiologic strain of submaximal exercise in patients with chronic obstructive bronchitis. Thorax 30:415–425, 1975.)

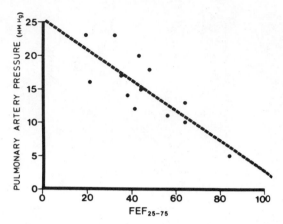

FIGURE 16–13. Changes in the pulmonary artery pressure as a function of changes in pulmonary function. The maximal midexpiratory flow rate is expressed as per cent predicted of maximal midexpiratory flow rate (FEF 25–75). (From Wright J, Lawson L, Pare P, et al. The structure and function of the pulmonary vasculature in mild chronic obstructive pulmonary disease. Am Rev Respir Dis 128:702–707, 1983.)

be pointed out that at maximal exertion, patients with obstructive lung disease do not reach their maximum predicted heart rate.

Several investigators have found a significant relationship between the maximal midexpiratory flow rate and the resting pulmonary artery pressure (Fig. 16–13).[10] In normal subjects, exercise causes a minor elevation in the pulmonary artery pressure and an increase in both right and left ventricular ejection fractions (Fig. 16–14). However, in patients with airway disease, exercise produces a much larger increase in pulmonary artery pressure, a variable change in right ventricular ejection fraction, and a normal increase in the left ventricular ejection fraction (Fig. 16–15). Thus, mild to moderate exercise will increase the pulmonary artery pressure, resulting in an increased pressure load on the right ventricle.[11]

Although the pulmonary capillary wedge pressure is generally normal in patients with airway disease at rest, with exercise it tends to increase. The interpretation of the changes in both pulmonary artery pressure and pulmonary capillary wedge pressure must be done carefully, because in patients with airway disease and in the case of air trapping, there is an increase in the mean intrathoracic pressure that can be transmitted to the pulmonary arteries. For patients in whom there is any doubt about the response in wedge pressure, and thereby the assessment of left ventricular dysfunction, CPX can be repeated with the measurement of pleural (esophageal) pressure.

Some patients with airway disease do develop an inappropriately low mixed venous oxygen saturation during exercise.[3] This suggests that there is inadequate oxygen delivery for the level of $\dot{V}O_2$. Considering that patients with airway disease have a ventilatory limitation to exercise at a very reduced work load, this would suggest that oxygen delivery was inappropriate. Inadequate oxygen delivery could be caused by either an inadequate increase in cardiac output or arterial oxygen desaturation, or both. Although this has not been well characterized, it is thought that there is an appropriate increase in the left ventricular ejection fraction and cardiac output in these patients. Thus, the low SvO_2 has been attributed to arterial oxygen desaturation.[9, 10] However, a low SvO_2 may also cause arterial hypoxemia.

EXERCISE TESTING IN RESTRICTIVE LUNG DISEASE

In general, the major indication for exercise evaluation of patients with known interstitial

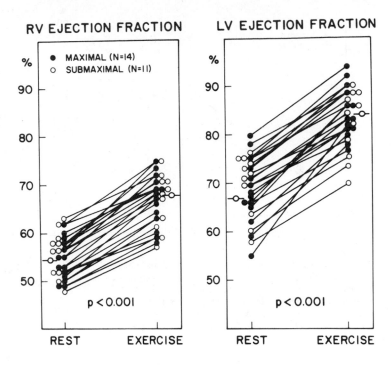

FIGURE 16–14. Right ventricular (*RV*) and left ventricular (*LV*) ejection fraction at rest and during exercise in 25 normal subjects. Both right and left ventricular ejection fractions increased by at least 5 per cent in all subjects. (From Matthay R, Berger, H, Davis R, et al. Right and left ventricular exercise performance in chronic obstructive pulmonary disease: Radionuclide assessment. Ann Intern Med 93:234–239, 1980.)

lung disease is the development of arterial oxygen desaturation. The evaluation of exercise performance may also be useful in patients who complain of dyspnea out of proportion to their pulmonary function studies or who have dyspnea and an abnormal chest x-ray but normal pulmonary function studies.[3]

Patients with interstitial lung disease tend to breathe at a higher respiratory rate and lower tidal volume than do normal subjects. Because they have a reduced FEV_1 and MVV, they are exercise-limited by ventilation. Figure 16–16 shows that patients with sarcoidosis or fibrosing alveolitis have a higher level of ventilation for a given $\dot{V}O_2$ than do

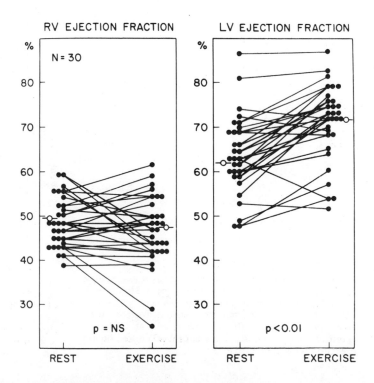

FIGURE 16–15. Right ventricular (*RV*) and left ventricular (*LV*) ejection fraction at rest and during exercise in 30 patients with COPD. Note that unlike the case with normal subjects (Fig. 16–14) there is no consistent increase in the right ventricular ejection fraction; in fact, in about one third of the patients there was even a decrease. (From Matthay R, Berger H, Davis R, et al. Right and left ventricular exercise performance in chronic obstructive pulmonary disease: Radionuclide assessment. Ann Intern Med 93:234–239, 1980.)

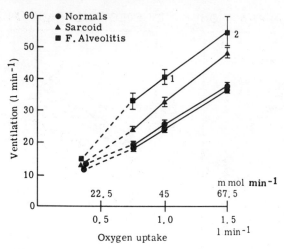

FIGURE 16–16. Relationship of minute ventilation at rest and at submaximal oxygen consumption in normal individuals and in patients with sarcoidosis or fibrosing alveolitis. (From Spiro S, Dowdeswell I, Clark T. An analysis of submaximal exercise response in patients with sarcoidosis and fibrosing alveolitis. Br J Dis Chest 75:169–180, 1981.)

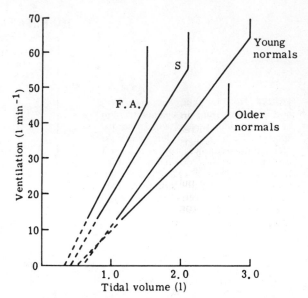

FIGURE 16–18. Relationship of tidal volume and ventilation during exercise in normal subjects and in patients with restrictive lung disease (*S*, sarcoidosis, *FA*, fibrosing alveolitis). The maximal tidal volumes reached are indicated by the inflexions, after which ventilation increased only by increasing the respiratory rate. (From Spiro S, Dowdeswell I, Clark T. An analysis of submaximal exercise response in patients with sarcoidosis and fibrosing alveolitis. Br J Dis Chest 75:169–180, 1981.)

normal individuals.[12] The exercise response of a 36 year old woman with advanced sarcoidosis and exertional dyspnea is shown in Figure 16–17. The increase in total ventilation is at least in part due to an increase in the physiologic dead space (VD/VT) both at rest and during exercise. Plots of VT against $\dot{V}_E$ demonstrate little or no increase in tidal volume with increasing $\dot{V}_E$ (Fig. 16–18). How-

ever, when corrected for differences in vital capacity, patients with interstitial lung disease fall within the range of normal individuals (Fig. 16–19).

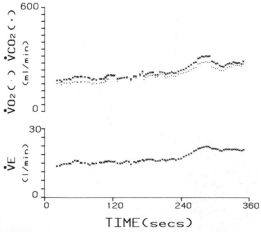

FIGURE 16–17. The response in respiratory gas exchange and ventilation to exercise is shown for a 36 year old woman with sarcoidosis and severe ventilatory dysfunction. A brief period of symptom-limited exercise (6.25 watts), which began after 4 minutes of rest, is shown. Arterial O_2 desaturation to 83 per cent was noted during exercise by ear oximetry.

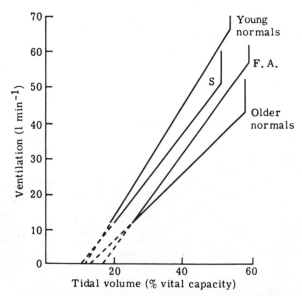

FIGURE 16–19. Relationship of tidal volume as a per cent of vital capacity and ventilation during exercise. The groups are the same as in Figure 16–18. (From Spiro S, Dowdeswell I, Clark T. An analysis of submaximal exercise response in patients with sarcoidosis and fibrosing alveolitis. Br J Dis Chest 75:169–180, 1981.)

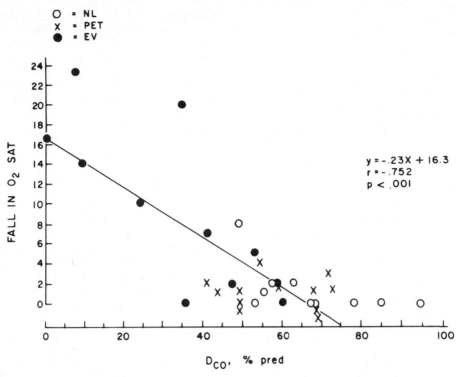

FIGURE 16–20. Resting diffusing capacity (D_{LCO} predicted) is compared with the fall in O_2 saturation during exercise in patients with interstitial lung disease who had either a normal exercise tolerance (*NL*), reduced maximal exercise tolerance (*PET*), or a reduced maximal exercise tolerance plus excessive ventilation during exercise (*EV*). (From Kelley MA, Daniele RP: Exercise testing in interstitial lung disease. Clin Chest Med 5:145–156, 1984.)

Patients with interstitial lung disease tend to have an abnormally elevated VD/VT at rest that does not decrease during exercise. Their $PaCO_2$ tends to remain normal or to decrease, suggesting adequate alveolar ventilation.[12] As in patients with airway disease, the D_{LCO} is a good predictor of arterial oxygen desaturation during exercise in patients with interstitial lung disease.[3] Figure 16–20 shows a graph of the resting D_{LCO} (per cent predicted) and the resulting fall in arterial oxygen saturation at maximal exercise. Most patients with a D_{LCO} below 60 per cent develop desaturation. Other studies have also demonstrated the fact that if a patient has a normal D_{LCO}, they are unlikely to develop exercise-induced arterial oxygen desaturation. Therefore, these results suggest that the D_{LCO} can be used to screen patients for exercise studies.[3]

Patients with interstitial lung disease tend to have a resting tachycardia.[12] With exercise, unlike patients with chronic cardiac failure, there is a disproportionate increase in the heart rate (Fig. 16–21). Other studies have demonstrated a normal cardiac output during constant work rate exercise in patients with interstitial lung disease. The reason for the resting and exercise high heart rates have not been explained completely but may be the result of an elevated pulmonary artery pressure or arterial oxygen desaturation.

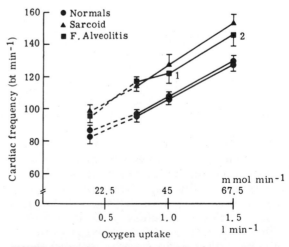

FIGURE 16–21. Mean values for cardiac frequency at rest and during submaximal levels of oxygen consumption in normal subjects and in patients with either sarcoidosis or fibrosing alveolitis. (From Spiro S, Dowdeswell I, Clark T. An analysis of submaximal exercise response in patients with sarcoidosis and fibrosing alveolitis. Br J Dis Chest 75:169–180, 1981.)

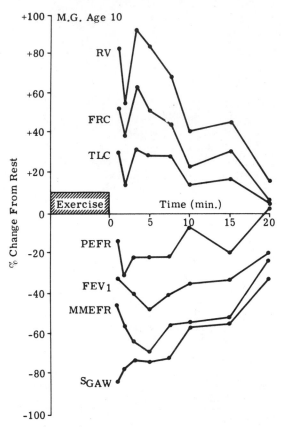

FIGURE 16–22. Time course of the changes in lung volumes and airway resistance (peak expiratory flow rate, PEFR); FEV_1; maximal midexpiratory flow rate (MMEFR); and specific airway conductance (S_{GAW}) after stopping exercise in a patient with exercise-induced bronchoconstriction. (From Anderson S, McEvoy J, Bianco S. Changes in lung volumes and airway resistance after exercise in asthmatic subjects. Am Rev Respir Dis *106*:30–36, 1973.)

EXERCISE TESTING IN REACTIVE AIRWAY DISEASE

Generally speaking, exercise testing is most commonly performed on patients with known asthma for research purposes. The main usefulness of CPX is for the patient who is not known to have asthma but who complains of mild dyspnea or coughing or both after moderate to strenuous exercise. Frequently, this will occur in the winter, when breathing cold, dry air, or following a viral upper respiratory tract infection. In these patients when a diagnosis cannot be made clinically, an exercise test may be indicated.

Conducting an exercise test to evaluate exercise-induced bronchoconstriction requires a slightly different protocol than that used for patients with airway or interstitial lung disease.[3, 13, 14] Running tends to produce more bronchospasm than does cycling; therefore, a treadmill should be used. The likelihood of bronchospasm, and the degree of bronchospasm can be maximized by having the patient breathe compressed air, which has zero per cent humidity. This, of course, may result in a severe episode of bronchospasm, which should be treated with inhaled beta$_2$ agonists. Generally, the exercise test must be fairly strenuous, consisting of 6 minutes of exercise at 80 to 90 per cent of the aerobic capacity. Pulmonary function testing with serial FEV_1 and forced vital capacity measurements are performed before the exercise test and then every 5 minutes after the exercise test for an additional 15 to 20 minutes. The rationale behind this approach is that exercise-induced bronchospasm occurs after stopping exercise.

Normally, exercise produces bronchodilatation. This is true even in patients with asthma. However, bronchoconstriction may develop anywhere from 1 to 15 minutes after the exercise has stopped (Fig. 16–22).[13] Furthermore, exercise also blunts the bronchoconstrictive effects of inhaled histamine.[14] This is illustrated in Figure 16–23. Figure 16–24 depicts flow-volume curves for eight patients with asthma immediately after exercise. All patients had a decrease in their FEV_1 that was reversible by an inhaled beta$_2$ agonist.[15] Furthermore, the postexercise–induced bronchoconstriction can be reversed by a second episode of exercise (Fig. 16–25).

Although extensively evaluated, the mechanism of exercise-induced bronchoconstriction has not been fully elucidated. It appears to be the result of respiratory heat loss or drying of the respiratory tract, or both. How this produces bronchoconstriction is unknown but may include mediator release, vagal and sympathetic neural mechanisms, conversion of beta receptors into alpha receptors, or decreased activity of the $Na^+ - K^+$ ATPase pump.[3]

CHEST WALL DEFORMITIES

In Chapter 1, the dynamic configuration of the thorax was reviewed. Inspiratory and expiratory changes in thoracic volume allow for corresponding lung expansion and deflation. The extent to which intrathoracic volume is altered by a given transthoracic gradient in pressure (between inside and outside of chest wall) is a function of the

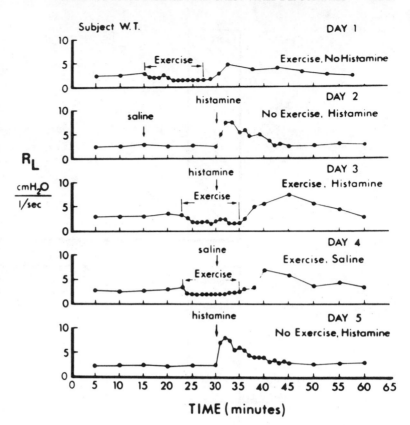

FIGURE 16–23. Effect of aerosolized histamine on pulmonary resistance (R_L) during exercise. Pulmonary resistance is plotted on the vertical axis and time on the horizontal axis. On day 1, measurements were made during a resting period, a 12 min exercise period, and then a 12 min resting period following completion of exercise. On day 2 there was no exercise, but aerosolized saline was inhaled at the 15 min point and aerosolized histamine at the 30 min point. On day 3, histamine was inhaled during exercise; on day 4, saline was inhaled during exercise; and on day 5, histamine was inhaled at rest. Notice that on day 3, aerosolized histamine during exercise failed to produce an increase in pulmonary resistance. (From Stirling DR, Cotton DJ, Graham BL, et al. Characteristics of airway tone during exercise in patients with asthma. J Appl Physiol 54:934–942, 1983.)

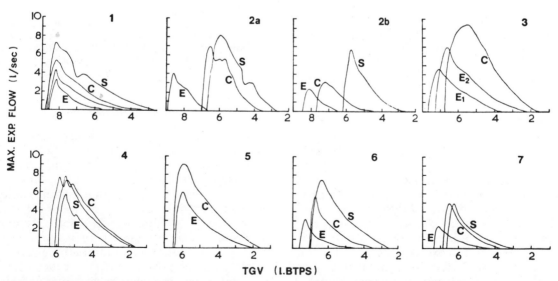

FIGURE 16–24. Maximum expiratory flow-volume curves obtained after exercise in eight patients with exercise-induced bronchoconstriction, plotted on an absolute lung volume scale (thoracic gas volume, *TGV*). *C*, control curve; *E*, postexercise; *S*, postaerosolized beta$_2$ agonist (salbutamol). (From Freedman S, Tattersfield AE, Pride NB. Changes in lung mechanics during asthma induced by exercise. J Appl Physiol 38:974–982, 1975.)

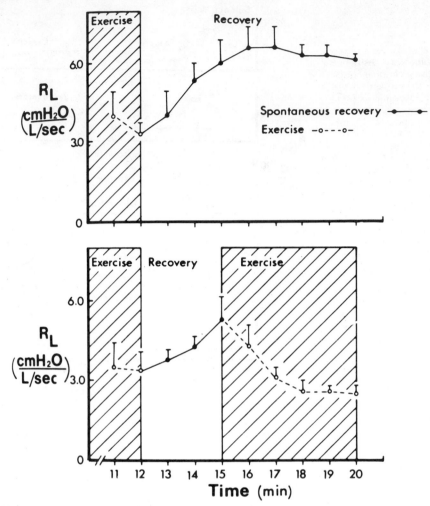

FIGURE 16–25. Reversal of exercise-induced increase in pulmonary resistance by a second episode of exercise in patients with exercise-induced bronchoconstriction. After exercise, there is an increase in pulmonary resistance (top), but this could be reversed by a second episode of exercise (bottom). (From Stirling DR, Cotton DJ, Graham BL, et al. Characteristics of airway tone during exercise in patients with asthma. J Appl Physiol 54:934–942, 1983.)

compliance of the thoracic cage. In children, the thorax is quite distensible in comparison to adults. In children or adults with congenital or acquired deformities of the thoracic cage, its compliance is decreased. Therefore, a larger respiratory muscle effort must be exerted to move air into the stiffer rib cage, which leads to exertional dyspnea. We have seen both gross and milder expressions of chest wall deformities interfere with the ventilatory response to exercise. Because the role of the chest wall deformity in causing exertional dyspnea is frequently underestimated and because these deformities are thought to limit exercise solely through circulatory causes, leaving the ventilatory component overlooked, we have reviewed this issue in this chapter.

Types of Deformities

Several different processes can lead to a deformity of the chest wall. *Kyphoscoliosis* is a term used to describe any abnormal degree of angulation between the spine and rib cage.[16] It may occur in the lateral plane, where it is mainly scoliosis, or in the forward or backward (kyphosis) direction. Kyphoscoliosis can be congenital, or it may occur during adolescence as an idiopathic process. It may follow poliomyelitis or tuberculosis (termed Pott's disease) or accompany Marfan's syndrome and neurofibromatosis.

Pectus excavatum is a congenital developmental anomaly in which the sternum, particularly its lower portion, is depressed toward the spine. Fibromuscular bands between the sternum and spine may be responsible for this deformity. This deformity will not only impair thoracic compliance but may also physically impede the filling and contraction of the heart. It is not uncommon to see patients with a straight spine who have "cardiomegaly" on chest radiograph because of the compression of the heart in the anteroposterior direction. Either a congenital deformity or ankylosing spondylitis, in which the vertebral joints become frozen or immobile, can lead to a "straight" spine.

Bergofsky, Turino, and Fishman have examined lungs for pathologic alterations in patients with kyphoscoliosis.[17] There was no evidence of emphysema unless the illness was accompanied by chronic bronchitis. On the other hand, Naeye[18] examined the pulmonary circulation in such cases and found medial hypertrophy and general dilatation of the pulmonary circulation. Certainly, pulmonary hypertension is known to accompany many of these cases and may represent the result of hypoxic pulmonary arteriolar vasoconstriction secondary to abnormal $\dot{V}/Q$ ratios within the lung. This may lead to cor pulmonale (right heart failure secondary to disease of the lung and/or pulmonary circulation). Patients with pectus excavatum or ankylosing spondylitis have shown no evidence of intrinsic or secondary lung disease. However, lung volumes, particularly the ventilatory reserve in vital capacity, is reduced in these patients typically to 3 liters or less, and $\dot{V}/Q$ abnormalities may be present in various lung segments; D_{LCO}, however, is preserved.

Exercise Response

Shneerson[19] has systematically studied the exercise response in 26 patients with scoliosis. He found that the aerobic work loads that the patients could accommodate during upright incremental cycle ergometry were lower than in age-matched control subjects. The average $\dot{V}O_2$ attained by the group was reduced to 25 ml/min/kg (range 11 to 34 ml/min/kg), and 16 (or 61 per cent) of the patients had a ventilatory impairment to exercise. Maximum $\dot{V}_E$ on exercise averaged 36 liters/min (range 13 to 76 liters/min), whereas the ratio of $\dot{V}_E$ max to MVV was 70 per cent. No differences were found between paralytic and nonparalytic groups having scoliosis. Figure 16–26 depicts the $\dot{V}_E$ to tidal volume and tidal volume to vital capacity ratio for normal subjects and Shneerson's patients with scoliosis. It can be seen that these patients were hyperventilating at each work load; $\dot{V}_E$ was at least 20 per cent greater than normal at each stage of exercise. Tidal volume increased linearly during exercise with the rise in $\dot{V}_E$ until the maximum tidal volume was attained; thereafter $\dot{V}_E$ rose solely through the response in respiratory frequency. The patients with scoliosis used over 50 per cent of their already reduced vital capacity in moving tidal air. Thus, their exercise is frequently ventilatory limited.

Of interest is the fact that, similar to other forms of lung disease, the heart rate response to exercise was greater than normal in both the men and women with scoliosis.

A 16 year old boy was referred to us

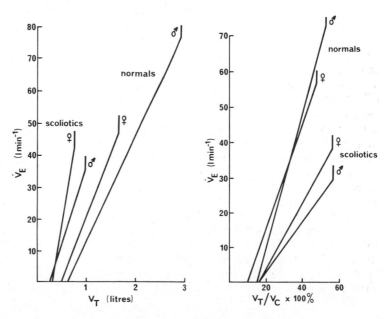

FIGURE 16–26. The response in $\dot{V}_E$, tidal volume (VT), and the VT to vital capacity ratio to upright cycle exercise in patients with scoliosis of the thoracic spine. (From Schneerson JM. The cardiorespiratory response to exercise in thoracic scoliosis. Thorax *33*:457–463, 1978.)

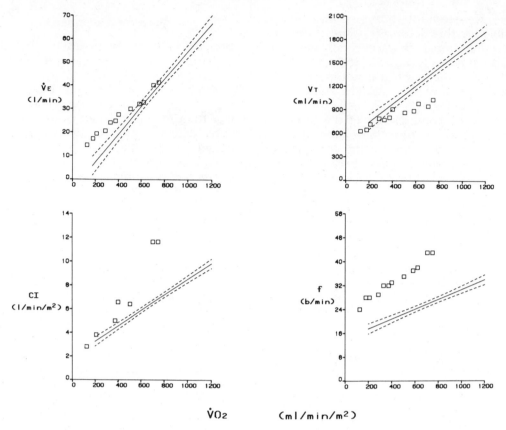

FIGURE 16–27. The response in minute ventilation ($\dot{V}_E$), cardiac index (*CI*), tidal volume (*VT*), and respiratory rate (*f*) to upright incremental treadmill exercise in a 16 year old boy with pectus excavatum. Exercise cardiac output was determined by thermodilution. There appeared to be no impairment in exercise cardiac output. A ventilatory limitation to exercise was present, however, as manifested by a pattern of rapid shallow breathing.

because of a marked pectus excavatum and exertional dyspnea. The issue before us was to determine whether or not this patient's limitation to exercise was ventilatory or circulatory in nature. Figure 16–27 depicts his cardiac index and ventilatory response to incremental treadmill exercise. The patient's cardiac output response to exercise was normal. On the other hand, his ventilatory response was abnormal and accounted for his effort intolerance and inability to achieve his aerobic capacity. The rise in tidal volume during exercise was subnormal, and respiratory rate was excessive at each work load. The poor compliance of the thorax accounted for this pattern of rapid shallow breathing. These findings resemble that reported by Shneerson[19] in patients with scoliosis.

Beiser and co-workers[20] have suggested that the major limitation to upright exercise in some patients with pectus excavatum is mediated by an impaired circulatory response that is the result of a direct compression on the heart by the decreased antero-posterior dimension of the thorax. As a result, ventricular filling is impaired and venous return is throttled. Respiratory gas exchange and ventilation, however, were not measured in this study. A circulatory limitation to exercise would appear to be operative in a smaller percentage of these cases; the majority of patients with chest wall deformity would have a ventilatory limitation to exercise.

REFERENCES

1. Bye PT, Farkas GA, Roussos C. Respiratory factors limiting exercise. Annu Rev Physiol 45:439–451, 1983.
2. Grimby G, Elgefors B, Oxhoj H. Ventilatory levels and chest mechanics during exercise in obstructive lung disease. Scand J Respir Dis 54:45–52, 1973.
3. Loke J (ed). Exercise: Physiology and clinical applications. Clin Chest Med 5:35–49, 145–156, 1984.
4. Rochester D, Arora N. Respiratory muscle failure. Med Clin North Am 67:573–597, 1983.
5. Owens G, Rogers R, Pennock B, Levin D. The

diffusing capacity as a predictor of arterial oxygen desaturation during exercise in patients with chronic obstructive pulmonary disease. N Engl J Med 310:1218–1221, 1984.

6. Jones N, Jones G, Edwards R. Exercise tolerance in chronic airway obstruction. Am Rev Respir Dis 103:477–491, 1971.

7. Marcus J, McLean R, Duffell G, Ingram R. Exercise performance in relation to the pathophysiologic types of chronic obstructive pulmonary disease. Am J Med 49:14–22, 1970.

8. Spiro S, Hahn H, Edwards R, Pride N. An analysis of the physiologic strain of submaximal exercise in patients with chronic obstructive bronchitis. Thorax 30:415–425, 1975.

9. Jones N. Pulmonary gas exchange during exercise in patients with chronic airway obstruction. Clin Sci 31:39–50, 1966.

10. Wright J, Lawson L, Pare P, Hooper R, Peretz D, Nelems J, Schulzer M, Hogg J. The structure and function of the pulmonary vasculature in mild chronic obstructive pulmonary disease. Am Rev Respir Dis 128:702–707, 1983.

11. Matthay R, Berger H, Davis R, Loke J, Mahler D, Gottschalk A, Zaret B. Right and left ventricular exercise performance in chronic obstructive pulmonary disease: Radionuclide assessment. Ann Intern Med 93:234–239, 1980.

12. Spiro S, Dowdeswell I, Clark T. An analysis of submaximal exercise response in patients with sarcoidosis and fibrosing alveolitis. Br J Dis Chest 75:169–180, 1981.

13. Anderson S, McEvoy J, Bianco S. Changes in lung volumes and airway resistance after exercise in asthmatic subjects. Am Rev Respir Dis 106:30–36, 1973.

14. Freedman S, Tattersfield AE, Pride NB. Changes in lung mechanics during asthma induced by exercise. J Appl Physiol 38:974–981, 1975.

15. Stirling DR, Cotton DJ, Graham BL, Hodgson WC, Cockcroft DW, Dosman JA. Characteristics of airway tone during exercise in patients with asthma. J Appl Physiol 54:934–942, 1983.

16. Bates DV, Christie RV. Respiratory Function in Disease. Philadelphia, WB Saunders Co, 1964, pp. 260–268.

17. Bergofsky EH, Turino GM, Fishman AP. Cardiorespiratory failure in kyphoscoliosis. Medicine 38:263–317, 1959.

18. Naeye RL. Kyphoscoliosis and cor pulmonale. A study of the pulmonary vascular bed. Am J Pathol 38:561–567, 1961.

19. Shneerson JM. The cardiorespiratory response to exercise in thoracic scoliosis. Thorax 33:457–463, 1978.

20. Beiser GD, Epstein SE, Stampfer M, Goldstein RE, Noland SP, Levitsky S. Impairment of cardiac function in patients with pectus excavatum, with improvement after operative correction. N Engl J Med 287:267–272, 1972.

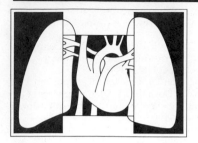

17

KARL T. WEBER
J. PETER SZIDON

Exertional Dyspnea

Normally, an individual is unaware of the act of breathing and of the fact that 500 ml of air enter and leave the lungs 15 times each minute at rest. Minute ventilation will increase secondary to normal or abnormal chemical stimuli (e.g., hypercapnia, hypoxemia, acidemia) or anxiety. Whenever breathing is perceived to be unpleasant, exaggerated, or inappropriate relative to the level of physical activity, it is considered an abnormal awareness of breathing. This sensation has been termed breathlessness, shortness of breath, or dyspnea. The issues surrounding the perception of dyspnea and the mechanisms that are thought to elicit this sensation are reviewed elsewhere.[1–6]

Dyspnea, and particularly dyspnea on exertion, is quite common in patients having heart disease, lung disease, pulmonary vascular disease, abnormalities of the chest wall, and weakness of the respiratory muscles. Because a sense of breathlessness may seriously hinder the patients' ability to perform muscular work and in turn compromise their quality of life, they seek medical attention. It is imperative that the physician obtain the requisite historic information that characterizes the nature, onset, and severity of dyspnea and its relationship to exercise and other symptoms.

The subjective sensation of dyspnea, as recounted by a patient to a physician, can be influenced by cognitive and affective factors. All too frequently, the physician finds that the patient's perception of dyspnea and subsequent recounting of the pertinent issues may be limited or its severity confounded by denial or overexaggeration (affective factors). The physician is also persuaded by his or her own perception and interpretation (cognitive factors) of the historic information. Care must

also be taken to place into perspective the sensation of breathlessness relative to the underlying physical condition of the patient. The patient's customary daily activity and adaptation to breathlessness must also be taken into account.

Given that therapeutic decisions are based on the extent to which the patient's quality of life is compromised by dyspnea (i.e., when dyspnea is the major morbid factor), it is mandatory that an objective and reliable estimate of its *nature* and *severity* be available. We characterize the nature or mechanism of exertional dyspnea by supplementing the history and physical examination with a cardiopulmonary exercise test in which the monitoring of blood pressure, heart rate, and the electrocardiogram are complemented by breath-by-breath measurements of respiratory gas exchange and airflow, and noninvasive arterial oxygen saturation. Borg and Noble[7] have suggested a method to grade the severity of dyspnea during exercise, as have Stark and co-workers.[8] Recently, Killian and Jones[6] have proposed an analytic method to assess the severity of exertional dyspnea in relationship to physiologic variables during exercise.

The purpose of this chapter is to review our approach to characterizing the mechanisms responsible for exertional dyspnea. We wish to indicate how this characterization can prove useful in identifying the organ system most likely to be involved in the genesis of dyspnea, by focusing therapeutic efforts in that direction in the dyspneic patient with heart disease, lung disease, pulmonary vascular disease, coexistent heart and lung disease, or diseases of the chest wall and respiratory muscles. First, however, the pathophysiologic responses that have been associated with the appearance of dyspnea during physical activity will be reviewed. No pretense is made to suggest that these responses are the fundamental signals that elicit this sensation. Nevertheless, this background information will provide a broader perspective of the pertinent issues.

THE PATHOPHYSIOLOGIC RESPONSES ASSOCIATED WITH EXERTIONAL DYSPNEA

Dyspnea is known to occur under the circumstances listed in Table 17–1. In each case, the work of breathing is increased when (1) ventilation is excessive relative to the degree of physical work, or $\dot{V}O_2$, and when $\dot{V}_E$ may be driven by chemical stimuli (e.g., by hypoxia or hypercapnia) or altered lung mechanics (e.g., lung disease, elevated pulmonary venous and capillary pressures, and chest wall deformity); or (2) $\dot{V}_E$ occupies an excessive proportion (>50 per cent) of the ventilatory reserve (i.e., maximum voluntary ventilation, MVV).

Dyspnea is experienced by normal individuals. A sense of breathlessness may appear during recovery from vigorous activity, such as running up stairs. Here, the level of $\dot{V}_E$ for the degree of activity during recovery (i.e., standing) is perceived to be excessive. Alternatively, a level of $\dot{V}_E$ to which the subject is unaccustomed may elicit the sensation of breathlessness (i.e., prolonged vigorous running in a normally sedentary individual). In either case, it is perhaps a chemical drive to respiration, mediated through the buffering of lactic acid and the

Table 17–1. *Circumstances in Which the Work of Breathing Is Increased, Predisposing to a Sense of Breathlessness*

Increased Work of Breathing	Circumstance
1) $\dot{V}_E$ inappropriately high (secondary to chemical stimuli or altered lung mechanics) relative to $\dot{V}O_2$ at rest or during exercise	Pulmonary emboli Interstitial lung disease Normal recovery from exercise Chronic cardiac failure Valvular heart disease Acute cardiac failure
2) $\dot{V}_E$ max on exercise is > 50% of maximal voluntary ventilation	Interstitial lung disease Obstructive lung disease Normal response

heightened carbon dioxide production and fall in arterial pH, that is responsible for the elevated $\dot{V}_E$. In patients with heart or lung disease or both, dyspnea may appear during routine physical activity if the load imposed on the respiratory muscles is increased or if there is an increased drive to breathe. As a result, daily living is interrupted and effort tolerance compromised. In patients with less severe disease dyspnea may occur only during moderately heavy work loads, whereas in more advanced disease the patient can be symptomatic even at rest.

Despite years of scientific inquiry into the mechanisms responsible for the perception of breathlessness, its explanation(s) remain uncertain. For interesting perspectives of the topic, the interested reader is referred elsewhere.[3, 5, 6] The sensation of dyspnea may arise not only because respiratory muscle work is increased or because chemical stimuli, such as hypoxia or hypercapnia, drive ventilation to excess, but also because of other factors that may be operative in the patient with heart or lung disease or both.[9] Juxtacapillary receptors located in the interalveolar interstitial space may be stimulated by fluid accumulation in the case of pulmonary venous and capillary hypertension. Alternatively, nerve spindles that sense respiratory muscle tension relative to muscle length may become malaligned, creating abnormal signals that the patient translates into an abnormal awareness of breathing.

Dyspnea in Heart Disease

It is well known that patients with pulmonary edema secondary to chronic mitral valve disease or left ventricular dysfunction have elevated pulmonary venous and capillary pressures. In the absence of long-standing heart disease, the transudation of fluid from the vascular compartment, first into the interalveolar interstitium and subsequently into the alveoli, takes place when capillary hydrostatic pressure exceeds 25 mm Hg, or the colloidal osmotic pressure of the capillaries. In patients with chronic interstitial edema secondary to chronic mitral, ischemic, or myopathic heart disease, higher levels of venous pressure (e.g., 30 to 40 mm Hg) are required to produce clinically apparent pulmonary congestion (e.g., rales). The higher level of hydrostatic pressure required to produce congestion under these circumstances is the result of two responses:[10] (1) the lymphatic drainage of the lung is enhanced secondary to chronic pulmonary venous hypertension; and (2) tissue and osmotic pressures of the lung that oppose the hydrostatic pressure are increased, as a result of chronic interstitial edema and enhanced lymphatic flow, respectively.

In either the acute or the chronic setting, pulmonary venous pressure is elevated, the lungs are "wet," their compliance is decreased, and the work of breathing is elevated. A pattern of rapid, shallow breathing is adopted to minimize respiratory muscle work. The patient who is dyspneic often prefers to sit upright or to elevate the head and upper thorax on several pillows. Dyspnea is relieved with the aggressive use of diuretics and venodilating agents, each of which reduce intravascular and intrapulmonary fluid volumes. Thus, it has been taken for granted that an elevated pulmonary venous pressure is the sole mechanism responsible for the appearance of dyspnea in these patients. Other factors, however, may also be operative.

Exertional dyspnea, for example, may occur in these patients for several reasons. We have observed patients with severe cardiac failure to have marked elevations in pulmonary venous pressure during upright exercise (see Chapter 11). These patients do not, however, necessarily stop exercising because of dyspnea. This important exception to the concept of elevated pulmonary venous pressure was clearly brought out during our experience with constant work rate exercise in these patients.[11] During aerobic exercise, we observed that patients with chronic cardiac failure could walk a full 20 minutes without dyspnea, despite occlusive wedge pressures of 30 mm Hg or more. For similar elevations in wedge pressure, but under conditions of anaerobic endurance exercise, these patients experienced dyspnea that caused them to terminate the exercise test prematurely.

What distinguished the constant work rate aerobic and anaerobic exercise responses was the pattern of ventilation. In the case of anaerobic exercise, a progressive and disproportionate rise in V_E relative to $\dot{V}O_2$ occurred, which was mediated by a given increment in tidal volume and a progressive rise in respiratory rate. With aerobic exercise, the ventilatory response was proportional to $\dot{V}O_2$. This difference in ventilation could be attributed to the difference in mixed venous lactate concentration between the two forms of exercise. In anaerobic exercise, there was a continuous rise in mixed venous lactate and

disproportionate elevation in $\dot{V}CO_2$ that led to hyperventilation and hyperpnea relative to the given work load. It would therefore appear that lactate production by anaerobic muscle, and its subsequent buffering by bicarbonate and the resultant enhanced $\dot{V}CO_2$, is responsible for a heightened chemical drive to respiration mediated by the carotid bodies.[12] It is this disproportionate ventilation relative to $\dot{V}O_2$ and not simply the elevated venous and capillary pressures in the lung that leads to the appearance of breathlessness.

It is also possible that under anaerobic conditions of muscular work, the $\dot{V}_E$ to MVV ratio may actually exceed 50 per cent and may therefore be difficult to sustain for any length of time (see Chapter 16) in patients with heart disease. One uncertainty surrounding this concept is knowing the true MVV that exists during exercise in these patients in the presence of enhanced pulmonary venous pressure. Exercise MVV, for example, may actually fall as pulmonary compliance is compromised. When exercise $\dot{V}_E$ at maximum exercise, however, is compared with the MVV measured during standard pulmonary function testing, this ratio does not exceed 50 per cent in these patients.

The reduced cardiac output response to exercise may also contribute to the dyspneic state in patients with heart disease because the oxygen delivery to respiratory muscles is compromised.[13] In patients with pulmonary vascular disease and pulmonary hypertension, a fixed or modest cardiac output response to exercise is observed that is similar to that seen in heart failure. Pulmonary venous and capillary pressures in these patients rise only modestly with exercise, rarely exceeding 18 mm Hg. Enhanced lactate production at low levels of work in these patients will result in hyperventilation relative to work load and the sense of dyspnea in the setting of inadequate respiratory muscle perfusion. The appearance of hypoxemia during exercise may add yet another chemical stimulus to ventilation in patients with pulmonary vascular disease, as we will discuss further on. Exercise hypoxemia, however, does not occur in patients with stable chronic cardiac failure.[14, 15]

In patients with chronic cardiac disease, the ventilatory response to progressive isotonic exercise is dependent on the severity of the disease, the secondary alteration in pulmonary compliance, and the aerobic capacity of the patient (Figs. 17–1 and 17–2). In

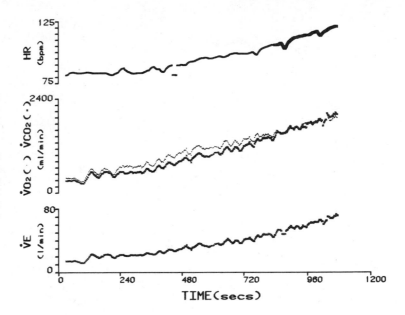

FIGURE 17–1. A cardiopulmonary exercise (CPX) test for a 62 year old man with aortic regurgitation. The patient had an anaerobic threshold at 23 ml/min/kg and a peak $\dot{V}O_2$ of 27 ml/min/kg. $\dot{V}O_2$ max was not achieved; however, the data are compatible with his being functional class A. Minute ventilation ($\dot{V}_E$) rose to 68 liters/min at peak exercise and was derived from increments in both tidal volume (VT) and respiratory rate (f).

class D patients, 30 per cent of the exercise tidal volume is wasted in the anatomic dead space[16–18] because of rapid, shallow breathing. Moreover, the maximum tidal volume and $\dot{V}_E$ that these patients achieve is generally <50 per cent of their ventilatory reserve measured during routine pulmonary function studies.[18]

Dyspnea in Lung Disease

Ventilatory mechanics during exercise are altered in patients having interstitial lung disease or obstructive airway disease. In the case of *interstitial lung disease*, pulmonary compliance is impaired and, as in the patient with stiff wet lungs secondary to heart disease, a pattern of rapid, shallow breathing is adopted to minimize the work of breathing (see Chapter 5) at the expense of greater dead-space ventilation.[19] Given that the ventilatory reserves (vital capacity and maximum voluntary ventilation) available to these patients are reduced, a large proportion (>50 per cent) of these reserves is used in generating a tidal volume and $\dot{V}_E$ during exercise, respectively (Fig. 17–3). This ventilatory effort poses a substantial work load on the respiratory muscles, increasing their need for oxygen. The enhanced respiratory muscle

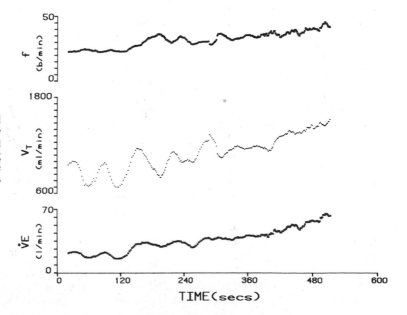

FIGURE 17–2. CPX for a 37 year old man with a dilated cardiomyopathy that was functional class D. He reached his anaerobic threshold at 6 ml/min/kg and a $\dot{V}O_2$ max of 9.8 ml/min/kg. The elevation in tidal volume (V_T) is less than the rise in respiratory rate (f).

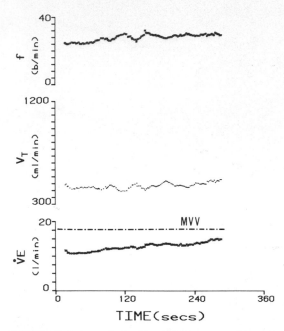

FIGURE 17–3. Record of a 72 year old woman with aortic regurgitation and chronic bronchitis whose exertional dyspnea was secondary to her ventilatory impairment. Her maximal voluntary ventilation (MVV) was only 18 liters/min. At end-exercise with marked dyspnea, she had used over 80 per cent of her MVV with $\dot{V}_E$, and she did not cross her anaerobic threshold.

work cannot be sustained for very long periods of time. It is known that an MVV maneuver cannot be sustained indefinitely and that more than 70 per cent of the MVV cannot be sustained by normal subjects for more than several minutes.[20, 21] Accordingly, it is not unreasonable to interpret the ventilatory response to exercise of the patient with interstitial lung disease as following a pattern of short-lived, near-maximum ventilation. What has been difficult to demonstrate, given the multiple venous drainage sites of the respiratory muscles and their relatively small muscle mass, is whether or not they are indeed anaerobic and actively producing lactate when this patient experiences dyspnea.

The patient with more advanced interstitial lung disease may be unable to sustain alveolar ventilation during exercise at a level that is commensurate with adequate arterial oxygen saturation. Consequently, hypoxemia may compound the patient's exercise response and be responsible for a heightened chemical drive to respiration. This is yet another potential mechanism for the exertional dyspnea that these patients so commonly experience.

In the case of *obstructive airway disease*, the need to move air through a partially ob-

structed bronchial tree creates an added work load on the respiratory pump. Airflow rates in these patients that are already compromised at rest must increase with exercise. Even though the drop in pleural pressure with inspiration increases luminal size of the airways, peak airflow rates generated during exercise in patients with obstructive airway disease approach the peak expiratory flow rate observed at maximal effort during pulmonary function testing (Fig. 17–4).[19, 22] This is in distinct contrast to normal subjects, who use 50 per cent or less of their maximal expiratory flow rate during exercise. Thus, the work of breathing is considerably increased in the patient with obstructive lung disease, prompting the use of a more efficient pattern of slow, deep breathing at rest and during exercise. In spite of these efforts of enhanced respiratory muscle efficiency, the patient is frequently dyspneic. In fact, disorders of airflow obstruction (e.g., emphysema, bronchitis, and asthma) are among the most common causes of exertional dyspnea.

Dyspnea in Pulmonary Vascular Disease

Patients with primary or secondary pulmonary hypertension frequently experience exertional dyspnea. In our experience (see Chapter 13), exertional dyspnea was the most common symptom that prompted these patients to seek medical attention.

Exertional dyspnea may occur in these pa-

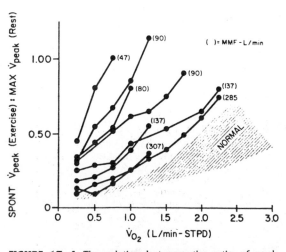

FIGURE 17–4. The relation between the ratio of peak airflow rate with exercise to maximum flow at rest and muscular work (or $\dot{V}O_2$) during exercise is shown for patients with chronic airway disease. (From Wasserman K, Whipp BJ. Exercise physiology in health and disease. Am Rev Resp Dis *112*:219–249, 1975.)

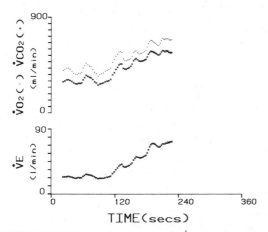

FIGURE 17–5. The marked increase in $\dot{V}_E$ seen during low level treadmill exercise in a 36 year old man with thromboembolic disease of the pulmonary circulation. Note the marked increase in $\dot{V}_E$ to 70 liters/min while walking 1 mph, 0 per cent grade. Despite this level of ventilation, the patient developed arterial hypoxemia.

tients for several reasons. On the one hand, the cardiac output response to exercise can be severely limited because of the elevated pulmonary vascular resistance. As a result, limb muscles convert to anaerobic glycolysis to derive their energy. The same may be true of respiratory muscles. The sense of breathlessness may be the result of a heightened chemical drive to respiration, which is mediated via the lactate production of anaerobic limb muscles and the resultant increased carbon dioxide production accompanying lactate buffering. Respiratory muscles may quickly fatigue under these circumstances of increased demand and poor perfusion.

In some dyspneic patients, and as a result of pulmonary vascular disease, arterial oxygen saturation falls during exercise, leading to another chemical drive to respiration. When pulmonary perfusion is reduced (e.g., large pulmonary emboli) a very large $\dot{V}_E$ is selected to sustain alveolar ventilation even at low levels of work (Fig. 17–5). When the defect is in the ventilatory portion of the response, a marked elevation in $\dot{V}_E$ also occurs with low-level exercise. Figure 16–17 depicts an example of this condition. In each of these patients exertional dyspnea was present.

Dyspnea in Chest Wall Deformities

The rib cage may be physically deformed by a congenital defect (e.g., pectus excavatum) or acquired disease (e.g., kyphoscoliosis). In either case, the ability of the respiratory pump to reduce intrathoracic pressure during exercise and to thereby move large quantities of air into and out of the lungs will be compromised by the abnormal compliance of the thorax. Respiratory muscle work is again increased, and major portions of the ventilatory reserves (>50 per cent) are used during exercise. This response is shown in Figure 16–26.

Exertional dyspnea can therefore be a common complaint of the patient with a chest wall deformity. The exercise response is characterized by a limited elevation in $\dot{V}_E$, a pattern of rapid, shallow breathing; and a propensity to develop arterial oxygen desaturation. Measurements of pleural (or esophageal) pressure in these patients would reveal a limited fall in intrapleural pressure during exercise.

In several cases, such as that seen with a severe pectus excavatum or in combination with a straight spine, the heart may be physically compressed, limiting its ability to be filled during isotonic exercise; thereby, the cardiac output response to exercise is compromised. The physical restraint on the cardiopulmonary unit may be greater than appreciated from physical examination or hemodynamic monitoring in the supine position. An upright cardiopulmonary exercise test may be more useful in assessing the constraint imposed by the deformity on the ventilatory and circulatory responses to exertion.

Dyspnea in Respiratory Muscle Weakness

Respiratory muscle weakness secondary to a specific neurologic disorder or disease of skeletal muscle can limit the patient's ability to bring air into the lungs. As a result, $\dot{V}_E$ will not rise appropriately during progressive isotonic exercise. Moreover, the patient selects a pattern of rapid, shallow breathing that minimizes the work load imposed on the weakened respiratory muscles. If respiratory muscle weakness is severe, alveolar ventilation may not be sustained at an appropriate level during exercise. The result is arterial oxygen desaturation. Figure 17–6 depicts the exercise response of a patient with respiratory muscle weakness.

AN APPROACH TO UNDERSTANDING THE NATURE OF DYSPNEA IN THE DYSPNEIC PATIENT

In each of the disease entities described earlier, we use a progressive, upright tread-

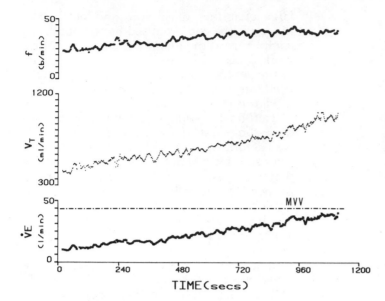

FIGURE 17–6. An 18 year old woman with a dilated cardiomyopathy and respiratory muscle weakness. During incremental treadmill exercise her $\dot{V}_E$ did not exceed 38 liters/min at a workload of 25 ml/min/kg, when she noted severe dyspnea.

mill, or bicycle exercise test to evaluate the physiologic mechanisms associated with the appearance of exertional dyspnea. Progressive isotonic exercise, together with noninvasive monitoring of breath-by-breath measurements of respiratory gas exchange and airflow, blood pressure, heart rate, and the electrocardiogram are used for this purpose. In selected circumstances, when lung disease or pulmonary vascular disease is suspected on clinical grounds, we also monitor arterial oxygen saturation by ear oximetry. Based on the noninvasive exercise test, we may elect to repeat the CPX in combination with the following invasive measures: (a) a flotation catheter positioned in the pulmonary artery to monitor the hemodynamic response of the right and left heart; (2) a catheter in the esophagus to monitor pleural pressure; and/or (3) a catheter in the radial artery to measure arterial oxygen saturation. The rationale behind each of these monitoring procedures is described hereafter, together with illustrative cases that highlight diagnostic issues that can be resolved by noninvasive and invasive CPX.

Progressive Isotonic Exercise

A defect within the cardiopulmonary unit can be elicited during exercise, particularly if the patient is symptomatic with physical activity. We generally prefer the patient's using the treadmill, as the treadmill represents a nonspecialized reproducible skill. The bicycle may be a better choice in obese patients, patients unable to walk, or patients with

severe disease in whom the rise in $\dot{V}O_2$ must of necessity be very modest. Mobile stairs have recently been manufactured and are an attractive though unproven method, particularly since many patients note dyspnea during or after climbing stairs. Finally, arm cranking can be used effectively in those patients who are unable to walk, pedal, or climb. The instrumentation needed to monitor the various responses described subsequently has been reviewed in Chapters 7 through 9.

VENTILATORY RESPONSE

One should measure tidal volume and respiratory rate on a breath-by-breath basis to assess the ventilatory response to exercise and specifically to assess the pattern of ventilation. The normal ventilatory response to progressive isotonic exercise for normal sedentary individuals consists of a rise in $\dot{V}_E$ that is mediated by an increase in tidal volume and a rise in respiratory rate (see Fig. 5–15).

Even with the most vigorous exercise, $\dot{V}_E$ will rarely exceed 90 per cent of MVV measured during routine pulmonary function studies, and rarely can it be sustained at this level for more than seconds. The MVV maneuver requires the patient's coordination and motivation and therefore may be difficult to obtain during routine pulmonary function studies. An approximation of maximum exercise ventilation can be derived by multiplying the FEV_1 by 35.

The maximum tidal volume during exercise will rarely exceed 80 per cent of vital capacity measured during pulmonary function studies. It should be apparent that it is valuable to obtain routine pulmonary function tests in all patients prior to CPX. Based on these results, it is possible to evaluate the ventilatory reserves and the fraction of these reserves that the ventilatory response to exercise occupies. For light, moderate, and even heavy work loads in untrained, normal individuals, $\dot{V}_E$ and tidal volume normally use less than 50 per cent of these respective reserves (Fig. 17–7).

In patients with more advanced expressions of *heart disease*, there is a pattern of rapid, shallow breathing that accompanies isotonic exercise. Table 11–4 depicts the ventilatory response for patients with mild, moderate, and severe heart failure relative to their ventilatory reserves. Even at maximal exercise, these patients rarely use more than 50 per cent of their ventilatory reserves. That is, their maximum tidal volume and $\dot{V}_E$ do not occupy more than 50 per cent of their forced vital capacity and maximum voluntary ventilation, respectively (Fig. 17–7). Moreover, they do not experience arterial oxygen desaturation during exercise. Finally, patients with cardiac or circulatory failure are able to cross their anaerobic threshold and exercise to the point of exhaustion, attaining their $\dot{V}O_2$ max without stopping because of dyspnea. By monitoring the breath-by-breath response in

$\dot{V}O_2$ and end-tidal oxygen relative to end-tidal carbon dioxide during exercise, the physician can immediately determine when the patient has achieved the anaerobic threshold and aerobic capacity. It should again be noted (see Chapters 11 and 12) that the dyspneic patient with predominant heart disease can in fact attain his or her anaerobic threshold and $\dot{V}O_2$ max, whereas this is much less likely in the patient with lung disease or the patient with coexistent heart and lung disease, in which the ventilatory system is the primary limitation to exercise.

In the patient with *lung disease*, a major (>50 per cent) portion of their ventilatory reserves is used during exercise (Fig. 17–7). It is not uncommon for these patients to use nearly all of their ventilatory reserve with exercise. When *restrictive* lung disease is the underlying disturbance, the ventilatory pattern is similar to that in heart failure; rapid, shallow breathing is the rule. In addition, these patients frequently experience arterial oxygen desaturation. Figure 17–8 illustrates the exercise response of such a patient, in whom tidal volume actually fell while respiratory rate rose markedly during exercise. Patients with *obstructive* lung disease generate excessive airflow rates to sustain their ventilatory response to exercise (see Fig. 17–4). These patients use 50 per cent or more of their peak expiratory flow rate with exer-

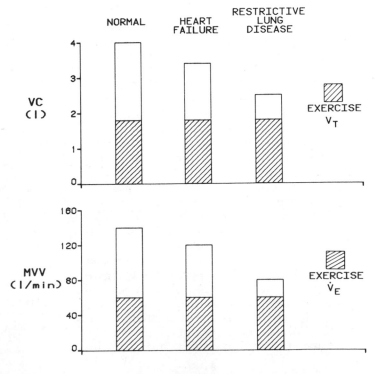

FIGURE 17–7. The fraction of the ventilatory reserves (vital capacity, *VC;* maximal voluntary ventilation, *MVV*) that are typically used at peak exercise in normal individuals and in patients with heart failure or restrictive lung disease. V_T, tidal volume; $\dot{V}_E$, minute ventilation.

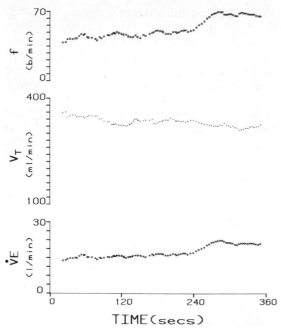

FIGURE 17–8. Record of a 38 year old woman with advanced interstitial lung disease who began to exercise after a rest period of 240 seconds. Note that the VT was invariant or actually fell during exercise. The increase in $\dot{V}_E$ with 6.25 watts of cycle exercise was mediated entirely by an increase in respiratory rate.

cise when they become dyspneic. The patient with emphysema frequently has a drop in arterial oxygen saturation. Finally, patients with either restrictive or obstructive lung disease are generally unable to achieve their anaerobic threshold and are rarely able to achieve $\dot{V}O_2$ max at symptomatic end point.

A more frequent dilemma confronted by the practicing physician presents itself in evaluating the dyspneic patient with *coexistent heart and lung disease*. Here again, the noninvasive exercise test will provide sufficient information from which to select additional studies and to seek consultation, as well as to derive the most appropriate therapeutic intervention. The proportion of the ventilatory reserves used in attaining symptomatic end point, the presence or absence of arterial oxygen desaturation, and the ability to achieve anaerobic threshold and aerobic capacity will determine which disease is dominant.

Patients with *nonhypoxic pulmonary vascular disease* and pulmonary hypertension will generally attain their $\dot{V}O_2$ max; their functional or aerobic capacity is similar to that of patients with cardiac disease or circulatory failure, but, unlike these patients, there may be evidence of arterial oxygen desaturation. In-

vasive hemodynamic monitoring with or without exercise is needed (1) when the physician must distinguish between patients with intrinsic pulmonary vascular disease (pulmonary vascular resistance >300 dynes · sec · cm^{-5}) and those with left heart disease, or (2) when a trial of vasodilators is anticipated for the treatment of pulmonary hypertension. Patients with pulmonary emboli or *hypoxic* pulmonary vasoconstriction, however, will stop exercising with a ventilatory impairment to exercise perceived as an excessive $\dot{V}_E$ relative to their work load; they rarely attain their anaerobic threshold or their $\dot{V}O_2$ max and commonly develop significant arterial oxygen desaturation. An example of such a case is given in Figures 17–9 and 17–10, for a patient with chronic lung disease, whose oxygen saturation fell to 77 per cent during exercise. The appearance of hypoxemia should signal the physician that the patient does not have cardiac disease; rather, the problem resides within the pulmonary circulation or the lungs, or both.

In the presence of a *chest wall deformity* or *respiratory muscle weakness*, there will be a limitation to the patient's ability to raise $\dot{V}_E$ with incremental exercise. Similarly, these patients have a depressed maximum voluntary ventilation during pulmonary function testing. Thus, despite the fact that treadmill work is increasing, $\dot{V}_E$ does not rise and represents >50 per cent of the MVV when the patient terminates exercise with dyspnea. The ventilatory response itself consists of rapid, shallow breathing. With a moderate to severe reduction in thoracic compliance or in

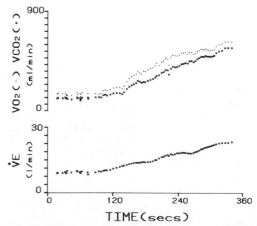

FIGURE 17–9. The response in respiratory gas exchange and ventilation for a 62 year old woman with chronic airway disease who developed marked arterial O_2 desaturation and dyspnea during low level treadmill exercise. Note that she did not cross her anaerobic threshold.

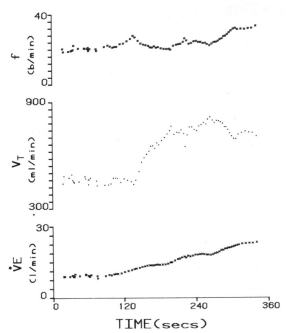

FIGURE 17–10. The ventilatory response to exercise for the patient shown in Figure 17–9, with the first 120 seconds at standing rest.

the presence of respiratory muscle weakness, it is not unusual to see respiratory rates of 40 to 50 bpm at low to moderate levels of work. In the case of respiratory muscle weakness, $\dot{V}_E$ may actually fall during exercise. Figure 16–27 depicts the response of a patient with pectus excavatum. Such patients will rarely reach their anaerobic threshold and do not achieve a $\dot{V}O_2$ max if the primary defect is ventilatory in nature. On the other hand, if the chest wall deformity primarily compromises the cardiac output response to exercise, these patients will behave as would any other patient with circulatory failure having a reduced anaerobic threshold and aerobic capacity, the severity of which can then be graded from the $\dot{V}O_2$ max determination. Hemodynamic monitoring may be necessary in this group to elucidate further the nature and severity of the circulatory impairment and to distinguish the ventilatory from the circulatory component in troublesome or puzzling cases.

The ventilatory response to exercise is rather predictable, with a rise in tidal volume and respiratory rate. Once anaerobic levels of exercise are achieved, there is a chemical drive to respiration that is difficult to control by volition. In an *emotionally disturbed* patient or in one seeking *disability*, an irregular ventilatory response to exercise may be seen that bears no resemblance to the normal response and will not be accompanied by arterial oxygen desaturation unless there is breath-holding, which can be detected from the air flow response.

We have observed an unusual or "saw-toothed" ventilatory response to exercise in some patients with heart disease (Fig. 17–11), which did not appear to be a Cheyne-Stokes pattern of breathing. Several of these patients had thromboembolic disease of the cerebral circulation. The saw-toothed response in $\dot{V}_E$ may be secondary to altered carbon dioxide sensitivity of central or peripheral chemoreceptors.

CIRCULATORY RESPONSE

In patients with cardiac or circulatory disorders who are dyspneic, invasive hemodynamic monitoring may be necessary for diagnosis, for evaluating the severity and nature of the disturbance, and for monitoring therapeutic response. This may also become necessary in patients with arterial oxygen

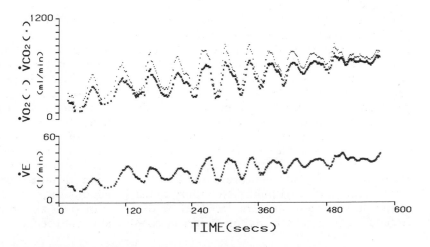

FIGURE 17–11. An abnormal ventilatory response to exercise, characterized as a saw-toothed pattern, in a 64 year old woman with a dilated cardiomyopathy. She did not cross her anaerobic threshold when she had to stop exercising with dyspnea.

desaturation and pulmonary hypertension, for assessing the severity and nature of the right heart pressure overload and its response to supplemental inspired oxygen. In the illustrative cases given subsequently, we wish to demonstrate the utility of this approach for the dyspneic patient who is referred for evaluation.

In patients with previously established heart disease of known etiology, invasive hemodynamic monitoring may be necessary to evaluate underlying severity of the disease, to distinguish between a disparity in clinical evaluation and effort tolerance, and to evaluate the response to medical therapy. In addition, hemodynamic monitoring can be used to establish proper drug dosage and the dosing interval.

Illustrative examples of these issues are presented next. In *valvular heart disease,* the severity of the hemodynamic overload placed on one or more cardiac chambers and the pulmonary circulation can be assessed by increasing venous return through exercise. As a result of this increase, blood flow through the heart and lungs will rise, producing elevations in pressure gradients between chambers to reflect the degree of valvular stenosis or incompetence. Importantly, the vascular resistance of the pulmonary circulation can be examined by deriving several pressure-flow points to construct this relation. A frequent dilemma arises in patients with mitral stenosis or mitral regurgitation, or both, in whom the severity of their hemodynamic overload on the heart and pulmonary circulation cannot be reliably gauged from data obtained in the supine, resting position via cardiac catheterization.

In Figure 17–12, we see the exercise hemodynamic response of an obese male patient with *alveolar hypoventilation* and systemic hypertension. An elevation in pulmonary artery pressure occurred during the transition from standing rest to walking on the treadmill (1 mph, 0 per cent grade) as pulmonary blood flow was increased and the patient developed hypoxemia with arterial oxygen saturation falling from 95 per cent at rest to 87 per cent with stage 1 of exercise. Echocardiography demonstrated a moderate enlargement of the right heart chambers that could not have been explained from the normal resting pulmonary artery and right ventricular pressures. It had been presumed that the patient had left heart failure secondary to his systemic hypertension. The fact that he did indeed have systemic hypertension is con-

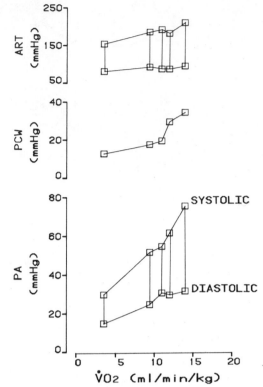

FIGURE 17–12. The hemodynamic response to treadmill exercise in a 52 year old man with obesity-related alveolar hypoventilation and systemic hypertension. Shown are the response in pulmonary artery (*PA*), wedge (*PCW*) and arterial (*ART*) pressures. See text.

firmed by the abnormal elevation in systemic arterial and wedge pressures with exercise. The abnormal rise in wedge pressure, which this man does not demonstrate until stage 4 of exercise when he develops mitral regurgitation, could not account for the disproportionate elevation in pulmonary artery pressure that was observed in stage 1. Later in exercise, the abnormal rise in arterial systolic pressure secondary to systemic hypertension and the accompanying elevation in wedge pressure indicated a second disorder that also required therapeutic intervention. A vascular-specific calcium channel blocker, nitrendipine, was administered to control his systemic hypertension and to ameliorate his pulmonary hypertension. Therapeutic response and drug dosage could be assessed and adjusted, respectively, with bedside hemodynamic monitoring. Moreover, it was possible to ensure that nitrendipine did not lead to a mismatch of ventilation relative to perfusion and the appearance of arterial oxygen desaturation secondary to enhanced venous oxygen admixture.

In patients with *systemic hypertension* and left ventricular hypertrophy, there is fre-

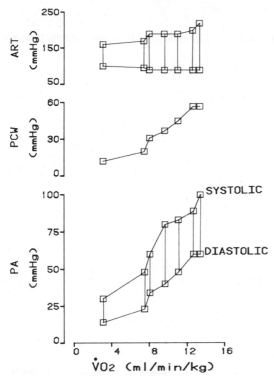

FIGURE 17–13. An illustration similar to that shown in Figure 17–12, for a 45 year old man with systemic hypertension who developed mitral regurgitation during treadmill exercise. See text.

quently the complaint of exertional dyspnea. Aside from an abnormality in left ventricular compliance that may accompany hypertrophy and lead to elevated pulmonary venous pressure, these patients may also develop mitral regurgitation during exercise, as was shown in Figure 17–12. Another example is depicted in Figure 17–13. The patient had actually been referred to us because of repeated bouts of cough, an interstitial infiltrate on chest x-ray, and a presumptive diagnosis of pneumonia with pulmonary hypertension.

REFERENCES

1. Cunningham DJC. Some quantitation aspects of the regulation of human respiration in exercise. Br Med Bull 19:25–30, 1963.

2. Cotes JE. Exercise limitation in health and disease. Br Med Bull 19:31–35, 1963.

3. Campbell EJM, Howell JBL. The sensation of breathlessness. Br Med Bull 19:36–40, 1963.

4. Turino GM, Fishman AP. The congested lung. J Chron Dis 9:510–524, 1959.

5. Killian KJ, Campbell EJM. Dyspnea and exercise. Annu Rev Physiol 45:465–479, 1983.

6. Killian KJ, Jones NL. The use of exercise testing and other methods in the investigation of dyspnea. Clin Chest Med 5:99–108, 1984.

7. Borg G, Noble B. Perceived exertion, *in* Wilmore JH (ed). Exercise and Sports Sciences Reviews. Academic Press, New York, 1974, pp 131–153.

8. Stark RD, Gambles SA, Chatlerjee SS. An exercise test to assess clinical dyspnea: estimation of reproducibility and sensitivity. Br J Dis Chest 76:269–278, 1982.

9. Murray JF. The lungs and heart failure. Hosp Practice 20:55–68, 1985.

10. Staub NC. Pulmonary edema. Physiol Rev 54:679–698, 1974.

11. Weber KT, Janicki JS. Lactate production during maximal and submaximal exercise in patients with chronic cardiac failure. J Am Coll Cardiol, 6:717–724, 1985.

12. Wasserman K, Whipp BJ, Casaburi R, Golden M, Beaver WL. Ventilatory control during exercise in man. Bull Eur Physiopathol Respir 15:27–47, 1979.

13. Macklem PT. Respiratory muscles: the vital pump. Chest 78:753–758, 1980.

14. Rubin SA, Brown HV, Swan HJC. Arterial oxygenation and arterial oxygen transport in chronic myocardial failure at rest, during exercise and after hydralazine treatment. Circulation 66:143–148, 1982.

15. Wilson JR, Ferraro N. Exercise intolerance in patients with chronic left heart failure: relation to oxygen transport and ventilatory abnormalities. Am J Cardiol 51:1358–1363, 1983.

16. West JR, Bliss HA, Wood JA, Richards DW. Pulmonary function in rheumatic heart disease and its relation to exertional dyspnea in ambulatory patients. Circulation 8:178–187, 1953.

17. Hayward GW, Knott JMS. The effect of exercise on lung distensibility and respiratory work in mitral stenosis. Br Heart J 17:303–311, 1955.

18. Weber KT, Kinasewitz GT, Janicki JS, Fishman AP. Oxygen utilization and ventilation in patients with chronic cardiac failure. Circulation 65:1213–1223, 1982.

19. Wasserman K, Whipp BJ. Exercise physiology in health and disease. Am Rev Respir Dis 112:219–249, 1975.

20. Shepard RJ. The maximum sustained voluntary ventilation in exercise. Clin Sci 32:167–176, 1967.

21. Freedman S. Sustained maximum voluntary ventilation. Respir Physiol 8:230–244, 1970.

22. Brown HV, Wasserman K. Exercise performance in chronic obstructive pulmonary disease. Med Clin North Am 65:525–547, 1981.

18

KARL T. WEBER

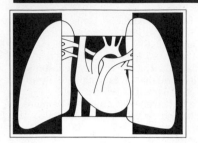

Illustrative Cases

In the preceding seven chapters, we have considered various cardiopulmonary disorders that can cause cardiac or circulatory failure or a ventilatory impairment and that can be examined and characterized by cardiopulmonary exercise testing. CPX provides the means to assess the nature of the disorder, its severity, and its course over time; moreover, CPX aids in identifying the choice of therapy and assessing therapeutic response. To conclude this section dealing with the clinical applications of CPX testing, illustrative cases have been selected from the files of our Cardiopulmonary Exercise Laboratory. Each case has been chosen to highlight the manner in which CPX served to address those issues that are relevant to the evaluation and management of cardiopulmonary disease.

IDENTIFYING THE NATURE OF CARDIOPULMONARY DISEASE

There is no substitute for a detailed patient interview and careful physical examination. Frequently, however, doubt exists as to the exact nature of the disorder that is responsible for the patient's symptoms, particularly when there are several coexistent diseases. The cases cited subsequently will identify how this frequent dilemma can be clarified by CPX testing.

Case 1

A 36 year old male chemical engineer was referred to our laboratory because of exertional dyspnea. The patient was in excellent health until 18 months prior to his referral, when he began to note the appearance of

dyspnea, at first while participating in recreational sports and later with normal daily activities. He noted "hyperventilation" with exertion that frequently was followed by near-syncope. His primary physician's initial evaluation did not indicate a cause of his exertional dyspnea. Bronchoscopy was unrewarding; pulmonary function studies revealed a mild restrictive defect; and a standard exercise tolerance test with electrocardiographic monitoring failed to demonstrate any evidence of myocardial ischemia or arrhythmia. The patient was forced to terminate this exercise test after 1 minute, at which point he was totally exhausted and near-syncopal, and had achieved a heart rate of 132 bpm.

The patient was thought to be anxious and a hyperventilator. Because a more definitive diagnosis was not forthcoming, the patient became depressed and required psychiatric care. Several months later because of persistent dyspnea the patient again sought medical attention. He was found to have an abnormal pulmonary ventilation/perfusion scan, demonstrating several segmental perfusion defects for which he received anticoagulant therapy for 1 year. Thereafter, however, he remained symptomatic and was referred to us for further evaluation. At the time of his presentation to our unit, there was clinical and laboratory evidence of an enlarged right ventricle and pulmonary hypertension.

The patient had a noninvasive CPX test with ear oximetry, the results of which are shown in Figure 18–1. Immediately upon commencing treadmill exercise (1 mph, 0 per cent grade), the patient's minute ventilation rose rapidly, reaching 70 liters/min within 2 minutes, while at the same time he devel-

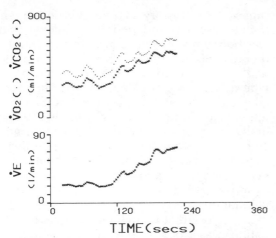

FIGURE 18–1. The response in breath-by-breath respiratory gas exchange and airflow to incremental treadmill exercise for a 36 year old man whose chief complaint was exertional dyspnea. Note the marked increment in minute ventilation ($\dot{V}_E$) with the onset of exercise. Despite a $\dot{V}_E$ of 70 liters/min, the patient developed arterial O_2 desaturation, as evidenced by both ear oximetry and arterial blood gas analysis.

oped significant arterial oxygen desaturation to 80 per cent. When the exercise test was terminated because of marked dyspnea, the patient had a respiratory rate and tidal volume of 45 bpm and 1700 ml, respectively.

It was apparent from CPX that there was a marked gas transfer abnormality with hypoxia, despite a marked level of $\dot{V}_E$. Moreover, the patient never crossed his anaerobic threshold and therefore never achieved his aerobic capacity. On the basis of these findings and a presumptive diagnosis of extensive thromboembolic disease and pulmonary hypertension, the patient was referred for right heart catheterization and pulmonary angiography from which massive thrombi

within the main pulmonary arteries and their branches were found.

Several points can be made from the patient's CPX test:

1. The patient's perceptions of dyspnea and "hyperventilation" were based on a clear pathophysiologic response to exercise, which, in all likelihood, could have been identified by CPX earlier in the course of his disease. Standard exercise testing, without respiratory gas exchange, airflow, or ear oximetry, was unable to properly discern the nature of this patient's problem.

2. The mechanism responsible for his dyspnea was identified as a gas transfer abnormality secondary to a major perfusion defect and large pulmonary emboli.

3. The appropriate direction for further diagnostic studies was identified.

Case 2

An 18 year old woman was admitted to Michael Reese Hospital because of exertional breathlessness, 3 months after an uneventful pregnancy and delivery; cardiomegaly was observed on chest radiograph. Her nuclear ejection fraction was 20 per cent, and an echocardiogram revealed left ventricular dilatation with generalized hypokinesia, although the valvular structures were normal. Endomyocardial biopsy was nondiagnostic. Based on the presumption that the patient's problem primarily was cardiac failure secondary to her dilated cardiomyopathy, she was sent to the exercise laboratory for a baseline functional evaluation.

Her CPX test results are shown in Figure 18–2. The patient stopped exercising with severe dyspnea at a $\dot{V}O_2$ of 25 ml/min/kg before she had crossed her anaerobic threshold or reached her $\dot{V}O_2$ max. Her exercise

FIGURE 18–2. The cardiopulmonary exercise (CPX) response for an 18 year old woman with dilated cardiomyopathy and biventricular failure. Note, however, that she does not cross her anaerobic threshold during this incremental treadmill test. She stopped exercising because of breathlessness. The limited rise in $\dot{V}_E$ (which approximates her MVV), despite a work load of 25 ml/min/kg, suggests respiratory muscle weakness. See text.

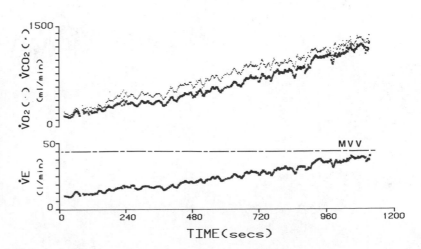

cardiac index exceeded 8 liters/min/m². At end exercise, her $\dot{V}_E$ was only 39 liters/min; this was achieved by a respiratory rate that had risen to 41 bpm at stage 5 and remained relatively constant until end exercise, while her exercise tidal volume rose from 466 ml at rest to only 768 ml at stage 5 and to 960 ml at end exercise. These findings were interpreted as indicating respiratory muscle weakness. Subsequent pulmonary function studies indicated that her MVV was only 44 liters/min, her forced vital capacity was 1.8 liter, and her lung volumes were reduced, compatible with muscular weakness. D_{LCO} was normal, and there was no evidence of an impairment in airflow. The patient refused to have either a repeat CPX with the monitoring of esophageal (pleural) pressure and inspiratory airflow rates or the measurement of maximum inspiratory pressure to further assess her presumed skeletal muscle disorder.

This case underscores several points:

1. One cannot predict the aerobic capacity or cardiac reserve from indices of resting left ventricular function, such as the ejection fraction, or from measurements of ventricular size.

2. The $\dot{V}O_2$ max, though not attained, predicts the maximum cardiac output and thereby the cardiac reserve.

3. Other illnesses (i.e., respiratory muscle weakness) may cause exertional dyspnea in patients with heart disease.

Case 3

A 52 year old unemployed, obese man was referred to our Heart Failure Program be-cause of his history of hypertension, exertional dyspnea, and peripheral edema that was poorly responsive to digoxin and diuretic therapy. Six months prior to his referral he had been admitted to another hospital, where he was treated for "pulmonary edema." The patient's medications included digoxin, 0.25 mg daily, furosemide, 40 mg orally twice daily, and isosorbide dinitrate, 40 mg orally four times daily. Despite these drugs, the patient still noted exertional dyspnea, orthopnea, and paroxysmal nocturnal dyspnea. He denied exertional chest pain, palpitations, syncope, or a history of previous myocardial infarction. Physical examination was notable only for a slightly increased pulmonary component to the second heart sound. Chest radiograph revealed a prominent main pulmonary artery but was otherwise normal.

An invasive CPX with ear oximetry was recommended because of the suspicion of obesity hypoventilation, pulmonary hypertension, and right heart failure. The results of the patient's invasive CPX are shown in Figures 18–3 and 18–4; the noninvasive portion of his exercise test is given in Figure 18–5. Immediately upon commencing exercise at 1 mph, 0 per cent grade, the patient's pulmonary artery pressure rose from its elevated level of 39/20 at standing rest to 45/24 (see Fig. 18–3). Coincident with his walking was the appearance of arterial oxygen desaturation. His arterial oxygen saturation at rest was 95 per cent and fell to 87 per cent with walking. By stage 4 (see Fig. 18–4), pulmonary artery pressure averaged 76/32 mm Hg

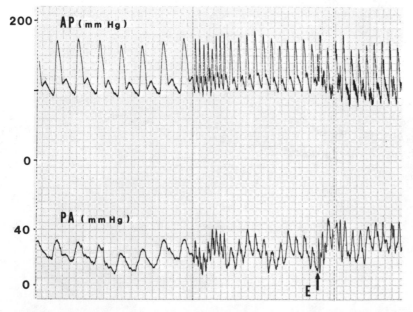

FIGURE 18–3. The response in pulmonary artery and radial artery pressure for case 3. Note that with the onset of exercise (*E*) there is an immediate rise in pulmonary artery pressure and a fall in arterial pressure.

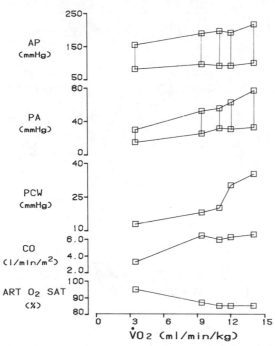

FIGURE 18–4. The hemodynamic response for each stage of treadmill exercise for the patient presented in Figure 18–3. See text.

when arterial saturation was 85 per cent; shortly thereafter, the patient stopped exercising. His resting wedge pressure was 13 mm Hg and arterial pressure, 150/82 mm Hg. During stage 4 of exercise, the patient's arterial pressure had risen to 214/98 mm Hg; simultaneously, his wedge pressure had risen to 35 mm Hg, and mitral regurgitation had appeared. Because of the hypoxemia and ventilatory abnormality, the CPX test was terminated prior to the patient's achieving

his anaerobic threshold or aerobic capacity. Nevertheless, several causes of a circulatory component to his exercise intolerance were also identified.

Highlights of the CPX response in this case include:

1. Right heart failure and pulmonary hypertension can be mistaken for or can coexist with left heart dysfunction.
2. With systemic hypertension, the rise in arterial pressure during exercise can be quite dramatic, even at low levels of work, and may be associated with mitral apparatus dysfunction.
3. Exercise-related hypoxemia can lead to pulmonary hypertension that is not apparent at rest. Moreover, a ventilatory impairment can coincide with cardiocirculatory disorders.

Case 4

A 72 year old woman with aortic regurgitation and left ventricular dilatation had had dyspnea on exertion for several years. As a result, she had been treated with digoxin and furosemide. She was referred to our Heart Failure Program for additional therapy. The patient also had a long history of cigarette smoking and a chronic cough. Pulmonary function studies had previously revealed her MVV to be 19 liters/min and her forced vital capacity, 2300 ml.

The results of her CPX test are shown in Figure 18–6. She became dyspneic when her $\dot{V}_E$ approximated her MVV. The patient did not cross her anaerobic threshold or attain her $\dot{V}O_2$ max, and there was no evidence of arterial oxygen desaturation. Thus, this pa-

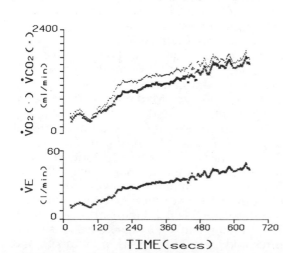

FIGURE 18–5. The CPX for a 52 year old obese man who was referred to the exercise laboratory because of presumed left ventricular failure secondary to systemic hypertension.

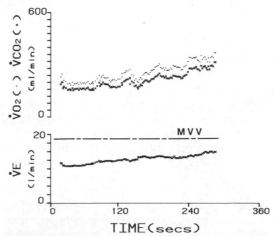

FIGURE 18–6. The noninvasive CPX for a 72 year old woman with aortic regurgitation and airway disease. Note that when she approached her maximal voluntary ventilation (MVV) she terminated the test with marked dyspnea. She did not develop hypoxemia during the test and did not cross her anaerobic threshold.

tient's primary limitation to exercise was not her chronic aortic regurgitation, but instead her ventilatory system. As a result, her therapeutic regimen was modified to include bronchodilators in accordance with these findings. The patient has felt somewhat improved, although she remains limited in her effort tolerance.

This case demonstrates the following points:

1. In patients with coexistent heart and lung disease, CPX testing will identify the mechanism responsible for the exertional dyspnea and the primary limitation to exercise.
2. Therapeutic guidelines can be logically formulated and former therapeutic regimens modified on the basis of CPX.

Case 5

A 45 year old male truck driver with systemic hypertension that was being treated with diuretics had presented with cough, dyspnea, and an infiltrate of unknown origin in the right lower lung field. A presumptive diagnosis of viral pneumonia was made and the patient given antibiotics. One month later, the patient again displayed these findings along with an accentuated pulmonic component of the second heart sound, suggesting the presence of pulmonary hypertension. His exercise tolerance remained impaired, and he was referred to our laboratory for evaluation.

His maximum oxygen uptake was 15 ml/min/kg. To evaluate the cause of the patient's reduced aerobic capacity, an invasive CPX test with hemodynamic monitoring was performed (Fig. 18–7). At standing rest *(upper panel)*, his pulmonary artery and capillary wedge pressures at end-expiration were 30/14 mm Hg and 12 mm Hg, respectively; systemic arterial pressure was 160/100 mm Hg. During stage 1 (1 mph, 0 per cent grade) of exercise, his arterial pressure was 190/90 mm Hg, and capillary wedge pressure rose to 30 mm Hg with the appearance of large *v* waves characteristic of mitral regurgitation *(middle panel)*. By stage 4 (2 mph, 7 per cent grade), his end-expiratory wedge pressure was 40 mm Hg *(lower panel)*. Left ventricular and mitral apparatus dysfunction were therefore identified as the cause of his compromised exercise cardiac output. A more aggressive approach to the management of his systemic hypertension was undertaken.

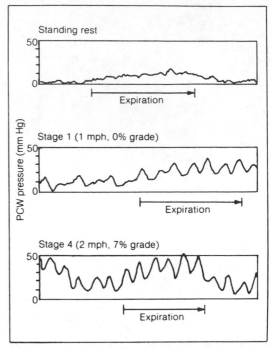

FIGURE 18–7. The results in pulmonary wedge pressure (*PCW*) monitored during exercise for a 45 year old man with systemic hypertension. Note the marked rise in PCW and the appearance of v waves and mitral regurgitation during stages 1 and 4 of treadmill exercise. (From Weber KT, Janicki JS. Pinpointing problems in cardiopulmonary circulation. J Resp Dis 4:71–76, 1983.)

Case 6

A 15 year old boy had been referred to Michael Reese Hospital because of exertional dyspnea that limited his participation in recreational activities (e.g., back-packing). He had previously been found to have a murmur of mitral regurgitation secondary to mitral valve prolapse. CPX was recommended to determine the severity of his functional impairment. On examination in the exercise laboratory, in addition to the presence of a mitral regurgitation murmur, it was apparent that the patient had a straight back and mild pectus excavatum. Marfanoid features were not present.

To further assess the severity of his mitral regurgitation and to consider the possibility that his chest wall deformity contributed to his exertional dyspnea, an invasive CPX with hemodynamic monitoring was performed, together with ear oximetry. The results of his CPX test are shown in Figures 18–8 and 18–9. The patient had approached his anaerobic threshold at a $\dot{V}O_2$ of 24 ml/min/kg, and shortly thereafter he had to stop exercising

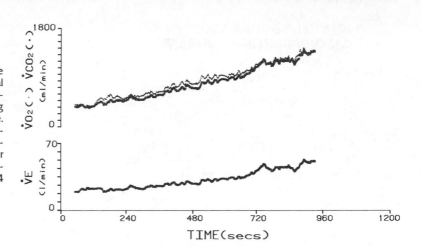

FIGURE 18–8. The exercise response for a 15 year old boy with mitral regurgitation at rest and the appearance of tricuspid regurgitation during moderate level treadmill exercise. His ventilatory response was the primary limitation to exercise. $\dot{V}_E$ remained invariant at 68 liters/min for two stages of exercise with the patient using a pattern of rapid (54 bpm), shallow (1260 ml) breathing.

because of breathlessness; there was evidence of mild arterial oxygen desaturation. His hemodynamic response to exercise indicated that his wedge pressure rose from 12 mm Hg at rest to 25 mm Hg throughout much of exercise, reaching 32 mm Hg at end exercise. Moreover, he developed tricuspid regurgitation during stage 4 of exercise, as manifested by a marked rise in right atrial pressure (from 5 mm Hg at rest to 18 mm Hg on exercise). Despite the abnormalities in

mitral and tricuspid valve function, the patient's cardiac output rose to 25 liters/min or 15 liters/min/m². His ventilatory response to exercise ($\dot{V}_E$ of 68 liters/min) was abnormal and was characterized by a pattern of rapid, shallow breathing, with a respiratory rate of 54 bpm and tidal volume of only 1260 ml. From these results, it appeared that the deformity of his thoracic cage and spine were primarily responsible for his exertional dyspnea at large work loads.

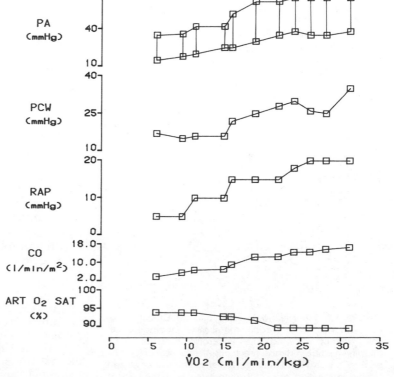

FIGURE 18–9. The hemodynamic response for the patient described in Figure 18–8.

IDENTIFYING THE SEVERITY OF CARDIOPULMONARY DISEASE

In Chapters 11 through 15, we identified how the determinations of aerobic capacity and anaerobic threshold are used to grade the severity of chronic cardiac or circulatory failure. Our objective here will be to indicate how CPX can be used to identify the severity of the impairment in functional status, which may not be apparent from clinical information or from laboratory tests, such as the ejection fraction or cardiac catheterization.

Case 7

This 62 year old man had a history of rheumatic mitral valve incompetence since age 8. He was clinically stable without evidence of heart failure until 2 weeks prior to admission, when he developed exertional dyspnea, orthopnea, and nocturnal dyspnea. He presented to the emergency room of this hospital short of breath, tachypneic, and with bibasilar rales. He was admitted and given intravenous furosemide, which subsequently relieved his dyspnea. Cardiac catheterization performed several days after admission indicated his wedge pressure to be 24 mm Hg with moderately severe mitral regurgitation. To define further the severity of his disease (including his cardiac reserve and operative candidacy), an invasive CPX test was performed on the fifth hospital day. The results of his CPX test are given in Figure 18–10.

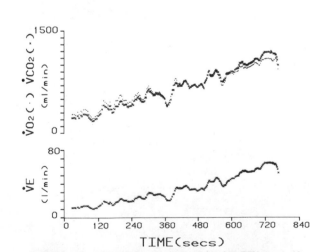

FIGURE 18–10. The noninvasive data for CPX in a 62 year old man with chronic mitral valve incompetence. The patient crossed his anaerobic threshold (15 ml/min/kg) but did not reach his aerobic capacity. His peak $\dot{V}O_2$ was 18 ml/min/kg. The fall in gas exchange and airflow at the end of exercise indicate where the patient discontinued using the mouthpiece.

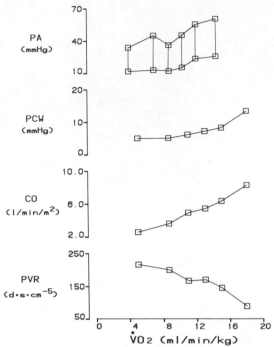

FIGURE 18–11. The hemodynamic response to treadmill exercise for the patient discussed in Figure 18–10. Abbreviations are the same as in previous figures. See text for discussions.

His anaerobic threshold was 15 ml/min/kg. He did not attain $\dot{V}O_2$ max, but his peak $\dot{V}O_2$ was 18 ml/min/kg. Even though he did not attain his $\dot{V}O_2$ max, his anaerobic threshold was compatible with functional class A and a predicted cardiac output of greater than 8 liters/min/m². These data supported his having a good cardiac reserve and indicated that he did not need valve replacement. By the fifth day of diuretic therapy, the patient's resting wedge pressure had fallen to 6 mm Hg and rose to only 18 mm Hg with maximum exercise (Fig. 18–11), suggesting there was little intrinsic left ventricular dysfunction. Pulmonary vascular resistance fell normally with exercise. Surgery was therefore not recommended. The patient has remained stable without failure over the subsequent 6 months of follow-up.

This experience once again indicates that:

1. Supine hemodynamic data and angiographic estimates of valvular incompetence may not indicate the true severity of mitral (or aortic) valvular incompetence or predict the cardiac reserve. These parameters, however, can be obtained by CPX.

2. The fact that left ventricular filling pressure did not rise substantially with exercise suggests that significant left ventricular dysfunction was not present.

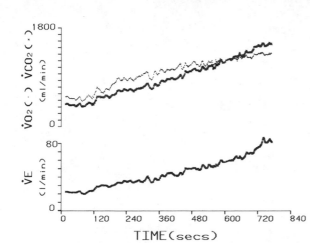

FIGURE 18–12. A 54 year old man with dilated cardiomyopathy and biventricular failure. His anaerobic threshold to incremental treadmill exercise was 12 ml/min/kg. At stage 5, his $\dot{V}O_2$ was 15.6 and at stage 6 it was 16.5 ml/min/kg, fulfilling our definition of $\dot{V}O_2$ max and class B status.

Case 8

A 54 year old member of the clergy had dilated cardiomyopathy and was referred to Michael Reese Hospital for further treatment and evaluation. He had been receiving daily doses of digoxin, furosemide, captopril, and nitrates but remained dyspneic and fatigued on exertion. His ejection fraction was 26 per cent. An echocardiogram performed at another hospital indicated he had a dilated left ventricle with diffuse hypokinesis and no segmental wall motion abnormality or anatomic defect of the valvular structures. Normal coronary arteries were found at coronary angiography. The patient was severely depressed, because his lifestyle had been significantly curtailed by his symptoms.

A CPX test was performed (Fig. 18–12), which indicated his anaerobic threshold to be 12 ml/min/kg; his $\dot{V}O_2$ max was 16.5 ml/min/kg. Based on his functional class B status with a predicted maximum cardiac output of 6 to 8 liters/min/m², the patient was given an exercise prescription of permissible physical activities. As a result, the patient's quality of life was substantially improved.

This case illustrates the facts that:

1. It is not possible to predict the severity of chronic cardiac failure or the cardiac reserve from indices of left ventricular function (e.g., the ejection fraction) obtained at rest.

2. Unlike the ejection fraction, CPX provides objective information on the patient's actual functional capacity.

3. Based on CPX testing, a rational program of physical activities (i.e., an exercise prescription) can be provided for the patient that does not unnecessarily restrict lifestyle. Similar to comparison of our present-day management of an uncomplicated acute myocardial infarction and its management in the past, we now know that bed rest is not mandatory in the patient with stable, chronic cardiac failure secondary to dilated cardiomyopathy.

Case 9

Owing to his dilated cardiomyopathy and ejection fraction of 36 per cent, a 36 year old postal worker was told by his primary physician that he would have to stop working and curtail his physical activities. He then presented to us for evaluation. These recommendations once again were made based on the presumed severity of his functional capacity.

The results of his CPX test using cycle ergometry are shown in Figure 18–13; it is evident that the patient had a good cardiac reserve achieving a peak $\dot{V}O_2$ max of 19 ml/min/kg.

A program of physical activities based on this patient's aerobic levels of work (<16 ml/min/kg) was provided. Over the years, we have been impressed with the fact that class A patients with dilated cardiomyopathy are likely to remain functionally stable for prolonged periods of time (years). Indeed, this patient has returned to his occupation and has been clinically stable 1 year since his initial evaluation.

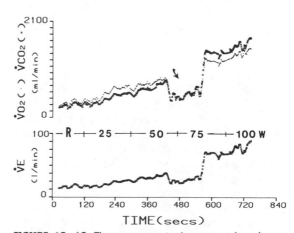

FIGURE 18–13. The response to incremental cycle ergometry of a 36 year old postman. Note that between 50 and 75 watts (w) of exercise his nose clip came off (arrow), which is the level at which he crossed his anaerobic threshold. His $\dot{V}O_2$ max was 19 ml/min/kg and represented a $\dot{V}O_2$ that he attained at 75 watts and sustained at 100 watts. See text for discussion.

MONITORING THE NATURAL COURSE OF CARDIOPULMONARY DISEASE

It is important for the practicing physician to be able to monitor the natural course of any cardiopulmonary disease and to identify any improvement or deterioration that occurs. This may not be apparent from bedside examination, historic information, or indices of ventricular function. In Chapters 11 and 12, we reviewed how CPX was useful in identifying a decline in the functional status of several patients. Herein, we will discuss a patient whose functional status improved over time.

Case 10

A 46 year old medical illustrator with insulin-dependent diabetes mellitus presented to the emergency room at Michael Reese Hospital with the chief complaints of dyspnea and weakness. On physical examination, she was found to have a blood pressure of 90/60 and pulmonary edema. She was promptly given intravenous furosemide and admitted to our cardiac care unit. Shortly thereafter, her low cardiac output state required the insertion of a triple-lumen flotation catheter and the administration of intravenous dobutamine, followed by intravenous dopamine to support her arterial pressure. Despite 20 mcg/kg/min of each catecholamine, her hemodynamic status continued to deteriorate, necessitating intra-aortic balloon counterpulsation. At this point, her cardiac output was only 1.8 liter/min/m²; her wedge pressure was 35 mm Hg with prominent *v* waves compatible with mitral regurgitation. Endomyocardial biopsy did not reveal an inflammatory process, and her coronary arteries were patent at coronary arteriography. The patient was felt to have a dilated cardiomyopathy of uncertain etiology. She was not considered to be a candidate for cardiac transplantation because of her insulin-dependent diabetes.

As a last resort, she was given an experimental cardiotonic agent, enoximone, whose mechanism of action is mediated by phosphodiesterase inhibition. A dramatic improvement in pump function followed, and within 48 hours it was possible to discontinue balloon counterpulsation and both catecholamines. The patient was discharged from the hospital 2 weeks after her admission, receiving oral enoximone and diuretics. Six weeks after discharge, she had her first CPX (Fig.

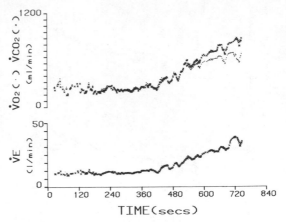

FIGURE 18–14. The incremental treadmill exercise test for a 46 year old woman with diabetes and a dilated cardiomyopathy. This CPX was performed 6 weeks after her discharge from the hospital. Her functional status was class C. See text for discussion.

18–14). Her aerobic capacity and anaerobic threshold were 13 and 8 ml/min/kg, respectively, and were compatible with moderately severe chronic cardiac failure (class C). Three months after this first CPX, her functional capacity was again assessed (Fig. 18–15); it had improved to class A status with a $\dot{V}O_2$ max of 22 ml/min/kg and an anaerobic threshold of 17 ml/min/kg. This improvement was verified 2 months later (Fig. 18–16). As a result, the patient was allowed to return to her full-time occupation. Without the objective information derived from CPX, it would not have been clear whether or not the patient could return to the work place. Her ejection fraction, which was 31 per cent on admission to the hospital, remained unchanged at 6 months of follow-up and therefore was of little value in monitoring the natural course of her illness.

SELECTING MANAGEMENT IN CARDIOPULMONARY DISEASE

The selection of a particular medical or surgical intervention for a disorder of the cardiopulmonary unit can be facilitated by the results obtained from CPX testing. Illustrative cases have appeared in earlier chapters as well as this chapter, to underscore the utility of CPX in this regard. We will not recount these specific issues further. In chapters that follow, the role of CPX in providing the requisite information to write an individualized exercise prescription will also be reviewed.

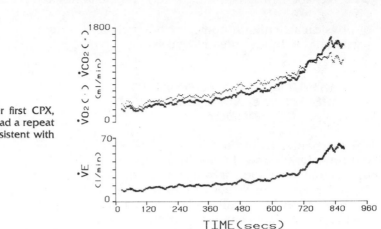

FIGURE 18–15. Three months after her first CPX, the patient presented in Figure 18–14 had a repeat test. Now her aerobic capacity was consistent with class A. See text.

Herein we will describe another facet of CPX that aids in the overall management of cardiopulmonary disease. The issue under consideration here is the use of a constant–work rate CPX test to provide patients with the tangible evidence and psychologic support that are necessary for them to participate in selected outpatient physical activities. By identifying a patient's actual effort tolerance, CPX can be invaluable in enhancing a patient's quality of life.

Case 11

A 64 year old man with several previous myocardial infarctions was referred to this hospital because of continued symptoms of chronic cardiac failure. His ejection fraction was 26 per cent, and he had electrocardiographic evidence of necrosis involving the anterior and inferior surfaces of the myocardium. The patient had been receiving digoxin

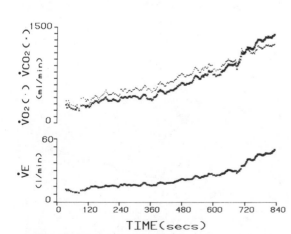

FIGURE 18–16. Two months after her second CPX, the patient described in Figures 18–14 and 18–15 had a third CPX, which again indicated her functional status to be stable at class A. See text.

and diuretics for over a year and had failed several trials with vasodilators because of hypotension and orthostasis. His baseline VO_2 max on CPX testing was 12 ml/min/kg, which was compatible with functional class C.

Oral enoximone (1.5 mg/kg three times daily) was added to the patient's regimen of digoxin and diuretics, resulting in a clear improvement in pump function demonstrable on hemodynamic monitoring. Subsequent CPX tests performed within 1 and 4 weeks of enoximone therapy indicated his aerobic capacity had improved to 16 ml/min/kg; this level was sustained for 12 weeks. The patient, however, denied that he had appreciated any outpatient improvement in his effort tolerance. He cited the fact that he could not walk more than a block with his wife without "becoming short of breath" and that he was unable to talk while walking because of breathlessness.

Owing to the disparity between his aerobic capacity and his symptoms, the patient underwent a constant–work rate treadmill exercise test (see Chapter 10) involving an aerobic work load to match the work load associated with walking at home (1.5 mph, 0 per cent grade). The patient completed the entire 20-minute protocol without dyspnea or fatigue. In discussing these findings with the patient, we ascertained that it was his voice that changed with exercise and this he perceived to be the early appearance of dyspnea. He previously had a tracheostomy following a myocardial infarction that was complicated by pulmonary edema and ventricular arrhythmia. Ever since, his voice would change spontaneously, particularly on exertion. After the aerobic endurance test the patient felt more confident that he was not impaired and he now enjoys a fuller range of physical activities at home, including light gardening, without "breathlessness."

MONITORING THE RESPONSE TO THERAPY IN CARDIOPULMONARY DISEASE

This chapter would not be complete without considering how the results of CPX serve to monitor the response to therapy. Chapter 21 will review our experience with CPX in the evaluation of vasodilator and cardiotonic agents in the management of chronic cardiac failure for groups of patients that participated in various clinical trials. In the remainder of this chapter, we will present several illustrative cases that deal with other forms of therapy in the individual patient.

Case 12

A 66 year old man with dilated cardiomyopathy was seen in consultation because of his chronic cardiac failure, which had not responded well to a regimen of digoxin and modest doses of furosemide. A CPX test was recommended, to establish his baseline functional status (Fig. 18–17) before a more aggressive diuretic program was initiated. One week after increasing his daily dose of furosemide from 40 mg to 80 mg and administering the drug on a twice-daily basis, the patient returned for a repeat CPX (Fig. 18–18). A clear improvement in his functional status was apparent, with anaerobic threshold and $\dot{V}O_2$ max increasing from 9 and 12 ml/min/kg

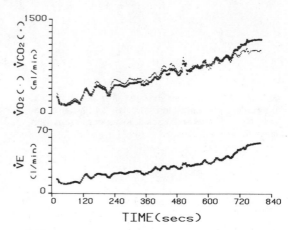

FIGURE 18–18. One week after enhanced diuresis, the patient described in Figure 18–17 was re-exercised. His anaerobic threshold and aerobic capacity had improved. See text for discussion.

to 11 and 16 ml/min/kg, respectively. His functional capacity remained stable at this new level for a minimum of 4 weeks before he was enrolled into a clinical trial involving a new cardiotonic agent.

CPX was useful here in documenting an improvement in functional status that accompanied diuretic therapy. This experience also underscores the need to obtain a constant aerobic capacity and stability in medical therapy before patients with chronic cardiac failure may be enrolled into clinical trials. If this is not done, erroneous conclusions can be drawn. Moreover, it should be stated that a true plateau in $\dot{V}O_2$ during an exercise test, or $\dot{V}O_2$ max, is a far superior parameter to monitor than is peak $\dot{V}O_2$ at symptomatic

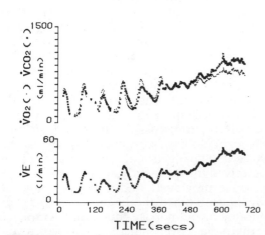

FIGURE 18–17. A baseline incremental treadmill response for a 66 year old man with a dilated cardiomyopathy who required larger doses of diuretics. See text for discussion.

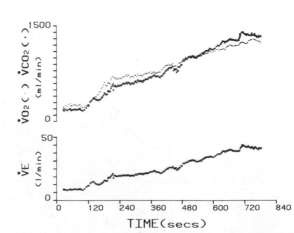

FIGURE 18–19. Twelve weeks after this 13 year old girl had received a cardiac transplantation, she underwent a CPX for baseline determination of her functional status.

end point, because VO_2 max is free of patient and physician bias. Peak $\dot{V}O_2$ should never be confused with or referred to as $\dot{V}O_2$ max, as is the case in many clinical trials.

Case 13

A 13 year old girl with dilated cardiomyopathy and severe heart failure underwent cardiac transplantation at another hospital. Several months after her return to Chicago and after she was actively participating in the recreational activities of her choice, her primary physician wished to establish her functional status for serial monitoring. CPX was performed (Fig. 18–19), revealing an anaerobic threshold and $\dot{V}O_2$ max of 15 and 23 ml/min/kg, respectively. These values, although not normal for a 13 year old girl (predicted $\dot{V}O_2$ max of over 40 ml/min/kg), did indicate an adequate cardiac reserve and established a "baseline" with which serial determinations could be compared. The value of CPX in predicting early transplant rejection remains to be defined but represents an intriguing possibility that merits consideration.

SECTION III

OTHER APPLICATIONS OF CPX TESTING

19

CAROL S. MASKIN

Aerobic Exercise Training in Cardiopulmonary Disease

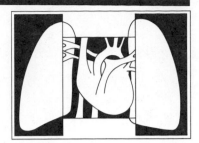

Improvement of functional capacity and hence quality of life are major goals in the management of patients with cardiovascular or pulmonary disease. Rational selection and titration of any therapy, including exercise training, necessitate consideration of the specific pathophysiologic mechanisms limiting exercise capacity and which may indeed differ as a function of the underlying disease and its severity.

Aerobic exercise training induces a complex series of systemic and regional adjustments (hemodynamic, metabolic, neuroendocrine, and musculoskeletal) that subserve improved cardiocirculatory efficiency during submaximal and maximal levels of activity in normal subjects. The question of whether the various physiologic adjustments induced by training are clinically relevant in cardiopulmonary disease states, and the extent to which they can be safely achieved and sustained, are of great interest.

As in the use of investigative pharmacologic interventions, before clinical application of training as a therapeutic modality, it is appropriate first to determine characterization of mechanism of action, dose-response relationship, duration of clinical effect, and safety. Hence, consideration of the limits of exercise capacity in normal subjects and of the mechanisms by which they are altered by aerobic exercise training is a logical first step toward understanding and making optimal clinical use of exercise as a therapeutic tool. To define the relationship between therapy and clinical response, an objective "assay" for the "dose" of exercise administered is necessary. Practical "dose" parameters include the duration of prescribed exercise, as well as the oxygen consumed ($\dot{V}O_2$, which can be measured), expressed as a percentage of the individual's maximal oxygen consumption ($\dot{V}O_2$ max). Quantification of the clinical response to training may, however, be more difficult; indeed, although changes in $\dot{V}O_2$ during maximal exercise can be measured, the appropriate end points during submaximal exercise are less clear.

An exhaustive review of exercise training and rehabilitation is beyond the intended scope of this chapter. For this purpose, the interested reader is referred to several excellent reviews.[1, 2] In this chapter, we will briefly discuss (1) the mechanisms limiting exercise capacity in normal subjects, as well as in patients with coronary artery disease, chronic left ventricular dysfunction, peripheral vascular disease, and systemic hypertension; (2) the physiologic adjustments induced by training in normal subjects; and (3) the potential value and limitations of training as therapy in cardiopulmonary disease.

LIMITATIONS OF EXERCISE CAPACITY

In healthy individuals, peak aerobic exercise is usually limited by the ability of the heart to augment cardiac output and deliver oxygen to the metabolically active limb(s) and by the capacity of skeletal muscle to extract and use oxygen (Fig. 19–1).[3] Moreover, the ability to endure a submaximal level of work for prolonged periods of time appears related to skeletal muscle metabolism, including the substrate source for oxidative metabolism and its availability,[4] the rate of skeletal muscle glycogen depletion and lactate accumulation, and the reduction of serum glucose concentration and its effect on the central nervous system.[5]

The increase in *cardiac output* during exer-

$$VO_2 = CO \times (A-V)O_2$$

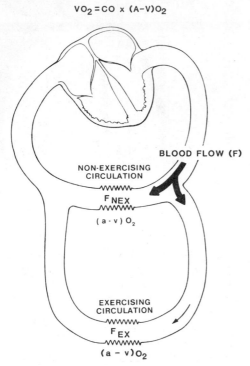

$$(A-V)O_2 = \left[NEx(a-v)O_2 \times \frac{F_{NEx}}{CO}\right] + \left[Ex\,(a-v)O_2 \times \frac{F_{Ex}}{CO}\right]$$

FIGURE 19–1. The central and regional circulatory and metabolic parameters involved in the exercise response. VO_2, systemic O_2 consumption; CO, cardiac output; $(A-V)O_2$, systemic arteriovenous O_2 difference; F, blood flow; $(a-v)O_2$, regional arteriovenous O_2 difference; NEx, nonexercising circulation; Ex, exercising circulation; ^FNEx and ^FEx, blood flow in the respective regional circulations; $NEx(a-v)O_2$ and $Ex(a-v)O_2$, arteriovenous O_2 difference in the respective regional circulations.

cise is coupled with *peripheral adjustments* aimed at supplying oxygenated blood to the limbs. The peripheral response to exercise, in turn, facilitates a parallel improvement in cardiac performance. For example, whereas vasodilatation in exercising skeletal muscle, consequent largely to locally accumulating metabolites, subserves the needed increase in regional blood flow, the resultant lowering of systemic vascular resistance reduces left ventricular afterload. In addition, augmentation of stroke volume during exercise is afforded, in accordance with the Frank-Starling mechanism, by increased venous blood return from contracting limb muscles.

Indeed, increased sympatho-adrenal activity, stimulated to a large extent by afferent signals from metabolically active skeletal muscles, induces vasoconstriction in nonexercising organs (e.g., gut and kidneys), thereby maintaining mean arterial pressure in the face of skeletal muscle vasodilatation. This results in an increased circulating blood volume (hence, left ventricular end-diastolic volume) and, specifically, in enhanced blood flow to the exercising muscles. The increased sympathetic activity during exercise further augments cardiac output by increasing heart rate and by increasing myocardial contractility.

The ability to increase cardiac output in response to exercise, however, may be impaired markedly in patients with chronic cardiac failure, owing to a limited ability to further augment stroke volume (see Chapter 11) in response to increased left ventricular filling pressure.[6] Moreover, in such patients the vasoconstricting effects of increased sympathetic activity during exercise may further jeopardize already reduced blood flow to the renal and mesenteric circulations.

The cardiac output response to exercise is also influenced by myocardial oxygen availability and by the relationship between myocardial oxygen supply and demand. Normally, a rise in coronary blood flow occurs with exercise to ensure myocardial oxygen availability sufficient to meet the enhanced metabolic demands imposed by increased blood pressure, heart rate, and left ventricular end-diastolic volume. This may not be the case, however, in the presence of coronary artery disease, wherein oxygen delivery to the myocardium is limited. Here, the aerobic capacity of cardiac muscle, rather than exercising skeletal muscle, limits exercise performance. Myocardial ischemia may be manifested by symptoms of angina at submaximal levels of work or by abnormalities in systolic and diastolic ventricular function, which compromise cardiac output and, hence, oxygen delivery to exercising skeletal muscle.

In addition to the ability of the heart to augment systemic blood flow, the aerobic capacity of exercising skeletal muscle is influenced by local factors that influence its oxygen availability: (1) oxygen *delivery*, which is influenced by the vasodilating capacity of the skeletal muscle circulation, the capillary–to–skeletal muscle fiber ratio, and the oxygen-carrying capacity of blood; (2) oxygen *extraction* within muscle, which is a function of the oxyhemoglobin dissociation curve and muscle concentration of myoglobin (a protein that enhances diffusion of oxygen through the cytoplasm to mitochondria, the site of oxidative metabolism); and (3) oxygen *utilization* within muscle, which is a function of skeletal muscle mass, fiber composition (fast versus slow twitch fibers), and oxidation capacity of the mitochondria.

The limitations of the periphery, independent of cardiac performance, are perhaps most obvious in patients with peripheral vascular disease, in whom peak aerobic power of the limb is limited by fixed arterial obstruction and manifested clinically by claudication.

Although fatigue is the predominant subjective symptom limiting exercise capacity in normal subjects, its physiologic basis is not well understood. Preliminary data from Le-Jemtel and co-workers[7] suggest, however, that peak aerobic power of the exercising limb in normals is not limited by the *vasodilating capacity* of its circulation. Indeed, in their study, the maximum femoral vein blood flow attained in a leg during exhaustive graded two-leg bicycle exercise could be further augmented when maximal exercise was performed with a single leg (hence, in response to an increased work load to that limb). This contrasts with the response observed by these investigators in patients with chronic severe heart failure (maximal $\dot{V}O_2$ <12 ml/kg/min). In these patients, the maximum femoral vein blood flow, and hence maximum limb oxygen consumption attained during two-leg exercise, could not be further augmented when work was performed by one leg alone. These data imply a relatively fixed and limited maximal vasodilating capacity in patients with severe heart failure. This may be consequent to increased vascular salt and water content, as previously suggested by Zelis and Mason.[8]

With regard to *oxygen extraction* in normal subjects performing two-leg exercise, the oxygen content of femoral venous blood at exhaustion averaged 4.5 ml/dl, and further extraction was not accomplished during one-leg maximal exercise; instead, increased limb oxygen consumption was attained by augmentation of local blood flow. In contrast, in the heart failure patients, femoral venous blood was already maximally desaturated during the two-leg bicycle exercise, with values as low as 1.5 ml/dl, depending on the severity of the disease.[9, 10] These findings are consistent with those of Donald and colleagues,[11] in normal subjects and in patients with cardiovascular disease. Pirnay and associates,[12] however, have demonstrated that in normal subjects, further desaturation of femoral venous blood can be induced when maximum cardiac output is acutely impaired by administration of a beta-blocking agent. Why oxygen extraction of such magnitude is not normally attained, thereby allowing greater aerobic exercise capacity, is unclear.

Hence, the performance of aerobic exercise is a multisystem endeavor, accomplished in an integrated manner. Moreover, it is clear that the limitations of exercise capacity are complex, reflecting the physiologic reserves of the heart and periphery in both health and disease.

AEROBIC EXERCISE TRAINING IN NORMAL SUBJECTS

In normal subjects, physiologic adjustments that subserve increased maximal oxygen consumption and improved cardiocirculatory efficiency are induced by performance of regular isotonic exercise. Although the optimal "dose" (intensity and duration) and the frequency of administration are controversial and may indeed differ with respect to functional status at the start of the training program,[13] it appears that to be effective isotonic exercise must be performed at least three times per week at an intensity sufficient to consume at least 50 per cent of maximal aerobic capacity for a minimum of 20 minutes.[14] Moreover, the rapidity of adaptation probably depends on the intensity and duration of initial work load and on the rate of progression to heavier work loads (Fig. 19–2).

During performance of *submaximal* levels of work, the most striking benefit induced by training in normal individuals, is a more efficient cardiocirculatory system. Efficiency, as defined in Chapter 4, refers to the work performed by muscle (skeletal or cardiac) relative to its consumption of energy, or

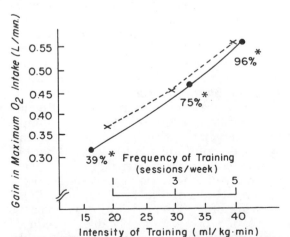

FIGURE 19–2. The influence of intensity (solid line) and frequency (dashed line) of training on improvement of $\dot{V}O_2$ max. Asterisks indicate the intensity of training expressed as per cent of maximum O_2 capacity. (From Shephard RJ. Insensity, duration and frequency of exercise as determinants of the response to a training regimen. Intern Z Agnew Physiol 26:272–278, 1968.)

Table 19–1. Effects of Aerobic Training on Hemodynamic, Metabolic, and Neuroendocrine Responses to Submaximal Levels of Exercise in Normal Subjects

Response	Submaximal Aerobic Training
Oxygen consumption	No change
Cardiac output	No change
Heart rate	Reduced
Stroke volume	No change or improved
Exercising limb blood flow	No change or reduced
Exercising limb O_2 extraction	Increased
Blood pressure	Reduced
Plasma norepinephrine	Reduced

oxygen. Indeed, as summarized in Table 19–1, improved oxygen extraction in the exercising limb supports performance of the same quantity of muscular work with greater efficiency. These benefits appear to be consequent to changes induced in trained skeletal muscle and, in fact, are not elicited when exercise is performed by untrained muscles (e.g., by the arms when the legs have been trained).[15]

Less cardiac work (e.g., decreased heart rate) and hence greater myocardial efficiency, also accompany exercise training. Reduced heart rate during submaximal levels of work appears related to both increased vagal tone and reduced sympatho-adrenal activity.[16] However, maximum lowering of heart rate during training occurs subsequent to maximum lowering of plasma catecholamines,[17] suggesting that other factors are involved. These may include changes in the metabolic and ionic milieu at sensory receptors in exercising muscle, as described subsequently, resulting in decreased nerve impulses and reduced adrenergic output by the autonomic nervous system. Moreover, as skeletal muscle fibers become stronger in response to physical training, the motor unit activity required to perform a given work load would be expected to decrease. Hence, the sympathetic nervous system, activated to the same extent as motor units in the limbs, would be stimulated to a lesser extent, thereby explaining many of the physiologic consequences of training. Indeed, the lower systolic blood pressure often observed during submaximal levels of work is probably due to reduced sympathetic tone in nonexercising circulations.

These changes in physiologic response to submaximal exercise occur in the presence of structural and metabolic adaptations in trained skeletal muscle.[18] Structural changes in skeletal muscle induced by training in normal individuals include an increased muscle mass that can be as great as 30 per cent and an increase in the proportion of "slow-twitch" muscle fibers, which are rich in enzymes involved in oxidative metabolism. Moreover, an increase in collateral blood vessels and an increased capillary–to–muscle fiber ratio allow an increased delivery of oxygen to a greater muscle mass and, once again, provide for greater efficiency.

The adaptations that appear within skeletal muscle as a result of aerobic training are outlined in Table 19–2. They appear to subserve an increased potential for oxidative metabolism, as well as a shift of carbon source for the citric acid cycle from glucose to fatty acids. Moreover, concomitant neuroendocrine adjustments to training, including increased circulating levels of insulin and growth hormone during submaximal levels of activity,[19] tend to enhance free fatty acid mobilization and thus their availability as an energy source. Increased oxidation of fat and reduced carbohydrate use during exercise may result in decreased muscle fatigue and improved endurance of submaximal levels of exercise, as a result of: (1) the glycogen-sparing effect afforded by increased use of fat; and (2) decreased lactate production consequent to reduced phosphorylation of glycogen. Moreover, a decreased rate of carbohydrate utilization may protect against the central nervous system manifestations of hypoglycemia, which may be produced by prolonged exercise. An increased skeletal muscle myoglobin content has also been observed with training and may contribute to improved peripheral oxygen extraction by facilitating oxygen diffusion through the cytoplasm to the mitochondria. Induction of such structural and metabolic changes within trained muscle might afford substantial ben-

Table 19–2. Metabolic Adaptations in Skeletal Muscle to Aerobic Exercise Training in Normal Subjects

1. Increased size and number of mitochondria
2. Increased activity of mitochondrial respiratory chain enzymes
3. Increased mitochondrial metabolism of free fatty acids
4. Reduced mitochondrial carbohydrate substrate metabolism
5. Decreased uptake of glucose
6. Increased myoglobin content

efits to patients with cardiopulmonary disease (e.g., severe chronic cardiac failure) in whom fatigue often limits performance at submaximal levels of exercise.

Indeed, the physiologic adjustments to submaximal exercise induced by training in healthy individuals offer potential benefits in a number of cardiovascular disorders. In peripheral vascular disease, for example, more efficient skeletal muscle might permit increased aerobic work despite a fixed arterial blood supply. In addition, in patients with coronary artery disease, reduced myocardial oxygen demand resulting from decreased heart rate, blood pressure, and inotropic stimulation, would improve myocardial efficiency and thereby ameliorate symptoms of angina or improve cardiac performance during exercise, or both. Moreover, reduced sympathetic activity and, hence, lower vasomotor tone in renal and mesenteric circulations may be particularly advantageous in patients with "intestinal angina," or in patients with heart failure in whom renal and mesenteric blood flow may be significantly impaired during exercise.[20]

Theoretically, such changes in neuroendocrine activity may be of special benefit in patients with ischemic heart disease who are at high risk for sudden cardiac death. Electrical stability of the heart has been found to be reduced by elevated sympathetic efferent activity and to be increased by a major rise in vagal efferent activity. Indeed, Billman and co-workers[21] recently reported that daily exercise prevented ventricular fibrillation, induced by acute myocardial ischemia, in a subpopulation of dogs previously identified as susceptible to sudden cardiac death. Whether these data can be extrapolated to the clinical setting is not known but is certainly intriguing.

In addition to the beneficial effects during submaximal exercise, *maximal oxygen consumption* and, hence, peak work load or aerobic capacity are significantly increased by training in healthy individuals, owing to increases in both oxygen delivery and oxygen extraction in active skeletal muscle (Table 19–3). Improved stroke volume and therefore cardiac output at peak exercise appear to result from an increased circulating blood volume, left ventricular end-diastolic volume, and in some cases myocardial mass, without augmentation of left ventricular ejection fraction.[22] Moreover, maximal systemic arterial pressure and cardiac work are increased. Whether intrinsic myocardial changes are induced by training and contrib-

Table 19–3. Effects of Aerobic Training on Hemodynamic, Metabolic, and Neuroendocrine Responses to Maximal Levels of Exercise in Normal Subjects

Response	Maximal Aerobic Training
Oxygen consumption	Increased
Cardiac output	Increased
Heart rate	No change
Stroke volume	Increased
Exercise limb blood flow (ml/min/gram)	No change
Exercising limb O_2 extraction	Increased
Blood pressure	Increased

ute to greater cardiac work capacity in the healthy adult human is unclear. The extent to which these cardiac adaptations can be attained may, however, limit the benefits at peak exercise derived by patients with cardiovascular disease. In chronic cardiac failure, for example, maximal cardiac output during exercise is limited by the inability of an already dilated left ventricle to further augment stroke volume in response to increased filling pressure. Moreover, in the presence of coronary artery disease, an inability to further increase myocardial blood flow may preclude an improvement in maximal cardiac performance and work and, therefore, in maximal exercise capacity.

In normal subjects, despite the increase in maximal cardiac output induced by training, maximal blood flow per gram of skeletal muscle does not change. This suggests that training results in augmented blood flow and oxygen delivery to an increased muscle mass, rather than increased oxygen delivery to the individual muscle cell, and is consistent with the structural adaptations described earlier. Thus, improvement of maximal vasodilatory response to exercise per se does not appear to be responsible for the improvement in oxygen delivery. The extent to which the described structural and metabolic skeletal muscle adaptations can be induced may greatly determine the benefits derived at peak exercise from training (e.g., in heart failure patients). Indeed, as previously noted, in many such patients femoral venous blood may already be almost maximally desaturated at peak exercise, potentially limiting the metabolic advantages induced by physical training.[9, 10]

The long-term effects of exercise training on factors other than exercise performance in normal subjects have been a focus of considerable interest and unresolved debate. Although a number of uncontrolled studies suggest a reduced incidence of "cardiac events" in physically active individuals, conclusive data and possible mechanisms for such benefits remain to be established. A number of studies in normal subjects have demonstrated reductions of serum cholesterol levels in response to aerobic exercise training; however, there is no consensus as to whether exercise has a significant independent effect on serum cholesterol level.[23] Whether such alterations prevent coronary atherogenesis or attenuate the progression of already established disease is unknown. Some studies have described an inverse relationship between high-density lipoprotein (HDL) levels and coronary risk,[24, 25] and it has been reported that vigorous exercise may actually increase HDL-cholesterol levels. It is postulated that HDL stimulates intracellular cholesterol acyl transferase, thereby facilitating cholesterol removal from the cell; that the HDL molecule interferes with low-density lipoprotein entry into the cell; and that HDL is preferentially transported to the liver for excretion and thus is less likely to be incorporated into atherosclerotic plaques. The role of aerobic exercise training in altering lipid metabolism, as well as the impact of such changes on atherogenesis or arrhythmia and on sudden death, are issues to be addressed by future investigation, in controlled prospective clinical trials.

The potential benefits of aerobic exercise training in cardiovascular disease will depend on the extent to which the physiologic adaptations achieved in healthy individuals can be induced in patients. Indeed, an inability to perform or sustain exercise at an intensity sufficient to stress the aerobic capacity of active skeletal muscle may preclude a training effect in patients limited by claudication or angina to very low levels of work. Also, it must be recognized that, perhaps with the exception of marked deconditioning (e.g., subsequent to prolonged bed rest),[26] exercise does not reverse the underlying cardiocirculatory abnormality; hence, training must be continued chronically to sustain the desired clinical benefits.

AEROBIC TRAINING IN CARDIOPULMONARY DISEASE

Coronary Artery Disease

Considerable interest has been focused on the potential benefits of exercise training in the rehabilitation of patients with coronary artery disease. As already pointed out, however, the limitations of exercise capacity differ with respect to the underlying cardiovascular pathophysiology; therefore, the variable responses reported in heterogeneous populations of patients with coronary artery disease are not at all surprising. Nor is it unexpected that the mechanisms by which improvements are induced appear to differ in these individuals. Moreover, the variable methods of titrating, administering, and quantifying the effects of exercise training, reported in the literature, confound generalization.

Nonetheless, most studies demonstrate that hemodynamic changes, consistent with a training effect, can be induced during submaximal levels of activity in patients with coronary artery disease who are without symptoms of cardiac failure. These changes generally include significant lowering of heart rate and systolic blood pressure, which are major determinants of myocardial oxygen demand (Fig. 19–3). Indeed, an increased threshold for angina is clearly the best documentation of training-induced benefits in patients with coronary artery disease. Moreover, Cooksey and colleagues[27] have shown that these adaptations to submaximal exercise are accompanied by significant reductions in circulating levels of norepinephrine, consistent with the neuroendocrine changes observed in normal subjects.

Training appears to induce an augmentation in stroke volume during submaximal levels of work in many patients with coronary artery disease; however, this response is quite variable[28–30] and may indeed reflect the heterogeneity of disease in most study populations. For example, important variables that may influence stroke volume response to exercise therapy include (1) presence of exercise-induced myocardial ischemia; (2) temporal relationship to the most recent myocardial infarction; (3) degree of left ventricular dysfunction; (4) history of coronary artery bypass surgery; and (5) concomitant medications. Mechanisms for improved stroke volume during training, which may be specific for such patients, include reduced myocardial ischemia, resulting from decreased myocardial oxygen demand during exercise; spontaneous improvement of asynchronous contraction and/or global left ventricular performance subsequent to myocardial infarction, as reported by Rousseau and associates;[31] or training-induced improve-

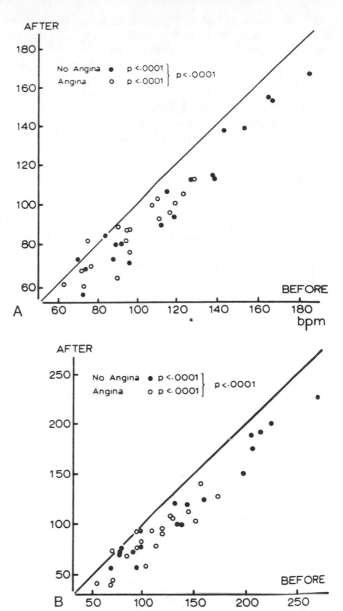

FIGURE 19–3. *A,* Effects of physical training on heart rate during the same absolute level of submaximal exercise in patients with coronary artery disease, with and without angina at maximum effort. *B,* Effects of physical training on pressure-rate product (mm Hg × 10⁻²/min). The reduced pressure-rate product after physical training results from both lower heart rate and systemic arterial pressure. The line of identity is shown in each graph. (From Detry JMR, Rousseau M, Vanderbroncke G, Kusumi F, Brasseur LA, Bruce RA. Increased arteriovenous oxygen difference after physical training in coronary heart disease. Circulation *44*:109–118, 1971.)

ment in myocardial blood flow, consequent to an increased density of collateral vessels, as described in animal models by Eckstein.[32]

There is little clinical evidence, however, to support the latter mechanism in humans. Indeed, Ferguson and co-workers[33] have reported that in patients with stable exertional angina, training reduced coronary sinus blood flow and myocardial oxygen demand at the same submaximal work load, concomitant with a reduction in heart rate and systolic blood pressure. Moreover, when compared with exercise during the baseline period, a greater work load could be performed without augmentation of coronary sinus blood flow or myocardial oxy-

gen consumption, but with a similar heart rate and blood pressure. Similarly, Nolewajka and colleagues,[34] evaluating myocardial perfusion studies with labeled microspheres, failed to demonstrate increased collateralization of the coronary circulation in patients with coronary artery disease, who were symptomatically improved subsequent to 7 months of exercise training. Thus, these data suggest that improved exercise tolerance in patients limited during submaximal activity by angina, is related to reduced myocardial oxygen requirement, rather than to augmented myocardial oxygen delivery. Indeed, it is likely that in humans the only clinically relevant stimulus for myocardial collateralization is ischemia, and even this response may be modulated by genetic predisposition.

Reduced myocardial oxygen demand during submaximal levels of work in normal subjects appears to be related to training-induced adaptations in exercising skeletal muscle which increases their efficiency, as discussed earlier. Similarly, in patients with coronary artery disease, Paterson,[30] Detry,[35] and co-workers have reported increases in systemic arteriovenous oxygen difference during both submaximal (Fig. 19–4) and maximal levels of exercise; in fact, the latter group of investigators has suggested that improvement in $\dot{V}O_2$ with training in patients with coronary artery disease is primarily consequent to increased oxygen ex-

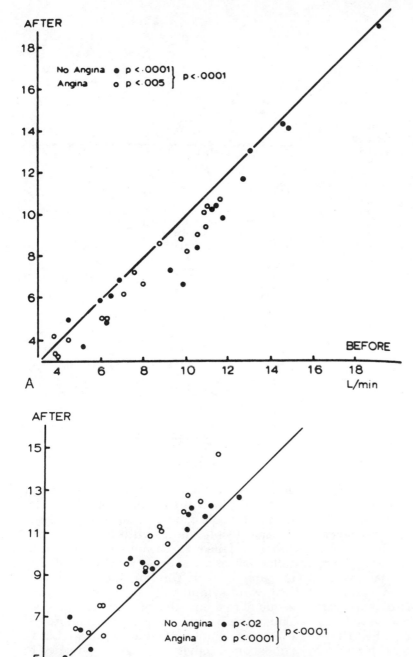

FIGURE 19–4. A, Effects of physical training on cardiac output during the same absolute level of submaximal exercise in patients with coronary artery disease, with and without angina at maximum effort. B, Effects of physical training on arteriovenous O_2 difference. (From Detry JMR, Rousseau M, Vanderbroncke G, Kusumi F, Brasseur LA, Bruce RA. Increased arteriovenous oxygen difference after physical training in coronary heart disease. Circulation 44:109–118, 1971.)

traction in exercising limbs, rather than to augmented cardiac output.

However, the limits of exercise tolerance differ in patients with variable degrees of coronary and myocardial reserves, or baseline levels of physical conditioning. Hence, it appears reasonable that the mechanisms by which training improves maximum exercise capacity may differ in individuals. For example, the response to training in patients post–complete myocardial revascularization may be most similar to changes observed with training in deconditioned normal subjects. In patients with exercise-induced myocardial ischemia, however, training may change the end point of exercise from angina (limiting factor being myocardial aerobic capacity) to generalized fatigue occurring at a higher work load (limiting factor being systemic aerobic capacity). Such physiologic and pathophysiologic heterogeneity helps to explain what would otherwise appear to be conflicting data regarding the ability of training to augment peak cardiac output and maximal exercise capacity in patients with coronary artery disease.

As in normal subjects, a training stimulus of adequate intensity, duration, and frequency is necessary to induce beneficial physiologic adaptations in patients with coronary artery disease with or without angina. Indeed, development of angina at low work levels (e.g., less than 50 per cent of maximal aerobic capacity) may preclude a significant training effect. Practically, it may not be possible to determine the actual maximal $\dot{V}O_2$ if angina is precipitated during aerobic work. In such individuals, more prolonged and/or more frequent work periods at the low work levels tolerated may represent an adequate stimulus for training. Moreover, treatment with nitrates immediately prior to each training session may allow the patient to train more effectively at a higher work load. Once peripheral adaptations become manifest, the intensity of the training work load can be increased to optimize results. Hence, attention to the limits of exercise capacity in any given disease state and individual adjustment of the training protocol are crucial.

The question has been raised as to whether the reduced maximal heart rate and cardiac output accompanying beta-blocking therapy in patients with ischemic heart disease might preclude sufficient end-organ stimulation to elicit a training effect. Several recent studies, however, have demonstrated reductions in heart rate and systolic blood pressure during submaximal levels of exercise, as well as significant increases in maximal oxygen consumption after 3 months of training at work loads requiring 70 per cent of maximal aerobic capacity.[36, 37] Although data from Vanhees and associates[38] suggest that improved tolerance of submaximal work loads was consequent to increased stroke volume as well as to increased oxygen extraction by the active limbs, the mechanisms underlying benefits at peak exercise are unclear. The variable resting heart rates in the aforementioned studies suggest that not all patients were receiving maximal beta blockade, and further investigation will be necessary to explore the potential synergistic benefits of these two interventions in the chronic management of ischemic heart disease. Nonetheless, exercise training of patients receiving beta-blocking therapy appears to be safe and potentially beneficial.

Since training, similar to most pharmacologic interventions, does not definitively alter the underlying cardiac disease, appropriate exercise must be continued chronically to sustain the desired beneficial changes in functional capacity. The long-term effects of exercise training on cardiovascular morbidity and mortality are, however, uncertain.

Although several descriptive reports suggest that regular exercise is beneficial and safe for patients following *myocardial infarction,* controlled prospective trials have been encouraging yet inconclusive. The recent National Exercise and Heart Disease Project[39] compared the clinical course of 651 patients with coronary artery disease, randomly assigned to a program of regular supervised exercise training or conventional medical therapy (control). It was observed that the cumulative 3-year mortality rates were 7.3 per cent and 4.6 per cent, and reinfarction rates were 7.0 per cent and 5.3 per cent, for the control and exercise groups, respectively. These differences, however, did not meet statistical significance. In another controlled prospective study by Wilhelmsen and colleagues,[40] a 22 per cent reduction in cardiovascular morbidity was noted, with 4-year cardiac mortality rates of 21 per cent and 14.6 per cent in their control and exercise groups, respectively. Problems in the interpretation of these studies are related to the heterogeneity of patient populations, as well as the design of training protocols (e.g., exercise intensity, compliance, and supervision). Nonetheless, extensive experience to date indicates that exercise training, when appropriately prescribed and monitored, is safe and induces physiologic changes that improve quality of life in patients with various clinical manifestations of coronary artery disease.

Indeed, at present, little more can be claimed for the use of various pharmacologic or surgical interventions in the long-term course of this disease.

Chronic Cardiac Failure

Improvement of exercise capacity is a major therapeutic objective in the management of patients with chronic left ventricular dysfunction complicated by chronic cardiac failure. Such patients may be markedly limited by symptoms of dyspnea and, perhaps more importantly, by fatigue. These symptoms are largely due to elevated pulmonary venous pressure, inadequate rise in cardiac output during exercise, and reduced vasodilating capacity in the metabolically active limbs. Hence, it appears logical that a more efficient cardiocirculatory system consequent to exercise training might be advantageous in this circumstance. Indeed, in patients with severe chronic cardiac failure in whom cardiac reserve is very limited, training-induced structural and metabolic adaptations in skeletal muscle that reduce either the cardiac output requirement at any given level of work or the rate of glycogen breakdown and lactate accumulation during prolonged effort, might tend to improve tolerance of submaximal levels of activity, and hence quality of life. Moreover, as suggested by the work of Detry and co-workers,[35] VO_2 may be improved significantly, without augmentation of peak cardiac output and cardiac work, by an increased oxygen extraction in the exercising limbs. However, depending in part on the severity of the disease, femoral venous blood may already be maximally desaturated at exhaustion thereby limiting the potential benefits of training.[10]

Although several investigators have postulated that the improvements in functional capacity noted during chronic vasodilator or inotropic therapy are related to peripheral training, very few clinical data are available describing the effects of physical training in patients with chronic cardiac failure.

Letac,[41] Lee,[42] and their colleagues have demonstrated an apparent training effect on heart rate and subjective improvements in functional capacity, after physical training in patients with coronary artery disease and modest left ventricular dysfunction at rest.

Data from Conn and associates,[43] on ten patients with coronary artery disease and left ventricular ejection fraction of less than 27 per cent, suggested that regular, supervised exercise could be performed safely and that improved tolerance of treadmill exercise can be induced in a subset of these patients. However, in this study left ventricular dysfunction was associated with cardiomegaly and chronic cardiac failure in only six patients, one of whom had exertional angina; the baseline functional status of these patients also varied considerably. Hence, the potential benefits and the role of exercise training in the management of patients with chronic cardiac failure remains to be established. Nonetheless, peripheral deconditioning consequent to prolonged bed rest and prescribed restriction of daily activity in these patients may be detrimental to functional capacity and should be avoided.

Peripheral Vascular Disease

In patients with peripheral vascular disease, the aerobic capacity of the exercising limb may be limited predominantly by fixed obstruction in the arterial circulation of the exercising extremity, rather than by reduced regional vasodilatory capacity or inability to augment cardiac output; it is manifested clinically by claudication. The effects of a 6-month exercise training program in patients with obliterative atherosclerotic disease of the legs and intermittent claudication were studied by Alpert and co-workers.[44] Using the xenon-133 clearance technique, these investigators demonstrated increases in calf muscle blood flow at the same submaximal level of work concomitant with improvements in symptom-limited exercise tolerance. The mechanisms responsible for these changes are unclear. Jonason and associates[45] have similarly reported improved walking distances in patients with initial capacities ranging from 25 to 1000 meters, without claudication at rest. Indeed, a very limited capacity to endure exercise may preclude stress of sufficient magnitude to induce the beneficial peripheral adaptations associated with training. Atherosclerotic disease of the femoral arterial system is frequently accompanied by coronary artery disease. Indeed, the beneficial effects of training on exercise capacity in such patients may be limited by development of claudication at higher work loads. Conversely, intermittent claudication during low levels of leg exercise may preclude training. In such patients, aerobic training of the upper extremities will induce beneficial cardiocirculatory responses to arm exercise and may therefore serve as an important adjunct to therapy.

Systemic Hypertension

The potential contribution of exercise training to the management of systemic hypertension may be a function of the stage of the underlying cardiac and vascular disease. For example, Wong and colleagues[46] suggest that in patients with labile or mild hypertension, abnormal blood pressure did not impose a limitation to exercise capacity; in patients with peripheral sequelae of long-standing hypertension, however, restricted transport of oxygen to skeletal muscle appeared to be a manifestation of end-organ disease (e.g., coronary artery disease, left ventricular dysfunction, congestive heart failure). Hence, in the labile or mild hypertension groups, therapy should be directed at altering the long-term course of the disease. A potential benefit of training in such patients might therefore be an attenuation of their heightened blood pressure response to exercise, accomplished by the reduction of sympathetic-mediated stimulation of inotropy or vasoconstriction or both in nonexercising circulations. Sannerstedt and associates[47] have observed tendencies toward reduced heart rate, cardiac output, and blood pressure, both at rest and during exercise, with concomitant widening of arteriovenous oxygen difference in men with borderline systemic hypertension, subsequent to 6 weeks of training. A number of investigators have observed reductions in resting and exercise blood pressure in more heterogeneous populations. Further controlled clinical studies will be helpful in establishing the independent effects of training on exercise tolerance and morbidity in this disease. Nonetheless, in formulating the prescription of exercise in hypertensive patients, particularly in patients with secondary end-organ damage, care must be taken to avoid the generation of very high and potentially harmful systemic arterial pressure during exercise. Titration of medical therapy and exercise testing prior to training are therefore indicated.

Chronic Airway Disease

Exercise capacity in patients with chronic obstructive pulmonary disease may be limited by symptoms of breathlessness, related to reduced ventilatory capacity or respiratory muscle fatigue or both, at work loads requiring less than maximal attainable cardiac output. However, prolonged disease-related inactivity and deconditioning may result in reduction of $\dot{V}O_2$ peak as well. Moreover, chronic airway disease is consequent to a variety of pulmonary diseases with varying severity and occurs most often in an older population with concomitant cardiovascular disease (e.g., coronary and peripheral arterial disease, heart failure, and hypertension). Hence, the end point of therapy must be individualized and may be facilitated by exercise testing. Reasonable goals of exercise training in such patients include (1) reduction of breathlessness and, hence, improved tolerance to a submaximal level of activity; and (2) prevention of the untoward physiologic consequences of prolonged physical inactivity. Theoretically, the latter goal may be accomplished by reducing the oxygen requirements of exercising muscle during submaximal workloads. In normal subjects, Milic-Emili and co-workers[48] have demonstrated a reduction in ventilation and work of breathing at any given level of $\dot{V}O_2$ in trained versus untrained individuals. However, in patients with severe airway disease, an inability to exercise at a work load of sufficient intensity to consume 50 per cent of $\dot{V}O_2$ max consequent to markedly impaired ventilatory capacity may preclude potential benefits of training. Nicholas and colleagues[49] have suggested that improved motivation and willingness to tolerate dyspnea, rather than true physiologic adaptations, could account for training-induced improvements in such patients. Indeed, typical changes in skeletal muscle enzymes were not observed after 6 weeks' training in patients with airway disease who did manifest improvements in exercise endurance; nor was there a reduction in ventilatory requirement at a given work load.[50] Nonetheless, investigators[51] have reported training-related improvements in exercise tolerance in patients with severe airway disease despite failure to improve pulmonary function. The addition of oxygen therapy to patients with arterial oxygen desaturation at rest or during exercise appears to improve their ability to tolerate training; however, the independent contributions of such combined therapy to improved exercise capacity are unclear.

Another approach to reducing symptoms of breathlessness during exercise in patients with lung disease has involved attempts to train respiratory muscle aerobically.[52–54] This approach is predicated on the supposition that the aerobic capacity of these muscles independently contributes to limited ventilatory and aerobic exercise capacity. In fact, the accessory muscles of ventilation are recruited when $\dot{V}_E$ exceeds 30 liters/min, or when tidal volume is large, thereby augmenting the oxygen cost of breathing. In normal subjects, the requirements of the respiratory muscles during exercise represent only a small proportion of the total $\dot{V}O_2$ and, therefore, is probably not a factor limiting exercise performance.[55] In patients with airway disease, however, there is a disproportionate increase in $\dot{V}_E$ at a given work load.[56] Hence, the greater metabolic requirement of the respiratory muscles accounts for a larger proportion of total $\dot{V}O_2$, leaving a lesser reserve for working skeletal muscle of the limbs. The effects of respiratory muscle training on exercise tolerance were studied by Pardy and associates[52] in patients with chronic airway disease. Training consisted of breathing through an inspiratory resistance for 15 minutes twice daily. The resistance selected was sufficient to increase the inspiratory pressure in the mouth to 40 per cent of the maximum attainable by each patient. Improvement in treadmill exercise performance was observed in the majority of these patients after 2 months of respiratory muscle training and coincided with amelioration of electromyographic evidence of diaphragmatic or scalene muscle fatigue during exercise. Indeed, further investigation of the role of respiratory muscle fatigue in limiting exercise capacity in patients with airway disease and of the potential benefits of specific training is necessary.

In summary, aerobic exercise training may substantially improve exercise capacity and quality of life in patients with a variety of cardiocirculatory and pulmonary disorders. Attention to the symptomatic and physiologic limits of exercise capacity in individuals facilitates formulating the appropriate exercise prescription for each patient and may therefore optimize the results of aerobic exercise training.

WRITING THE INDIVIDUALIZED EXERCISE PRESCRIPTION

The design of a prescription for exercise training in a given individual with cardiopulmonary disease must be based on a recognition of the underlying symptomatic and pathophysiologic limitations to his or her exercise response. Defects within the cardiocirculatory and ventilatory systems that will compromise the exercise response can be identified through the use of incremental isotonic exercise testing, as described in Chapters 7–10, wherein respiratory gas exchange and airflow are monitored (Fig. 19–5). In so doing, we have the basic information

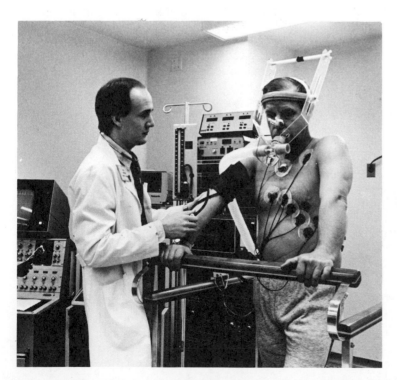

FIGURE 19–5. Oxygen consumption is determined during graded maximal exercise performed on a treadmill with continuous monitoring of 12 electrocardiogram leads and blood pressure. Methodology for graded testing and respiratory gas exchange analysis is detailed in Chapters 7–10. The patient shown here is resting in the standing position.

with which to design a prescription for exercise training as well as to assess the individual's response to this therapy.

The exercise training response is elicited when patients exercise at aerobic work loads near their anaerobic threshold. The anaerobic threshold, or work load coincident with the appearance of lactate in working muscle, is normally reached when exercise is performed at a level requiring 50 to 60 per cent of the maximal aerobic capacity. This relationship, however, is variable, depending on the baseline level of conditioning or the presence of chronic cardiac failure. Hence, only guidelines, as opposed to a general formula, for exercise prescription are herein proposed; moreover, it is important to recognize that the individual's exercise prescription may require revision, to achieve best results. Repeat exercise testing, as previously described, facilitates such adjustments.

The Exercise Prescription

Having established aerobic capacity and the symptomatic limitations of exercise, patients are provided with ranges of physical activity that should be well tolerated. This recommendation of nonsupervised activity helps the patient to set rational limits and to avoid the hazards of overexertion. It is not designed to represent a supervised training program for the patient with cardiopulmonary disease. A list of recommended physical activities and those that should be avoided is provided in Table 19–4; these are based on the maximal oxygen consumption achieved by a patient during the exercise testing.

Our program in Cardiac Rehabilitation at Michael Reese Hospital is designed to provide supervised training for patients with various cardiopulmonary disorders, using various arm and leg exercises (Fig. 19–6) that are relevant to daily living. The electrocardiogram is monitored for heart rate, rhythm, and ST segment response in each patient who performs arm exercise, or leg exercise, or both. Work intensity, duration, and progression differ among patients in accordance with the principles described earlier. We periodically monitor the $\dot{V}O_2$ attained during these training sessions with the Waters Instrument, to assure ourselves that the prescribed level of work is indeed being performed (Fig. 19–7). We do not rely on the heart rate response to determine the appropriate level of exercise, since, as noted earlier, the heart rate response will vary according

Table 19–4. *The Individualized Exercise Prescription: Recommendations for Household, Recreational, and Sports Activities*

$\dot{V}O_2$ **3.5–10 ml/min/kg**
 cooking, standing
 hobby painting
 sweeping floors, light
 gardening, light
 polishing furniture
 light ironing, standing
 driving car
 dusting
 horseback riding, slow
 vacuum cleaning
 sweeping or raking
 walking normal pace,
  1 mile in 24 min
 scrubbing floors
 cleaning windows

$\dot{V}O_2$ **10–16 ml/min/kg**
 mowing lawn, power
 making beds
 mopping
 waxing floors
 bowling
 cycling 5.5 mph,
  1 mile in 11 min
 straight leg raises
 swimming, 20 yds/min
 walking briskly,
  1 mile in 20 min
 golf, walking with caddie
 carrying 20 lbs
 cycling 10 mph,
  1 mile in 6 min
 gardening, moderate

$\dot{V}O_2$ **16–20 ml/min/kg**
 rowing, alone
 walking moderately fast,
  1 mile in 15 min
 golf, pulling cart or
  carrying bag
 ice skating
 table tennis
 washing and waxing car
 carrying 50 lbs
 carpentry
 swimming, 30 yds/min
 tennis, doubles
 walking briskly uphill,
  5% grade

$\dot{V}O_2$ **20–25 ml/min/kg**
 mowing lawn, hand
 walking fast, 1 mile in
  12.5 min
 canoeing
 deep knee bends, 30/
  min
 push-ups, 30/min

$\dot{V}O_2$ **25–30 ml/min/kg**
 skiing, downhill
 squash
 walking, level,
  2.5 inches of snow
 running 1 mile in 11
  min
 cycling 13 mph,
  1 mile in 4.5 min
 walking 5 mph,
  1 mile in 12 min

$\dot{V}O_2$ **30–35 ml/min/kg**
 shoveling moderately
  wet snow
 swimming fast,
  50 yds/min
 skiing, cross-country
 walking briskly
  uphill,
  10% grade

$\dot{V}O_2$ **> 35 ml/min/kg**
 running 1 mile in 7.5
  min

to the level of training and the initial level of conditioning.

Following 12 weeks of supervised aerobic training (three times per week), exercise testing is repeated and the prescription is revised accordingly. Subsequently, in appropriate patients an unmonitored, unsupervised but structured program of aerobic training and rehabilitation may be recommended; whereas in other, more high-risk patients, ECG-

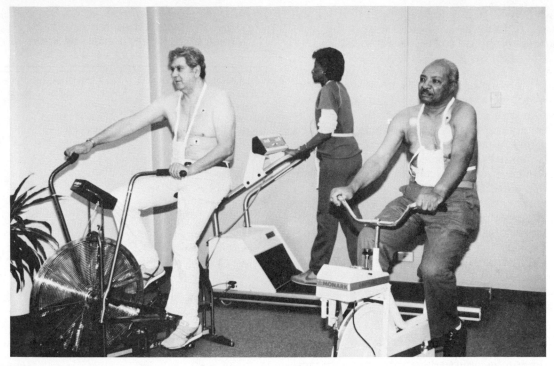

FIGURE 19–6. Patients are performing isotonic exercise with continuous electrocardiographic monitoring by telemetry. From left to right, equipment includes a Schwinn Air-Dyne ergometer, which allows arm and leg exercise to be performed at a variable work load as prescribed; a Quinton treadmill; and a Monark bicycle ergometer for leg exercise.

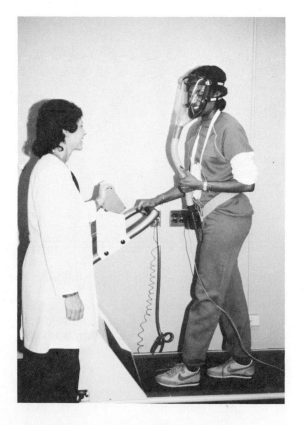

FIGURE 19–7. Oxygen consumption is being determined with the portable Waters Instrument during a training session, while a patient exercises on a treadmill. Accordingly, the work load is adjusted such that the patient's oxygen consumption approximates a prescribed proportion of maximal oxygen consumption.

monitored training is continued in the hospital's rehabilitation program.

REFERENCES

1. Pollock ML, Wilmore JH, Fox SM (eds). Exercise in Health and Disease. Philadelphia, WB Saunders, 1984.
2. Wenger NK, Hellerstein HK (eds). Rehabilitation of the Coronary Patient. New York, John Wiley & Sons, 1978.
3. Ekblom B, Astrand PO, Saltin B, Stenberg J, Wallstram B. Effect of training on the circulatory response to exercise. J Appl Physiol 24:518–528, 1968.
4. Issekutz B, Miller HI, Paul P, Rodahl K. Aerobic work capacity and plasma FFA turnover. J Appl Physiol 20:293–296, 1965.
5. Pruett EDR. Glucose and insulin during prolonged work stress in men living on different diets. J Appl Physiol 28:199–208, 1970.
6. Weber KT, Kinasewitz GT, Janicki JS, Fishman AP. Oxygen utilization and ventilation during exercise in patients with chronic cardiac failure. Circulation 65:1213–1223, 1982.
7. LeJemtel TH, Maskin CS, Sinoway L, Chadwick B. Fixed vasodilating capacity in exercising leg muscles: a limitation of aerobic capacity in heart failure (abstr). Clin Res 31:200A, 1983.
8. Zelis R, Mason DT. Diminished forearm arteriolardilator capacity produced by mineralocorticoid-induced salt retention in man. Implications concerning congestive heart failure and vascular stiffness. Circulation 41:589–593, 1970.
9. Kugler J, Maskin CS, Frishman WH, Sonnenblick EH, LeJemtel TH. Regional and systemic metabolic effects of angiotensin converting enzyme inhibition during exercise in patients with severe heart failure. Circulation 66:1256–1261, 1982.
10. LeJemtel TH, Maskin C, Chadwick B, Sinoway L. Near maximal oxygen extraction by exercising muscles in patients with severe heart failure: a limitation to benefits of training (abstr). JACC 2:662, 1983.
11. Donald KW, Wormald PN, Taylor SH, Bishop JM. Changes in the oxygen content of femoral venous blood and leg blood flow during leg exercise in relation to cardiac output response. Clin Sci 16:567–591, 1957.
12. Pirnay F, Lamy M, Dujardin J, Deroanne R, Petit JM. Analysis of femoral venous blood during maximum muscular exercise. J Appl Physiol 33:289–292, 1972.
13. Saltin B, Hartley L, Kilbom A, Astrand P. Physical training in sedentary middle-aged men, II. Scand J Clin Lab Invest 24:323–334, 1969.
14. Shephard RJ. Intensity, duration and frequency of exercise as determinants of the response to a training regimen. Intern Z Agnew Physiol 26:272–278, 1968.
15. Clausen JP, Trap-Jensen J, Lassen NA. The effects of training on the heart rate during arm and leg exercise. Scand J Clin Lab Invest 26:295–301, 1970.
16. Ekblom B, Kilbom A, Soltysiak J. Physical training, bradycardia and the autonomic nervous system. Scand J Clin Lab Invest 32:251–256, 1973.
17. Winder WW, Hagberg JM, Hickson RC, Ehsani AA, McLane JA. Time course of sympathoadrenal adaptation to endurance exercise training in man. J Appl Physiol 45:370–374, 1978.
18. Holloszy JO. Adaptations of muscular tissue to training. Prog Cardiovasc Dis 18:445–458, 1976.
19. Hartley LH, Mason JW, Hogan RP, Jones LG, Lotchen TA, Mougey EH, Wherry FE, Pennington LL, Ricketts PT. Multiple hormonal responses to prolonged exercise in relation to physical training. J Appl Physiol 33:607–610, 1972.
20. Clausen JP, Trap-Jensen J. Effects of training on the distribution of cardiac output in patients with coronary artery disease. Circulation 42:611–624, 1970.
21. Billman GE, Schwartz PJ, Stone HL. The effects of daily exercise on susceptibility to sudden cardiac death. Circulation 69:1182–1189, 1984.
22. Rerych SK, Scholz PM, Sabiston DC, Jones RH. Effects of exercise training on left ventricular function in normal subjects: a longitudinal study by radionuclide angiography. Am J Cardiol 45:244–252, 1980.
23. Holloszy JO, Skinner JS, Toro G. Effects of a six-month program of endurance exercise on the serum lipids of middle-aged men. Am J Cardiol 14:753–760, 1964.
24. Rhoads GG, Gulbrandsen CL, Kagan A. Serum lipoproteins and coronary heart disease in a population of Hawaiian Japanese men. N Engl J Med 294:293–298, 1976.
25. Castelli WP, Doyle JT, Gordon T. HDL cholesterol and other lipids in coronary heart disease. Circulation 55:767–772, 1977.
26. Saltin B, Blomqvist G, Mitchell JH, Johnson RL Jr, Wildenthal K, Chapman GB. Response to exercise after bed rest and after training. Circulation 37(Suppl 7):1–78, 1968.
27. Cooksey JD, Reilly P, Brown S, Bromze H, Cryer PE. Exercise training and plasma catecholamines in patients with ischemic heart disease. Am J Cardiol 42:372–376, 1978.
28. Verani MS, Hartung GH, Hoepfel-Harris J, Welton DE, Pratt CM, Miller RR. Effects of exercise training on left ventricular performance and myocardial perfusion in patients with coronary artery disease. Am J Cardiol 47:797–803, 1981.
29. Hagberg JM, Ehsani AA, Holloszy JO. Effect of 12 months of intense exercise training on stroke volume in patients with coronary artery disease. Circulation 67:1194–1199, 1983.
30. Paterson DH, Shephard RJ, Cunningham D, Jones NL, Andrew G. Effects of physical training on cardiovascular function following myocardial infarction. J Appl Physiol 47:482–489, 1979.
31. Rousseau MF, Degree S, Messin R, Brasseur LA, Denolin H, Detry JMR. Hemodynamic effects of early physical training after acute myocardial infarction. Comparison with a control untrained group. Eur J Cardiol 2(1):39–45, 1974.
32. Eckstein RW. Effects of exercise and coronary artery narrowing on coronary collateral circulation. Circ Res 5:230–239, 1957.
33. Ferguson RJ, Cote P, Gauthier P, Bourassa MG. Changes in exercise coronary sinus blood flow with training in patients with angina pectoris. Circulation 58:41–47, 1978.
34. Nolewajka AJ, Kostuk WJ, Rechnitzer PA, Cunningham DA. Exercise and human collateralization. An angiographic and scintigraphic assessment. Circulation 60:114–121, 1979.
35. Detry JMR, Rousseau M, Vanderbroncke G, Kusumi

F, Brasseur LA, Bruce RA. Increased arteriovenous oxygen difference after physical training in coronary heart disease. Circulation 44:109–118, 1971.

36. Pratt CM, Welton DE, Squires WG Jr, Kirby TE, Hartung H, Miller RR. Demonstration of training effect during chronic β-adrenergic blockade in patients with coronary artery disease. Circulation 64:1125–1129, 1981.

37. Laslett LF, Paumer L, Scott-Baier P, Amsterdam EA. Efficacy of exercise training in patients with coronary artery disease who are taking propranolol. Circulation 68:1029–1034, 1983.

38. Vanhees L, Fagard R, Amery A. Influence of beta-adrenergic blockade on the hemodynamic effects of physical training in patients with ischemic heart disease. Am Heart J 108:270–275, 1984.

39. Shaw LW. Effects of a prescribed supervised exercise program on mortality and cardiovascular morbidity in patients after a myocardial infarction: the National Exercise and Heart Disease Project. Am J Cardiol 48:39–46, 1981.

40. Wilhelmsen L, Ganne H, Elmfeldt D, Grimby G, Tibbin G, Wedel H. A controlled trial of physical training after myocardial infarction. Prev Med 4:491–508, 1975.

41. Letac B, Cribier A, Desplanches JF. A study of left ventricular function in coronary patients before and after physical training. Circulation 56:374–378, 1978.

42. Lee AP, Ice R, Blessey R, Sanmarco ME. Long term effects of physical training in coronary patients with impaired ventricular function. Circulation 60:1519–1526, 1969.

43. Conn EH, Williams RS, Wallace AG. Exercise responses before and after physical conditioning in patients with severely depressed left ventricular function. Am J Cardiol 49:296–300, 1982.

44. Alpert JS, Larsen OA, Lassen NA. Exercise and intermittent claudication. Blood flow in the calf muscle during walking studied by the xenon-133 clearance method. Circulation 39:353–359, 1969.

45. Jonason T, Jonzon B, Ringquist I, Oman-Rudberg A. Effect of physical training on different categories of patients with intermittent claudication. Acta Med Scand 206:253–258, 1979.

46. Wong HO, Kasser IS, Bruce RA. Impaired maximal exercise performance with hypertensive cardiovascular disease. Circulation 39:633–638, 1969.

47. Sannerstedt R, Wasir H, Henning R, Werko L. Systemic hemodynamics in mild arterial hypertension before and after physical training. Clin Sci Mol Med 45(Suppl 1):145–150, 1973.

48. Milic-Emili G, Petit JM, Deroanne R. The effects of respiratory rate on the mechanical work of breathing during muscular exercise. Intern Z Agnew Physiol 18:330–339, 1960.

49. Nicholas JJ, Gilbert R, Grobe R, Auchincloss JH Jr. Evaluation of exercise therapy program for patients with chronic obstructive pulmonary disease. Am Rev Respir Dis 102:1–9, 1970.

50. Belman MJ, Kendregan BA. Exercise training fails to increase skeletal muscle enzymes in patients with chronic obstructive pulmonary disease. Am Rev Respir Dis 123:256–261, 1977.

51. Pierce AK, Taylor HF, Archer RK, Miller WF. Response to exercise training in patients with emphysema. Arch Intern Med 113:28–36, 1964.

52. Pardy RL, Rivington RN, Despas PJ, Macklem PT. The effects of inspiratory muscle training on exercise performance in chronic air flow limitation. Am Rev Respir Dis 123:426–433, 1981.

53. Peress L, McLean P, Woolf CR, Zamel N. Ventilatory muscle training in obstructive lung disease. Bull Eur Physiopathol Respir 15:91–94, 1979.

54. Keens TG, Krastins IR, Wannamaker EM, Levison H, Crozier DN, Bryan AC. Ventilatory muscle endurance training in normal subjects and patients with cystic fibrosis. Am Rev Respir Dis 116:853–860, 1977.

55. Stubbing DG, Pengelly LD, Morse JLC, Jones NL. Pulmonary mechanics during exercise in normal males. J Appl Physiol 49:506–510, 1980.

56. Stubbing DG, Pengelly LD, Morse JLC, Jones NL. Pulmonary mechanics during exercise in subjects with chronic airflow obstruction. J Appl Physiol 49:511–515, 1980.

DAVID A. MEYERSON

20

The Role of Predischarge Exercise Testing for Risk Stratification Postmyocardial Infarction

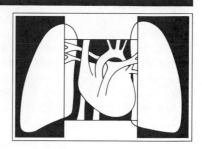

The goals of risk stratification following acute myocardial infarction include more efficient and effective means of patient management. This is particularly underscored by the fact that patients at lesser risk for subsequent cardiac events often have little to gain from empiric and perhaps expensive prophylactic drug therapy, coronary angiography, percutaneous transluminal coronary angioplasty, or coronary artery bypass surgery. These patients, however, clearly are candidates for early rehabilitation, reassurance, and return to gainful existence within the nation's work force.

With half or perhaps more of the year-1 deaths following acute myocardial infarction occurring within the first 8 to 12 weeks, the earlier a patient can be risk stratified, the sooner the physician can design and implement an appropriate regimen for the patient. Predischarge risk stratification, based on prehospital discharge and limited treadmill exercise testing, can be provided and is recommended. With the aid of this exercise test, patients at higher risk can be identified by three major independent predictors of morbidity and mortality. These include (1) residual myocardial ischemia, (2) ventricular arrhythmia, and (3) left ventricular dysfunction.

The overall goals of therapy are to prolong life, relieve symptoms of angina or heart failure, and preserve functional capacity. However, it is still unclear as to whether more aggressive therapies, such as coronary angioplasty or surgery or anti-ischemic and antiarrhythmic medications, will in fact prevent disabling symptoms, prevent reinfarction, or prolong life in the high-risk patient. Given our current understanding, aggressive therapy for the high-risk patient post-myo-

cardial infarction appears warranted and the value of predischarge exercise testing justified. The purposes of this chapter are to outline the central studies that established the utility of this approach, to detail the pertinent information that can be obtained from the noninvasive exercise test relevant to risk stratification, and to identify an overall approach to patient management. We begin by reviewing the rationale, efficacy, and safety of the limited, predischarge treadmill exercise test.

THE RATIONALE, EFFICACY, AND SAFETY OF THE PREDISCHARGE EXERCISE TEST

From the time of hospital discharge after an acute myocardial infarction through the following 12-month period, the overall mortality is approximately 10 to 12 per cent. Importantly, more than half of these deaths may occur within the first 3 months. In a prospective postmyocardial infarction study of 759 patients reported by Moss and coworkers,[1] 42 posthospital deaths occurred within the first 6 months. Almost 60 per cent of the 6-month mortality occurred within the first 2 months. Based on this distribution, they and others[2, 3] have suggested that considerable potential exists for reducing cardiac death in the early posthospital phase of myocardial infarction if the high-risk subset of patients could be identified. Furthermore, the development of unstable angina pectoris and acute myocardial reinfarction appears to be clustered even earlier than are the deaths in the postinfarction period (Fig. 20–1). These observations provide a compelling argument for the predischarge risk stratification of postinfarction patients. If this can be accomplished successfully, such a screening procedure will have a far-reaching impact both on the individual's long-term well being and on our national economy through health care cost containment and patient productivity. The prevention of avoidable hospital readmissions, recurrent infarction, and premature cardiac death are important goals that may be addressed with this approach.

High-Risk Stratification

Pierre Theroux and co-workers[4] from the Montreal Heart Institute evaluated 210 consecutive postinfarction patients who had no evidence of heart failure or recent chest pain (within 4 days). In essence, they selected a group of postinfarction patients who had heretofore been thought of as a low-risk population. In accordance with a recurring theme expressed in this text, the physiologic stress of exercise was used to examine abnormalities within the cardiopulmonary unit. These "low-risk" patients underwent early postinfarction limited treadmill testing (as described subsequently) on the day prior to discharge and were followed for 1 year.

The overall mortality for the year after discharge was 9.5 per cent. Thirty per cent of these deaths occurred within the first 12 weeks. ST segment depression (>0.1 mV) on the exercise electrocardiogram was highly predictive of mortality in the follow-up year. For those patients with ST segment depres-

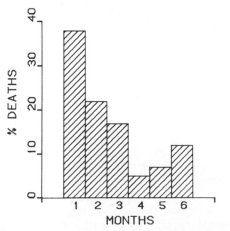

FIGURE 20–1. Distribution of cardiac deaths in the early posthospital period, postmyocardial infarction. Note the higher incidence of death within the first 3 months. (Adapted from Moss AJ, DeCamilla J, Davis H. Cardiac death in the first 6 months after myocardial infarction: Potential for mortality reduction in the early post-hospital period. Am J Cardiol *39:* 816–820, 1977.)

sion during the exercise test, there was a 27 per cent 1-year mortality. This was strikingly contrasted with a 2.1 per cent 1-year mortality in those patients without exercise-induced ST segment depression. The risk of sudden cardiac death was 23 times higher in those patients with ST segment depression than in their counterparts with normal ST segment response to exercise (Fig. 20–2). Additionally, in patients with exercise-induced ST segment depression, the risk of death due to recurrent infarction was 11 times greater than in those with normal ST segment responses. In this study, the development of angina alone without ST segment changes was not predictive of subsequent mortality. They also found that the development of angina along with ST segment depression did not add to the predictive value of ST segment depression alone.

Two critical points must therefore be emphasized. First, within the "traditional" low-risk group of patients sustaining uncomplicated myocardial infarction, there exists a high-risk subset. This subset has approximately 13 times the overall 1-year cardiac mortality and 23 times the incidence of sudden cardiac death compared with that of the "true" low-risk group. Second, this subset of patients at higher risk after uncomplicated myocardial infarction can be identified easily, safely, and inexpensively by electrocardiographic monitoring during a limited exercise test performed prior to hospital discharge.

DeBusk and Haskell[5] have also emphasized the importance of early exercise testing. Of 12 patients suffering cardiac events between the 3rd and 11th weeks postinfarction in their experience, seven had ischemic ST segment changes >0.1 mV during an exercise test. More importantly, all patients experiencing fatal or near-fatal events in the 11 weeks postinfarct demonstrated marked ST segment depression (>0.2 mV) at a maximum heart rate of less than 130 bpm. The powerful predictive value of markedly ischemic ST segment changes induced at low levels of exercise has been confirmed by others. Sami and co-workers[6] reported that the risk of recurrent myocardial infarction and death in the 24 months following an uncomplicated myocardial infarction was 40 per cent if >0.2 mV ST segment depression was present, as opposed to 25 per cent if <0.2 mV was present during heart rate–limited early postinfarction exercise testing.

The Multicenter Post-infarction Research Group[7] recently reported the usefulness of low-level exercise testing after myocardial

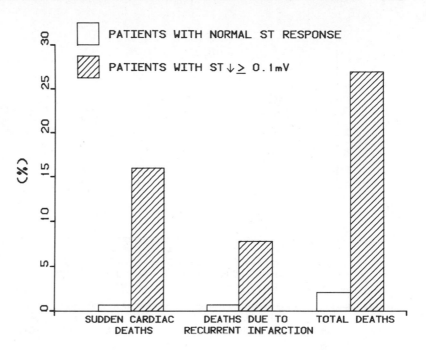

FIGURE 20–2. Incidence of cardiac death as related to the ST segment response in predischarge postinfarction exercise testing. (Adapted from Theroux P, Waters DD, Halphen C, Debaisieux JC, Mizgala HF. Prognostic value of exercise testing soon after myocardial infarction. N Engl J Med *301*:341–345, 1979.)

infarction in enhancing clinical risk stratification. Of the 866 patients enrolled in this study, 667 patients were able to undergo early exercise testing. Just the ability to take the low-level exercise test effectively stratified the patients into high- and low-risk groups. There was a 17 per cent 1-year mortality in the 192 patients who could not take the test, and a 6 per cent 1-year mortality in the 667 who could. Importantly, almost half (38 of 77) of the deaths in their cardiac care unit survivors occurred in the "lower-risk" group. Three features of the exercising low-risk group were identified as likely to cause cardiac death in these patients within the first year. These were (1) impaired exercise performance, defined as an inability to achieve systolic blood pressures of 110 mm Hg or to complete their 9-minute low-level test; (2) evidence of myocardial ischemia, or angina developing during the test; and (3) evidence of instability in cardiac rhythm, such as arrhythmias that were noted at rest, during exercise, or in the recovery period. In contrast, the study also identified a large proportion of postinfarction patients with little likelihood of death in the subsequent year. A group of 298 patients with 0 per cent cardiac mortality in the ensuing year was identified by the combination of (1) an exercise systolic blood pressure response of greater than 110 mm Hg, (2) absence of pulmonary congestion observed on the admission chest radiograph, and (3) the ability to complete the low-level exercise test (Fig.

20–3). It is this true low-risk group (approximately half of all exercising patients in this study) that is unlikely to benefit, in terms of longevity, from prophylactic drug therapy, angioplasty, or coronary artery bypass surgery.

Exercise Thallium-201 Scintigraphy

Thallium-201 scintigraphy is frequently combined with predischarge low-level exercise testing postmyocardial infarction, for many of the same reasons that it has been added to conventional maximal exercise testing. Postinfarction patients frequently have electrocardiographic abnormalities or are receiving drugs that may complicate electrocardiographic interpretation of the exercise response. For example, the heart rate of those patients on beta-blocking drugs may not be able to elevate sufficiently, even to the 70 per cent age-predicted level, whereas other patients taking digitalis or certain antiarrhythmic agents may have uninterpretable ST segment changes during their exercise test.

The sensitivity and specificity in combined exercise thallium-201 scintigraphy and electrocardiography is considerably better than in exercise electrocardiography alone. The presence of both a positive exercise test by electrocardiographic criteria and a reversible perfusion defect with stress thallium-201 scintigraphy is said to convey a predictive accuracy of significant coronary artery dis-

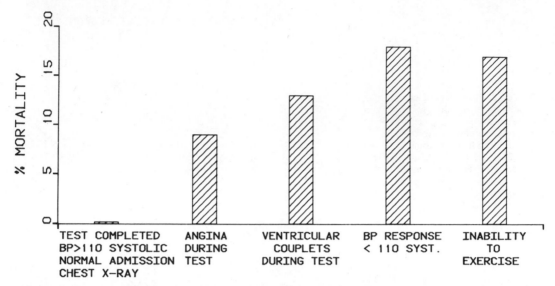

FIGURE 20–3. One year mortality postinfarction. See text. (Adapted from data of Krone RJ, Gillespie JA, Weld FM, Miller JP, Moss AJ, and The Multicenter Post-infarction Research Group: Low-level exercise testing after myocardial infarction: Usefulness in enhancing clinical risk stratification. Circulation 71:80–89, 1985.)

ease approaching 100 per cent. Gibson and co-workers[8] prospectively examined predischarge, heart rate–limited treadmill testing, stress thallium-201 scintigraphy, and coronary angiography in postinfarction patients. They found that each type of test predicted mortality with equivalent accuracy. They further reported that thallium-201 defects in more than one discrete region of the myocardium, the presence of delayed redistribution, or increased lung thallium-201 uptake were more sensitive predictors of subsequent cardiac events, such as recurrent myocardial infarction or development of NYHA class III or IV angina pectoris, than were ST segment depression, exercise-induced angina pectoris, or the extent of angiographically determined disease. Scintigraphy also predicted low-risk status better than did exercise electrocardiography or coronary angiography (Fig. 20–4). Low-risk patients were defined by a thallium-201 defect in a single region without redistribution or evidence of increased lung uptake or both.

Cardiopulmonary Exercise Testing

As described in Chapter 10, the noninvasive measurement of respiratory gas exchange can be performed during the predischarge exercise test to determine a patient's anaerobic threshold,[9] which occurs at approximately 60 to 70 per cent of $\dot{V}O_2$ max. The role of cardiopulmonary exercise testing in patients postmyocardial infarction has yet

to be defined, and its usefulness in determining risk stratification postmyocardial infarction requires further study. CPX will, however, identify the $\dot{V}O_2$ response to limited exercise testing and will generate an objective and individualized exercise prescription that the patient can use at home or in a structured program of rehabilitation (see Chapter 19).

Safety

It has taken years of clinical and experimental study to dispel the misconception that early mobilization after acute myocardial infarction may be associated with infarct extension, the appearance of lethal arrhythmias, aneurysm formation, and myocardial rupture. As this intuitive fear was dispelled, so too was the clinician's reticence to exercise a patient in the early postinfarction period. It was only recently that official publications of the American Heart Association listed recent myocardial infarction as an absolute contraindication to exercise testing. Of interest, and as an aside, chronic heart failure is still given as an exemption to a supervised exercise test by the Association. The consensus in the literature over the past 8 years has placed the risk of an untoward event (such as major arrhythmia, myocardial infarction, and death) occurring during limited early postinfarction exercise testing at less than one-fourth of 1 per cent. There is little doubt that early postinfarction limited exercise testing is safe.

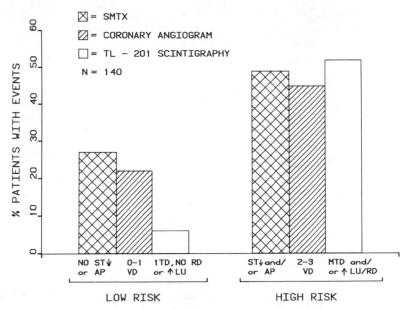

FIGURE 20—4. Proportion of patients with a subsequent cardiac event related to the results of submaximal treadmill exercise testing (SMTX), coronary angiography, and ^{201}Tl scintigraphy. 1TD, thallium defect in one vascular region; RD, redistribution; MTD, thallium defects involving multiple vascular regions; LU, increased lung uptake of ^{201}Tl; ST, exercise-induced ST segment depression; AP, exercise-induced angina pectoris. Cardiac events defined as cardiac death, recurrent myocardial infarction, and development of NYHA class III or IV angina pectoris. (From Gibson RS, Watson DD, Craddock GB, Crampton RS, Kaiser DL, Denny MJ, Beller GA: Prediction of cardiac events after uncomplicated myocardial infarction: A prospective study comparing predischarge exercise thallium-201 scintigraphy and coronary angiography. Circulation 68:321–336, 1983.)

In order to justify any level of risk, no matter how small, potentially significant benefits should be realized by the patient and physician. The benefits of predischarge postinfarction exercise testing also focus on the identification of those patients who are at low risk for subsequent cardiac events. A reassessment of the data from the Beta-blocker Heart Attack Trial Study[10] of the effect of propranolol after myocardial infarction suggests that benefit is confined to patients who suffered complicated infarctions. This is wholly consistent with the concept of risk stratification, suggesting that low-risk patients might perhaps be spared unnecessary prophylactic drug therapy. It has been estimated that in the low-risk subset of post-infarct patients, approximately 700 patients would have to receive prophylactic beta-blockade in order to benefit only one patient.[11] These are dramatic cost and side effect issues. Additionally, the patient might be spared unnecessary, expensive, and perhaps risky diagnostic and therapeutic procedures. These low-risk patients would best be candidates for reassurance, accelerated rehabilitation, and an early readjustment to their premorbid life style. Certainly a successful predischarge exercise test may provide a po-

tent psychologic advantage on which the patient can build an emotionally satisfying recovery.

In those patients whose postinfarction predischarge treadmill performance is not satisfactory, we would hope to at least translate prognostication into effective secondary prevention. Perhaps we can significantly alter the early clustering of sudden cardiac death and recurrent infarction by knowing a patient's ischemic threshold before discharge (Table 20–1). It would seem unwise to send patients home to care for themselves if we

Table 20–1. *Benefits of Predischarge Postinfarction Exercise Testing*

Identification of Low-Risk Patients
- Physician observation of patient's work load response
- Reassurance
- Accelerated rehabilitation program
- No angiography
- No prophylactic drug therapy

Identification of High-Risk Patients
- Determine safety of discharge
- Physician observation of patient's workload response
- Concentrate therapeutic efforts to alter early postinfarction morbidity/mortality.

have not objectively proved that they are safely capable of reaching the modest energy expenditure necessary to perform limited activities of daily living. It has been said with some wisdom that failing to perform a predischarge postinfarction limited exercise test is asking the patient to do the stress test by himself at home!

THE PREDISCHARGE EXERCISE TEST

In order to maintain the one-quarter of 1 per cent or less risk level in performing the postinfarction predischarge limited exercise test, one should be careful to exclude those patients who, in essence, have already identified themselves as being "high risk." In most series, patients who have reported chest pain within 3 or 4 days have generally been excluded. Those with clinical evidence of significant decompensated left ventricular dysfunction, which may be manifested by hypotension, pulmonary congestion, or persistent resting sinus tachycardia, should also not be expected to perform. Additional exclusions include patients with uncontrolled rhythm disturbances; an unstable resting electrocardiogram, as evidenced by spontaneous ST-T wave changes or by spontaneous alterations in intraventricular conduction; uncontrolled hypertension; significant valvular stenosis; physical disability; or advanced age (Table 20–2). Finally, the patient should be capable of walking unaided approximately 100 feet on a level surface (e.g., 1 mph, 0 per cent grade).

Those patients with uncomplicated myo-cardial infarction not falling into any of the above categories are candidates for predischarge limited exercise testing. We recommend that the test be performed on the day prior to projected discharge, so that the patient has had a reasonable period of time to ambulate in the hospital and effectively to begin the early phases of reconditioning.

Protocol

Of the many limited treadmill exercise protocols for screening the general postinfarction population, a modification of that proposed by Naughton and Haider[12] appears to be most widely adopted. A constant speed of 2 mph is used throughout the test and can be easily and safely tracked by most patients. From a baseline grade of 0 per cent, the treadmill elevation is increased by 2.5 per cent grade every 2 minutes, and, in the absence of untoward signs or symptoms (vide infra), the increase in elevation is continued until the patient reaches 70 per cent of the age-predicted maximum heart rate (Table 20–3). This allows a moderately slow progression of $\dot{V}O_2$, permitting the physician to monitor the patient's response to work loads commensurate with and somewhat above the activities of daily living that the patient will perform upon discharge. Cuff blood pressure and 12-lead electrocardiogram are performed both at rest and during the latter portion of each stage. These recordings, along with the clinical appearance and symptomatology of the patient, constitute the basis for clearing the patient to proceed into the next stage. When thallium-201 scintigraphy is added to the protocol, the physician must essentially anticipate the patient's capability to continue exercising and must inject a bolus

Table 20–2. Exclusions to Predischarge Postinfarction Exercise Testing

Postinfarct Angina or Symptoms at Rest

Left Ventricular Dysfunction
- Hypotension
- Pulmonary rales
- Persistent resting sinus tachycardia

Uncontrolled Rhythm Disturbances
- Ventricular tachycardia
- Other arrhythmias
- Supraventricular rhythm disturbances with uncontrolled ventricular response

Uncontrolled Hypertension

Significant Valvular Stenosis

Unstable Resting Electrocardiogram

Physical Disability

Table 20–3. Predischarge Treadmill Test Protocol for Patients Postmyocardial Infarction

Stage	Speed (mph)	Grade (%)	Duration (min)
1	2.0	0	2.0
2	2.0	2.5	2.0
3	2.0	5.0	2.0
4	2.0	7.5	2.0
5	2.0	10.0	2.0
6	2.0	12.5	2.0
7	2.0	15.0	2.0
8	2.0	17.5	2.0

Adapted from Naughton and Haider.[12]

of intravenous thallium-201 at or near peak exercise. That level of exercise should continue for at least 1 minute for the isotope to be adequately absorbed by the myocardium. Once the test has been terminated and the physician is confident that no evidence of ongoing ventricular arrhythmias, chest pain, ST segment changes, or hemodynamic instability exists, thallium-201 imaging should promptly begin. After the immediate postexercise images have been performed, the redistribution or rest imaging is performed approximately 4 hours later.

End Points

In heart rate–limited exercise testing in the early postinfarction period, 70 per cent of the age-predicted maximum heart rate (i.e., target heart rate) is generally between 120 and 130 bpm. Evidence of significant myocardial ischemia, arrhythmias, and left ventricular dysfunction should be firm end points. Signs and symptoms of these include severe chest pain, undue dyspnea, fatigue, dizziness, lightheadedness, confusion, and a hypotensive response to exercise. The development of rapid supraventricular arrhythmias, or of other arrhythmias, evidenced by ventricular tachycardia (generally viewed as three or more repetitive ventricular depolarizations) or by frequent isolated ventricular depolarizations, are recommended end points. Electrocardiographic ST segment criteria for termination of the test would include the development of flat and downsloping ST segment depression >0.4 mV for three consecutive beats. A hypertensive response to exercise (e.g., systolic blood pressure >200 mm Hg) is an additional frequently employed end point, especially in early postinfarct exercise testing. Last, there remains some controversy regarding the rare patient who develops ST segment elevation during exercise. In those segments of myocardium having previously sustained transmural infarction, ventricular dyskinesia has been implicated as the cause of ST segment elevation, as opposed to acute transmural myocardial ischemia. Nevertheless, it would appear prudent to select the development of ST segment elevation associated with chest pain as an end point to exercise. Although some advocate allowing a patient with ST segment elevation in the absence of chest pain to continue, the fact that significant ischemia may occur in the absence of chest pain makes this unwise as a uniform recommendation (Table 20–4).

Table 20–4. Reasons for Termination of Exercise Test

Patient Response
- Severe chest pain
- Undue dyspnea or fatigue
- Lightheadedness
- Confusion

Blood Pressure Alterations
- Hypotensive response to exercise (>10 mm Hg drop in systolic pressure from resting value)
- Hypertensive response to exercise (>200 mm Hg systolic pressure)

Rhythm Disturbances
- Ventricular tachycardia
- High-frequency ventricular premature beats
- New-onset rapid nonsinus supraventricular rhythms

Electrocardiographic Changes
- ST segment depression >0.4 mV (flat or downsloping, ST segment for 3 consecutive beats)
- ST segment elevation >0.2 mV (without chest pain, >0.1 mV with chest pain)

In addition to the aforementioned clinical parameters, selected end points derived from cardiopulmonary exercise testing (CPX) would be based on the patient's reaching anaerobic threshold. Given that this occurs at 60 to 70 per cent of patients' aerobic capacity, there is little reason to advise them to engage in physical activity that exceeds their anaerobic threshold at home or in a program of supervised rehabilitation.

MANAGEMENT CONSIDERATIONS
(Figure 20–5)

Within a large cross section of patients once believed to be at low risk after an uncomplicated myocardial infarction, there exists a high-risk subset with morbidity and mortality approaching 30 per cent in the first year post–hospital discharge (Table 20–5). This subset can be safely identified prior to hospital discharge by limited exercise testing and by limited stress thallium-201 scintigraphy. With the distribution of cardiac death and recurrent myocardial infarction skewed toward the early postdischarge period (i.e., within 12 weeks of infarction), predischarge risk stratification of postinfarction patients is strongly recommended. Most patients can be effectively risk stratified using limited stress electrocardiography complemented by evaluation of clinical variables. At this time, cost considerations suggest that predischarge, postinfarction, limited stress thallium-201

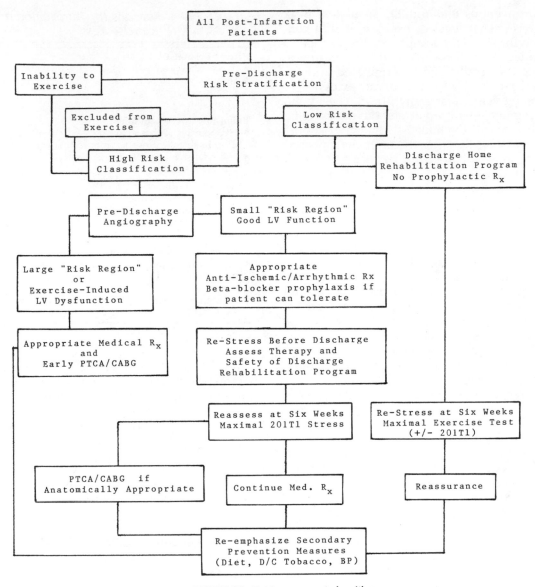

FIGURE 20–5. Management algorithm.

scintigraphy be used somewhat selectively and that it not be the initial screening tool of choice for all postinfarction patients. The usefulness of cardiopulmonary exercise testing to determine anaerobic threshold in this special subset of patients remains to be determined. However, from a management standpoint, it would seem wise to establish the postinfarction patient's capacity for home activities, thereby verifying that he or she is capable of safely expending given levels of energy required for self-care. We have heretofore taken this important aspect of rehabilitation for granted.

Although it is beyond the intended scope of this chapter, we strongly advocate predischarge 24-hour ambulatory Holter monitor-

ing at this hospital, as well as obtaining an index of ventricular function and regional wall motion, such as that provided by 2D echocardiography or radionuclide ventriculography.

Medical and Surgical Therapy

We have thus identified a major clinical challenge: to preserve functional capacity and prevent recurrent myocardial infarction and premature cardiac death in high-risk patients within weeks to months postmyocardial infarction. It remains unclear as to whether effective prognostication can be translated into equivalent effective secondary prevention in this subset of patients by applying

Table 20–5. Summary of High-Risk Indices from Predischarge Postinfarction Exercise Testing

Low-Level Exercise Electrocardiography
- ST segment depression >0.1 mV
- Angina at heart rate <130 bpm
- Exercise-induced hypotension
- Exercise-induced ventricular tachycardia
- Failure to complete low-level exercise test
- Failure to achieve exercise systolic blood pressure >110 mm Hg
- Inability to perform exercise test (secondary to cardiovascular status)

Low-Level Exercise Thallium-201 Scintigraphy
- Multiple thallium-201 perfusion defects (>1 vascular territory)
- Delayed thallium-201 redistribution
- Increased thallium-201 uptake in the lung

maximal stress thallium-201 scintigraphy be performed in this group of patients 6 weeks after hospital discharge (see Figure 20–5). The incidence of cardiac events and sudden death in those patients whose postinfarction stress test normalizes with medical therapy is unknown and represents a major gap in our knowledge. Therefore, it remains unclear whether prognostication has been translated into prevention.

aggressive early medical management and early coronary angiography, angioplasty, or bypass surgery.

Those patients who are incapable of exercising have stratified themselves as being at high risk. Most of these patients will be candidates for predischarge cardiac catheterization. With current data from the Coronary Artery Surgery Study (CASS)[13] indicating divergent survival curves in favor of surgery for those patients with triple-vessel coronary artery disease and poor left ventricular function, early revascularization may be the treatment of choice. Philosophically, although these patients may have a somewhat higher surgical risk pursuant to impaired ventricular function, they are also the least capable of supporting further loss of functional myocardium. Newer myocardial preservation techniques may improve survival in this group of patients.

In patients capable of exercising, those manifesting an early positive predischarge treadmill test generally should undergo coronary arteriography during that admission. Appropriate medical therapy should then be added and the patient re-evaluated for improved functional capacity and risk. Those who have large myocardial segments at risk in spite of medical therapy and those with evidence of early exercise-induced left ventricular dysfunction should then undergo coronary angioplasty or bypass surgery if these are anatomically appropriate. Patients who stratify at high risk during initial screening and whose second predischarge exercise test normalizes after medical therapy generally can be discharged and begin participating in a cautious rehabilitation program, as described in Chapter 19. We recommend that

REFERENCES

1. Moss AJ, DeCamilla J, Davis H: Cardiac death in the first 6 months after myocardial infarction: Potential for mortality reduction in the early post-hospital period. Am J Cardiol 39:816–820, 1977.
2. Weinblatt E, Shapiro S, Frank CW, et al: Prognosis of men after myocardial infarction: Mortality and first recurrence in relation to selected parameters. Am J Public Health 58:1329–1347, 1968.
3. Bigger JT Jr, Heller CA, Wenger TL, Weld FM: Risk stratification after acute myocardial infarction. Am J Cardiol 42:202–210, 1978.
4. Theroux P, Waters DD, Halphen C, Debaisieux JC, Mizgala HF: Prognostic value of exercise testing soon after myocardial infarction. N Engl J Med 301:341–345, 1979.
5. DeBusk RF, Haskell W: Symptom limited vs. heart rate limited exercise testing soon after myocardial infarction. Circulation 61:738–743, 1980.
6. Sami M, Kraemer H, DeBusk RF: The prognostic significance of serial exercise testing after myocardial infarction. Circulation 60:1238–1246, 1979.
7. Krone RJ, Gillespie JA, Weld FM, Miller JP, Moss AJ, and the Multicenter Post-infarction Research Group. Low-level exercise testing after myocardial infarction: usefulness in enhancing clinical risk stratification. Circulation 71:80–89, 1985.
8. Gibson RS, Watson DD, Craddock GB, Cramptom RS, Kaiser DL, Denny MJ, Beller GA: Prediction of cardiac events after uncomplicated myocardial infarction: a prospective study comparing predischarge exercise thallium-201 scintigraphy and coronary angiography. Circulation 68:321–336, 1983.
9. Weber KT, Kinasewitz GT, Janicki JS, Fishman AP: Oxygen utilization and ventilation during exercise in patients with chronic cardiac failure. Circulation 65:1213–1223, 1982.
10. Furburg CD, Hawkins CM, Lichstein E, for the Beta-blocker Heart Attack Trial Study Group. Effect of propranolol in post-infarction patients with mechanical or electrical complications. Circulation 69:761–765, 1984.
11. Ahumada GG: Identification of patients who do not require beta antagonists after myocardial infarction. Am J Med 76:900–904, 1984.
12. Naughton JP, Haider R: Methods of exercise testing, in Naughton JP, Hellerstein HK, Mohler LC (eds). Exercise testing and exercise training in coronary heart disease. Academic Press, New York, 1973, pp 89–91.
13. CASS Principal Investigators and their Associates: Coronary Artery Surgery Study (CASS): A randomized trial of coronary artery bypass surgery. Survival data. Circulation 68:939–950, 1983.

21

KARL T. WEBER

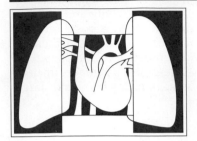

Monitoring the Response to Medical Therapy in Chronic Cardiac Failure

Diseases of the heart and lungs frequently lead to right or left heart failure or both and to the appearance of dyspnea or fatigue or both during activity. The presence of these symptoms and the accompanying level of exercise that is required to elicit these symptoms (effort tolerance) are used by the practicing physician to grade the severity of heart and lung disease. These symptoms also guide therapy, when expected end points include the amelioration or abolition of these symptoms, with a view toward improving the patient's quality of life. It is therefore not unexpected that clinical trials designed to evaluate the efficacy of new therapies for the long-term treatment of heart failure (e.g., vasodilators, cardiotonic agents) have focused on whether or not the agent in question improves exercise performance. In this connection, objective measurements of exercise performance, such as aerobic capacity and anaerobic threshold obtained by incremental cardiopulmonary exercise (CPX) testing, have been monitored in several open and placebo-controlled clinical trials.

From the discussion on chronic cardiac failure in Chapter 11, it should be apparent that in order for a vasodilator or inotropic agent to improve exercise performance it should alter favorably the following pathophysiologic responses of the cardiopulmonary unit to exercise: (a) resting and exercise cardiac output, (2) oxygen delivery to working muscle, and (3) resting and exercise work of breathing.

The noninvasive monitoring of aerobic capacity and anaerobic threshold can be used to assess the degree to which a drug will accomplish the first two of these objectives. These parameters also represent objective measures that are devoid of patient or phy-

sician bias. The disadvantage of this methodology is that it requires incremental exercise testing to exhaustion. This is not directly representative of normal daily living activities in these patients. We[1] have begun to investigate the usefulness of a constant–work rate anaerobic treadmill exercise test to provide the requisite objective information relating to submaximal effort tolerance. This test, however, has not been used in clinical trials, and therefore we cannot recommend it at the present time. We do occasionally use a constant low–work rate (aerobic) treadmill exercise test to reinforce or restore a patient's confidence in walking as a recreational activity.

Finally, the measurement of airflow and its integral (volume of air) can be assessed during an incremental exercise test, to assess the ventilatory response. The ventilatory pattern used by a patient during exercise is an indirect measure of respiratory muscle work and would be indicative of alterations in lung compliance that accompany an improvement in pulmonary congestion on medical therapy (see Chapter 11). To date, a systematic analysis of this issue has not been undertaken and therefore remains to be examined.

The purpose of this chapter is to review our experience and those of others when placebo-controlled trials were carried out over the past decade using vasodilator or cardiotonic agents in the long-term management of patients with chronic cardiac failure. In many cases, CPX was used to determine the efficacy and to monitor response to therapy. We do so in order to provide the practicing physician with an approach we have found useful for this purpose and to indicate the conclusions we have drawn about various therapies. We begin by reviewing the nonspecific and specific vasodilators, followed by a discussion of experimental agents with positive inotropic properties. In the vast majority of these clinical trials, whether multicentric in design or not, our incremental treadmill exercise test protocol, described in Chapter 9, was used to measure serially the effort tolerance, and specifically the aerobic capacity, of a patient.

EVALUATING VASODILATOR THERAPY FOR CHRONIC CARDIAC FAILURE

The concept of systemic vasodilation as a means to counteract the heightened resistance of the systemic arterioles that accompanies heart failure, in order to improve pump function, has been recognized since the turn of the century. Vasodilation may be accomplished in a variety of ways. Warm baths with a moving current was a popular form of treatment in 1897 to create cutaneous vasodilation and "unload" the heart.[2] Today, a variety of pharmacologic methods, including nonspecific vascular smooth muscle relaxation (e.g., hydralazine); stimulation of the vascular beta$_2$ receptor (e.g., dobutamine, pirbuterol); blockade of the vascular alpha receptor (e.g., trimazosin, prazosin); or the inhibition of naturally occurring vasoactive substances like angiotensin II (e.g., captopril) have received their share of attention and support.[3, 4]

Additional salutary hemodynamic benefits can be achieved by venous vasodilation (e.g., the nitrates). These include (1) a reduction in venous return and thus in right ventricular volume, which serves to decompress the left ventricle and increase its distensibility;[5] and (2) a reduction in left ventricular chamber size, which serves to attenuate systolic loading on this muscular pump and to improve its efficiency (see Chapters 3 and 4).

If long-term vasodilator therapy is to be considered effective in the overall management of patients with chronic cardiac failure of diverse severity, it would be reasonable to expect a reduction in the size of the failing heart as well as an improvement in exercise performance, particularly if vasodilator therapy were introduced early in the course of the disease. The indications for the early introduction of such therapy, however, remain to be clarified. Ideally, the selection of a vasodilating agent for any given patient should be based on the degree of cardiac failure and the relative contribution of neu-

rohumoral and adrenergic mechanisms and of the kidney. Unfortunately, our limited understanding of the pathophysiologic characteristics of heart failure and its compensatory mechanisms in each patient prohibits our developing an individualized prescription at the present time. Despite these limitations, vasodilator therapy has provided an effective method to treat many patients with chronic cardiac failure. We have examined a variety of vasodilating agents, each having a different nonspecific or specific mode of action.

Nonspecific Vasodilators

Nonspecific pharmacologic vasodilation promotes a reduction in vascular resistance that is mediated through a drug's mechanism of action, which is not directed at counteracting a specific vasoconstrictor process that has been activated (e.g., alpha receptor blockade when plasma norepinephrine is increased). Nonspecific vasodilators include hydralazine, minoxidil, and the nitrates.

The arteriolar smooth muscle dilation induced by *hydralazine* has been shown to increase resting cardiac output in patients with chronic cardiac failure.[6] In general, however, right and left ventricular filling pressures are not affected, which suggests that hydralazine has little influence on the venous circulation. We have participated in a multicenter controlled trial of hydralazine (200 mg daily versus placebo) in the treatment of chronic cardiac failure.[7, 8] Nineteen patients with medically refractory failure were followed in our laboratory for an average period of 20 weeks. Maximal treadmill exercise capacity (duration of exercise) at the time of enrollment into the study was not improved by the administration of either hydralazine (ten patients) or placebo (nine patients) at 5, 12, 20, or 28 weeks of therapy (Fig. 21–1). Moreover, the clinical status of those patients receiving hydralazine was not improved. The experience of Franciosa combined with our own (Fig. 21–2)[8] and with that of Rubin and co-workers[9] also showed no improvement in effort tolerance.

This apparent disparity between augmented resting cardiac output with hydralazine and the lack of improvement in exercise capacity may be explained in part by an attenuation in the vasoreactivity of skeletal muscle[10] that occurs in patients with chronic cardiac failure. As a result, hydralazine may lead to the vasodilation of other, more re-

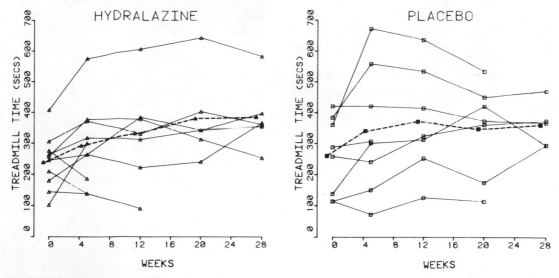

FIGURE 21–1. Response in exercise capacity, or the duration of symptom-limited treadmill exercise, for patients receiving either hydralazine or placebo during a 28 week clinical trial. (From Weber KT, Andrews V, Kinasewitz, GT, Janicki JS, Fishman AP. Vasodilator and inotropic agents in treatment of chronic cardiac failure: Clinical experience and response in exercise performance. Am Heart J *102*:569–577, 1981.)

sponsive, circulatory beds (e.g., splanchnic). Thus, even though systemic blood flow is increased and systemic arteriovenous oxygen difference declines with hydralazine,[9] aerobic capacity remains unchanged, because skeletal muscle blood flow is not increased. Hence, maximal exercise tolerance remains unchanged. More recently, Wilson and colleagues[11] have examined the response in femoral venous blood flow and aerobic capacity of the exercising limb before and after hydralazine administration. Even though cardiac output and limb blood flow were improved by the use of the drug, aerobic capacity and onset of lactate production by the limb during exercise were unchanged, sug-

gesting that a shunting of limb blood flow to nonworking muscle was present.

Another factor contributing to hydralazine's lack of efficacy in the long-term management of heart failure may be the fact that hydralazine does not promote venodilation. Consequently, venous return is not reduced, the right and left ventricles are not "decompressed," and left ventricular distensibility is not improved. This may explain why Packer and co-workers[12] have found patients with chronic cardiac failure and elevated right atrial pressure (>14 mm Hg) to have less of a hemodynamic response to usual doses of the drug; daily doses in excess of 300 mg were therefore required.

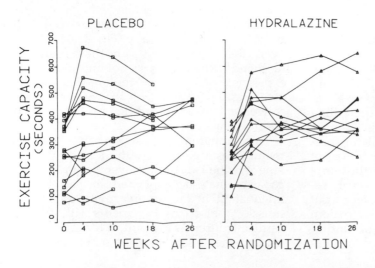

FIGURE 21–2. Effects of long-term hydralazine and placebo on symptom-limited treadmill exercise. (From Franciosa JA, Weber KT, Levine TB, Kinasewitz GT, Janicki JS, West J, Harris MM, Cohn JN. Hydralazine in the long-term treatment of chronic heart failure: Lack of difference from placebo. Am Heart J *104*:587–594, 1982.)

We have concluded that hydralazine is not effective as a sole vasodilator in improving clinical status or maximal exercise capacity in patients with chronic cardiac failure.

In a controlled trial comparing patients with chronic cardiac failure receiving another nonspecific arterial vasodilator, *minoxidil,* for 12 weeks with those receiving placebo, Franciosa and colleagues[13] found no improvement in aerobic capacity above baseline for either form of treatment. Moreover, a poorer clinical course, manifested by increased need for diuretics, ventricular arrhythmias, and worsening heart failure, was noted with the administration of minoxidil.

Although we have not examined patients' response in exercise capacity to the *nitrates,* other laboratories have. For example, Franciosa and co-workers[14] have found that patients receiving 12 weeks of oral isosorbide dinitrate (40 mg four times daily) improved their aerobic capacity in comparison to those receiving placebo (Fig. 21–3). Leier and co-workers[15] have monitored the response in exercise capacity to oral nitrate therapy (i.e., 40 to 60 mg four times daily) in patients with chronic cardiac failure. Like Franciosa and co-workers,[13] these investigators could not demonstrate an early improvement in exercise capacity with the drug. However, after 4 weeks of therapy, there was a significant improvement in symptom-limited exercise duration (Fig. 21–4) that was not apparent in their placebo control group. The mechanism(s) by which chronic nitrate therapy im-

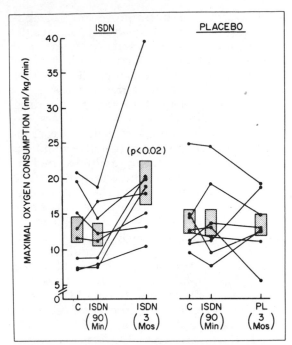

FIGURE 21–3. Response in aerobic capacity, or O_2 uptake, during chronic oral isosorbide dinitrate (*ISDN*) therapy versus placebo (*PL*). The shaded areas represent mean ± SEM. (From Franciosa JA, Goldsmith SR, Cohn JN. Contrasting immediate and long-term effects of isosorbide dinitrate on exercise capacity in congestive heart failure. Am J Med *69*:559–566, 1980.)

proves exercise tolerance is not clear. Several possibilities include the venodilating effects of the nitrates, which may serve to unload the right and left heart during exercise as well as to reduce pulmonary venous hyper-

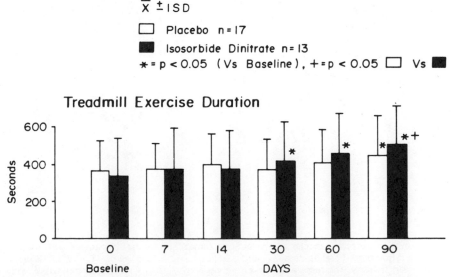

FIGURE 21–4. The response in exercise capacity to chronic oral isosorbide dinitrate versus placebo therapy. (From Leier CV, Huss P, Magorien RD, Unverferth DV. Improved exercise capacity and differing arterial and venous tolerance during chronic isosorbide dinitrate therapy for congestive heart failure. Circulation *67*:817–822, 1983.)

tension and thereby improve lung compliance and the work of breathing. As a result, patients are less symptomatic to submaximal exercise and therefore may be able to train themselves by engaging in greater levels of physical work on a more frequent basis.

One point relevant to monitoring drug response relates to the merits of measuring the duration of symptom-limited treadmill exercise test versus the actual determination of aerobic capacity. In the controlled hydralazine trial,[7, 8] treadmill time to symptomatic end point was used to estimate effort tolerance. As we have indicated several times elsewhere in this text, exercise time correlates poorly with aerobic capacity. A closer examination of Figures 21–1 and 21–2 indicates the variability in exercise time that is observed with symptom-limited exercise in these patients, as well as the "marked improvements" that can be seen in patients receiving placebo. A true determination of aerobic capacity, however, when $\dot{V}O_2$ remains invariant despite increments in work, is not likely to be changed. This experience further emphasizes the need for objective end points to exercise, such as $\dot{V}O_2$ max, which is free of patient and investigator bias.

Specific Vasodilators

Pharmacologic agents that counteract a particular vasoconstrictor response mediated by either the adrenergic or the renin-angiotensin pressor systems can be considered specific in their mechanism of action. Because of these specific pharmacologic effects, a more targeted approach to vasodilation may occur, favoring regional blood flow to skeletal muscle or to the kidney, or both.

Trimazosin, a quinazoline derivative with alpha$_1$ receptor blockade properties, has a balanced vasodilatory effect on the systemic arterial and venous circulations.[16] We have examined the efficacy of long-term trimazosin therapy in 27 patients with chronic heart failure of varying severity (5 class B, 11 class C, and 11 class D) and of varying etiology.[17] We also purposely chose to include not only patients refractory to standard therapy, but also those with less severe cardiac dysfunction, to examine the attractive though unproved assumption that long-term vasodilator therapy may be useful in the latter patients.

Following two reproducible baseline exercise tests and a 1-week single-blind placebo period, 23 patients were randomized, 10 to trimazosin (150 to 900 mg daily) and 13 to placebo, for 6 weeks. Four patients were given trimazosin directly at the request of their referring physicians. Twelve of the 13 patients given placebo were then transferred to treatment with trimazosin, and the 13 patients randomized to trimazosin continued to receive that therapy. The patients were re-exercised after 2 and 6 weeks of double-blind therapy and at 4, 12 to 18, and 52 weeks of open trimazosin therapy. These results are given in Figures 21–5 and 21–6. It can be seen that in the majority (89 per cent) of patients, peak exercise $\dot{V}O_2$ was significantly

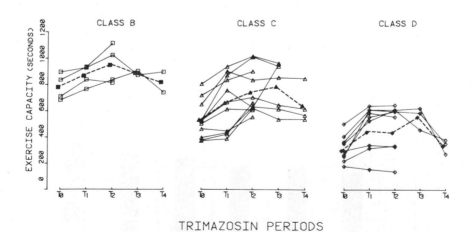

FIGURE 21–5. Response in exercise capacity to chronic oral trimazosin therapy in patients with moderate to severe chronic cardiac failure. Shown are baseline data (T_0), and data following 4 to 6 weeks (T_1), 12 to 18 weeks (T_2) and 52 weeks (T_3) of trimazosin therapy. The response in exercise capacity 2 to 6 weeks after trimazosin withdrawal (T_4) is also shown. (From Weber KT, Andrews V, Kinasewitz GT, Janicki JS, Fishman AP. Vasodilator and inotropic agents in treatment of chronic cardiac failure: Clinical experience and response in exercise performance. Am Heart J *102*:569–577, 1981.)

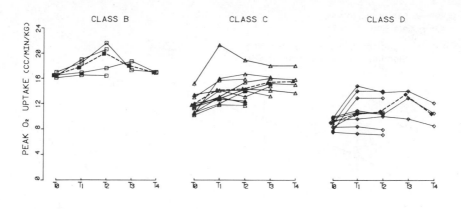

TRIMAZOSIN PERIODS

FIGURE 21–6. Response in O_2 uptake to long-term oral trimasozin therapy. Time intervals are the same as those in Figure 21–5. (From Weber KT, Andrews V, Kinasewitz GT, Janicki JS, Fishman AP. Vasodilator and inotropic agents in treatment of chronic cardiac failure: Clinical experience and response in exercise performance. Am Heart J *102*:569–577, 1981.

increased with trimazosin. This was not the case for the placebo group (not shown). The appearance of anaerobic metabolism was also delayed by trimazosin. With trimazosin, the patients were able to engage in a broader range of physical activities not possible previously; symptomatic clinical status of 24 patients improved.

After completing 1 year of therapy, trimazosin was withheld and exercise performance was re-examined 2 to 6 weeks later in nine patients. In five of these patients, exercise performance returned toward or declined below baseline values; in four others, exercise capacity remained improved.

Based on this experience, we would conclude that alpha$_1$ receptor blockade with trimazosin is an exceedingly effective vasodilator for treating patients with chronic cardiac failure of marked or moderate severity. The fact that all aspects of exercise performance were increased with alpha$_1$ receptor blockade suggests that both cardiac performance and skeletal muscle blood flow were improved during exercise. These findings may have important implications to the natural history and progression of cardiac disease and require further investigation in controlled clinical trials. Regrettably, and for reasons that are not apparent, the manufacturer of trimazosin has elected not to pursue further trials with this compound to establish its efficacy and safety in the treatment of chronic cardiac failure.

In a more limited trial, prazosin, another quinazoline derivative, was found to be more effective than placebo in improving exercise capacity.[18] Unlike trimazosin, however, prazosin is associated with weight gain and the need for increased diuretic dosage secondary to an increase in plasma renin concentration and a tolerance to its pharmacologic effects.[19] We have found the addition of captopril or spironolactone to be helpful in counteracting hyper-reninemia, whereas others have recommended increasing the daily dose of prazosin to achieve this end.[20]

Captopril

The efficacy of the angiotensin-converting enzyme inhibitor, captopril, in the treatment of chronic cardiac failure has been demonstrated in a multicenter randomized trial,[21] in which treadmill exercise tolerance to the drug was monitored and compared with a cohort of patients receiving placebo. The results of this study indicated a significant increase in treadmill exercise tolerance above baseline at 2, 4, 8, and 12 weeks of captopril therapy. In comparison to placebo, captopril increased exercise duration by an average of 119 seconds at 12 weeks (Fig. 21–7). As a result of these findings, the Food and Drug Administration approved the use of captopril in chronic cardiac failure. It is the only vasodilator to date that has received approval for this condition. The influence of captopril on more .specific measurements of aerobic capacity, however, remains to be clarified.

EVALUATING CARDIOTONIC AGENTS IN THE TREATMENT OF CHRONIC CARDIAC FAILURE

Positive inotropic agents augment myocardial contractility by enhancing the interaction

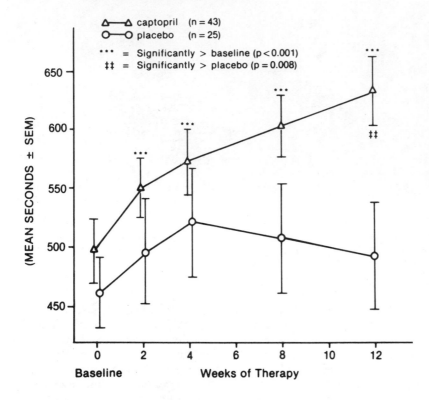

FIGURE 21–7. Results in exercise capacity, or the duration of symptom-limited treadmill exercise, are shown for patients receiving captopril or placebo over a 12 week period. (From Captopril Multicenter Research Group. A placebo-controlled trial of captopril in refractory chronic congestive heart failure. J Am Coll Cardiol 2:755–763, 1983.)

of calcium with the contractile proteins actin and myosin. They do so through a variety of mechanisms[22] depicted in Figure 21–8, which include the following: raising intracellular cyclic AMP to open calcium channels in the sarcolemma (e.g., stimulation of the beta adrenergic receptor, activation of adenylate cyclase); and inhibiting phosphodiesterase, which prevents the breakdown of cyclic AMP. In some cases, the mechanism of action of these drugs remains to be clarified. We will subdivide our review of these agents and their influence on exercise performance according to these various mechanisms of action, beginning with the beta adrenergic receptor agonists.

Beta Adrenergic Receptor Agonists

Because the intravenous catecholamines have been the clinical standard for judging inotropic potency over the years, it was only natural that a variety of orally active beta receptor agonists were developed. Their efficacy in the long-term management of chronic cardiac failure was then examined. Most of these agents stimulated beta$_1$ adrenergic receptors in the myocardium, as well as the beta$_2$ receptors of vascular smooth muscle that mediate vasodilation. Several of these compounds, such as *butopamine*, the

oral analog of dobutamine, never reached extensive clinical trials because of their propensity to induce ventricular arrhythmias.[22] Other agents, such as *pirbuterol* and *prenalterol*, however, entered more extensive clinical trials, only to be withdrawn later because of drug-induced ventricular arrhythmias.

Nevertheless, several important lessons emerged from this experience, including those pertinent to exercise performance. In the case of *pirbuterol*, a catecholamine whose hemodynamic effects are mediated via stimulation of both beta$_1$ and beta$_2$ adrenergic receptors, several trials have demonstrated a dose-dependent, acute improvement in ventricular function.[23–26] This hemodynamic response, however, abated after several weeks of therapy.[27] In a controlled trial, in which pirbuterol was compared with placebo over a 12-week period, no improvement in exercise performance was noted.[26] These results are shown in Figure 21–9, where the response in $\dot{V}O_2$ max is depicted for 12 patients who participated in the controlled trial. These results, however, do provide additional evidence supporting the reproducibility of the aerobic capacity determination.

Colucci and coworkers[27] observed that the loss of clinical efficacy and hemodynamic response was associated with a down regulation (decreased number or affinity of recep-

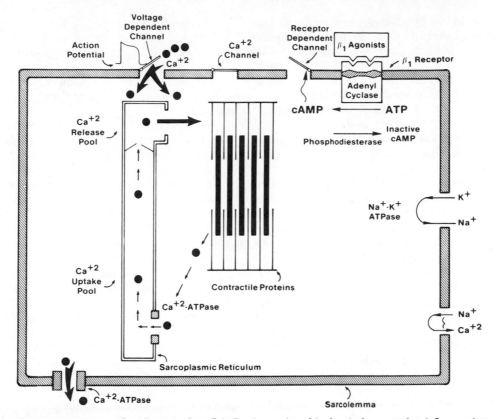

FIGURE 21—8. A representation of cardiac muscle cell, indicating various biochemical events that influence intracellular calcium. Calcium will be increased and myocardial contractility enhanced by beta adrenergic receptor agonists, adenylate cyclase activators, phosphodiesterase inhibitors, Na^+-K^+ ATPase inhibitors, and mechanisms that remain to be identified (e.g., enhanced calcium uptake by sarcoplasmic reticulum). (From Weber KT. New hope for the failing heart. Am J Med 72:665–671, 1982.)

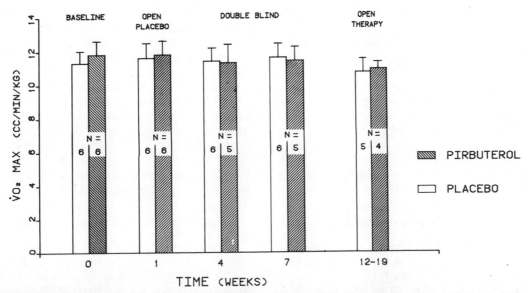

FIGURE 21—9. Response in aerobic capacity to treadmill exercise in patients randomly placed on pirbuterol or placebo during a controlled clinical trial. See text. (From Weber KT, Janicki JS, Maskin CS. Effects of new inotropic agents on exercise performance. Circulation 73:in press, 1986.)

tors or both) of beta adrenergic receptors on circulating lymphocytes. Whether a similar down regulation occurs within myocardial and/or vascular beta receptors to chronic pirbuterol therapy is not known. Like pirbuterol, *prenalterol* is no longer in clinical trial. Recently reported placebo-controlled results with the drug[28, 29] suggested that it too did not provide a sustained improvement in ventricular function or an enhanced level of effort tolerance.

In addition, Maskin and co-workers[30] have demonstrated that although intravenous administration of the beta adrenergic agonist dobutamine can significantly improve cardiac output both at rest and during exercise in patients with severe cardiac failure, aerobic capacity is not acutely improved during dobutamine infusion. Wilson and associates[31] noted a similar response. These findings imply that although the beta$_1$ agonist effect of dobutamine may augment cardiac performance, its beta$_2$ agonist effects permit a shunting of systemic blood flow to nonexercising circulations rather than to metabolically active muscle—a concept similar to that described for nonspecific vasodilators earlier in this chapter.

Of further interest, Maskin and co-workers[32] observed, in contrast to dobutamine, that dopamine, a catecholamine largely devoid of beta$_2$ agonist activity, increases cardiac output at rest but not during maximal exercise. These data suggest that the augmented cardiac output observed during maximal exercise with dobutamine predominantly resulted from the drug's vasodilatory effect. Indeed, during maximal exercise, when myocardial beta adrenergic receptors may already be maximally saturated by the increased levels of endogenous catecholamines, administration of a beta agonist may induce little additional inotropic effect. Bristow and colleagues[33] have recently reported a reduction in myocardial beta receptor density and responsiveness in the chronically failing human heart, which may further limit the effectiveness of beta$_1$ adrenergic agonists during maximal exercise.

Phosphodiesterase Inhibitors

Two phosphodiesterase (PDE) inhibitors, *enoximone* (MDL 17,043) and *piroximone* (MDL 19,205), have recently entered clinical trials. Several centers have reported that each drug improves ventricular pump function in patients with chronic heart failure.[34–36] An improvement in perceived effort tolerance has also been reported;[35] however, the study population was small, and objective parameters of exercise performance in these patients could not be ascertained because of the advanced severity of their symptomatic heart failure.

In on-going open clinical trials involving each of these compounds in our laboratory, we have found an improvement in exercise performance. To date, *enoximone* in average unit doses of 1.5 mg/kg has been given to 24 patients with chronic cardiac failure of varying severity (classes A through C) in whom exercise performance could be monitored before and after initiation of drug therapy. The aerobic capacity of these patients was followed from baseline levels, before enoximone administration and while the patient was receiving stable doses of oral digoxin and one or more diuretics, and then periodically thereafter when the new drug was given in addition to digoxin and diuretics. Our preliminary results indicate that, for the entire group of patients representing mild to moderately severe heart failure, an improvement in VO$_2$ max was observed after 2 weeks of enoximone therapy and was sustained for 16 weeks of continued treatment.

Piroximone, a congener of enoximone, has been administered to date in our laboratory to 12 patients having moderately severe and severe cardiac failure. Our preliminary results suggest that average unit doses of piroximone of 1.5 mg/kg, plus digoxin and diuretics, provide an early improvement in aerobic capacity over baseline for the group that was sustained for 16 weeks of therapy.

No major side effects have been noted with either of these phosphodiesterase inhibitors when unit doses of the drugs were kept between 1 and 2 mg/kg. Similar to our earlier experience,[35] these doses were found to produce a moderate (>30 per cent) improvement in resting cardiac output and left ventricular filling pressure. It is worth noting that it is not necessary to use excessive doses of an inotropic agent to improve either ventricular function or exercise performance.

Unknown Mechanisms of Action

Amrinone and its analog *milrinone* are bipyridine derivatives whose mechanisms of action have not been fully elucidated. Both drugs, however, do not behave like the digitalis glycosides or catecholamines.[37]

In a controlled clinical trial,[38] unit doses of

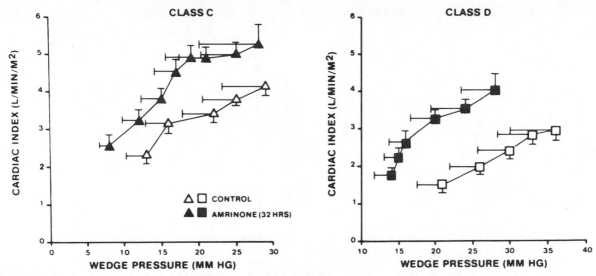

FIGURE 21–10. The response of the exercise left ventricular function curve to oral amrinone. (From Likoff MJ, Weber KT, Andrews V, Janicki JS, St. John-Sutton M, Wilson H, Rocci ML. Amrinone in the treatment of chronic cardiac failure. JACC 3:1282–1290, 1984.)

approximately 1.5 mg/kg of oral *amrinone*, in combination with digoxin and diuretics, have been shown to improve resting and exercise pump function in patients having moderately severe and severe heart failure. In Figure 21–10, it can be seen that the ventricular function curve to exercise shifted to the left with amrinone therapy, so that at any level of exercise there is a higher cardiac output generated from a lesser left ventricular filling pressure. Siskind and co-workers[39] have reported that the amrinone-induced improvement in cardiac output delayed the appearance of lactate during upright cycle ergometry and prolonged the symptomatic end point of exercise in a similar population of patients. We have noted a similar response to amrinone during incremental treadmill exercise.[1]

The acute improvement (within 32 hours) in resting and exercise cardiac performance with the administration of amrinone was accompanied by an increase in aerobic capacity to incremental treadmill exercise. This acute improvement in $\dot{V}O_2$ max, shown in Figure 21–11, was sustained for up to 28 weeks. When amrinone was withdrawn for placebo in a double-blind fashion after 28 weeks of amrinone therapy (see Figure 21–12), a deterioration in clinical status and exercise performance was observed.[38] However, as in our experience with trimazosin, the rate of this deterioration was entirely unpredictable and appeared to be a function of sustained improvements in the heart and periphery consequent to the drug-

dependent improvement in cardiac performance achieved during the drug treatment portion of the trial.

In a multicenter randomized withdrawal trial,[40] patients initially responsive to 4 weeks of oral amrinone therapy were randomly assigned to placebo or amrinone. No significant difference in symptoms of failure or treadmill exercise duration was observed after the introduction of placebo. A major adverse effect, primarily gastrointestinal in nature, was observed, which led to a discontinuation of the drug's further development as an oral preparation.

Milrinone, a more potent inotropic agent than amrinone, has recently been introduced to clinical trials. It too has been shown to improve right and left ventricular pump function,[41, 42] in patients with chronic cardiac failure who are still symptomatic despite medical therapy with digoxin, diuretics, and vasodilators. In these patients, chronic oral milrinone therapy has been reported to be associated with symptomatic improvement without major adverse effects or drug tolerance,[42] and therefore oral milrinone may be an effective alternative to oral amrinone.

In an early controlled trial with milrinone,[43] 12 patients with mild to moderate failure were randomly given either placebo or milrinone; the latter, in the majority of cases, was given in doses of 5 mg every 4 to 6 hours. Aerobic capacity was not improved in either treatment group over an 8-week follow-up period. A controlled withdrawal trial

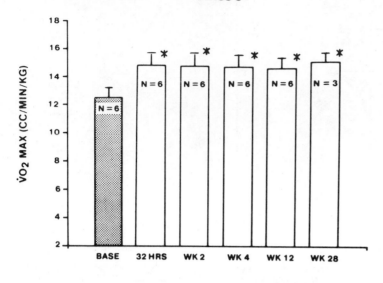

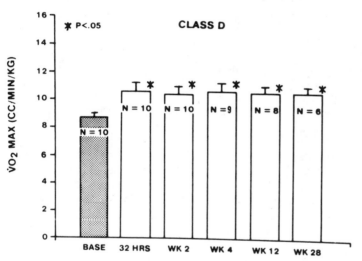

TIME DURING AMRINONE THERAPY

FIGURE 21–11. The response in aerobic capacity to 28 weeks of oral amrinone therapy. (From Likoff MJ, Weber KT, Andrews V, Janicki JS, St. John-Sutton M, Wilson H, Rocci ML. Amrinone in the treatment of chronic cardiac failure. JACC 3:1282–1290, 1984.)

compared effects of larger doses of milrinone with those of placebo. Ribeiro and associates[44] have found that after 10 weeks of oral milrinone therapy, milrinone withdrawal resulted in a decline in the aerobic capacity and the anaerobic threshold in a group of nine patients with chronic heart failure.

Maskin and co-workers[45] had the opportunity to follow 39 patients with moderate to severe heart failure who were treated on a long-term basis with this drug. Although most patients reported subjective improvements, the exercise response was variable. In a subset of these patients, milrinone improved exercise performance within 2 weeks of therapy, and clinical improvements were sustained for periods as long as 20 weeks. In other patients, milrinone administration did not enhance $\dot{V}O_2$ max despite acute and sustained augmentation of cardiac output. In almost all patients, a worsening of congestive symptoms and aerobic capacity was observed during long-term follow-up; although the rate and severity of deterioration varied in individuals, withdrawal of chronic milrinone therapy has demonstrated sustained drug-dependent hemodynamic efficacy, suggesting that such deterioration may result from a progression of the underlying disease and not from tolerance to the drug.

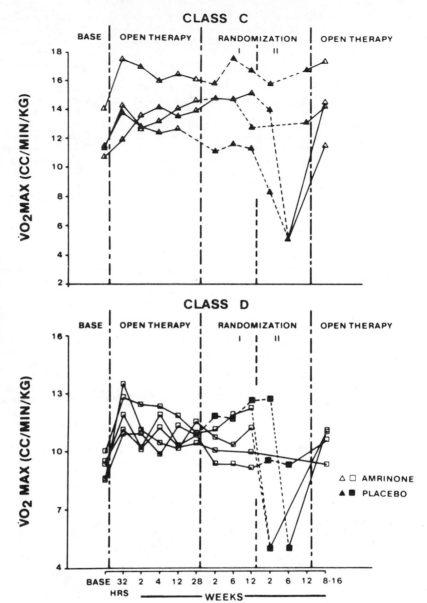

FIGURE 21–12. The deterioration in aerobic capacity following oral amrinone withdrawal was quite variable and unpredictable. Following the reinstitution of amrinone therapy, aerobic capacity improved over time. (From Likoff MJ, Weber KT, Andrews V, Janicki JS, St. John-Sutton M, Wilson H, Rocci ML. Amrinone in the treatment of chronic cardiac failure. JACC 3:1282–1290, 1984.)

REFERENCES

1. Weber KT, Janicki JS. Lactate production during maximal and submaximal exercise in patients with chronic cardiac failure. JACC 6:717–724, 1985.
2. Coupland S. Diseases of the heart and circulation, in The Yearbook of Treatment for 1897. Philadelphia, 1897, Lea Brothers and Co, pp 1–26.
3. Chatterjee K, Parmley WW. The role of vasodilator therapy in heart failure. Prog Cardiovasc Dis 19:301–325, 1977.
4. Cohn JN, Franciosa JA. Vasodilator therapy of cardiac failure. N Engl J Med 297:27–31; 255–258, 1977.
5. Weber KT, Janicki JS, Shroff S, Fishman AP. Contractile mechanics and interaction of the right and left ventricles. Am J Cardiol 47:685–695, 1981.
6. Franciosa JA, Pierpont G, Cohn JN. Hemodynamic improvement after oral hydralazine in left ventricular failure. Ann Intern Med 86:388–393, 1977.
7. Weber KT, Andrews V, Kinasewitz GT, Janicki JS, Fishman AP. Vasodilator and inotropic agents in treatment of chronic cardiac failure: clinical experience and response in exercise performance. Am Heart J 102:569–577, 1981.
8. Franciosa JA, Weber KT, Levine TB, Kinasewitz GT, Janicki JS, West J, Harris MM, Cohn JN. Hydralazine in the long term treatment of chronic heart failure: lack of difference from placebo. Am Heart J 104:587–594, 1982.
9. Rubin SA, Chatterjee K, Ports TA, Gelberg HJ,

Brundage BH, Parmley WW. Influence of short-term oral hydralazine therapy on exercise hemodynamics in patients with severe chronic heart failure. Am J Cardiol 44:1183–1189, 1979.

10. Zelis R, Mason DT, Braunwald E. A comparison of the effects of vasodilator stimuli on peripheral resistance vessels in normal subjects and in patients with congestive heart failure. J Clin Invest 47:960–970, 1968.

11. Wilson JR, Martin JL, Ferraro N, Weber KT. Effect of hydralazine on perfusion and metabolism in the leg during upright bicycle exercise in patients with heart failure. Circulation 68:425–432, 1983.

12. Packer M, Meller J, Medina N, Gorlin R, Herman MV. Dose requirements of hydralazine in patients with severe chronic congestive heart failure. Am J Cardiol 45:655–660, 1980.

13. Franciosa JA, Jordan RA, Wilen MM, Leddy CL. Minoxidil in patients with chronic left heart failure: contrasting hemodynamics and clinical effects in a controlled trial. Circulation 70:63–68, 1984.

14. Franciosa JA, Goldsmith SR, Cohn JN. Contrasting immediate and long-term effects of isosorbide dinitrate on exercise capacity in congestive heart failure. Am J Med 69:559–566, 1980.

15. Leier CV, Huss P, Magorien RD, Unverferth DV. Improved exercise capacity and differing arterial and venous tolerance during chronic isosorbide dinitrate therapy for congestive heart failure. Circulation 67:817–822, 1983.

16. Awan NA, Hermanovich J, Whitcomb C, Skinner P, Mason DT. Cardio-circulatory effects of afterload reduction with oral trimazosin in severe chronic congestive heart failure. Am J Cardiol 44:126–131, 1979.

17. Weber KT, Kinasewitz GT, West JS, Janicki JS, Reichek N, Fishman AP. Long term vasodilator therapy with trimazosin in chronic cardiac failure. N Engl J Med 303:242–250, 1980.

18. Aronow WS, Lurie M, Turbow M, Whittaker K, Van Camp S, Hughes D. Effect of prazosin vs placebo on chronic left ventricular heart failure. Circulation 59:344–350, 1979.

19. Packer M, Meller J, Gorlin R, Herman MV. Hemodynamic and clinical tachyphylaxis to prazosin-mediated afterload reduction in severe congestive heart failure. Circulation 59:531–539, 1979.

20. Awan NA, Miller RR, DeMaria AN, Maxwell KS, Neumann A, Mason DR. Efficacy of ambulatory systemic vasodilatory therapy with oral prasozin in chronic refractory heart failure: concomitant relief of pulmonary congestion and elevation of pump output demonstrated by improvements in symptomatology, exercise tolerance, hemodynamics and echocardiography. Circulation 56:346–354, 1977.

21. Captopril Multicenter Research Group. A placebo-controlled trial of captopril in refractory chronic congestive heart failure. JACC 2:755–763, 1983.

22. Weber KT. New hope for the failing heart. Am J Med 72:665–671, 1982.

23. Rude RE, Turi Z, Brown EJ, Lorell BH, Colucci WS, Mudge GH Jr, Taylor CR, Grossman W. Acute effects of oral pirbuterol on myocardial oxygen metabolism and systemic hemodynamics in chronic congestive heart failure. Circulation 64:139–145, 1981.

24. Awan NA, Evenson MK, Needham KE, Evans TO, Hermanovich J, Taylor CR, Amsterdam E, Mason DT. Hemodynamic effects of oral pirbuterol in chronic severe congestive heart failure. Circulation 63:96–101, 1981.

25. Sharma B, Hoback J, Francis GS, Hodges M, Asinger RW, Cohn JN, Taylor CR. Pirbuterol: a new oral sympathomimetic amine for the treatment of congestive heart failure. Am Heart J 102:533–541, 1981.

26. Weber KT, Andrews V, Janicki JS, Likoff M, Reichek N. Pirbuterol, an oral beta adrenergic receptor agonist, in the treatment of chronic cardiac failure. Circulation 66:1262–1267, 1982.

27. Colucci WS, Alexander RW, Williams GH, Rude RE, Holman BL, Konstam MA, Wynee J, Mudge GH Jr, Braunwald E. Decreased lymphocyte beta-adrenergic-receptor density in patients with heart failure and tolerance to the beta-adrenergic agonist pirbuterol. N Engl J Med 305:185–190, 1981.

28. Lambertz H, Meyer J, Erbel R. Long term hemodynamic effects of prenalterol in patients with severe congestive heart failure. Circulation 69:298–305, 1984.

29. Roubin GS, Choong CYP, Devenish-Meares S, Sadick NN, Fletcher PJ, Keller DT, Harris PJ. β-adrenergic stimulation of the failing ventricle: a double-blind, randomized trial of sustained therapy with prenalterol. Circulation 69:955–962, 1984.

30. Maskin CS, Forman R, Sonnenblick EH, Frishman WH, LeJemtel TH. Failure of dobutamine to increase exercise capacity despite hemodynamic improvement in severe chronic heart failure. Am J Cardiol 51:177–182, 1983.

31. Wilson JR, Martin JL, Ferraro N. Impaired skeletal muscle nutritive flow during exercise in patients with congestive heart failure: role of cardiac pump dysfunction as determined by the effect of dobutamine. Am J Cardiol 53:1308–1315, 1984.

32. Maskin CS, Kugler J, Sonnenblick EH, LeJemtel TH. Acute inotropic stimulation with dopamine in severe congestive heart failure: beneficial hemodynamic effect at rest but not during maximal exercise. Am J Cardiol 52:1028–1035, 1983.

33. Bristow MR, Ginsberg R, Minobe W, Cubieceiotti RS, Sageman WS, Lurie K, Billingham ME, Harrison DC, Stinson EB. Decreased catecholamine sensitivity and β-adrenergic-receptor density in failing human hearts. N Engl J Med 307:205–211, 1982.

34. Uretsky BF, Generalovich T, Reddy PS, Spangenberg RB, Follansbee WP. The acute hemodynamic effects of a new agent, MDL 17,043, in the treatment of congestive heart failure. Circulation 67:823–828, 1983.

35. Martin JL, Likoff MJ, Janicki JS, Laskey WK, Hirschfeld JW, Weber KT. Myocardial energetics and clinical response to the cardiotonic agent MDL 17,043 in advanced heart failure. JACC 4:875–883, 1984.

36. Petein M, Levine TB, Cohn JN. Hemodynamic effects of a new inotropic agent, piroximone (MDL 19,205), in patients with chronic heart failure. JACC 4:364–371, 1984.

37. Alousi AA, Farah AE, Lesher GY, Opalka CJ. Cardiotonic activity of amrinone-Win 40680 [5-amino-3,4'-bipyridin-6 (IH)-one]. Circ Res 45:666–677, 1979.

38. Likoff MJ, Weber KT, Andrews V, Janicki JS, St John-Sutton M, Wilson H, Rocci ML. Amrinone in the treatment of chronic cardiac failure. JACC 3:1282–1290, 1984.

39. Siskind SJ, Sonnenblick EH, Forman R, Scheuer J,

LeJemtel TH. Acute substantial benefit of inotropic therapy with amrinone on exercise hemodynamics and metabolism in severe congestive heart failure. Circulation 64:966–973, 1981.

40. DiBianco R, Chabetai R, Silverman BD, Leier CV, Benotti JR. Oral amrinone for the treatment of congestive heart failure: results of a multicenter randomized double-blind and placebo-controlled withdrawal study. JACC 4:855–866, 1984.

41. Maskin CS, Sinoway L, Chadwick B, Sonnenblick EH, LeJemtel TH. Sustained hemodynamic and clinical effects of a new cardiotonic agent WIN 47203 in patients with severe congestive heart failure. Circulation 67:1065–1070, 1983.

42. Baim DS, McDowell AV, Cherniles J, Monrad ES, Parker JA, Edelson J, Braunwald E, Grossman W. Evaluation of a new bipyridine inotropic agent— milrinone—in patients with severe congestive heart failure. N Engl J Med 309:748–756, 1983.

43. Likoff MJ, Weber KT, Andrews V, Janicki JS, Wilson H, Rocci ML. Milrinone in the treatment of chronic cardiac failure: a controlled trial. Am Heart J 110:1035–1042, 1985.

44. Ribeiro JP, White HD, Arnold JMD, Hartley LH, Wright RF, Fifer MA, Jaski BE, Colucci WS. Chronic milrinone therapy: differential effects of maximal and submaximal metabolic responses to exercise in heart failure (Abstr). Circulation 70:II-11, 1984.

45. Maskin CS, Mancini D, Chadwick B, Sonnenblick EH, LeJemtel TH. Clinical response to long-term milrinone therapy in severe chronic heart failure: two year experience (Abstr). Circulation 70:II-168, 1984.

Index

Note: Page numbers in *italics* refer to illustrations; page numbers followed by (t) refer to tables.

357